MW00561144

Paramedic Lab Manual

SUE CAMPBELL, RN/EMT-P, A.S. EMS
Clinical Coordinator
Brevard Community College
Health Sciences Paramedic Program
Cocoa, Florida

MELISSA B. ROBINSON, RN/EMT-P, B.S.H.
Program Director
Brevard Community College
Health Sciences Paramedic Program
Cocoa, Florida

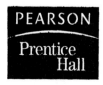

PEARSON

Prentice
Hall

Upper Saddle River, New Jersey 07458

Publisher: Julie Levin Alexander
Publisher's Assistant: Regina Bruno
Executive Editor: Marlene McHugh Pratt
Senior Acquisitions Editor: Stephen Smith
Senior Managing Editor for Development: Lois Berlowitz
Associate Editor: Monica Moosang
Editorial Assistant: Diane Edwards
Executive Marketing Manager: Katrin Beacom
Director of Marketing: Karen Allman
Marketing Coordinator: Michael Sirinides
Director of Production and Manufacturing: Bruce Johnson
Managing Production Editor: Patrick Walsh
Production Liaison: Julie Li
Production Editor: Karen Fortgang, bookworks
Manufacturing Manager: Ilene Sanford
Manufacturing Buyer: Pat Brown
Senior Design Coordinator: Cheryl Asherman
Cover Designer: Christopher Weigand
Composition: The GTS Companies/York, PA Campus
Printing and Binding: Courier Westford
Cover Printer: Phoenix Color Corporation

Copyright © 2006 by Pearson Education, Inc., Upper Saddle River, New Jersey 07458.
Pearson Prentice Hall. All rights reserved. Printed in the United States of America. This
publication is protected by Copyright and permission should be obtained from the publisher
prior to any prohibited reproduction, storage in a retrieval system, or transmission in any
form or by any means, electronic, mechanical, photocopying, recording, or likewise. For
information regarding permission(s), write to: Rights and Permissions Department.

Pearson Prentice Hall™ is a trademark of Pearson Education, Inc.
Pearson® is a registered trademark of Pearson plc
Prentice Hall® is a registered trademark of Pearson Education, Inc.

Pearson Education LTD
Pearson Education Singapore, Pte. Ltd
Pearson Education Canada, Ltd
Pearson Education—Japan

Pearson Education Australia PTY, Limited
Pearson Education North Asia Ltd
Pearson Educación de Mexico, S.A. de C.V.
Pearson Education Malaysia, Pte. Ltd
Pearson Education, Upper Saddle River, New Jersey

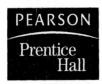

10 9 8 7 6 5 4 3
ISBN 0-13-119437-2

Contents

©2006 Prentice-Hall Inc.

©2006 Prentice-Hall Inc.

©2006 Prentice-Hall Inc.

©2006 Prentice-Hall Inc.

©2006 Prentice-Hall Inc.

©2006 Prentice-Hall Inc.

©2006 Prentice-Hall Inc.

©2006 Prentice-Hall Inc.

PREFACE

Welcome to the stimulating and challenging world of EMS education. This lab manual was devised to aid you in the pursuit of your educational goals. Developed to document compliance with the 1998 DOT National Standard Curriculum (NSC) psychomotor and affective domain objectives, completion of the skills (one sheet per skill) and all the scenarios ensures that programs meet CAAHEP/CoAEMSP Joint Review for National Accreditation.

The understanding that lab experiences are an integral part of your educational experience needs to be embraced. Prepare for your labs beforehand by reading the required skills, Daily Discussions and Pertinent Points, and the corresponding chapter(s) in your textbook. The lab manual is designed to be used in coordination with the Brady text for explanations of the procedures and theories behind the skills. Fabulous Factoids make interesting reading—trivia gleaned from the Brady text, books, and programs aired on The Learning Channel and Discovery. The Pathophysiologies section covers all the 1998 NSC pathophysiology objectives, and the scenarios assigned to each section meet the diagnosis-based patient assessment requirements of the curriculum.

The manual itself is a comprehensive compilation of the psychomotor and affective domain objectives required by the 1998 NSC. It also meets many of the cognitive domain objectives. If utilized as designed by the authors, students and educators can be assured that they are in compliance with the psychomotor, affective domain, and pathophysiology essentials in the NSC. Please understand, however, that no hands-on (psychomotor) skill is learned from reading a book. Competence in performing these skills will be achieved under the guidance of the experienced, qualified instructors your program provides in your classroom, lab, and clinical areas.

It is our sincere hope that this manual becomes a valuable resource in your EMS education.

THANK YOU!

We would very much like to thank the following:

- Brevard Community College paramedic students of the past several years for all their input and suggestions. They are the most wonderful "brats" and we couldn't have done this without them.
- Ms. Debbie Tchorz, for her invaluable help with the Chronic Care/Home Health revisions (and teaching the lab). The students love her as an instructor and we agree.
- Mrs. Shirley R. Watson, for her numerous hours of proofreading and editing.
- Our families, Shirley Watson (Sue's mom), Brienne Petcher (Sue's daughter), James Michael Robinson (Melissa's husband), and Mesilla Brookley Watson (Melissa's daughter), for living without us for many hours and days during this process, and the constant disruptions of our relationships. It's finally complete!
- Our reviewers: Brenda M. Beasley, RN, BS, EMT-P, Department Chair, Allied Health, Calhoun Community College, Decatur, Alabama; Nita Ham, EMT-P, Grady Memorial Hospital, Atlanta, Georgia; John J. Heiser, FF/EMT-P, Coconut Creek, Florida; Bill J. Hufford, REMT-P, P.I., EMS Director, FMH EMS, Connersville, Indiana; Scott Karr, M.Ed., NREMT-P, Paramedic Program Director, Bevill

State Community College, Sumiton, Alabama; Nikhil Natarajan, NREMT-P, CCEMT-P, I/C, Instructor, Paramedic Program, Stone Ridge, New York; Mac Snead, BS, NREMT-P, Assistant Director/Instructor, Emergency Health Sciences—Paramedic Program, Roanoke, Virginia; and E. Ray Werts, EMT-P/PI, Flight Paramedic, PHI Air Medical, Indianapolis, Indiana. Thank you for the discerning eye and constructive input to make this a more beneficial educational adjunct.

©2006 Prentice-Hall Inc.

INTRODUCTION AND INSTRUCTIONS

This manual is assembled in 10 sections. Sections 1–8 contain the student skill sheets (core skills listed in bold), Fabulous Factoids, the correlating EMS drugs (from the Emergency Drug Quiz Key), and the correlating pathophysiologies (from the Pathophysiologies section). Sections 9 and 10 include a paramedic review section and the glossary. At the end of each section are the scenarios[1] and Daily Discussions and Pertinent Points. Depending on the length of your course, labs will be spread out to cover the material (one section does NOT mean it will be covered in one lab). It is suggested that programs assign the drug quizzes and pathophysiologies every week (one drug and five or six pathophysiologies). Completing all sheets for each section will assure completion of NSC psychomotor and affective domain objectives. Please note there are skill sheets for intubation, IV insertion, radio report, and written patient care report (PCR) for many of the scenarios throughout the manual. The authors believe that comfort and competence in these skills is mandatory, and they have attempted to provide as much practice as possible. The NSC and CAAHEP/CoAEMSP Joint Review for National Accreditation do not require documentation of skill repetition (if successful on initial try). This is at the discretion of the program. However, the diagnosis-based assessments (scenarios) that are duplicated, such as Dyspnea or Behavioral, ARE required. There are twelve required Trauma scenarios, two of which are the instructor's choice. All scenarios are mandatory, and each student must be the lead medic in at least one diagnosis group per scenario category. All students must be exposed to all required diagnoses.

In the first weeks of lab, we suggest a review of all required EMT skills and an introduction of the students to scenario management. Included in this section are many scenario sheets and scenario-related skill sheets for practice. None of these scenarios are required by the NSC, but would be beneficial because the transition from an EMT level skills-oriented method to a paramedic level scenario-based level is often confusing to incoming students. As a new paramedic student, completing a scenario at the EMT level can build confidence, yet initiate critical thinking. Incorporating the basic skills into scenarios can be a fun-filled way to accomplish the skills required in the section.

Included here is a summary of the 10 sections. Please refer to the table of contents for specific skill sheets for each section. Examples of paperwork and student completion records are in this introductory section.

Section 1
- Fabulous Factoids
- EMT Skills—Basic/Advanced/Special Operations[2]

All objectives of the official 1998 USDOT National Standard Curriculum for paramedic training courses are available for download (have two very large binders and three reams of paper on hand) at the following site: www.nhtsa.dot.gov/people/injury/ems/EMT-P/

[1]Scenarios are based on a 6:1 student-to-instructor ratio. Smaller groups may need to have students take the lead and other positions more than once for each scenario category. Instructions follow the Student Scenario Completion Record. Scenarios at the EMT level are not included in the Student Scenario Completion Record because they are for practice only.

[2]The Special Operations section (under EMT) is not meant to be accomplished during one lab session, but in several mandatory outdoor specialty labs (Extrication, High-Angle Rescue, Water Rescue, Hazardous Materials, Mass Casualty Incident, etc.).

- Patient assessment scenario sheets
- Daily Discussions and Pertinent Points

Section 2
- Fabulous Factoids
- **ADVANCED AIRWAY MANAGEMENT**
- **Patient assessment scenario sheets**
- Daily Discussions and Pertinent Points

Section 3
- Fabulous Factoids
- **PATIENT ASSESSMENT and RESPIRATORY**
- **Patient assessment scenario sheets**
- Daily Discussions and Pertinent Points

Section 4
- Fabulous Factoids
- **IV THERAPY AND MEDICATION ADMINISTRATION**
- **Patient assessment scenario sheets**
- Daily Discussions and Pertinent Points

Section 5
- Fabulous Factoids
- **TRAUMA**
- **Patient assessment scenario sheets**
- Daily Discussions and Pertinent Points

Section 6
- Fabulous Factoids
- **MEDICAL**
- **Patient assessment scenario sheets**
- Daily Discussions and Pertinent Points

Section 7
- Fabulous Factoids
- **CARDIOLOGY**
- **Patient assessment scenario sheets**
- Daily Discussions and Pertinent Points

Section 8
- Fabulous Factoids
- **SPECIALTY: GYN/OB/NEONATAL/PEDS/CHRONIC CARE/HOME HEALTH**
- **Patient assessment scenario sheets**
- Daily Discussions and Pertinent Points

Section 9
- **PERTINENT POINTS FOR PARAMEDIC REVIEW**
- Paramedic Review Section

Section 10
- **PATHOPHYSIOLOGIES**
- Pathophysiology Checklist
- Glossary

©2006 Prentice-Hall Inc.

STUDENT SKILLS VERIFICATION

SAMPLE Student Scenario Completion Record

Student Scenario Completion Record

Scenario Diagnoses Chart

Paramedic Master Skills Log

Patient Data Sheet (PDS)

SAMPLE Student Scenario Completion Record

Student: *Ima Parafetus*

Scenario Category	LEAD	Airway	IV	Hospital Radio	Scribe	Assist	Date	Instructor
SECTION 3: Respiratory								
Dyspnea (1st scenario)	A	B	C	D	E	F	1/1/08	*Jack Ofalltrades*
Dyspnea (2nd scenario)	D	F	E	A	C	E	1/1/08	*Jack Ofalltrades*
Allergy (1st scenario)	F	A	B	C	D	E	1/1/08	*Jack Ofalltrades*
Allergy (2nd scenario)	A	C	B	E	D	F	1/1/08	*Jack Ofalltrades*
Anaphylaxis								

Jack was the instructor who checked off the first four scenarios—all on 1/1/08. (See Scenario Diagnoses Chart for scenarios.)
Ima was the LEAD on the Dyspnea (1st scenario) for the diagnosis A—spontaneous pneumothorax. She did the airway management for B—SARS, and the IV for the C—COPD patient. On D—pulmonary embolus, she answered the team leader's radio report to the hospital, and she scribed for the E—tuberculosis scenario. For the 6th diagnosis of F—cystic fibrosis, Ima was the assistant. This verifies that Ima actively participated in all the Dyspnea (1st scenario) patients.
Ima could have kept her same order (A-B-C-D-E-F) for the second Dyspnea group, but she was the LEAD for D—neoplasm, instead.
As the team LEAD, Ima has to give the radio report AND write up the patient care report (PCR). Each student should be sure to get the chance to do one intubation and one peripheral IV insertion each lab day. Not all scenarios require these interventions, but it is the student's responsibility to do the skill once each week (not every scenario).

Student Scenario Completion Record

Student: _____

Students will participate as team members in all scenarios. Each student must be the team leader for a minimum of one scenario in each assessment category (per National Standard Curriculum). Other students in the group will be team members (1) in charge of the airway, (2) responsible for the IV insertion, (3) scribing the scenario (team leader will need these notes to do a PCR/patient care report), and (4) will "answer" the radio (hospital radio) when the team leader calls in the radio report. Other students can participate by giving meds as needed, performing CPR, holding C-spine, and so on. All students must participate in all six scenarios in each category. The diagnoses are required by 1998 NSC (you will notice some, such as Dyspnea, require TWO scenarios). The team leader is graded on the assessment/treatment, radio report, patient care report, and management of the overall scenario. An example of the completion record precedes this form. No EMT scenarios are mandatory. They are good for practice or to include if you are using the beginning of this manual as an EMT skills manual.

Scenario Category	LEAD	Airway	IV	Hospital Radio	Scribe	Assist	Date	Instructor
SECTION 3: RESPIRATORY								
Dyspnea (1st scenario)								
Dyspnea (2nd scenario)								
Allergy (1st scenario)								
Allergy (2nd scenario)								
Anaphylaxis								
SECTION 5: TRAUMA								
Abdominal								
Abuse/Assault								
Burn								
Geriatric								
Head/Facial/Neck								
Musculoskeletal								
Shock/Hemorrhage								
Soft Tissue								
Spinal								
Thoracic								
Trauma Mix (1st scenario)								
Trauma Mix (2nd scenario)								
Trauma Arrest								
SECTION 6: MEDICAL								
Abdominal (1st scenario)								
Abdominal (2nd scenario)								

Scenario Category	LEAD	Airway	IV	Hospital Radio	Scribe	Assist	Date	Instructor
Altered LOC								
Behavioral (1st scenario)								
Behavioral (2nd scenario)								
Behavioral (3rd scenario)								
Chest Pain								
Diabetic								
Environmental/Thermal								
GI Bleeding								
Seizure								
Toxicologic/Hazardous Material								
SECTION 7: CARDIOLOGY								
Asystole								
VF								
VT								
PEA								
AMI								
Bradycardia								
Cardiogenic Shock								
Medical Arrest								
Pulmonary Edema								
Renal Dialysis Code								
Stable Tachycardia								
Syncope								
Unstable Tachycardia								
SECTION 8: GYN/OB/NEONATAL/PEDS								
Vaginal Bleeding								
Childbirth								
Pediatric Medical (1st scenario)								
Pediatric Medical (2nd scenario)								
Pediatric Trauma								

Scenario Diagnoses Chart

Scenario Category	A	B	C	D	E	F
			SECTION 3: RESPIRATORY			
Dyspnea (1st scenario)	spontaneous pneumothorax	SARS or other contagious resp.	COPD	pulmonary embolus	tuberculosis	cystic fibrosis
Dyspnea (2nd scenario)	asthma	hyperventilation	URI	neoplasm	CHF	geriatric pneumonia
Allergy (1st scenario)	skin rash—topical	medication reaction	poison ivy	red tide or mold/dust	food allergy	EPS—dystonic reaction
Allergy (2nd scenario)	man-of-war stings or local allergen	periorbital cellulitis	bee sting	hay fever	perfume	iodine
Anaphylaxis	bee sting	home medication	food	drug given in rescue	party dip	latex
			SECTION 5: TRAUMA			
Abdominal	ruptured spleen	lacerated liver	stab wound	pelvic fracture	72-hour-old spleen injury/rupture	uterine rupture
Abuse/Assault	refusal of transport	child abuse	elderly abuse	domestic assault	sexual assault	assault with baseball bat
Burn	blast injury with burn	scald	house fire with burn and inhalation	steam inhalation	circumferential chest	acid burn
Geriatric	GI bleed with fall	AAA with fall	hip fracture	subdural hematoma	HTN with dizziness and head laceration	extremity fracture with decubiti/gangrene
Head/Facial/Neck	fractured larynx	geriatric fall with closed head inj. & LeFort fx.	diffuse axonal injury	cerebral contusion	basilar skull fx.	lacerated jugular vein
Musculoskeletal	open fracture	down and under hip dislocation	back injury with spasm	fractured femur	elbow fracture with neurovascular compromise	tendon laceration
Shock/Hemorrhage	MVC entrapped off-road/hypothermia	geriatric on beta blocker in shock	toxic shock syndrome or septic foreign body	geriatric with urosepsis (shock)	spinal injury	cardiogenic
Soft Tissue	road rash	impaled wire to thigh	contusions/refusal, geriatric with poor environment	plate glass laceration	crush trauma	hand amputation
Spinal	spinal shock	thoracic spine step-off	cervical fx. MVC	hanging/cervical fx.	GSW with spinal cord injury	axial load trauma (off roof)
Thoracic	open pneumothorax	myocardial contusion	ruptured diaphragm	thoracic aorta tear (leaking)	pulmonary contusion	flail chest
Trauma Mix (1st scenario)	(all instructor's choice)					
Trauma Mix (2nd scenario)						
Trauma Arrest	traumatic asphyxia	geriatric osteoporosis with rib fx. from CPR	GSW to head of geriatric	arm amputation with hypovolemia	head trauma	chest trauma in arrest

Scenario Category	A	B	C	D	E	F
			SECTION 6: MEDICAL			
Abdominal (1st scenario)	acute gastroenteritis	colitis	appendicitis	pancreatitis	cholecystitis	UTI
Abdominal (2nd scenario)	Crohn's	diverticulitis	hepatitis	sickle cell crisis, abdominal pain	renal calculi	small bowel obstruction
Altered LOC	stroke with speech impairment	intracranial hemorrhage	TIA	hyperglycemia	GHB use	postictal
Behavioral (1st scenario)	head trauma	geriatric with cerebral vascular disease	developmental disability	dementia	delirium	ETOH withdrawal
Behavioral (2nd scenario)	Alzheimer's	Parkinson's	hypoglycemia	ETOH	drug-induced	bipolar
Behavioral (3rd scenario)	posttraumatic stress disorder	paranoid schizophrenia	speaks Spanish only, uncooperative	suicidal	organic brain syndrome	obsessive-compulsive disorder
Chest Pain	pulmonary embolus	cocaine	unstable angina	esophagitis	pleuritis	costochondritis
Diabetic	DKA	conscious, hypoglycemia	unresponsive, hypoglycemia	diabetic with peripheral vascular disease	combative, hypoglycemia	diabetic MI
Environmental/Thermal	frostbite/nip	near drowning	POPS	high-altitude pulmonary edema	heatstroke	snakebite
GI Bleeding	geriatric with arthritis taking ASA, has UGI	lower GI bleed	geriatric with cirrhosis, esophageal varices	hemorrhoids, rectal bleeding	ulcerative colitis	peptic ulcer disease
Seizure	hypoglycemia	obese hypoxia	VF/AED in use	neoplasm of brain	epilepsy	status epilepticus
Toxicological/ Hazardous Materials	organophosphate	Sarin or nerve agent	thyroid OD	Phenol exposure	train derail/gas	anthrax or smallpox
			SECTION 7: CARDIOLOGY			
Asystole	hypothermia	potassium OD	electrocution	cardiac	DNR patient	hypoxia
VF	sudden death	lightning	drowning	seizure	unknown down	hypothermia
VT	looks like CHF but lungs clear	asymptomatic	morbidly obese/ no IV alert—use cough conversion	stopped taking meds	stable to unstable	VF conversion to VT with a pulse
PEA	cardiac tamponade	tension pneumothorax	hypovolemia	hypoxia (FBAO)	DKA	ventricular pacer with no pulse
AMI	cocaine	silent MI diabetic female	wakes up with pain	anterior wall MI	CHF	inferior MI/vomiting
Bradycardia	organophosphates	digoxin OD	calcium channel blocker OD	athlete asymptomatic	hypoxia	2nd degree type 2 block
Cardiogenic Shock	complete heart block	SVT	AMI	Lasix patient who took whole bottle of potassium	magnesium OD	pericarditis
Medical Arrest	geriatric heart failure	geriatric sepsis pneumonia	acute renal failure	OD	meningitis	SVT convert to code

Scenario Diagnoses Chart (continued)

Scenario Category	A	B	C	D	E	F
Pulmonary Edema	fire extinguisher inhalation	CHF	submersion/near drowning	hypertension	pulmonary contusion	left ventricular failure/fulminating
Renal Dialysis Code	missed dialysis	septic AV shunt	chest pain on machine	patient cuts into shunt—hemorrhage	MI before dialysis	trauma MVC on way to dialysis
SECTION 7: CARDIOLOGY						
Stable Tachycardia	ST asymptomatic	anxiety	SVT	caffeine OD	pain	SVT responds to vagal
Syncope	Stokes-Adams	hypovolemic	hypertensive crisis	myocardial contusion dysrhythmias	vasovagal from seeing own blood	sinus and ear infection
Unstable Tachycardia	SVT	VT	A Fib/dehydrated	hx PSVT—can't "break" this one	asthma—multiple MDI sprays	palpitations/weak sudden A Fib RVR
SECTION 8: GYN/OB/NEONATE/PEDs						
Vaginal Bleeding	Muslim female with ectopic	placenta previa	MVC with abruptio placenta	vaginal trauma	postpartum fistula/infected episiotomy	sexual assault
Childbirth	preeclamptic abruptio with meconium	postpartum hemorrhage	prolapsed cord	breech	uterus prolapses after delivery	eclamptic seizing
Pediatric Medical (1st scenario)	FBAO	respiratory distress	SIDS	seizure	opiate OD	blind peds with meningitis
Pediatric Medical (2nd scenario)	special needs on PEEP needs suction	sickle cell	epiglottitis	croup	deaf/vomiting with dehydration/shock	neglect/low blood sugar
Pediatric Trauma	head/fall off bike	abuse/abdominal trauma	chest—run over by vehicle	electrocution	burns	near drowning

Paramedic Master Skills Log

Name: _____

Lab Date	Skill	Instructor
	CPR	
	Combi-tube	
	ET Intubation**	
	Nasal Intubation**	
	ET Suction/Oral	
	BVM/BVT**	
	Chest Decompression	
	Cricothyrotomy	
	Peripheral IV**	
	EJ Cannulation	
	Glucose Check	
	IO Insertion	
	Nebulizer**	
	IVP Meds**	
	IVPB Meds**	
	IM Meds**	
	ET Meds**	
	SQ Meds**	
	PO/SL Meds**	
	Rectal Meds**	
	Synch Cardioversion	
	Defibrillation	
	TCP	
	Spinal Immobilization	
	KED	
	MAST	
	Scoop Stretcher	
	Dressing/Bandage	
	Traction Splint	

Lab Date	Skill	Instructor
	NG Tube	
	Delivery	
	Neonate/APGAR	
	Adult Assessment**	
	Child Assessment**	
	Infant Assessment**	
	Foley Insertion	
	IV Pump	
	Transport Ventilator	

Students must be signed off on skill before they can perform it on a clinical.

Carry the Master Skills Log to all clinicals.

All skills required by the 1998 National Standard Curriculum and Joint Review Committee (for CAAHEP/CoAEMSP National Accreditation) are marked with ** and need to be tracked (along with age groups and diagnosis groups) on patient data sheet (PDS), FISDAP, or program's choice for documentation.

©2006 Prentice-Hall Inc.

Patient Data Sheet

Name: _____

Term: _____

Preceptor Signature: _____

Location/station: _____

Clinical/Agency: _____

Date: _____

Patient Number	Age Group	Gender	Diagnosis #1	Diagnosis #2	Diagnosis #3	Assess	IV Initiatd	IVP Med	IVPB Med	SQ Med	IM Med	SL/PO Med	ET Med	Rectal Med	Nebulizer	Intubation	BVM	BVT	Preceptor Initials

1 **Trauma** **A** = Arrest **B** = HEENT **C** = Thoracic/Back **D** = Abdominal **E** = Pelvic **F** = Extremity **G** = ≥ 2
2 **Chest Pain** **A** = Arrest **B** = Cardiac **C** = Non-cardiac
3 **Dyspnea** **P** = Pediatric (<18 y.o.)
4 **Altered LOC** **A** = CVA/TIA **B** = Seizure **C** = Diabetic **D** = Overdose
5 **Abdominal** **A** = GI **B** = GYN **C** = GU/Renal
6 **Psych/Behavioral**
7 **Syncope**
8 **OB 8N** = Neonate
9 **Toxicological** **A** = Allergy **B** = Environmental **C** = Communicable
10 **Hemodynamics** **A** = Hypertension **B** = Hypotension
11 **WRITE-IN complaint**

Age Groups
1 Neonate -30 days
2 1 - 11mos (Infant)
3 12 - 36 mos (Toddler)
4 3 - 5 yr (Preschool)
5 6–12 yr (School-age)
6 13–18 yr (Adolescent)
7 19–40 yr (Early Adult)
8 41–60 yr (Middle Adult)
9 Over 60 (Late Adult

Emergency Drug Quiz Key

Trade Name	Generic	Actions	Uses	Side Effects	Contraindications	Average Dose	Routes
Oxygen	"O"s	gas making up 21% room air that enables aerobic metabolism, required for proper breakdown of glucose	1. hypoxia 2. chest pain 3. nausea 4. potential hypoxia 5. hypovolemia	apnea in patients on hypoxic drive	NONE in emergency Exception: Paraquat	per device—dependent on patient condition	NC NRBM BVM ATV
Normal Saline	NS	1. isotonic crystalloid fluid 2. 0.9% NaCl in water	1. replace volume 2. flush meds 3. irrigation	1. FLUID OVERLOAD 2. CHF/pulmonary edema	pulmonary edema caution with rate	TKO/KVO to WO dependent on patient condition	IV IVP
Versed	midazolam	1. sedative 2. short-acting benzodiazepine 3. NO ANALGESIA	1. induce sedation/amnesia 2. seizures (nasal)	1. drowsiness 2. hypotension 3. N/V 4. respiratory arrest	1. ETOH 2. glaucoma 3. shock	1–2.5 mg slow IVP usual dose 5 mg	IVP IM Nasal
Amidate	etomidate	1. hypnotic 2. general anesthetic 3. acts at level of reticular activating system (RAS) 4. NO ANALGESIA	1. induction 2. sedation with RSI	1. tachy- or bradycardia 2. hypotension 3. hypertension 4. tonic movements 5. LARYNGOSPASM 6. apnea	pregnancy (term)	0.1–0.3 mg/kg over 15–30 seconds	IVP
Anectine	succinylcholine	1. depolarizing neuromuscular blocker 2. affinity for ACh sites 3. skeletal muscle relaxant 4. adjunct to anesthesia 5. paralytic/NO ANALGESIA	1. facilitate intubation 2. assist mechanical ventilation 3. orthopedic manipulations	1. apnea 2. hypotension	1. penetrating eye injuries 2. hypotension 3. hyperkalemia	1–2 mg/kg IVP	IVP IM
Norcuron	vecuronium "vec"	1. nondepolarizing skeletal muscle relaxant 2. "intermediate acting paralytic" 3. neuromuscular blocker binds with ACh	with INTUBATED patients	1. apnea 2. malignant hyperthermia	UNSECURED AIRWAY	0.1 mg/kg	IVP
Proventil Ventolin	albuterol	1. sympathomimetic 2. beta-2 stimulator	bronchodilation	1. arrhythmias 2. dizziness 3. palpitations 4. chest pain	symptomatic tachyarrhythmia	HHN—2.5 mg/ 2–3 ml MDI—1–2 puffs	Inhaled

Emergency Drug Quiz Key (continued)

Trade Name	Generic	Actions	Uses	Side Effects	Contraindications	Average Dose	Routes
Epinephrine	adrenalin "epi"	1. alpha and beta adrenergic agonist 2. natural catecholamine (SNS) 3. ↑HR/↑force of contraction 4. ↑automaticity/↑conduction 5. ↑excitability 6. bronchodilation	1. allergic reaction to reverse bronchospasm from histamine 2. replace natural epi 3. enhance CPR, coronary artery, and cerebral perfusion DEAD PEOPLE NEED 4. drip for symptomatic brady	1. tachycardia 2. shakiness 3. palpitations 4. hypertension 5. V Fib 6. pulmonary edema	none in emergency situations	1. allergy: 0.3– 0.5 mg of 1:1000 subQ 2. anaphylaxis: 0.3– 0.5 mg of 1:10,000 IVP 3. code: 1 mg of 1:1000 or 1:10,000 q 3–5 minute IVP 4. DRIP: 2–10 mcg/ min 5. ET 2–2½ × dose 6. Peds ET—10X	IVP IO ET SQ IVPB— 1 mg/ 250 cc or 2 mg/ 250 cc ET alternate route
Benadryl	diphenhydra-mine	1. antihistamine (H₁ receptor antagonist) 2. binds with histamine receptors 3. decreases cough reflex 4. inhibits mast cell damage 5. sedative 6. anticholinergic/antiemetic 7. antipruritic	1. allergic reactions 2. anaphylaxis 3. antidote for EPS	1. sedation/confusion 2. hypotension 3. dry mouth/nose 4. thickened bronchial secretions 5. wheezing 6. chest tightness	1. ETOH 2. ASTHMA	1. allergy/ anaphylaxis: 50–100 mg 2. EPS: 10–25 mg 3. Peds: 1–2 mg/ kg up to 50 mg for allergy up to 25 mg for EPS	IVP IM PO
Narcan	naloxone	narcotic antagonist	1. CNS depression 2. coma of unknown origin 3. narcotic OD	none unless patient has narcotic addiction	FULL DOSE may precipitate acute withdrawal in addict	0.4–2 mg q 3 minutes usually max 10 mg if not effective	IVP IM SQ IO Nasal ET alternate route
Pitressin	vasopressin	1. vasoconstriction (pressor) 2. possesses ADH properties to increase sodium reabsorption	1. increase PVR during cardiac arrest 2. may be useful hemodynamic support in vasodilatory shock 3. used to control bleeding from esophageal varices	1. increase PVR may provoke cardiac ischemia/angina	1. ischemic heart disease 2. pulmonary edema (relative)	1. During arrest: 40 units IV/IO to replace 1ˢᵗ or 2ⁿᵈ dose of epi 2. esophageal varices: IVPB 0.2-0.4 units/min	1. IVP 2. IVPB 250u/250c c ET alternate route in CPR
Cardizem	Dilitiazem	1. calcium channel blocker 2. coronary artery dilator	1. control ventricular rate in atrial fib or flutter 2. after adenosine for refractory SVT 3. increase coronary perfusion in angina	1. hypotension 2. bradycardia 3. heart blocks	1. Wide complex tachycardias 2. WPW 3. Caution with beta blocker use	1. 15-20 mg over 1-2 mins 2. may repeat in 15 mins at 20-25 mg 3. Maintenance . Drip 5-15 mg/hr	IVP IVPB 100mg/ 250 cc

Trade Name	Generic	Actions	Uses	Side Effects	Contraindications	Average Dose	Route
Levophed	norepinephrine	1. natural catecholamine 2. primarily alpha qualities 3. sympathomimetic 4. peripheral vasoconstriction 5. decreased renal blood flow	1. hypotension— systolic BP <70 mmHg 2. neurogenic shock	1. ↑myocardial ischemia 2. tachycardia 3. dysrhythmias 4. hypertension 5. oliguria/anuria	1. hypovolemia 2. mesenteric or peripheral thrombosis	0.5–30 mcg/min	IVPB— 4 mg/ 250 cc
D$_{50}$	50% dextrose	1. 25 g dextrose in 50 cc water 2. carbohydrate (50%) 3. principal form of sugar to body 4. enables cellular metabolism	1. sugar replacement in hypoglycemia 2. coma of unknown origin	1. osmotic diuresis 2. NECROSIS if infiltrates 3. use with Thiamine 100 mg in ETOH	1. hyperglycemia 2. intracranial hemorrhage 3. NONE with documented hypoglycemia	1. 25–50 g depends on BGL 2. 25% for Peds 3. 10–12.5% for neonate	IVP PO rectal
Glucagon	glucagon	natural pancreatic hormone to convert glycogen to glucose in the liver	when unable to administer glucose to hypoglycemic patient	none in documented hypoglycemia	cirrhotic patients/ETOH needs Thiamine	1 mg	IM
Atropine	atropine sulfate	1. parasympatholytic 2. anticholinergic 3. antagonizes acetylcholine receptors causing ↑HR 4. decreases GI effects	1. symptomatic brady 2. asystole 3. PEA with brady 4. organophosphate OD	1. tachycardia 2. ↑myocardial oxygen demand 3. dry mouth 4. flushed skin 5. blurred vision 6. BRADYCARDIA IF PUSHED SLOWLY	1. tachycardia 2. MI 3. CHF 4. glaucoma	1. 0.5 mg rapid IVP if perfusing 2. 1 mg rapid IVP if nonperfusing q 3–5 minutes up to 3 mg cardiac 3. organophosphate: 2 mg rapid IVP q 3–5 minutes until sx subside	rapid IVP ET IM eye ET alternate route
Intropin	dopamine	1. sympathomimetic—natural catecholamine with dopaminergic, alpha and beta properties 2. precursor of norepinephrine 3. ↑contractility and ↑HR(beta) 4. skeletal vasoconstriction (alpha) 5. ↑SV and CO (+inotropic) 6. ↑renal and mesenteric blood flow (dopaminergic)	1. to ↑renal and mesenteric bld flow 2. to ↑BP 3. symptomatic brady refractory to Atropine and TCP	1. ventricular ectopy 2. tachycardia 3. NECROSIS if infiltrates	1. deactivated with bicarb 2. hypertension 3. hypotension if too low dose 4. uncorrected hypovolemia	1. 2–4 mcg/kg/min = dopaminergic 2. 5–20 mcg/kg/min = beta to alpha progressively 3. beta = 5– 10 mcg/kg/min 4. Alpha = 10– 20 mcg/kg/min	IVPB— 400 mg/ 250 cc or 800 mg/ 250 cc
Lasix	furosemide	1. sulfonamide distal loop diuretic 2. inhibits reabsorption of Na$^+$ and Cl$^-$ 3. peripheral venodilator 4. reverses ischemic kidney response	1. CHF with pulmonary edema 2. acute cerebral edema 3. hypertension 4. renal failure	1. hypotension 2. hypovolemia 3. HYPOKALEMIA 4. transient deafness if pushed too fast	1. hypotension 2. dehydration 3. anuria 4. electrolyte imbalance 5. caution with sulfa allergy	0.5–1 mg/kg	IVP PO IM
Lidocaine	xylocaine	1. antidysrhythmic (sodium channel blocker) 2. depresses ventricular automaticity 3. RAISES V Fib threshold	1. in NONbradycardic PVCs 2. unifocal >6/min 3. multifocal 4. couplets 5. "R on T" PVC 6. salvos 7. V Fib/V Tach 8. Local anesthetic	1. confusion 2. seizures 3. hypotension 4. bradycardia 5. heart blocks	1. Stokes-Adams 2. WPW 3. heart blocks 4. bradycardia 5. torsades 6. caution with liver failure and elderly	1. 1–1.5 mg/kg up to 3 mg/kg followed by drip: 2–4 mg/min 2. Reduce drip 50% in shock, CHF, ↓hepatic flow, age >70	IVP ET IO IVPB–1 g/250 cc local anesth. ET alternate route

Emergency Drug Quiz Key (continued)

Trade Name	Generic	Actions	Uses	Side Effects	Contraindications	Average Dose	Routes
Morphine	morphine sulfate (MS and MSO_4 are NOT acceptable abbreviations per JCAHO)	1. opium derivative analgesic 2. CNS depressant 3. respiratory and cough depressant 4. stimulates vomiting center in medulla 5. ↓PVR	1. drug of choice pain and anxiety of AMI 2. burns/trauma 3. CHF/acute pulmonary edema	1. hypotension 2. respiratory depression 3. vomiting	1. undiagnosed abdominal pain 2. coma 3. hypotension 4. RR < 12	1–3 mg (usually 2 mg) q 5 minutes slow IVP/max 10 mg	IVP PO IM SQ
Haldol	haloperidol	1. antipsychotic that blocks dopamine receptors in brain 2. similar to phenothiazines 3. anticholinergic	acute psychotic episodes	1. EPS 2. sedation 3. hypotension 4. dry mouth 5. LONG TERM: Tardive dyskinesia	Talwin use coma	2–5 mg IM	IM PO rare IVP
Valium	diazepam	1. anticonvulsant-sedative 2. benzodiazepine 3. skeletal muscle relaxant 4. RAISES seizure threshold	1. grand mal seizures 2. sedation	1. slurred speech 2. drowsiness 3. bradycardia 4. hypotension 5. RESP. DEPRESSION	1. resp. depression 2. shock 3. coma 4. head injury 5. hypotension	1. 2–10 mg in 2 mg increments SLOW IVP 2. Peds: 0.1–0.3 mg/kg IVP	IVP Rectal PO IM Nasal
Calcium Chloride	CaCl	1. electrolyte 2. increases myocardial contractility 3. may slow impulse conduction 4. important mineral for skeletal system, enzyme activity, and coagulation	1. reverse mag sulfate 2. Ca^{++} channel blocker OD 3. hypocalcemia 4. hyperkalemia 5. renal dialysis codes	1. hypotension 2. bradycardia 3. necrosis if infiltrates 4. RAPID IVP can cause cardiac arrest	1. ↑calcium 2. hypokalemia 3. V Fib 4. digitalis toxicity	1. Reverse mag = 200 mg/min up to 1 g 2. Calcium channel OD = 8–16 mg/kg SLOW IVP (Peds 5–7 mg/kg) 3. Dialysis Codes = up to 10 g depending on frequency of dialysis	Slow IVP IO
Sodium Bicarbonate	bicarb	1. electrolyte 2. alkalinizing agent 3. reacts with hydrogen ion to form water and carbon dioxide to buffer metabolic acidosis	1. severe met. acidosis if ventilation verified 2. long cardiac arrest 3. symptomatic TCA OD 4. hyperkalemia 5. renal dialysis codes	1. fluid retention 2. metabolic alkalosis	none in emergency setting	1. 1 mEq/kg 2. 2–5 × normal dose for renal dialysis codes	IVP IO
ASA	acetylsalicylic acid	1. ↓platelet aggregation 2. antipyretic 3. anti-inflammatory 4. analgesic	1. AMI/angina 2. A Fib 3. fever 4. mild to moderate pain arthritis 5. TIA/ischemic stroke 6. arthritis	1. bleeding 2. thrombocytopenia 3. Reyes syndrome 4. tinnitus 5. GI distress	1. active bleeding 2. children <12 y.o.	81–650 mg	PO Rectal

Trade Name	Generic	Actions	Use	Side Effects	Contraindications	Average Dose	Routes
NTG/Tridil	nitroglycerin	1. vasodilator 2. smooth muscle dilator 3. postcapillary dilator promoting venous pooling 4. decreases myocardial oxygen demand 5. reduces preload 6. dilates coronaries 7. releases vasospasm and ↑blood flow	1. angina/chest pain 2. AMI 3. severe hypertension 4. pulmonary edema	1. headache 2. hypotension	1. ↑ICP 2. hypotension 3. Viagra or other performance enhancers in last 24–72 hours, depending on the drug	0.3–0.6 mg SL usually—0.4 mg SL q 5 minutes × 3 doses DRIP (Tridil): 1–50 mcg/min dependent on BP	SL paste IVPB—50 mg/100 cc or 100 mg in 250 cc
Adenocard	adenosine	1. antidysrhythmic (ATP—the energy source necessary for cellular function) 2. vasodilation of coronary beds and inhibits calcium flow 3. acts directly on AV junction to slow conduction 4. restores sinus function in SVT	1. stable or unstable SVT/PSVT including those with WPW 2. diagnostic tool for wide complex tachycardia to rule out atrial aberrancies	1. hypotension 2. chest pain/pressure 3. heart blocks 4. brady—usually transient 5. transient asystole 6. dyspnea 7. bronchospasm	1. heart blocks 2. sick sinus syndrome (SSS)	1. 6 mg RAPID IVP (follow w/20 cc NS) 2nd dose 12 mg × 2 2. Peds: 0.1–0.2 mg/kg up to 12 mg dose	RAPID IVP
Cordarone	amiodarone	1. antidysrhythmic 2. prolongs duration of action potential 3. ↑PRI and QT interval 4. ↓ sinus rate	1. severe V Tach 2. SVT 3. A Fib 4. V Fib 5. PRO-dysrhythmic when used with other antidysrhythmics	1. hepatotoxicity 2. sinus arrest 3. CHF 4. halos/blurred vision 5. photophobia 6. pulmonary fibrosis 7. hypo- or hyperthyroid 8. salivation 9. tremors	1. goiter 2. sinus node dysfunction 3. heart blocks 4. electrolyte imbalance 5. pregnancy 6. bradycardia	1. nonperfusing/load: 300 mg in 30 cc over 30 seconds 2. perfusing: 150 mg in 50–100 cc over 10 minutes (15 mg/min) q 10 minutes	IVP IVPB
Procardia	nifedipine	1. calcium channel blocker 2. dilates coronary arteries 3. decreases PVR	1. hypertension 2. tachycardia 3. angina	1. hypotension 2. dyspnea	1. hypotension 2. compensatory hypertension	10 mg SL (puncture or bite and swallow)	SL PO
Retavase	retaplase	fibrinolytic	1. acute MI 2. thrombotic stroke 3. use with heparin and ASA	1. hemorrhage 2. allergic reaction 3. hypotension 4. reperfusion dysrhythmias	fibrinolytic exclusion criteria	1. initial bolus: 10 units over 2 minutes 2. 2nd bolus 30 minutes later: 10 units over 2 minutes	IV slow bolus
Magnesium Sulfate	magnesium/mag (MgSO₄ NOT acceptable abbreviation per JCAHO)	1. electrolyte 2. CNS depressant 3. anticonvulsant 4. prevent release of ACh at neuromuscular junction 5. "physiological" Ca⁺⁺ channel blocker 6. negative chrono- and dromotrope 7. peripheral vasodilation 8. inhibit uterine contractions 9. enhance uterine blood flow	1. torsades de pointes 2. refractory V Fib and pulseless V Tach 3. eclamptic seizures 4. preeclampsia seizure prevention	1. hypotension 2. resp. depression 3. bradycardia 4. heart blocks 5. reverse with CaCl	1. resp. depression 2. hypotension 3. renal failure	1. torsades: 1–2 g over 1–2 minutes IVP followed by drip: 500 mg/hr 2. Seizures: 2–5 g	IVP IVPB
Pitocin	oxytocin	1. produces uterine contractions 2. stimulates milk ejection	1. induction of labor—NOT prehospital 2. postpartum hemorrhage	1. HTN 2. convulsions 3. tetanic contractions 4. hypotension 5. dysrhythmias	ANY time PRIOR to delivery	10 units/1000 cc run at 2–4 cc/min	IVPB

Emergency Drug Quiz Key *(continued)*

Section 1

EMT and Special Operations

Part 1: Basic EMT Skills

Fabulous Factoids

Skill Sheets

Proper Hand Washing
PPE Removal
Proper Lifting Techniques
Stretcher Operation
Scoop Stretcher Operation
Stair Chair Operation
Spinal Motion Restriction (SMR) Exercise
Spinal Motion Restriction (SMR)—Supine Long Backboard (LBB)
Spinal Motion Restriction (SMR)—Standing Long Backboard (LBB)
Seated Spinal Motion Restriction (SMR)
Rapid Extrication
BLS Skills (Locally Accepted Certification Standards)
Fixation Splint
Traction Splint
Vital Signs
Oxygen Administration
Blow-by Oxygen
Manual Airway Maneuvers
Nasopharyngeal/Oropharyngeal Airway Insertion
Bag-Valve-Mask Ventilation
Bag-Valve-Tube Ventilation
Pulse Oximetry
Glucometer
Patient Restraints

FABULOUS FACTOIDS—BASIC EMT SKILLS LAB

One beer permanently destroys 10,000 brain cells—they do NOT regenerate.

An average American consumes 22 GALLONS of beer in a year.

Two and one-half million RBCs die each SECOND and are replaced just as quickly.

RBCs live for 4 months and make 75,000 trips to the lungs and back.

Shock, or hypoperfusion, has been described as a "momentary pause in the act of death."

The brain is a greedy 3-pound organ, demanding 17% of cardiac output and 20% of all available oxygen.

Every second your senses send about 100 million different messages to your brain.

On average, an adult has about 2.4 yards of skin weighing 9 pounds.

The thickest skin on your body is on the soles of your feet.

Your feet have the most sweat glands in your body.

The average person sheds a complete layer of skin every 28 days.

Your skin accounts for 16% of your body weight.

An average adult body produces 300 billion new cells daily.

The largest cell in the human body is the female egg.

The smallest cell in the human body is the male sperm.

There are no reliable ways to determine which patients are infectious. Take appropriate PPE on all calls. If it is wet and not yours—don't touch it without protection.

If your patient says, "I'm going to die," take him or her seriously.

How strong are your bones? For its weight, bone is as strong as steel and four times stronger than the same amount of reinforced concrete.

You use 200 muscles to take a step.

You have about 650 muscles, with over 50 muscles in the face alone. You use 17 muscles to smile—but over 40 to frown. So smile—it's less work.

Muscle cells live as long as you do, but skin cells live less than 24 hours.

Because of the increased risk of TB in nursing homes, consider your PPE.

The common housefly can carry more than 25 different diseases.

Every 3 months you replace your eyelashes.

You blink an average of 17,000 times each day.

Brain waves have been used to run electric trains.

The average adult has 5 million hair follicles.

Ducks can get the flu and snakes can get malaria.

Drug of the Section: Oxygen (see Emergency Drug Quiz Key, p. xxxi)

Pathophysiologies of the Section: 1.01–1.05 (see Checklist, p. 595)

©2006 Prentice-Hall Inc.

SKILL SHEETS

Proper Hand Washing

Student: _____   **Examiner:** _____

Date: _____

	Done ✓	Not Done
Assesses the environment		
Assesses own hands		
Removes jewelry and pushes up sleeves of uniform or shirt		
Assesses hands for hangnails, cuts or breaks in skin, and heavily soiled areas		
Accesses towel or dryer		
Turns on water and adjusts flow and temperature		
Wets hands and lower forearms thoroughly by holding under running water, keeping hands and forearms in downward position with elbows straight		
Applies about 5 ml (1 tsp) of liquid soap and lathers thoroughly		
Thoroughly rubs hands together for 10–15 seconds, washing *between fingers*		
Rinses with hands in the downward position, elbows straight, forearm to wrist to fingers		
Blots hands and forearms to dry thoroughly in direction of fingers to wrist to forearms		
Uses towels to turn off faucets and accesses more towels if necessary		
Student exhibits competence with skill		

There are no "mandatory" points for this skill—it **must** be performed correctly in all aspects to be successful. The student **must** be aware of safety and protection. Examiners will "dust" hands of candidate with glitter (germs) and have candidate apply gloves for other skills in this lab (or short period of time). At appropriate time, examiner will have candidate remove gloves, verifying that candidate has not "scattered" glitter (germs) in the removal process. Candidate will then proceed to wash hands following above procedure. Examiner will inspect hands for presence of glitter (germs) and direct candidate to reattempt hand washing if indicated.

☐ Successful   ☐ Unsuccessful   Examiner Initials: _____

PPE Removal

Student: _____   **Examiner:** _____

Date: _____

NOTE: Examiner should "contaminate" outer gloves and front of gown with glitter (germs).

Gloves and Goggles	Done ✓	Not Done
Dons minimum EMS personal protective equipment/PPE (gloves and goggles)		*
Grasps any contaminated materials in one gloved hand and with other hand peels glove from inside, rolling over to enclose contaminated items (if more contaminated items than can hold in hand, cleans up area prior to removing gloves)		
Places this "peeled glove package" in remaining gloved hand and with ungloved hand, peels (from inside) contaminated glove off, rolling contaminated materials to inside		
Disposes in appropriate container		*
Washes hands		*
Student exhibits competence with skill		

Gloves, Gown, Goggles, and Mask	Done ✓	Not Done
Puts on mask, goggles, and one pair of gloves		
Puts on gown		
Puts on SECOND pair of gloves so glove cuff comes over sleeve ends of gown		
Provides patient care (instructor contaminates gloves)		
Unties waist tie of gown (if neck tie done, has assistant untie neck tie)		
Touching only FRONT of gown, pulls forward and off shoulders in rolling movement		
Removes gown AND outside pair of gloves as a unit, rolling in upon itself		
Rolls completed unit so ALL contamination to inside—if at all uncertain or gown is wet, immediately places in contaminated linen or disposal bag (inside pair of gloves is now contaminated)		*
Grasps any contaminated materials in one gloved hand and with other hand peels glove from inside, rolling over to enclose contaminated items (if more contaminated items than can hold in hand, cleans up area prior to removing gloves)		*
Places this "peeled glove package" in remaining gloved hand and with ungloved hand, peels (from inside) contaminated glove off, rolling contaminated materials to inside		
Disposes in appropriate container		*
Puts on clean gloves and unties mask		
Removes goggles by using bows on side of goggles (or elastic)		
Removes mask, rolling contaminated surface area inward		
Disposes of mask in proper disposal container		
Cleanses goggles and removes gloves as before		
Cleanses hands		*
Student exhibits competence with skill		

Any items in the Not Done column that are marked with an * are mandatory for the student to complete. A check mark in the Not Done column of an item with an * indicates that the student was unsuccessful and must attempt the skill again to assure competency. Examiners should use a different-color ink for the second attempt.

☐ Successful   ☐ Unsuccessful   Examiner Initials: _____

                    ©2006 Prentice-Hall Inc.

Proper Lifting Techniques

Student: _____   **Examiner:** _____

Date: _____

	Done ✓	Not Done
Utilizes appropriate PPE		*
Assesses access and need for additional personnel/equipment in removal of patient		*
Reduces or removes obstacles prior to lifting patient		*
Verifies patient is secured to lifting device (LBB, stretcher, sheet, chair, etc.)		*
Maintains low center of gravity by bending at hips and knees, not at waist		
Squats down rather than bends over to lift and/or lower patient		*
FEMALES ONLY: Tucks pelvis forward as performs squatting maneuver		
Establishes wide base of support with feet spread apart		*
Adjusts lift technique to size of partner—smaller person places hands in "curling" position		
Lifts stretcher—stops midway for hand position change to overhand PRN		
Verifies that patient is secure (stretcher is locked, or other personnel "set" for carry)		*
Uses feet to move, not a twisting or bending motion from waist		
When pushing or pulling, stands near object and staggers one foot partially ahead		
When pushing object, leans into it, applying continuous light pressure		
When pulling object, leans away and grasps with light pressure		
Never jerks or twists body to force an object to move		
When stooping to move an object, maintains wide base, flexes knees, keeps back straight		
When lifting, squats down, takes firm hold and stands, using leg muscles (back straight)		*
When rising from squat, arches back slightly, keeps buttocks and abdomen tucked in		
When lifting/carrying heavy objects, keeps weight as close to center of gravity as possible		
When reaching for an object, keeps back straight		
Uses safety aids, equipment, and extra personnel as needed to protect back		
Does not endanger patient or team member		*
Student exhibits competence with skill		

Any items in the Not Done column that are marked with an * are mandatory for the student to complete. A check mark in the Not Done column of an item with an * indicates that the student was unsuccessful and must attempt the skill again to assure competency. Examiners should use a different-color ink for the second attempt.

☐ Successful   ☐ Unsuccessful   Examiner Initials: _____

Stretcher Operation

Student: _____   **Examiner:** _____

Date: _____

	Done ✓	Not Done
Utilizes appropriate PPE		*
Performs or verbalizes proper securing of patient to stretcher		*
Adjusts head portion to accommodate patient or maneuver into elevator/around corners		
Able to place patient into Trendelenberg position		
Raises and lowers stretcher smoothly, using multiple levels and safe body mechanics		
Places stretcher into unit using proper techniques and body mechanics		
Secures or verbalizes method of securing stretcher to unit		*
Demonstrates how to remove a patient from an ambulance/rescue unit		
Student exhibits competence with skill		

Any items in the Not Done column that are marked with an * are mandatory for the student to complete. A check mark in the Not Done column of an item with an * indicates that the student was unsuccessful and must attempt the skill again to assure competency. Examiners should use a different-color ink for the second attempt.

☐ Successful   ☐ Unsuccessful   Examiner Initials: _____

©2006 Prentice-Hall Inc.

Scoop Stretcher Operation

Student: _____   **Examiner:** _____

Date: _____

	Done ✓	Not Done
Utilizes appropriate PPE		*
Assesses distal PMS (pulse, movement, sensation)		*
Positions scoop alongside patient		
Measures and adjusts scoop to proper length if adjustable		
Student at head slowly closes head end of scoop ensuring scoop doesn't pinch patient		
Student at foot slowly closes foot end of scoop ensuring scoop doesn't pinch patient		
Students check to be certain patient tissue not caught in scoop stretcher		*
Student(s) strap patient to scoop providing safe transfer to the stretcher		
Scoop is transferred to stretcher with proper lifting techniques		
Secures patient to stretcher (removes scoop if not fractured hip)		
Reassesses distal PMS (pulse, movement, sensation)		*
Assesses patient's response to intervention		*
Student exhibits competence with skill		

Any items in the Not Done column that are marked with an * are mandatory for the student to complete. A check mark in the Not Done column of an item with an * indicates that the student was unsuccessful and must attempt the skill again to assure competency. Examiners should use a different-color ink for the second attempt.

☐ Successful   ☐ Unsuccessful   Examiner Initials: _____

Stair Chair Operation

Student: _____   Examiner: _____

Date: _____

	Done ✓	Not Done
Utilizes appropriate PPE		*
Unfolds stair chair and locks into sitting position		
Properly secures patient to stair chair		*
Able to carefully move patient down stairs and direct partner in assist		
Performs all skills with proper body mechanics		
Transfers patient to stretcher and secures		*
Places stretcher into unit using proper techniques and body mechanics		
Secures or verbalizes method of securing stretcher to unit		*
Folds stair chair and secures for transport		
Student exhibits competence with skill		

Any items in the Not Done column that are marked with an * are mandatory for the student to complete. A check mark in the Not Done column of an item with an * indicates that the student was unsuccessful and must attempt the skill again to assure competency. Examiners should use a different-color ink for the second attempt.

☐ Successful   ☐ Unsuccessful   Examiner Initials: _____

©2006 Prentice-Hall Inc.

Spinal Motion Restriction (SMR) Exercise

Spinal motion restriction (SMR) of the elderly may require additional padding underneath the head to provide proper cervical spine motion restriction. In actuality, many patients require at least a small amount of padding beneath the head.

Instructor: Have students arrange themselves in groups of three. Two students of the group are to stand with their backs to the wall and HEELS touching the wall (just as a patient's heels touch a long backboard [LBB]). Have students stand up STRAIGHT, but without leaning heads back. Most students will not have their head against the wall.

The third student of the group places fingers, one at a time, behind a standing student's head to see how much padding would be appropriate to achieve in-line neutral positioning (no hyperextension of cervical spine). Repeat with the other student and then rotate members.

Now place a "hump" between shoulder blades of students to simulate loss of flexibility and "hunching" of an elderly patient and repeat exercise.

Very interesting and enlightening. Have FUN!

Spinal Motion Restriction (SMR)—Supine Long Backboard (LBB)

Student: _____   **Examiner:** _____

Date: _____

	Done ✓	Not Done
Utilizes appropriate PPE		*
Directs assistant to place/maintain head in neutral in-line position		*
Directs assistant to maintain manual spinal motion restriction (SMR) of the head		*
Assesses distal PMS (pulse, movement, sensation) in extremities		*
Applies appropriately sized extrication collar		
Positions the long backboard (LBB) beside the patient		
Directs second assistant to kneel at patient's hip on side opposite LBB and places self, kneeling, at level of patient's chest next to second assistant		
Directs rescuer maintaining C-spine motion restriction to count to 3 when ready to log roll, places hands across patient, staggering hands with second assistant, and log rolls patient		
Inspects and palpates patient's back, buttocks, and legs while maintaining spinal alignment		
Scoots LBB (or has third assistant slide LBB) under patient and at count of person in control of head, log rolls patient onto LBB		
If adjustment needed to center patient, directs team to move patient along axial line (not slide to the side), angling patient up and down at count of person controlling C-spine		*
Secures the patient's torso to the LBB BEFORE the head		*
Evaluates and pads behind the patient's head as necessary, then secures the patient's head with a cervical spinal motion restriction (CID/SMR) device		
Secures the patient's legs to the device		
Reassesses distal PMS in extremities		*
Assesses patient's response to intervention		*
Student exhibits competence with skill		

Any items in the Not Done column that are marked with an * are mandatory for the student to complete. A check mark in the Not Done column of an item with an * indicates that the student was unsuccessful and must attempt the skill again to assure competency. Examiners should use a different-color ink for the second attempt.

☐ Successful   ☐ Unsuccessful   Examiner Initials: _____

©2006 Prentice-Hall Inc.

Spinal Motion Restriction (SMR)—Standing Long Backboard (LBB)

Student: _____   **Examiner:** _____

Date: _____

	Done ✓	Not Done
Utilizes appropriate PPE		*
Directs assistant to place/maintain head in neutral in-line position		*
Directs assistant to maintain manual SMR of the head		*
Assesses distal PMS (pulse, movement, sensation) in extremities		*
Applies appropriately sized extrication collar		
Positions the long backboard (LBB) behind the patient		
Secures the device to the patient's torso using hands and arms of rescuers, and ensures that the arms are placed to prevent sliding of the patient		
Directs lowering of board and patient, ensuring that rescuers use their legs instead of their back		
Secures the patient's torso to the backboard BEFORE the head		*
Evaluates and pads behind the patient's head as necessary, then secures the patient's head with a cervical SMR device		*
Secures the patient's legs to the device		
Reassesses distal PMS in extremities		*
Assesses patient's response to intervention		*
Student exhibits competence with skill		

Any items in the Not Done column that are marked with an * are mandatory for the student to complete. A check mark in the Not Done column of an item with an * indicates that the student was unsuccessful and must attempt the skill again to assure competency. Examiners should use a different-color ink for the second attempt.

☐ Successful   ☐ Unsuccessful   Examiner Initials: _____

Seated Spinal Motion Restriction (SMR)

Student: _____   **Examiner:** _____

Date: _____

	Done ✓	Not Done
Utilizes appropriate PPE		*
Directs assistant to place/maintain head in neutral in-line position		*
Directs assistant to maintain manual motion restriction of the head		*
Assesses distal PMS (pulse, movement, sensation) in each extremity		*
Applies appropriately sized extrication collar		
Places the SMR device behind the patient		
Secures the device to the patient's torso (M-B-L-H-T)		
Evaluates torso fixation and adjusts as necessary		
Applies leg straps		
Evaluates and pads behind the patient's head as necessary		
Secures the patient's head to the device		*
Tightens chest straps—last		*
Verbalizes moving the patient to a long backboard (LBB), holding legs up until they can be released simultaneously and lowered to LBB		*
Relaxes/loosens chest fixation		*
Secures patient to LBB—head last		*
Reassesses distal PMS in each extremity		*
Assesses patient's response to intervention		*
Student exhibits competence with skill		

Any items in the Not Done column that are marked with an * are mandatory for the student to complete. A check mark in the Not Done column of an item with an * indicates that the student was unsuccessful and must attempt the skill again to assure competency. Examiners should use a different-color ink for the second attempt.

☐ Successful   ☐ Unsuccessful   Examiner Initials: _____

©2006 Prentice-Hall Inc.

Rapid Extrication

Student: _____ **Examiner:** _____

Date: _____

	Done ✓	Not Done
Ensures scene safety and utilizes appropriate PPE		*
Directs assistant to place/maintain head in a neutral in-line position from behind		*
Assesses distal PMS		
Directs same assistant to maintain manual SMR of the head/cervical spine		*
Does a rapid survey, then applies the appropriately sized cervical collar		
Slides LBB slightly beneath patient's buttocks with 2nd assistant/PD supporting end of LBB		
Directs 3rd assistant to enter vehicle from opposite side to support legs during swivel		
Maintaining right arm down axial spine and left arm laterally angled across chest, swivels patient approximately 45° until C-spine motion restriction can be taken by either 2nd or 3rd assistant (after moving around), then transferred back after C-spine person moves out from behind patient		
Swivels patient (as a unit) remainder of distance and, still supporting axial spine, lowers to LBB		
Directs team to carefully slide the patient completely onto the LBB with axial movement only		
Directs/assists with careful movement of LBB to stretcher		
Secures patient to LBB, then LBB to stretcher		*
Reassesses distal PMS		*
Assesses patient's response to intervention		*
Student exhibits competence with skill		

Any items in the Not Done column that are marked with an * are mandatory for the student to complete. A check mark in the Not Done column of an item with an * indicates that the student was unsuccessful and must attempt the skill again to assure competency. Examiners should use a different-color ink for the second attempt.

☐ Successful   ☐ Unsuccessful   Examiner Initials: _____

BLS Skills (Locally Accepted Certification Standards)

Student: _____   **Examiner:** _____

Date: _____

	Pass	Fail
FBAO Adult		
FBAO Child		
FBAO Infant		
Respiratory Arrest Rescue Breathing Adult		
Respiratory Arrest Rescue Breathing Child		
Respiratory Arrest Rescue Breathing Infant		
One-Rescuer CPR Adult		
One-Rescuer CPR Child		
One-Rescuer CPR Infant		
Two-Rescuer CPR Adult		
Two-Rescuer CPR Child		
Two-Rescuer CPR Infant		

Students MUST be able to perform ANY BLS skill according to current regionally accepted organization guidelines.

☐ Pass   ☐ Fail   Examiner Initials: _____

Document area of skill(s) student performed incorrectly in the area below.

                                    ©2006 Prentice-Hall Inc.

Fixation Splint

Student: _____   Examiner: _____

Date: _____

NOTE: Student should be advised patient has isolated simple fracture of humerus, radius/ulna, or tibia/fibula.

	Done ✓	Not Done
Utilizes appropriate PPE		*
Directs assistant to manually stabilize involved extremity		
Assesses distal pulse, movement, sensation (PMS) in extremity		*
Prepares splint (ladder, foam, board, pillow, air, available equipment)		
Applies splint (according to type and manufacturer's recommendations)		
Immobilizes joint above and below the fracture site		*
Secures entire injured extremity to body or LBB		
Reassesses distal PMS in extremity		*
Assesses patient's response to intervention		*
Student exhibits competence with skill		

Any items in the Not Done column that are marked with an * are mandatory for the student to complete. A check mark in the Not Done column of an item with an * indicates that the student was unsuccessful and must attempt the skill again to assure competency. Examiners should use a different-color ink for the second attempt.

☐ Successful   ☐ Unsuccessful   Examiner Initials: _____

Traction Splint

Student: _____   Examiner: _____

Date: _____

NOTE: Student should be advised patient has closed fracture of midshaft femur.

	Done ✓	Not Done
Utilizes appropriate PPE		*
Directs assistant to manually stabilize the fracture		
Assesses distal PMS (pulse, movement, sensation)		*
Applies ankle hitch or alternative		
Directs assistant to apply manual traction until pain relief		*
Prepares and adjusts splint to proper length		
Positions splint beside injured leg		
Directs assistant maintaining traction to elevate the leg as 2nd assistant applies light support under fracture (if using Hare)		
Nestles base of Hare into gluteal fold if using Hare or positions Sager for securing device		*
Applies proximal securing device (e.g., ischial strap) using padding when necessary		*
Applies mechanical traction WITHOUT releasing manual traction until mechanical in place		*
Positions and secures supporting straps		
Reassesses distal PMS		*
Immobilizes hip joint to LBB		*
Secures patient and splint to long backboard (LBB)		*
Reassesses distal PMS		*
Assesses patient's response to intervention		*
Student exhibits competence with skill		

Any items in the Not Done column that are marked with an * are mandatory for the student to complete. A check mark in the Not Done column of an item with an * indicates that the student was unsuccessful and must attempt the skill again to assure competency. Examiners should use a different-color ink for the second attempt.

☐ Successful   ☐ Unsuccessful   Examiner Initials: _____

©2006 Prentice-Hall Inc.

Vital Signs

Student: _____   **Examiner:** _____

Date: _____

Blood Pressure by AUSCULTATION	Done ✓	Not Done
Utilizes appropriate PPE		*
Applies proper size cuff to proximal extremity (upper arm)		
Places level of sphygmomanometer at level of right atrium, if possible		
Palpates arterial point and applies stethoscope diaphragm to arterial point		
Pumps up cuff to above level of top Korotkoff sound		
SLOWLY releases air at 2–4 mmHg per heartbeat		
Accurately identifies systolic and diastolic Korotkoff points (checked by examiner)		
Records results but does NOT verbalize		
Student exhibits competence with skill		

Examiners will now have partners swap and take BP of new partner by PALPATION, comparing results to previously checked auscultated BP.

Blood Pressure by PALPATION		
Utilizes appropriate PPE		*
Applies proper size cuff to proximal extremity (upper arm)		
Places level of sphygmomanometer at level of right atrium, if possible		
Palpates radial arterial point and lightly holds with index and middle fingers		
Pumps up cuff to approximately 10 mmHg above loss of radial pulse		
SLOWLY releases air until palpation of radial arterial pulse possible		
Accurately identifies systolic pressure (checked against BP obtained by examiner)		
Records results		
Student exhibits competence with skill		

Pulse		
Utilizes appropriate PPE		*
Palpates arterial point at radial artery in wrist		
Counts regular pulse for 15 seconds and multiplies by 4 (irregular for 30 sec × 2)		
Records pulse rate		
Checks pulse rate recorded against apical rate for one full minute (examiner checks also)		
Student exhibits competence with skill		

Respirations		
Utilizes appropriate PPE		*
Places hand over diaphragm or watches chest rise and fall		
Counts regular respirations for 30 seconds and multiplies by 2 (irregular for full minute)		
Records respiratory rate		
Checks respiratory rate recorded against rate obtained by examiner		
Student exhibits competence with skill		

Any items in the Not Done column that are marked with an * are mandatory for the student to complete. A check mark in the Not Done column of an item with an * indicates that the student was unsuccessful and must attempt the skill again to assure competency. Examiners should use a different-color ink for the second attempt.

☐ Successful   ☐ Unsuccessful   Examiner Initials: _____

Oxygen Administration

Student: _____   **Examiner:** _____

Date: _____

	Done ✓	Not Done
Utilizes appropriate PPE		*
Assembles regulator to tank		
Opens tank		
Checks for leakage		
Verbalizes evaluation for leak and technique for "O" ring replacement, if applicable		
Attaches nonrebreather mask (NRBM) to regulator		
Prefills reservoir, then places NRBM on patient—elastic behind patient's head		*
Adjusts liter flow to keep reservoir inflated during patient respirations (usually 12–15 LPM)		*
Examiner informs student that patient now needs a nasal cannula applied instead of the NRBM.		
Removes NRBM from patient PRIOR to disconnecting from oxygen source		*
Attaches nasal cannula to oxygen source and adjusts liter flow (2–6 LPM) PRIOR to placing on patient		*
Places nasal cannula, prongs upward and curving in toward patient and tubing around back of each ear (pad if necessary)—not around head		
Adjusts slide mechanism under patient's chin to make cannula snug		
Assesses patient's response to intervention		*
Examiner informs student that patient care has been transferred to ED and needs to return to service.		
Shuts off the regulator		*
Relieves pressure within the regulator		*
Student exhibits competence with skill		

Any items in the Not Done column that are marked with an * are mandatory for the student to complete. A check mark in the Not Done column of an item with an * indicates that the student was unsuccessful and must attempt the skill again to assure competency. Examiners should use a different-color ink for the second attempt.

☐ Successful   ☐ Unsuccessful   Examiner Initials: _____

©2006 Prentice-Hall Inc.

Blow-by Oxygen

Student: _____   **Examiner:** _____

Date: _____

	Done ✓	Not Done
Utilizes appropriate PPE		*
Connects oxygen tubing and turns liter flow to 5 LPM		
Partially cups one hand over infant's nose and mouth approximately 2 in. away		
With other hand, holds oxygen tubing steady and directs oxygen flow against cupped hand		*
Verifies flow from tubing is not directed at infant's eyes or directly into mouth/nose		*
Reassesses infant for improvement or need for further resuscitation		*
Student exhibits competence with skill		

Any items in the Not Done column that are marked with an * are mandatory for the student to complete. A check mark in the Not Done column of an item with an * indicates that the student was unsuccessful and must attempt the skill again to assure competency. Examiners should use a different-color ink for the second attempt.

☐ Successful   ☐ Unsuccessful   Examiner Initials: _____

Manual Airway Maneuvers

Student: _____   Examiner: _____

Date: _____

NOTE: Students should perform each of these skills on the manikin and then on each other.

Head-Tilt/Chin-Lift	Done ✓	Not Done
Utilizes appropriate PPE		*
Places patient supine and positions self at side of patient's head		
Places one hand on forehead—using firm downward pressure with the palm, tilts the head back		*
Puts two fingers under bony part of chin and lifts jaw anteriorly to open airway		*
Assesses patient's response to intervention		*
Student exhibits competence with skill		

Any items in the Not Done column that are marked with an * are mandatory for the student to complete. A check mark in the Not Done column of an item with an * indicates that the student was unsuccessful and must attempt the skill again to assure competency. Examiners should use a different-color ink for the second attempt.

☐ Successful   ☐ Unsuccessful   Examiner Initials: _____

Trauma Jaw-Thrust	Done ✓	Not Done
Utilizes appropriate PPE		*
Places patient supine and positions self at top of patient's head		
Applies fingers to each side of jaw at the mandibular angles		*
Elevates jaw anteriorly without tilting head		*
Assesses patient's response to intervention		*
Student exhibits competence with skill		

Any items in the Not Done column that are marked with an * are mandatory for the student to complete. A check mark in the Not Done column of an item with an * indicates that the student was unsuccessful and must attempt the skill again to assure competency. Examiners should use a different-color ink for the second attempt.

☐ Successful   ☐ Unsuccessful   Examiner Initials: _____

©2006 Prentice-Hall Inc.

Nasopharyngeal/Oropharyngeal Airway Insertion

Student: _____   **Examiner:** _____

Date: _____

Nasopharyngeal Airway	Done ✓	Not Done
Utilizes appropriate PPE		*
Places patient's head in sniffing position if no history of trauma		
Directs preoxygenation if indicated		*
Measures NPA from tip of nose to angle of jaw and checks diameter of nostril		*
Lubricates exterior of tube with water-soluble jelly		
Pushes gently upward on tip of nose and passes NPA into nostril, bevel toward septum		
Verifies appropriate position of airway, breath sounds, chest rise, and airflow		*
Ventilates with 100% oxygen		
Assesses patient's response to intervention		*
Student exhibits competence with skill		

Any items in the Not Done column that are marked with an * are mandatory for the student to complete. A check mark in the Not Done column of an item with an * indicates that the student was unsuccessful and must attempt the skill again to assure competency. Examiners should use a different-color ink for the second attempt.

☐ Successful   ☐ Unsuccessful   Examiner Initials: _____

Oropharyngeal Airway (unresponsive)	Done ✓	Not Done
Utilizes appropriate PPE		*
Places patient's head in sniffing position if no history of trauma		
Opens mouth and removes any visible obstructions		*
Directs preoxygenation if indicated		*
Measures OPA from corner of mouth to earlobe		*
Grasps patient's jaw and lifts anteriorly		
With other hand, holds OPA at proximal end and inserts into patient's mouth with curve reversed and tip pointing to roof of mouth **OR** uses tongue blade correctly to assist insertion		*
As tip reaches level of soft palate, gently rotates 180° advancing to proper depth		*
Verifies appropriate position of airway, breath sounds, and chest rise		*
Ventilates with 100% oxygen		
Assesses patient's response to intervention		*
Student exhibits competence with skill		

Any items in the Not Done column that are marked with an * are mandatory for the student to complete. A check mark in the Not Done column of an item with an * indicates that the student was unsuccessful and must attempt the skill again to assure competency. Examiners should use a different-color ink for the second attempt.

☐ Successful   ☐ Unsuccessful   Examiner Initials: _____

Bag-Valve-Mask Ventilation

Student: _____   **Examiner:** _____

Date: _____

	Done ✓	Not Done
Determines scene safety and utilizes appropriate PPE		*
Manually opens the airway using technique appropriate to patient condition		*
Checks mouth for blood or foreign matter		
Suctions or removes loose oral debris		
Determines patient is apneic/inadequately ventilating and unresponsive		
Properly inserts simple airway adjunct		*
Fits appropriately sized mask to bag-valve device		
Creates tight mask-to-face seal		*
Obtains adequate ventilation in less than 30 seconds		*
Observes chest rise/fall and evaluates compliance		*
Connects oxygen reservoir and adjusts flow rate to fill reservoir		
Turns ventilation over to assistant and bilaterally auscultates over lungs		*
Creates tight mask-to-face seal with two hands		*
Instructs assistant to resume ventilation		
Provides adequate tidal volume for at least 30 seconds		
Assesses patient's response to intervention		*
Student exhibits competence with skill		

Any items in the Not Done column that are marked with an * are mandatory for the student to complete. A check mark in the Not Done column of an item with an * indicates that the student was unsuccessful and must attempt the skill again to assure competency. Examiners should use a different-color ink for the second attempt.

☐ Successful   ☐ Unsuccessful   Examiner Initials: _____

©2006 Prentice-Hall Inc.

Bag-Valve-Tube Ventilation

Student: _____   **Examiner:** _____

Date: _____

	Done ✓	Not Done *
Determines scene safety and utilizes appropriate PPE		*
Manually opens the airway using technique appropriate to patient condition		*
Checks mouth for blood, foreign material, or loose teeth that may become airway obstruction		*
Suctions or removes foreign matter if needed		
Properly inserts simple airway adjunct		
Fits appropriately sized mask to bag-valve device		
Creates tight mask-to-face seal		*
Obtains adequate ventilation in less than 30 seconds		*
Observes chest rise/fall and evaluates compliance		
Connects oxygen reservoir and adjusts flow rate to fill reservoir		
Turns ventilation over to assistant and auscultates bilateral breath sounds		*
Student is advised paramedic has successfully intubated patient and student needs to ventilate.		
Removes mask from bag-valve device		*
Places one hand on ET tube to stabilize and, using other hand, attaches bag-valve device		*
Keeps one hand on ET tube and resumes ventilation		*
Provides adequate tidal volume for at least 30 seconds		*
Assesses patient's response to intervention		*
Student exhibits competence with skill		

Any items in the Not Done column that are marked with an * are mandatory for the student to complete. A check mark in the Not Done column of an item with an * indicates that the student was unsuccessful and must attempt the skill again to assure competency. Examiners should use a different-color ink for the second attempt.

☐ Successful   ☐ Unsuccessful   Examiner Initials: _____

Pulse Oximetry

Student: _____   **Examiner:** _____

Date: _____

	Done ✓	Not Done
Utilizes appropriate PPE		*
Explains procedure to patient		*
Removes nail polish, if present, from index, middle, or ring finger		
Removes earring if using earlobe		
Turns on pulse oximeter and calibrates		
Applies pulse oximeter probe to prepared area		*
Monitors reading for trends		*
Evaluates patient condition correlation to readings and treats appropriately		*
Student exhibits competence with skill		

Any items in the Not Done column that are marked with an * are mandatory for the student to complete. A check mark in the Not Done column of an item with an * indicates that the student was unsuccessful and must attempt the skill again to assure competency. Examiners should use a different-color ink for the second attempt.

☐ Successful   ☐ Unsuccessful   Examiner Initials:_____

                                   ©2006 Prentice-Hall Inc.

Glucometer

Student: _____   **Examiner:** _____

Date: _____

	Done ✓	Not Done
Utilizes appropriate PPE		*
Prepares equipment according to manufacturer's recommendations		*
Obtains finger stick blood or blood from IV catheter upon IV insertion		
Applies blood drop to appropriate site (chemstrip or glucometer), initiates timing mechanism		*
Checks IV for patency or places DSD over finger stick site (with pressure)		*
Reads and RECORDS results		*
Disposes of used items per protocols		*
Assesses patient's response to intervention		*
Student exhibits competence with skill		

Any items in the Not Done column that are marked with an * are mandatory for the student to complete. A check mark in the Not Done column of an item with an * indicates that the student was unsuccessful and must attempt the skill again to assure competency. Examiners should use a different-color ink for the second attempt.

☐ Successful   ☐ Unsuccessful   Examiner Initials: _____

Patient Restraints

Student: _____   **Examiner:** _____

Date: _____

	Done ✓	Not Done
Utilizes appropriate PPE		*
Verbalizes proper indications for use of restraints		*
Calmly explains procedure to patient		

Prepares equipment
   Soft wrist restraints for unresponsive patient
   Leather four-point restraints for combative patient		

Assures adequate personnel available for restraint application		*
Places patient supine		
Applies soft wrist restraints, checking distal PMS before and after application, OR pads beneath leather restraint one extremity at a time, checking distal PMS before and after		*
Places sheet restraint or padded strap across chest securing combative patient to stretcher		
Reassesses patient after restraints in place		*
Monitors restrained patient continuously		*
Documents indications, assessment findings, and continuous monitoring		*
Student exhibits competence with skill		

Any items in the Not Done column that are marked with an * are mandatory for the student to complete. A check mark in the Not Done column of an item with an * indicates that the student was unsuccessful and must attempt the skill again to assure competency. Examiners should use a different-color ink for the second attempt.

☐ Successful   ☐ Unsuccessful   Examiner Initials: _____

©2006 Prentice-Hall Inc.

Bleeding Control and Shock Management

Student: _____   Examiner: _____

Date: _____

NOTE: Student should be advised that patient has a bleeding laceration on an extremity.

	Done ✓	Not Done
Utilizes appropriate PPE		*
Applies direct pressure to the wound		*
Elevates the extremity		*
Student should be advised that the wound continues to bleed.		
Applies an additional dressing, maintains pressure to the wound, and elevates extremity		*
Assesses patient's response to intervention		*
Student should be advised that the wound still continues to bleed.		
Locates and applies pressure to appropriate arterial pressure point		*
Assesses patient's response to intervention		*
Student should be advised that the bleeding is controlled.		
Bandages the wound		
Assesses patient's response to intervention		*
Student should be advised that the patient is pale, cool, clammy, with rapid pulse and dropping BP.		
Properly positions the patient		*
Administers high-concentration oxygen		*
Indicates steps to prevent heat loss from the patient		
Indicates the need for immediate transportation		*
Assesses patient's response to intervention		*
Student exhibits competence with skill		

Any items in the Not Done column that are marked with an * are mandatory for the student to complete. A check mark in the Not Done column of an item with an * indicates that the student was unsuccessful and must attempt the skill again to assure competency. Examiners should use a different-color ink for the second attempt.

☐ Successful   ☐ Unsuccessful   Examiner Initials: _____

Pneumatic Anti-Shock Garment (PASG)

Student: _____   Examiner: _____

Date: _____

NOTE: Student should be advised that patient's BP is <80 mmHg and Medical Control ordered the PASG.

	Done ✓	Not Done
Utilizes appropriate PPE		*
Directs assistant in helping slide PASG under patient		
Assesses lung sounds for pulmonary edema		*
Assesses for relative contraindications (i.e., impaled objects, pregnancy, head or chest trauma)		*
Inflates leg compartments of PASG until Velcro crackle		*
Assesses BP		*
Student should be advised that patient's systolic BP is still less than 80 mmHg.		
Inflates abdominal compartment until Velcro crackle		*
Assesses BP		*
Student should be advised that patient's systolic BP is greater than 90 mmHg.		
Assesses lung sounds and distal PMS (pulse, movement, sensation)		*
Assesses patient's response to intervention		*
Student exhibits competence with skill		

Any items in the Not Done column that are marked with an * are mandatory for the student to complete. A check mark in the Not Done column of an item with an * indicates that the student was unsuccessful and must attempt the skill again to assure competency. Examiners should use a different-color ink for the second attempt.

☐ Successful   ☐ Unsuccessful   Examiner Initials: _____

©2006 Prentice-Hall Inc.

Radio Skills

Student: _____   **Examiner:** _____

Date: _____

	Done ✓	Not Done
Verifies/requests open channel		
Presses transmit button 1 second before speaking		
Holds microphone 2–3 in. from mouth		*
Speaks slowly and clearly		
Speaks in a normal voice, avoiding emotion		
Is brief, but transmits PERTINENT patient information		*
Does not waste airtime		
Protects privacy of patient—even if asked for patient name over a "private line" channel		*
Echoes dispatch information or physician orders		*
Writes down dispatch information or physician orders		
Confirms that message is received		*
Demonstrates/verbalizes ability to troubleshoot basic equipment malfunction		
Student exhibits competence with skill		

Any items in the Not Done column that are marked with an * are mandatory for the student to complete. A check mark in the Not Done column of an item with an * indicates that the student was unsuccessful and must attempt the skill again to assure competency. Examiners should use a different-color ink for the second attempt.

☐ Successful   ☐ Unsuccessful   Examiner Initials: _____

DAILY DISCUSSIONS AND PERTINENT POINTS—BASIC EMT SKILLS LAB

Student: _____   **Date:** _____

Instructor: _____

	Instructor Initials
Serve as a role model for others relative to professionalism in EMS in classroom, labs, and clinical areas.	
Value the need to serve as the patient advocate inclusive of those with special needs, alternate lifestyles, and cultural diversity.	
Defend the importance of continuing medical education and skills retention.	
Assess personal attitudes and demeanor that may distract from professionalism.	
Value the role that family dynamics play in the total care of patients.	
Advocate the need for injury prevention, including abusive situations.	
Exhibit professional behaviors in the following areas: integrity, empathy, self-motivation, appearance and personal hygiene, self-confidence, communications, time management, teamwork and diplomacy, respect, patient advocacy, and careful delivery of service in classroom, labs, and clinical areas.	
Discuss how cardiovascular endurance, muscle strength, and flexibility contribute to physical fitness.	
Discuss the concept of wellness and its benefits.	
Define the components of wellness.	
Advocate the benefits of working toward the goal of total personal wellness.	
Defend the need to treat each patient as an individual, with respect and dignity.	
Value the need to assess his or her own lifestyle.	
Challenge him or herself to each wellness concept in his or her role as an EMS provider.	
Assess his or her own prejudices related to the various aspects of cultural diversity.	
Serve as a role model for other EMS providers in regard to a total wellness lifestyle.	
Improve personal physical well-being through achieving and maintaining proper body weight, regular exercise, and proper nutrition.	
Promote and practice stress management techniques.	
Defend the need to respect the emotional needs of dying patients and their families.	
Advocate and practice the use of personal safety precautions in all scene situations, labs, or any patient contact.	
Advocate and serve as a role model for other EMS providers relative to PPE/BSI practices.	
Document primary and secondary injury prevention data.	
Value and defend tenets of prevention in terms of personal safety and wellness.	
Value and defend tenets of prevention for patients and communities being served.	
Value the contribution of effective documentation as one justification for funding of prevention programs.	
Value personal commitment to the success of prevention programs.	
Value the patient's autonomy in the decision-making progress.	
Defend the following ethical positions: a. The EMS provider is accountable to the patient. b. The EMS provider is accountable to the medical director. c. The EMS provider is accountable to the EMS system. d. The EMS provider is accountable for fulfilling the standard of care.	
Given a scenario, defend or challenge an EMS provider's actions concerning a patient who is treated against his or her own wishes.	
Given a scenario, defend or challenge an EMS provider's actions in a situation in which a physician orders therapy the EMS provider feels to be detrimental to the patient's best interests.	
Serve as a role model for an effective communication process in classroom, labs, and clinical areas.	
Advocate the importance of external factors of communication.	
Promote proper responses to patient communications.	
Exhibit professional nonverbal behaviors in classroom, labs, and clinical areas.	
Advocate development of proper patient rapport.	
Value strategies to obtain patient information.	
Exhibit professional behaviors in communicating with patients in special situations.	
Exhibit professional behaviors in communicating with patients from different cultures.	
Describe the purpose of verbal communication of patient information to the hospital.	
Advocate the need to show respect for the rights and feelings of patients.	
Assess his or her personal commitment to protecting patient confidentiality.	
Value the importance of presenting the patient (to the ED) accurately and clearly.	
Assess personal practices relative to ambulance/rescue operations that may affect the safety of the crew, the patient, and bystanders.	
Serve as a role model for others relative to the operation of ambulances/rescue units in classroom, labs, and clinical areas.	

©2006 Prentice-Hall Inc.

Part 2: Advanced EMT Skills

Fabulous Factoids
   Initial Assessment Algorithm

Skill Sheets
   Scene Size-up and Initial Assessment
   Rapid Trauma Assessment
   Helmet Removal
   Infant/Child Car Seat Spinal Motion Restriction (SMR)
   Glasgow Coma Score (GCS) Evaluation
   Rule of Nines
   Pregnant Patient to LBB (Supine Patient)
   Performing a General Patient Survey
   "SAMPLE" History
   Obtaining a Patient History
   EMT: Stroke Exam—Speech, Droop, Drift
   Stethoscope Placement
   Breath Sounds Identification
   Nasopharyngeal/Oropharyngeal Suction
   Dual Lumen (Biluminal) Airway Insertion
   BLS Emergency Ventilation via Tracheostomy Tube
   BLS Emergency Ventilation via Stoma
   Automated External Defibrillator (AED)
   Lead Placement
   IV Solution Setup
   Discontinuing an IV
   Auto-Injector
   EMT: Prolapsed Cord Presentation
   EMT: Breech Presentation
   APGAR Score
   EMT: Childbirth
   Neonatal Resuscitation Equipment
   EMT: Postpartum Hemorrhage
   Pediatric Manual Airway Maneuvers
   Pediatric Nasopharyngeal/Oropharyngeal Airway Insertion
   Humidified Oxygen
   EMT: Emergency Care for Heat Disorders
   EMT: Recognition and Treatment of Hypothermia
   Documentation Skills: Patient Care Report (PCR)
   Radio Report

Daily Discussions and Pertinent Points

FABULOUS FACTOIDS—ADVANCED EMT SKILLS LAB

Patient assessment is the one important skill that an EMS provider uses on every call and with every patient.

Abandonment is the number-one reason for legal suits against EMS.

> Document mental capacity
> Reason for refusal
> Understanding of consequences
> Advice given

DNR and pronouncement of death.

> Who/what time

Sloppy/incomplete recording will imply sloppy/incomplete care. You may have to review a PCR 5–10 years from now. Write it so it will be legible at that time. Remember, lawyers LOVE discrepancies and disagreement.

Four uses for PCR = medical, administrative, research, LEGAL.

If you don't know how to spell a word, look it up or use another word.

Document any medical advice or orders you receive and the results of implementing that advice or those orders.

Document *all* findings of assessment, even those that are normal.

Be aware of your body language and the message it sends.

Patient body language is important. The quieter patients lie, the more ill they are.

Inflating the abdominal section of the PASG may cause up to a 50% reduction in diaphragmatic movement.

Einstein couldn't read until the age of 9.

Einstein failed his college entrance exam.

Einstein slept 10 hours a night. (He obviously wasn't in EMS.)

The average American sleeps 7 hours, 20 minutes per night.

The kidneys weigh about 5 ounces each, but process about 425 gallons of blood in a day.

Forty-five percent of all prescription drugs contain ingredients originating in the rain forest.

The liver—largest organ in the torso—processes about a quart of blood every minute.

The world's longest human foot is 27 inches long.

Drug of the Section: Review Oxygen (the most frequently used drug in emergency medicine) (see Emergency Drug Quiz Key, p. xxxi)

©2006 Prentice-Hall Inc.

Initial Assessment Algorithm

Initial Assessment "Memory Jogger"

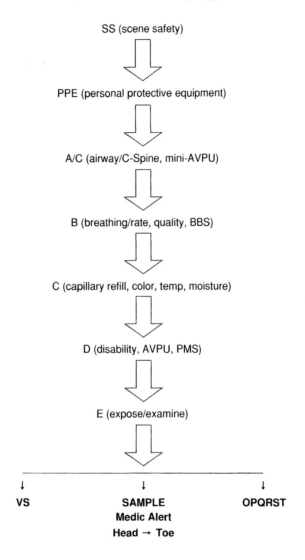

SS (scene safety)

PPE (personal protective equipment)

A/C (airway/C-Spine, mini-AVPU)

B (breathing/rate, quality, BBS)

C (capillary refill, color, temp, moisture)

D (disability, AVPU, PMS)

E (expose/examine)

VS	SAMPLE	OPQRST
	Medic Alert	
	Head → Toe	

©2006 Prentice-Hall Inc.

SKILL SHEETS

Scene Size-up and Initial Assessment

Student: _____   Examiner: _____

Date: _____

	Done ✓	Not Done
Utilizes appropriate PPE		*
Evaluates and ensures scene safety		*
Locates all patients		*
Determines mechanism of injury/nature of illness		*
Forms general impression (visual general survey) of patient		*
Stabilizes cervical spine as needed		*
Assesses baseline level of response		
Manually opens the airway with appropriate maneuver for patient condition		*
Looks, listens, and feels for air movement		*
Immediately corrects obstructed airway		*
Properly inserts simple airway adjunct as needed		
Assesses breathing rate and quality		*
Inspects chest and back		
Palpates chest and back		
Auscultates bilaterally for equality/adequacy of ventilation/heart sounds		*
Immediately corrects injuries that may compromise airway/breathing		*
Administers oxygen, assists ventilation as needed		*
Checks radial pulses for rate and quality		*
Checks skin color, temperature, and condition		*
Checks capillary refill time in children		*
Controls gross hemorrhage		*
Elevates legs and keeps patient warm as needed		
Assigns priority for transport		
Student exhibits competence with skill		

Any items in the Not Done column that are marked with an * are mandatory for the student to complete. A check mark in the Not Done column of an item with an * indicates that the student was unsuccessful and must attempt the skill again to assure competency. Examiners should use a different-color ink for the second attempt.

☐ Successful   ☐ Unsuccessful   Examiner Initials: _____

©2006 Prentice-Hall Inc.

Rapid Trauma Assessment

Student: _____   **Examiner:** _____

Date: _____

	Done ✓	Not Done
Utilizes appropriate PPE		*
Assures C-spine SMR is being maintained		*
In assessing areas students may use DCAP-BTLS* or DCAP-BLS-TIC*		
HEAD: Palpates the head and facial bones		*
Periodically examines gloves for blood		*
NECK: Inspects and palpates anterior neck		*
Checks for tracheal deviation		
Checks for subcutaneous emphysema		
Checks for jugular vein distention		*
Inspects and palpates posterior neck for tenderness, irregularity, or edema		
CHEST: Inspects and palpates the chest		*
Checks for subcutaneous emphysema		
Auscultates both lungs		*
ABDOMEN: Inspects and palpates abdomen		*
PELVIS: Evaluates the pelvic ring		*
EXTREMITIES: Inspects and palpates all four extremities		*
Evaluates distal neurovascular function—PMS (pulse, movement, sensation)		*
POSTERIOR: Inspects and palpates posterior trunk, buttocks		*
Student exhibits competence with skill		

Any items in the Not Done column that are marked with an * are mandatory for the student to complete. A check mark in the Not Done column of an item with an * indicates that the student was unsuccessful and must attempt the skill again to assure competency. Examiners should use a different-color ink for the second attempt.

☐ Successful   ☐ Unsuccessful   Examiner Initials: _____

- DCAP-BTLS: Deformities, Contusions, Abrasions, Penetrations, Burns, Tenderness, Lacerations, Swelling

- DCAP-BLS-TIC: Deformities, Contusions, Abrasions, Penetrations, Burns, Lacerations, Swelling, Tenderness, Instability, Crepitus

Helmet Removal

Student: _____   Examiner: _____

Date: _____

	Done ✓	Not Done
Utilizes appropriate PPE		*
Positions self above or behind the victim, stabilizes the head and neck by holding the helmet and the patient's neck		
Directs assistant to remove the chin strap		
Directs assistant to assume stabilization by placing one hand under neck and occiput, the other on anterior neck with thumb on one angle of the mandible, index and middle fingers on other angle of mandible		*
Removes the helmet by pulling out laterally on each side to clear the ears and then up to remove. Tilts full-face helmet back to clear the nose		*
After removal of helmet, assumes motion restriction of neck by grasping head on either side with fingers holding one angle of jaw and occiput		*
Directs placement of properly sized cervical collar		
Assesses patient's response to intervention		*
Student exhibits competence with skill		

Any items in the Not Done column that are marked with an * are mandatory for the student to complete. A check mark in the Not Done column of an item with an * indicates that the student was unsuccessful and must attempt the skill again to assure competency. Examiners should use a different-color ink for the second attempt.

☐ Successful   ☐ Unsuccessful   Examiner Initials: _____

©2006 Prentice-Hall Inc.

Infant/Child Car Seat Spinal Motion Restriction (SMR)

Student: _____   **Examiner:** _____

Date: _____

	Done ✓	Not Done *
Assesses scene safety and utilizes appropriate PPE		*
Takes or directs manual cervical SMR		*
Performs ABCD, including distal PMS		*
Checks car seat integrity		*
Performs visual and palpation body survey for glass and DCAP-BLS-TIC/DCAP-BTLS		*
Resecures restraining straps		
Restricts motion of head and shoulders with towel roll or blanket roll as appropriate		*
Reassesses ABCD and distal PMS		*
Secures car seat to rescue unit		*
Monitors infant/child at all times		*
Student exhibits competence with skill		

Any items in the Not Done column that are marked with an * are mandatory for the student to complete. A check mark in the Not Done column of an item with an * indicates that the student was unsuccessful and must attempt the skill again to assure competency. Examiners should use a different-color ink for the second attempt.

☐ Successful   ☐ Unsuccessful   Examiner Initials: _____

Glasgow Coma Score (GCS) Evaluation

Student: _____   **Examiner:** _____

Date: _____

	Done ✓	Not Done
Utilizes appropriate PPE		*
Properly demonstrates and scores EYE OPENING: Spontaneous (4)		
Properly demonstrates and scores EYE OPENING: To speech (3)		
Properly demonstrates and scores EYE OPENING: To pain (2)		
Properly demonstrates and scores EYE OPENING: No response (1)		
Properly demonstrates and scores VERBAL: Oriented (5)		
Properly demonstrates and scores VERBAL: Confused (4)		
Properly demonstrates and scores VERBAL: Inappropriate (3)		
Properly demonstrates and scores VERBAL: Garbled (2)		
Properly demonstrates and scores VERBAL: No verbal response (1)		
Properly demonstrates and scores MOTOR: Obeys command (6)		
Properly demonstrates and scores MOTOR: Localizes pain (5)		
Properly demonstrates and scores MOTOR: Withdraws from pain (4)		
Properly demonstrates and scores MOTOR: Flexion to pain (3)		
Properly demonstrates and scores MOTOR: Extension to pain (2)		
Properly demonstrates and scores MOTOR: No response to pain (1)		
Properly scores four simulated patients		*
Student exhibits competence with skill		

Any items in the Not Done column that are marked with an * are mandatory for the student to complete. A check mark in the Not Done column of an item with an * indicates that the student was unsuccessful and must attempt the skill again to assure competency. Examiners should use a different-color ink for the second attempt.

☐ Successful   ☐ Unsuccessful   Examiner Initials: _____

©2006 Prentice-Hall Inc.

Rule of Nines

Student: _____   **Examiner:** _____

Date: _____

	Done ✓	Not Done
Properly scores an infant's arm (9%)		
Properly scores an adult's back (18%)		
Properly scores an infant's leg (14%)		
Properly scores an adult's chest and abdomen (18%)		
Properly scores an infant's head (18%)		
Properly scores an adult's head (9%)		
Properly scores an infant's back (18%)		
Properly scores an adult's leg (18%)		
Properly scores an infant's genitalia (1%)		
Properly scores an adult's arm (9%)		
Properly scores an infant's chest and abdomen (18%)		
Properly scores an adult's genitalia (1%)		
Properly scores three simulated patients with 100% accuracy		*
Student exhibits competence with skill		

Any items in the Not Done column that are marked with an * are mandatory for the student to complete. A check mark in the Not Done column of an item with an * indicates that the student was unsuccessful and must attempt the skill again to assure competency. Examiners should use a different-color ink for the second attempt.

☐ Successful   ☐ Unsuccessful   Examiner Initials: _____

Pregnant Patient to LBB (Supine Patient)

Student: _____   Examiner: _____

Date: _____

	Done ✓	Not Done *
Assesses scene safety and utilizes appropriate PPE		*
Directs assistant to place/maintain head in neutral in-line position		*
Performs initial assessment		
Checks perfusion status, manually displacing gravid uterus to left if compromised		*
Assesses distal PMS (pulse, movement, sensation) in each extremity		*
Applies appropriately sized extrication collar		
Positions the motion restriction device (LBB) appropriately		
Log rolls patient and checks back/buttocks		
Directs movement of the patient onto the device without compromising the integrity of the spine		
Applies padding to voids between the torso and the device as necessary		*
Secures the patient's torso to the device		*
Evaluates and pads behind the patient's head as necessary		*
Secures the patient's head to the device		
Secures the patient's legs to the device		
Secures the patient's arms to the device		
Reassesses distal PMS in each extremity		*
Recognizes potential for SHS (supine hypotensive syndrome)		*
Tilts board to left, relieving pressure of gravid uterus on vena cava		*
Reassesses perfusion status, SMR, and distal PMS		*
Assesses patient's response to intervention		*
Student exhibits competence with skill		

Any items in the Not Done column that are marked with an * are mandatory for the student to complete. A check mark in the Not Done column of an item with an * indicates that the student was unsuccessful and must attempt the skill again to assure competency. Examiners should use a different-color ink for the second attempt.

☐ Successful   ☐ Unsuccessful   Examiner Initials: _____

©2006 Prentice-Hall Inc.

Performing a General Patient Survey

Student: _____   Examiner: _____

Date: _____

NOTE: Bold italicized items should be evaluated as student is approaching patient.

	Done ✓	Not Done
Utilizes appropriate PPE		*
Evaluates level of consciousness		*
Evaluates for obvious signs of distress		*
Evaluates apparent state of health		
Evaluates vital statistics		
Evaluates skin color and obvious lesions		*
Evaluates posture, gait, and motor activity, if ambulating		
Evaluates dress, grooming, and personal hygiene		
Evaluates odors of breath or body		*
Evaluates airway and respirations		*
Evaluates pulse (notes skin temperature, moisture, color, and turgor)		*
Evaluates blood pressure		
Evaluates pulse oximetry		
Evaluates cardiac monitor pattern		
Evaluates blood glucose level		
Student exhibits competence with skill		

Any items in the Not Done column that are marked with an * are mandatory for the student to complete. A check mark in the Not Done column of an item with an * indicates that the student was unsuccessful and must attempt the skill again to assure competency. Examiners should use a different-color ink for the second attempt.

☐ Successful   ☐ Unsuccessful   Examiner Initials: _____

"SAMPLE" History

Student: _____   **Examiner:** _____

Date: _____

	Done ✓	Not Done
Assesses scene safety and utilizes appropriate PPE		*
Asks patient/caregiver for his or her Symptoms		*
Asks patient/caregiver for his or her Allergies		*
Asks patient/caregiver for a list of Medications patient takes and if they are being taken as directed		*
Asks patient/caregiver for his or her Past (pertinent) medical history		*
Asks patient/caregiver for time of the Last oral intake (including water)		*
Asks patient/caregiver for information on the Event that initiated the 9-1-1 call		*
Student exhibits competence with skill		

Any items in the Not Done column that are marked with an * are mandatory for the student to complete. A check mark in the Not Done column of an item with an * indicates that the student was unsuccessful and must attempt the skill again to assure competency. Examiners should use a different-color ink for the second attempt.

☐ Successful   ☐ Unsuccessful   Examiner Initials: _____

©2006 Prentice-Hall Inc.

Obtaining a Patient History

Student: _____   **Examiner:** _____

Date: _____

	Done ✓	Not Done
Utilizes appropriate PPE		*
Establishes patient rapport and trust; gets down to eye level with shorter patients		
Performs proper introductions		
Asks appropriate open-ended questions		*
Asks appropriate close-ended questions		
Demonstrates active listening skills		*
Obtains preliminary data (age, overall condition)		
Obtains chief complaint		*
Obtains SAMPLE (if on medications, finds out if they are being taken as directed)		*
Obtains history of present illness or injury (if a fall, what was the CAUSE of the fall?)		*
Obtains information on pertinent past history (cardiac, diabetic, CVA)		*
Obtains information on current health status		
Performs a review of body systems		*
Handles special challenges appropriately		
Student exhibits competence with skill		

Any items in the Not Done column that are marked with an * are mandatory for the student to complete. A check mark in the Not Done column of an item with an * indicates that the student was unsuccessful and must attempt the skill again to assure competency. Examiners should use a different-color ink for the second attempt.

☐ Successful   ☐ Unsuccessful   Examiner Initials: _____

EMT: Stroke Exam—Speech, Droop, Drift

Student: _____   **Examiner:** _____

Date: _____

	Done ✓	Not Done
Assesses scene safety and utilizes appropriate PPE		*
During assessment, notes facial droop and altered level of consciousness		*
Prepares to do stroke exam—speech, droop, drift		
Asks patient to repeat the phrase "You can't teach an old dog new tricks"		*
Evaluates if patient slurs words, can't repeat, jumbles words, etc.		*
Asks patient to smile and observes face for unilateral facial droop		*
Evaluates symmetry and movement of mouth and cheeks		*
Explains to patient the need to close his or her eyes and hold his or her arms out straight		*
Takes patient's arms and places them out straight in front of the patient at the level of the shoulders, and tells patient to hold them there and close his or her eyes		*
Evaluates for one arm drifting downward when patient closes eyes		*
Verbalizes that ANY of the above tests being abnormal can indicate stroke in progress		*
Student exhibits competence with skill		

Any items in the Not Done column that are marked with an * are mandatory for the student to complete. A check mark in the Not Done column of an item with an * indicates that the student was unsuccessful and must attempt the skill again to assure competency. Examiners should use a different-color ink for the second attempt.

☐ Successful   ☐ Unsuccessful   Examiner Initials: _____

©2006 Prentice-Hall Inc.

Stethoscope Placement

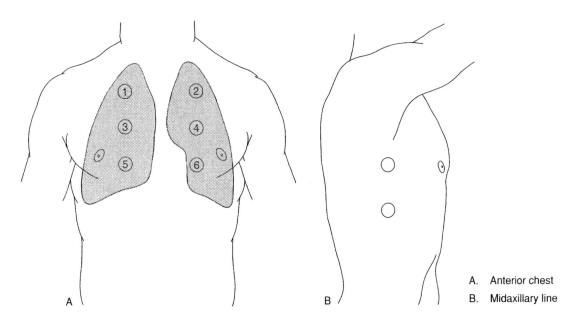

A. Anterior chest
B. Midaxillary line

Student: _____   **Examiner:** _____

Date: _____

	Done ✓	Not Done
Utilizes appropriate PPE		*
Explains procedure to the patient		
Instructs the patient to open his or her mouth and take slow, deep breaths after each placement of the stethoscope		*
Identifies all 16 points of auscultation		
Identifies where each type of lung sound is normally auscultated (tracheal, bronchial, bronchovesicular, vesicular)		*
Student exhibits competence with skill		

Any items in the Not Done column that are marked with an * are mandatory for the student to complete. A check mark in the Not Done column of an item with an * indicates that the student was unsuccessful and must attempt the skill again to assure competency. Examiners should use a different-color ink for the second attempt.

☐ Successful   ☐ Unsuccessful   Examiner Initials: _____

Breath Sounds Identification

Student: _____   Examiner: _____

Date: _____

NOTE: Lung sounds should be identified by use of generator, video, or audiotape for consistency.

	Done ✓	Not Done *
Identifies rhonchi		*
Identifies wheezes		*
Identifies friction rub		
Identifies stridor		*
Identifies rales (also known as crackles)		*
Identifies absent lung sounds		*
Student exhibits competence with skill		

Any items in the Not Done column that are marked with an * are mandatory for the student to complete. A check mark in the Not Done column of an item with an * indicates that the student was unsuccessful and must attempt the skill again to assure competency. Examiners should use a different-color ink for the second attempt.

☐ Successful   ☐ Unsuccessful   Examiner Initials: _____

©2006 Prentice-Hall Inc.

Nasopharyngeal/Oropharyngeal Suction

Student: _____

Examiner: _____

Date: _____

	Done ✓	Not Done
Washes hands		*
Utilizes appropriate PPE (goggles, gown, mask, gloves)		*
Gathers supplies and explains procedure to patient		
Positions patient in high or semi-Fowler's		
Adjusts suction control to between 110 and 120 mmHg		
Opens suction kit, using inside of wrapper as sterile field		
Puts sterile lubricant on field and sterile solution into container		
Carefully lifts wrapped gloves from kit without contaminating field or gloves		
Opens wrapper and applies sterile gloves		
Designates one hand clean and one sterile		
Uses sterile hand to pick up catheter and coils tip around fingers		
Picks up extension tubing and connects to catheter		
Has assistant preoxygenate patient		*
Positions thumb of clean hand over port and dips catheter into sterile solution to check suction		
Oropharyngeal: Asks patient to open mouth, and advances catheter, suctioning as withdraws		
Nasopharyngeal: Lubricates catheter and measures from nose to earlobe		
Inserts and advances with downward tilt and slight rotation		
Occludes port and suctions while withdrawing—NO LONGER than 15 seconds		*
Repeats both as needed		
Dips catheter into solution to clean and disconnects from extension tubing		
Removes glove by pulling over catheter		
Disposes of soiled items appropriately		*
Reassesses patient and washes hands		*
Documents correctly		
Student exhibits competence with skill		

Any items in the Not Done column that are marked with an * are mandatory for the student to complete. A check mark in the Not Done column of an item with an * indicates that the student was unsuccessful and must attempt the skill again to assure competency. Examiners should use a different-color ink for the second attempt.

☐ Successful   ☐ Unsuccessful   Examiner Initials: _____

Dual Lumen (Biluminal) Airway Insertion

Student: _____   Examiner: _____

Date: _____

	Done ✓	Not Done
Utilizes appropriate PPE		*
Opens the airway manually—assures unresponsiveness		*
Opens mouth and checks for blood, loose teeth, or foreign matter		
Suctions or removes potential airway debris as needed		
Inserts simple airway adjunct (oropharyngeal or nasopharyngeal airway)		
Ventilates patient immediately (with room air)		
Obtains effective patient ventilation in less than 30 seconds		*
Attaches oxygen to bag-valve-mask at high flow and uses reservoir if available		
Effectively ventilates patient for 30 seconds		*
Auscultates over bilateral lung fields for baseline lung sounds		*
Directs assistant to take over preoxygenation		*
Checks/prepares airway device		*
Lubricates distal tip of the device (may be verbalized)		
Positions head properly and removes airway adjunct if inserted		
Assures unresponsiveness and performs a tongue-jaw lift		
Inserts dual lumen airway according to manufacturer's instructions		*
Inflates cuffs and secures airway device in sequence recommended for device		*
Removes syringes		*
Attaches bag-valve device to first lumen (esophageal) and ventilates		*
Auscultates over epigastrium to confirm placement		*
If hears gurgling over epigastrium, verbalizes that tube is in trachea		
Changes bag-valve device to second (tracheal) lumen and ventilates		
Auscultates over epigastrium and bilateral lungs to verify effective ventilations		*
Observes for rise and fall of chest, patient color change, and improvement		*
Secures device or confirms that the device remains properly secured		*
Student exhibits competence with skill		

Any items in the Not Done column that are marked with an * are mandatory for the student to complete. A check mark in the Not Done column of an item with an * indicates that the student was unsuccessful and must attempt the skill again to assure competency. Examiners should use a different-color ink for the second attempt.

☐ Successful   ☐ Unsuccessful   Examiner Initials: _____

©2006 Prentice-Hall Inc.

BLS Emergency Ventilation via Tracheostomy Tube

Student: _____

Date: _____

Examiner: _____

	Done ✓	Not Done
Utilizes appropriate PPE		*
Attempts ventilation by bag-valve device to trach tube		
Attempts BVM ventilation while setting up for suction		
Suctions through tracheostomy tube		
If still unable to ventilate and trach tube has inner cannula, removes inner cannula		
Attempts to suction through outer cannula		
If STOMA without tube—attempts to ventilate via BVM using infant mask		
Asks assistant to ventilate while one person holds mask to stoma for good seal		
If unable to ventilate via stoma, suctions through stoma (no longer than 15 seconds)		*
Attempts to ventilate—if still unable to ventilate, attempts BVM via mouth/nose as usual		
Ventilates and confirms effectiveness with auscultation, chest rise and fall, and pulse oximeter		*
Assesses patient's response to intervention		*
Student exhibits competence with skill		

Any items in the Not Done column that are marked with an * are mandatory for the student to complete. A check mark in the Not Done column of an item with an * indicates that the student was unsuccessful and must attempt the skill again to assure competency. Examiners should use a different-color ink for the second attempt.

☐ Successful   ☐ Unsuccessful   Examiner Initials: _____

BLS Emergency Ventilation via Stoma

Student: _____   **Examiner:** _____

Date: _____

	Done ✓	Not Done
Utilizes appropriate PPE		*
Attempts to ventilate using mouth-to-mask with one-way valve while equipment set up **OR** Attempts BVM ventilation via mask over mouth and nose		*
Hooks up infant mask (with inflatable/soft mask) to bag-valve device with 100% oxygen and reservoir		
Attempts to seal mask over trach stoma with both hands and has assistant compress bag		
If unable to ventilate, verbalizes patient may need suction and directs suction to be set up with a soft "whistle-tip" catheter (keeps sterile)		*
Does NOT suction longer than 15 seconds		
Ventilates and confirms ventilation by auscultation and observation of chest rise and fall		*
Removes mask intermittently to aid exhalation of carbon dioxide		
Assesses patient's response to intervention		*
Student exhibits competence with skill		

Any items in the Not Done column that are marked with an * are mandatory for the student to complete. A check mark in the Not Done column of an item with an * indicates that the student was unsuccessful and must attempt the skill again to assure competency. Examiners should use a different-color ink for the second attempt.

☐ Successful   ☐ Unsuccessful   Examiner Initials: _____

©2006 Prentice-Hall Inc.

Automated External Defibrillator (AED)

Student: _____   **Examiner:** _____

Date: _____

	Done ✓	Not Done
Determines scene safety and utilizes appropriate PPE		*
Briefly questions rescuer about events witnessed/done by rescuer		
Directs cessation of CPR		
Checks pulse and (if absent) directs rescuers to resume CPR		*
Turns on AED power		
Properly attaches AED to patient		
Stops CPR and verifies nobody is touching patient (visually AND verbally)		*
Pushes AED "Analyze" button		*
Delivers shock if advised		*
Immediately resumes CPR (start with compressions)		*
Checks with bystanders/family for SAMPLE history		
Checks for pulse and ventilations WITH CPR (ventilation and compression)		*
Inserts simple airway adjunct (OPA/NPA) if not done previously		
Attaches reservoir to BVM and verifies high-flow oxygen		
Assures CPR continues without unnecessary/prolonged interruption		
Reevaluates patient after 5 cycles (2 mins)		*
Repeats AED analysis following advice of AED		*
Prepares patient for transport		
Verbalizes continuing sequence to be followed during transport		
Student exhibits competence with skill		

Any items in the Not Done column that are marked with an * are mandatory for the student to complete. A check mark in the Not Done column of an item with an * indicates that the student was unsuccessful and must attempt the skill again to assure competency. Examiners should use a different-color ink for the second attempt.

☐ Successful   ☐ Unsuccessful   Examiner Initials: _____

©2006 Prentice-Hall Inc.

Lead Placement

Student: _____   **Examiner:** _____

Date: _____

	Done ✓	Not Done
Utilizes appropriate PPE		*
Preps the skin		
Places electrodes according to manufacturer's recommendations for 3 lead cable		*
Places four limb leads according to manufacturer's recommendations for 12 lead		*
Places lead V1		*
Places lead V2		*
Places lead V4		*
Places lead V3		*
Places lead V6		*
Places lead V5		*
Ensures that all leads are attached		
Checks quality of tracing being received		
Can verbalize troubleshooting of poor-quality tracing		
Records tracing		*
Assesses patient's response to intervention		
Student exhibits competence with skill		

Any items in the Not Done column that are marked with an * are mandatory for the student to complete. A check mark in the Not Done column of an item with an * indicates that the student was unsuccessful and must attempt the skill again to assure competency. Examiners should use a different-color ink for the second attempt.

☐ Successful   ☐ Unsuccessful   Examiner Initials: _____

©2006 Prentice-Hall Inc.

IV Solution Setup

Student: _____   **Examiner:** _____

Date: _____

	Done ✓	Not Done
Washes hands		*
Selects correct IV fluid		*
Removes protective cover and checks fluid, clarity, and expiration date		*
Selects proper tubing for fluid and rate of infusion		*
Removes safety cover from IV bag port		
Removes safety cover from IV tubing "spike" keeping spike sterile		*
Inverts fluid bag and inserts spike so it pierces membrane		*
Clamps off tubing and pinches drip chamber PRIOR to turning upright		*
Flips IV bag and tubing upright, releasing drip chamber only		*
Fills drip chamber to appropriate level		*
Opens clamp and runs IV fluid through to end of tubing		*
Checks IV line for presence of bubbles		*
Labels IV bag with date and time of setup		
Student exhibits competence with skill		

Any items in the Not Done column that are marked with an * are mandatory for the student to complete. A check mark in the Not Done column of an item with an * indicates that the student was unsuccessful and must attempt the skill again to assure competency. Examiners should use a different-color ink for the second attempt.

☐ Successful   ☐ Unsuccessful   Examiner Initials: _____

Discontinuing an IV

Student: _____   **Examiner:** _____

Date: _____

	Done ✓	Not Done
Utilizes appropriate PPE		*
Explains procedure to patient		
Clamps the infusion tubing		*
Holds catheter firmly and loosens tape or transparent dressing from venipuncture site		*
Places a DSD over insertion site		
Pulls catheter gently in reverse direction of insertion until removed, without "spraying" blood		*
Holds pressure to site firmly until good hemostasis obtained (elevates arm if needed)		*
Applies dressing to puncture site		
Disposes of used catheter in proper container		
Student exhibits competence with skill		

Any items in the Not Done column that are marked with an * are mandatory for the student to complete. A check mark in the Not Done column of an item with an * indicates that the student was unsuccessful and must attempt the skill again to assure competency. Examiners should use a different-color ink for the second attempt.

☐ Successful   ☐ Unsuccessful   Examiner Initials: _____

©2006 Prentice-Hall Inc.

Auto-Injector

Student: _____

Date: _____

Examiner: _____

	Done ✓	Not Done
Utilizes appropriate PPE		*
Contacts medical direction as needed		
Checks medication for correctness		*
Checks for expiration date		*
Checks for cloudiness or discoloration (if medication is visible)		*
Rechecks patient for indications he or she needs medication		
Removes safety cap from injector		
Selects appropriate injection site (thigh or shoulder) and cleanses site		
Pushes injector firmly against site		
Holds injector firmly against site for a minimum of 10 seconds		*
Properly discards equipment		
Assesses patient's response to intervention		*
Monitors patient for desired effect or potential complications		*
Student exhibits competence with skill		

Any items in the Not Done column that are marked with an * are mandatory for the student to complete. A check mark in the Not Done column of an item with an * indicates that the student was unsuccessful and must attempt the skill again to assure competency. Examiners should use a different-color ink for the second attempt.

☐ Successful   ☐ Unsuccessful   Examiner Initials: _____

EMT: Prolapsed Cord Presentation

Student: _____   **Examiner:** _____

Date: _____

	Done ✓	Not Done
Utilizes appropriate PPE		*
Checks perineum and evaluates cord for pulsation		*
Places mother in knee-chest position		
Places sterile hand into vagina to relieve pressure on cord by gently pressing against presenting part and elevating part off the cord		*
Administers high-flow oxygen to mother		*
Rapid transport		
Calls for ALS		*
If baby begins to deliver, provides airway for neonate while in birth canal		*
Student exhibits competence with skill		

Any items in the Not Done column that are marked with an * are mandatory for the student to complete. A check mark in the Not Done column of an item with an * indicates that the student was unsuccessful and must attempt the skill again to assure competency. Examiners should use a different-color ink for the second attempt.

☐ Successful   ☐ Unsuccessful   Examiner Initials: _____

©2006 Prentice-Hall Inc.

EMT: Breech Presentation

Student: _____   **Examiner:** _____

Date: _____

	Done ✓	Not Done
Utilizes appropriate PPE		*
Checks perineum for imminent delivery		*
Suspects breech presentation from presenting part and pregnancy history		
Positions mother and prepares for delivery during rapid transport		
Inserts hand beside torso of neonate and attempts to extract BOTH legs, enabling sterile hand to provide airway for neonate while still in birth canal (fingers in V framing nose)		*
Calls for ALS		*
Maintains airway throughout rapid transport if infant does not deliver		*
Student exhibits competence with skill		

Any items in the Not Done column that are marked with an * are mandatory for the student to complete. A check mark in the Not Done column of an item with an * indicates that the student was unsuccessful and must attempt the skill again to assure competency. Examiners should use a different-color ink for the second attempt.

☐ Successful   ☐ Unsuccessful   Examiner Initials: _____

APGAR Score

Student: _____   **Examiner:** _____

Date: _____

	Done ✓	Not Done
Utilizes appropriate PPE		*
Scores neonate using APGAR criteria below at 1 minute after birth		*
Appropriately cares for neonate		*
Scores neonate using APGAR criteria below at 5 minutes		*
Student exhibits competence with skill		

Sign	0	1	2
Appearance (skin color)	Blue, pale	Body pink, extremities blue	Completely pink
Pulse (heart rate)	Absent	Less than 100/minute	Greater than 100/minute
Grimace (irritability)	No response	Grimace	Cough, sneeze, cry
Activity (muscle tone)	Limp	Some flexion	Active motion
Respirations (effort)	Absent	Slow, irregular	Good, crying

Any items in the Not Done column that are marked with an * are mandatory for the student to complete. A check mark in the Not Done column of an item with an * indicates that the student was unsuccessful and must attempt the skill again to assure competency. Examiners should use a different-color ink for the second attempt.

☐ Successful   ☐ Unsuccessful   Examiner Initials: _____

©2006 Prentice-Hall Inc.

EMT: Childbirth

Student: _____   Examiner: _____

Date: _____

	Done ✓	Not Done
Determines scene safety and utilizes appropriate PPE		*
Obtains prenatal history		
Examines for crowning (present) and prepares for imminent delivery		*
Explains to patient and family both situation and expectations, takes appropriate PPE		
Positions the patient		
Takes/verbalizes sterile technique, opens OB Kit, and drapes patient		
Supports perineum to prevent tearing, gentle pressure to head to prevent explosive delivery		*
As head delivers feels for nuchal cord, gently removing if necessary		*
After head delivers, suctions mouth, then nose of infant until clear		*
Rotates shoulder as body delivers, tips as necessary to ease baby out		*
Dries, warms, and wraps infant, then places on firm surface at level of mother		*
Notes time of birth		
Evaluates infant's airway status if not briskly crying, suction PRN		*
Evaluates infant's breathing and circulatory status		*
Feels cord for absence of pulsations		
Places umbilical clamps at approximately 6 and 10 in. from infant		
Cuts, or directs father to cut, cord with scalpel—between the clamps		
Checks cord ends for bleeding (applies second clamp if bleeding)		
Evaluates infant for 1-minute APGAR		*
Allows placenta to deliver spontaneously, bags all tissue, and takes to hospital		*
Massages fundus/puts baby to breast to control bleeding		
Examines mother for hemorrhage and places sterile pad to perineum		*
Evaluates infant for 5-minute APGAR		*
Reassesses mother and infant en route to hospital		*
Student exhibits competence with skill		

Any items in the Not Done column that are marked with an * are mandatory for the student to complete. A check mark in the Not Done column of an item with an * indicates that the student was unsuccessful and must attempt the skill again to assure competency. Examiners should use a different-color ink for the second attempt.

☐ Successful   ☐ Unsuccessful   Examiner Initials: _____

Neonatal Resuscitation Equipment

Student: _____   **Examiner:** _____

Date: _____

	Done ✓	Not Done
Demonstrates familiarity with neonatal BVM		*
Demonstrates familiarity with neonatal EKG monitoring		
Demonstrates familiarity with neonatal diapering		*
Demonstrates familiarity with neonatal Broselow (or other brand) tape use		
Demonstrates familiarity with neonatal blood glucose level		*
Demonstrates familiarity with dilution for neonatal glucose and bicarbonate administration		
Demonstrates familiarity with neonatal umbilical clamp and tape		*
Demonstrates familiarity with neonatal intubation equipment		
Student exhibits competence with skill		

Any items in the Not Done column that are marked with an * are mandatory for the student to complete. A check mark in the Not Done column of an item with an * indicates that the student was unsuccessful and must attempt the skill again to assure competency. Examiners should use a different-color ink for the second attempt.

☐ Successful   ☐ Unsuccessful   Examiner Initials: _____

©2006 Prentice-Hall Inc.

EMT: Postpartum Hemorrhage

Student: _____   Examiner: _____

Date: _____

	Done ✓	Not Done
Utilizes appropriate PPE		*
Administers high-flow oxygen		*
Massages fundus		*
Places patient in Trendelenberg		*
Keeps patient warm		*
Calls for ALS		*
Replaces perineal pads as needed to evaluate blood loss		
Verifies placenta has delivered		
Rapid transport		
Monitors for blood loss		*
Student exhibits competence with skill		

Any items in the Not Done column that are marked with an * are mandatory for the student to complete. A check mark in the Not Done column of an item with an * indicates that the student was unsuccessful and must attempt the skill again to assure competency. Examiners should use a different-color ink for the second attempt.

☐ Successful   ☐ Unsuccessful   Examiner Initials: _____

Pediatric Manual Airway Maneuvers

Student: _____   **Examiner:** _____

Date: _____

Head-Tilt/Chin Lift	Done ✓	Not Done
Utilizes appropriate PPE		*
Places patient supine and positions self at side of patient's head		
Places one hand on forehead—uses soft hand pressure to forehead, tilts the head back **slightly**		*
Puts two fingers under bony part of chin and gently lifts jaw anteriorly to open airway		*
Verifies ventilation		*
Assesses patient's response to intervention		*
Student exhibits competence with skill		

Any items in the Not Done column that are marked with an * are mandatory for the student to complete. A check mark in the Not Done column of an item with an * indicates that the student was unsuccessful and must attempt the skill again to assure competency. Examiners should use a different-color ink for the second attempt.

☐ Successful   ☐ Unsuccessful   Examiner Initials: _____

Trauma Jaw-Thrust	Done ✓	Not Done
Utilizes appropriate PPE		*
Places patient supine and positions self at top of patient's head		
Applies fingers to each side of jaw at the mandibular angles		*
Gently elevates jaw anteriorly without tilting head		*
Verifies ventilation		*
Assesses patient's response to intervention		*
Student exhibits competence with skill		

Any items in the Not Done column that are marked with an * are mandatory for the student to complete. A check mark in the Not Done column of an item with an * indicates that the student was unsuccessful and must attempt the skill again to assure competency. Examiners should use a different-color ink for the second attempt.

☐ Successful   ☐ Unsuccessful   Examiner Initials: _____

©2006 Prentice-Hall Inc.

Pediatric Nasopharyngeal/Oropharyngeal Airway Insertion

Student: _____   Examiner: _____

Date: _____

Nasopharyngeal Airway	Done ✓	Not Done
Utilizes appropriate PPE		*
Places head in "sniffing" position if no history of trauma		
Ventilates patient with high-flow oxygen (hyperventilates if indicated)		*
Measures NPA from tip of nose to angle of jaw and diameter of nostril		*
Lubricates exterior of tube with water-soluble jelly		
Pushes gently upward on tip of nose and passes NPA into nostril, bevel toward septum, and directed posteriorly (NOT upward to follow septum)		*
Verifies appropriate position of airway, breath sounds, chest rise, and airflow		*
Ventilates with 100% oxygen		
Assesses patient's response to intervention		*
Student exhibits competence with skill		

Any items in the Not Done column that are marked with an * are mandatory for the student to complete. A check mark in the Not Done column of an item with an * indicates that the student was unsuccessful and must attempt the skill again to assure competency. Examiners should use a different-color ink for the second attempt.

☐ Successful   ☐ Unsuccessful   Examiner Initials: _____

Oropharyngeal Airway (unresponsive)	Done ✓	Not Done
Utilizes appropriate PPE		*
Places head in "sniffing" position if no history of trauma		
Opens mouth, checks for loose or foreign objects, and removes if present		*
Ventilates with high-flow oxygen (hyperventilates if indicated)		*
Measures OPA from corner of mouth to earlobe		*
Gently grasps patient's jaw and lifts anteriorly		*
With other hand, holds proximal end of OPA and inserts into patient's mouth with curve reversed and tip pointing to roof of mouth **OR** uses tongue blade correctly to assist insertion		*
As tip reaches level of soft palate, gently rotates 180° advancing to proper depth		*
Verifies appropriate position of airway, breath sounds, chest rise, and airflow		*
Ventilates with 100% oxygen		
Assesses patient's response to intervention		*
Student exhibits competence with skill		

Any items in the Not Done column that are marked with an * are mandatory for the student to complete. A check mark in the Not Done column of an item with an * indicates that the student was unsuccessful and must attempt the skill again to assure competency. Examiners should use a different-color ink for the second attempt.

☐ Successful   ☐ Unsuccessful   Examiner Initials: _____

Humidified Oxygen

Student: _____   **Examiner:** _____

Date: _____

	Done ✓	Not Done
Utilizes appropriate PPE		*
Attaches flow regulator with oxygen humidifier "Christmas tree" adapter to wall		*
Opens patient humidifier bottle and checks for color, clarity, and expiration date		*
Screws bottle onto flow regulator, being careful to pierce bottle and thread correctly		*
Turns on flow meter appropriate for delivery adjunct		*
Applies oxygen delivery device to patient		*
Reassesses patient		*
Removes humidifier bottle at end of transport and takes with patient		
Replaces usual flow regulator into wall of rescue/ambulance		*
Verifies that connection and oxygen flow are ready for next patient		*
Reports to ED on patient response and documents correctly		*
If no humidifier bottle available, hooks up in-line nebulizer with only water/saline in chamber		
Assesses patient's response to intervention		*
Student exhibits competence with skill		

Any items in the Not Done column that are marked with an * are mandatory for the student to complete. A check mark in the Not Done column of an item with an * indicates that the student was unsuccessful and must attempt the skill again to assure competency. Examiners should use a different-color ink for the second attempt.

☐ Successful   ☐ Unsuccessful   Examiner Initials: _____

©2006 Prentice-Hall Inc.

EMT: Emergency Care for Heat Disorders

Student: _____   Examiner: _____

Date: _____

Heat Cramps

	Done ✓	Not Done
Utilizes appropriate PPE		*
Removes patient from hot environment		*
Places patient in a cool, shaded, or air-conditioned environment		
Administers oral fluids if patient is alert and able to swallow		
Assesses patient's response to intervention		*
Student exhibits competence with skill		

Heat Exhaustion

	Done ✓	Not Done
Utilizes appropriate PPE		*
Removes patient from hot environment		*
Places patient in a cool, shaded, or air-conditioned environment		
Administers oral fluids if patient is alert and able to swallow		
Places patient in supine position		*
Removes some clothing and fans the patient, but does not chill the patient		*
Treats for shock if shock is suspected		
Assesses patient's response to intervention		*
Student exhibits competence with skill		

Heatstroke

	Done ✓	Not Done
Utilizes appropriate PPE		*
Removes patient from hot environment		*
Places patient in a cool, shaded, or air-conditioned environment		
Initiates rapid active cooling en route to hospital by removing patient's clothing		*
Covers patient with sheets soaked in tepid water		*
Cools body temperature to no lower than 102°F/30°C		*
Administers high-flow oxygen by nonrebreather mask		*
Administers oral fluids if patient is alert and able to swallow		
Calls for ALS and treats for shock		*
Assesses patient's response to intervention		*
Student exhibits competence with skill		

Any items in the Not Done column that are marked with an * are mandatory for the student to complete. A check mark in the Not Done column of an item with an * indicates that the student was unsuccessful and must attempt the skill again to assure competency. Examiners should use a different-color ink for the second attempt.

☐ Successful   ☐ Unsuccessful   Examiner Initials: _____

EMT: Recognition and Treatment of Hypothermia

Student: _____   Examiner: _____

Date: _____

Mild Hypothermia	Done ✓	Not Done
Utilizes appropriate PPE		*
Recognizes mild hypothermia/verbalizes core temperature greater than 90°F/32°C		*
Observes for shivering		
Verbalizes checking level of consciousness as may be lethargic and somewhat dulled or AAO × 4		
Observes for uncoordinated or stiff and stumbling gait		
Removes from environment (heat on) and removes any wet clothing/wraps in DRY blankets		*
Gives warm liquids, avoiding caffeine, stimulants, or alcohol		*
Assesses patient's response to intervention		*
Student exhibits competence with skill		

Severe Hypothermia		
Utilizes appropriate PPE		*
Recognizes severe hypothermia/verbalizes core temperature less than 90°F/32°C		*
Verbalizes shivering will usually stop by this stage and physical activity will be uncoordinated		*
Checks level of consciousness as patient will be stuporous and complete coma will follow		*
Removes from environment (heat on) and removes any wet clothing/wraps in dry blankets		*
Places patient in supine position		*
Initiates rapid transport for active rewarming in the hospital environment		x
Calls for ALS and treats for shock		*
Does NOT allow rough handling as may initiate ventricular fibrillation		*
Monitors core temperature with hypothermia thermometer		
Assesses patient's response to intervention		*
Student exhibits competence with skill		

Any items in the Not Done column that are marked with an * are mandatory for the student to complete. A check mark in the Not Done column of an item with an * indicates that the student was unsuccessful and must attempt the skill again to assure competency. Examiners should use a different-color ink for the second attempt.

☐ Successful   ☐ Unsuccessful   Examiner Initials: _____

©2006 Prentice-Hall Inc.

Documentation Skills: Patient Care Report (PCR)

Student: _____   **Examiner:** _____

Date: _____

	Done ✓	Not Done
Records all pertinent dispatch/scene data, using a consistent format		
Completely identifies all additional resources and personnel		
Documents chief complaint, signs/symptoms, position found, age, sex, and weight		
Identifies and records all pertinent, reportable clinical data for each patient		
Documents SAMPLE and OPQRST if applicable		
Records all pertinent negatives		
Records all pertinent denials		
Records accurate, consistent times and patient information		
Includes relevant oral statements of witnesses, bystanders, and patient in "quotes" when appropriate		
Documents initial assessment findings: airway, breathing, and circulation		
Documents any interventions in initial assessment with patient response		
Documents level of consciousness, GCS (if trauma), and VS		
Documents rapid trauma assessment if applicable		
Documents any interventions in rapid trauma assessment with patient response		
Documents focused history and physical assessment		
Documents any interventions in focused assessment with patient response		
Documents repeat VS (every 5 minutes for critical; every 15 minutes for stable)		
Repeats initial assessment and documents findings		
Records ALL treatments with times and patient response(s) in treatment section		
Documents field impression		
Documents transport to specific facility and transfer of care WITH VERBAL REPORT		
Uses correct grammar, abbreviations, spelling, and terminology		
Writes legibly		
Thoroughly documents refusals, denials of transport, and call cancellations		
Documents patient GCS of 15 PRIOR to signing refusal		
Documents advice given to refusal patient, including "call 9-1-1 for further problems"		
Properly corrects errors and omissions		
Writes cautiously, avoids jargon, opinions, inferences, or any derogatory/libelous remarks		
Signs run report		
Uses EMS supplement form if needed		
Student exhibits competence with skill		

Any items in the Not Done column should be evaluated with student. Check marks in this column do not necessarily mean student was unsuccessful as all lines are not completed on all patients. Evaluation of each PCR should be based on the scenario given.

Student must be able to write an EMS report with consistency and accuracy.

☐ Successful   ☐ Unsuccessful   Examiner Initials: _____

Radio Report

Student: _____   Examiner: _____

Date: _____

	Done ✓	Not Done
Requests and checks for open channel before speaking		
Presses transmit button 1 second before speaking		
Holds microphone 2–3 in. from mouth		
Speaks slowly and clearly		*
Speaks in a normal voice		
Briefly transmits: Agency, unit designation, identification/name		*
Briefly transmits: Patient's age, sex, weight		*
Briefly transmits: Scene description/mechanism of injury or medical problem		*
Briefly transmits: Chief complaint with brief history of *present* illness		*
Briefly transmits: Associated symptoms (unless able to be deferred to bedside report)		
Briefly transmits: Past medical history (usually deferred to bedside report)		
Briefly transmits: Vital signs		*
Briefly transmits: Level of consciousness/GCS on trauma		*
Briefly transmits: General appearance, distress, cardiac rhythm, blood glucose, and other pertinent findings unable to be deferred to bedside report		
Briefly transmits: Interventions by EMS AND response(s)		*
ETA (the more critical the patient, the earlier you need to notify the receiving facility)		
Does not waste airtime		
Protects privacy of patient		*
Echoes dispatch information and any physician orders		*
Writes down dispatch information or physician orders		
Confirms with facility that message is received		
Demonstrates/verbalizes ability to troubleshoot basic equipment malfunction		
Student exhibits competence with skill		

Any items in the Not Done column that are marked with an * are mandatory for the student to complete. A check mark in the Not Done column of an item with an * indicates that the student was unsuccessful and must attempt the skill again to assure competency. Examiners should use a different-color ink for the second attempt.

☐ Successful   ☐ Unsuccessful   Examiner Initials: _____

©2006 Prentice-Hall Inc.

DAILY DISCUSSIONS AND PERTINENT POINTS— ADVANCED EMT SKILLS LAB

Student: _____   **Date:** _____

Instructor: _____

	Instructor Initials
Discuss analyzing disease risk.	
Describe environmental risk factors.	
Discuss combined effects and interaction among risk factors.	
Advocate the need for supporting and participating in research efforts aimed at improving EMS systems.	
Advocate the need to understand and apply the knowledge of pathophysiology to patient assessment and treatment.	
Discuss medical asepsis and the difference between clean and sterile techniques.	
Describe the use of antiseptics and disinfectants.	
Compare the physiological and psychosocial characteristics of an infant with those of an early adult.	
Compare the physiological and psychosocial characteristics of a toddler with those of an early adult.	
Compare the physiological and psychosocial characteristics of a preschool child with those of an early adult.	
Compare the physiological and psychosocial characteristics of a school-aged child with those of an early adult.	
Compare the physiological and psychosocial characteristics of an adolescent with those of an early adult.	
Summarize the physiological and psychosocial characteristics of an early adult.	
Compare the physiological and psychosocial characteristics of a middle-aged adult with those of an early adult.	
Compare the physiological and psychosocial characteristics of a person in late adulthood with those of an early adult.	
Value the uniqueness of infants, toddlers, preschool, school-aged, adolescent, early adulthood, middle-aged, and late adulthood physiological and psychosocial characteristics.	
Evaluate the benefits and shortfalls of protocols, standing orders, and patient care algorithms.	
List factors that impede effective verbal communications.	
List factors that enhance verbal communications.	
Identify the importance of proper verbal communications during an EMS event.	
Identify the importance of proper written communications during an EMS event.	
List factors that impede effective written communications.	
List factors that enhance written communications.	
Show appreciation for proper terminology when describing a patient or patient condition.	
Evaluate the confidential nature of an EMS report.	
Advocate among peers the relevance and importance of properly completed documentation.	
Resolve the common negative attitudes toward the task of documentation.	
Given a scenario in which equipment and supplies have been exposed to body substances, plan for the proper cleaning, disinfection, and disposal of the items.	
Discuss the physiologic changes associated with the pneumatic anti-shock garment (PASG).	
Discuss the indications and contraindications for the application and inflation of the PASG.	
Demonstrate the proper use of the PASG in a patient with suspected abdominal trauma, in a simulated lab patient.	
Demonstrate the proper use of the PASG in a patient with suspected pelvic fracture, in a simulated lab patient.	
Discuss the usefulness of the PASG in the management of fractures.	

Part 3: EMT Patient Assessment Sheets

All assessment forms have skill sheets included for a radio report, a patient care report (PCR), and overall scenario management. Instructors will choose which scenarios student is "lead" and which skills are to be completed based on length of program and the number of labs to be spent on EMT assessment review. If the first section of this manual is to be used as an EMT lab manual, the section should be completed in its entirety.

Skill Sheets

EMT Patient Assessment: Medical—Abdominal
Radio Report (EMT Medical—Abdominal)
Documentation Skills: Patient Care Report (PCR) (EMT Medical—Abdominal)
Overall Scenario Management (EMT Medical—Abdominal)
EMT Patient Assessment: Medical—Allergy
Radio Report (EMT Medical—Allergy)
Documentation Skills: Patient Care Report (PCR) (EMT Medical—Allergy)
Overall Scenario Management (EMT Medical—Allergy)
EMT Patient Assessment: Medical—Cardiac
Radio Report (EMT Medical—Cardiac)
Documentation Skills: Patient Care Report (PCR) (EMT Medical—Cardiac)
Overall Scenario Management (EMT Medical—Cardiac)
EMT Patient Assessment: Medical—Diabetic
Radio Report (EMT Medical—Diabetic)
Documentation Skills: Patient Care Report (PCR) (EMT Medical—Diabetic)
Overall Scenario Management (EMT Medical—Diabetic)
EMT Patient Assessment: Medical—Medical Shock
Radio Report (EMT Medical—Medical Shock)
Documentation Skills: Patient Care Report (PCR) (EMT Medical—Medical Shock)
Overall Scenario Management (EMT Medical—Medical Shock)
EMT Patient Assessment: Medical—Respiratory
Radio Report (EMT Medical—Respiratory)
Documentation Skills: Patient Care Report (PCR) (EMT Medical—Respiratory)
Overall Scenario Management (EMT Medical—Respiratory)
EMT Patient Assessment: Medical—Stroke
Radio Report (EMT Medical—Stroke)
Documentation Skills: Patient Care Report (PCR) (EMT Medical—Stroke)
Overall Scenario Management (EMT Medical—Stroke)
EMT Patient Assessment: Medical—Examiner's Choice
Radio Report (EMT Medical—Examiner's Choice)
Documentation Skills: Patient Care Report (PCR) (EMT Medical—Examiner's Choice)
Overall Scenario Management (EMT Medical—Examiner's Choice)
EMT Patient Assessment: Trauma—Burn Trauma
Radio Report (EMT Trauma—Burn Trauma)
Documentation Skills: Patient Care Report (PCR) (EMT Trauma—Burn Trauma)
Overall Scenario Management (EMT Trauma—Burn Trauma)
EMT Patient Assessment: Trauma—Chest Trauma
Radio Report (EMT Trauma—Chest Trauma)
Documentation Skills: Patient Care Report (PCR) (EMT Trauma—Chest Trauma)

©2006 Prentice-Hall Inc.

Overall Scenario Management (EMT Trauma—Chest Trauma)
EMT Patient Assessment: Trauma—Extremity Trauma
Radio Report (EMT Trauma—Extremity Trauma)
Documentation Skills: Patient Care Report (PCR) (EMT Trauma—Extremity Trauma)
Overall Scenario Management (EMT Trauma—Extremity Trauma)
EMT Patient Assessment: Trauma—Fractured Femur
Radio Report (EMT Trauma—Fractured Femur)
Documentation Skills: Patient Care Report (PCR) (EMT Trauma—Fractured Femur)
Overall Scenario Management (EMT Trauma—Fractured Femur)
EMT Patient Assessment: Trauma—Head Injury
Radio Report (EMT Trauma—Head Injury)
Documentation Skills: Patient Care Report (PCR) (EMT Trauma—Head Injury)
Overall Scenario Management (EMT Trauma—Head Injury)
EMT Patient Assessment: Medical—Pediatric
Radio Report (EMT Medical—Pediatric)
Documentation Skills: Patient Care Report (PCR) (EMT Medical—Pediatric)
Overall Scenario Management (EMT Medical—Pediatric)
EMT Patient Assessment: Trauma—Shock/Hemorrhage
Radio Report (EMT Trauma—Shock/Hemorrhage)
Documentation Skills: Patient Care Report (PCR) (EMT Trauma—Shock/Hemorrhage)
Overall Scenario Management (EMT Trauma—Shock/Hemorrhage)

SKILL SHEETS

EMT Patient Assessment: Medical—*Abdominal*

Student: _____   **Examiner:** _____

Date: _____

	Done ✓	Not Done
Assesses scene safety and utilizes appropriate PPE		*
OVERALL SCENE EVALUATION		
Medical—determines nature of illness/if trauma involved determines MOI		*
Determines the number of patients, location, obstacles, and requests any additional resources as needed		
Verbalizes general impression of the patient as approaches		*
Considers stabilization/spinal motion restriction of spine if trauma involved		*
INITIAL ASSESSMENT		
Determines responsiveness/level of consciousness/AVPU		*
Opens airway with appropriate technique and assesses airway/ventilation		*
Manages airway/ventilation and applies appropriate oxygen therapy in less than 3 minutes		*
Assesses circulation: radial/carotid pulse, skin color, temperature, condition, and turgor		*
Controls any major bleeding		*
Makes rapid transport decision if indicated		
Obtains BGL, GCS, and complete vital signs		
FOCUSED HISTORY AND PHYSICAL EXAMINATION/RAPID ASSESSMENT		
Obtains SAMPLE history		
Obtains OPQRST for differential diagnosis		
Obtains associated symptoms, pertinent negatives/denials		
Evaluates decision to perform focused exam or completes rapid assessment		*
Vital signs including AVPU (and GCS if trauma)		*
Assesses cardiovascular system including heart sounds, peripheral edema, and peripheral perfusion		*
Assesses pulmonary system including reassessing airway, ventilation, breath sounds, pulse oximetry, chest wall excursion, accessory muscle use, or other signs of distress		*
Assesses neurological system including speech, droop, drift, if applicable, and distal movement and sensation		*
Assesses musculoskeletal and integumentary systems		
Assesses behavioral, psychological, and social aspects of patient and situation		
States field impression of patient—abdominal problem (states suspected cause)		*
Verbalizes treatment plan for patient and calls for appropriate intervention(s)		*
Reevaluates transport decision		
ONGOING ASSESSMENT		
Repeats initial assessment		*
Repeats vital signs and evaluates trends		*
Evaluates response to treatments		*
Repeats focused assessment regarding patient complaint or injuries		
Gives radio report to receiving facility		
Turns over patient care with verbal report		*
Student exhibits competence with skill		

Any items in the Not Done column that are marked with an * are mandatory for the student to complete. A check mark in the Not Done column of an item with an * indicates that the student was unsuccessful and must attempt the skill again to assure competency. Examiners should use a different-color ink for the second attempt.

☐ Successful   ☐ Unsuccessful   Examiner Initials: _____

©2006 Prentice-Hall Inc.

Radio Report (EMT Medical—Abdominal)

Student: _____   **Examiner:** _____

Date: _____

	Done ✓	Not Done
Requests and checks for open channel before speaking		
Presses transmit button 1 second before speaking		
Holds microphone 2–3 in. from mouth		
Speaks slowly and clearly		*
Speaks in a normal voice		
Briefly transmits: Agency, unit designation, identification/name		*
Briefly transmits: Patient's age, sex, weight		*
Briefly transmits: Scene description/mechanism of injury or medical problem		*
Briefly transmits: Chief complaint with brief history of *present* illness		*
Briefly transmits: Associated symptoms (unless able to be deferred to bedside report)		
Briefly transmits: Past medical history (usually deferred to bedside report)		
Briefly transmits: Vital signs		*
Briefly transmits: Level of consciousness/GCS on trauma		*
Briefly transmits: General appearance, distress, cardiac rhythm, blood glucose, and other pertinent findings unable to be deferred to bedside report		
Briefly transmits: Interventions by EMS AND response(s)		*
ETA (the more critical the patient, the earlier you need to notify the receiving facility)		
Does not waste airtime		
Protects privacy of patient		*
Echoes dispatch information and any physician orders		*
Writes down dispatch information or physician orders		
Confirms with facility that message is received		
Demonstrates/verbalizes ability to troubleshoot basic equipment malfunction		
Student exhibits competence with skill		

Any items in the Not Done column that are marked with an * are mandatory for the student to complete. A check mark in the Not Done column of an item with an * indicates that the student was unsuccessful and must attempt the skill again to assure competency. Examiners should use a different-color ink for the second attempt.

☐ Successful   ☐ Unsuccessful   Examiner Initials: _____

Documentation Skills: Patient Care Report (PCR)
(EMT Medical—Abdominal)

Student: _____   Examiner: _____

Date: _____

	Done ✓	Not Done
Records all pertinent dispatch/scene data, using a consistent format		
Completely identifies all additional resources and personnel		
Documents chief complaint, signs/symptoms, position found, age, sex, and weight		
Identifies and records all pertinent, reportable clinical data for each patient		
Documents SAMPLE and OPQRST if applicable		
Records all pertinent negatives		
Records all pertinent denials		
Records accurate, consistent times and patient information		
Includes relevant oral statements of witnesses, bystanders, and patient in "quotes" when appropriate		
Documents initial assessment findings: airway, breathing, and circulation		
Documents any interventions in initial assessment with patient response		
Documents level of consciousness, GCS (if trauma), and VS		
Documents rapid trauma assessment if applicable		
Documents any interventions in rapid trauma assessment with patient response		
Documents focused history and physical assessment		
Documents any interventions in focused assessment with patient response		
Documents repeat VS (every 5 minutes for critical; every 15 minutes for stable)		
Repeats initial assessment and documents findings		
Records ALL treatments with times and patient response(s) in treatment section		
Documents field impression		
Documents transport to specific facility and transfer of care WITH VERBAL REPORT		
Uses correct grammar, abbreviations, spelling, and terminology		
Writes legibly		
Thoroughly documents refusals, denials of transport, and call cancellations		
Documents patient GCS of 15 PRIOR to signing refusal		
Documents advice given to refusal patient, including "call 9-1-1 for further problems"		
Properly corrects errors and omissions		
Writes cautiously, avoids jargon, opinions, inferences, or any derogatory/libelous remarks		
Signs run report		
Uses EMS supplement form if needed		
Student exhibits competence with skill		

Any items in the Not Done column should be evaluated with student. Check marks in this column do not necessarily mean student was unsuccessful as all lines are not completed on all patients. Evaluation of each PCR should be based on the scenario given.

Student must be able to write an EMS report with consistency and accuracy.

☐ Successful   ☐ Unsuccessful   Examiner Initials: _____

    ©2006 Prentice-Hall Inc.

Overall Scenario Management (EMT Medical—Abdominal)

Student: _____   Examiner: _____

Date: _____   Scenario: _____

NOTE: This skill sheet is to be done after the student completes a scenario as the TEAM LEADER. It is to let the student know if he or she is beginning to "put it all together" and use critical thinking skills to manage an EMS call. PLEASE notice that it is graded on a different basis than the basic lab skill sheet.

	Done ✓	Needs to Improve
SCENE MANAGEMENT		
Recognized hazards and controlled scene—safety, crowd, and patient issues		
Recognized hazards, but did not control the scene		
Unsuccessfully attempted to manage the scene	*	
Did not evaluate the scene and took no control of the scene	*	
PATIENT ASSESSMENT		
Performed a timely, organized complete patient assessment		
Performed complete initial, focused, and ongoing assessments, but in a disorganized manner		
Performed an incomplete assessment	*	
Did not perform an initial assessment	*	
PATIENT MANAGEMENT		
Evaluated assessment findings to manage all aspects of patient condition		
Managed the patient's presenting signs and symptoms without considering all of assessment		
Inadequately managed the patient	*	
Did not manage life-threatening conditions	*	
COMMUNICATION		
Communicated well with crew, patient, family, bystanders, and assisting agencies		
Communicated well with patient and crew		
Communicated with patient and crew, but poor communication skills	*	
Unable to communicate effectively	*	
REPORT AND TRANSFER OF CARE		
Identified correct destination for patient transport, gave accurate, brief report over radio, and provided full report at bedside demonstrating thorough understanding of patient condition and pathophysiological processes		
Identified correct destination and gave accurate radio and bedside report, but did not demonstrate understanding of patient condition and pathophysiological processes		
Identified correct destination, but provided inadequate radio and bedside report	*	
Identified inappropriate destination or provided no radio or bedside report	*	
Student exhibits competence with skill		

Any items that are marked with an * indicate the student needs to improve and a check mark should be placed in the right-hand column. A check mark in the right-hand column indicates that the student was unsuccessful and must attempt the skill again to assure competency. Examiners should use a different-color ink for the second attempt.

☐ Successful   ☐ Unsuccessful   Examiner Initials: _____

©2006 Prentice-Hall Inc.

EMT Patient Assessment: Medical—*Allergy*

Student: _____   Examiner: _____

Date: _____

	Done ✓	Not Done
Assesses scene safety and utilizes appropriate PPE		*
OVERALL SCENE EVALUATION		
Medical—determines nature of illness/if trauma involved determines MOI		*
Determines the number of patients, location, obstacles, and requests any additional resources as needed		
Verbalizes general impression of the patient as approaches		*
Considers stabilization/spinal motion restriction of spine if trauma involved		*
INITIAL ASSESSMENT		
Determines responsiveness/level of consciousness/AVPU		*
Opens airway with appropriate technique and assesses airway/ventilation		*
Manages airway/ventilation and applies appropriate oxygen therapy in less than 3 minutes		*
Assesses circulation: radial/carotid pulse, skin color, temperature, condition, and turgor		*
Controls any major bleeding		*
Makes rapid transport decision if indicated		
Obtains BGL, GCS, and complete vital signs		*
FOCUSED HISTORY AND PHYSICAL EXAMINATION/RAPID ASSESSMENT		
Obtains SAMPLE history		
Obtains OPQRST for differential diagnosis		
Obtains associated symptoms, pertinent negatives/denials		
Evaluates decision to perform focused exam or completes rapid assessment		*
Vital signs including AVPU (and GCS if trauma)		*
Assesses cardiovascular system including heart sounds, peripheral edema, and peripheral perfusion		*
Assesses pulmonary system including reassessing airway, ventilation, breath sounds, pulse oximetry, chest wall excursion, accessory muscle use, or other signs of distress		*
Assesses neurological system including speech, droop, drift, if applicable, and distal movement and sensation		*
Assesses musculoskeletal and integumentary systems		
Assesses behavioral, psychological, and social aspects of patient and situation		
States field impression of patient—allergic reaction (states suspected cause)		*
Verbalizes treatment plan for patient and calls for appropriate intervention(s)—calls for ALS		*
Reevaluates transport decision		
ONGOING ASSESSMENT		
Repeats initial assessment		*
Repeats vital signs and evaluates trends		*
Evaluates response to treatments		*
Repeats focused assessment regarding patient complaint or injuries		
Gives radio report to receiving facility		
Turns over patient care with verbal report		*
Student exhibits competence with skill		

Any items in the Not Done column that are marked with an * are mandatory for the student to complete. A check mark in the Not Done column of an item with an * indicates that the student was unsuccessful and must attempt the skill again to assure competency. Examiners should use a different-color ink for the second attempt.

☐ Successful   ☐ Unsuccessful   Examiner Initials: _____

©2006 Prentice-Hall Inc.

Radio Report (EMT Medical—Allergy)

Student: _____   **Examiner:** _____

Date: _____

	Done ✓	Not Done
Requests and checks for open channel before speaking		
Presses transmit button 1 second before speaking		
Holds microphone 2–3 in. from mouth		
Speaks slowly and clearly		*
Speaks in a normal voice		
Briefly transmits: Agency, unit designation, identification/name		*
Briefly transmits: Patient's age, sex, weight		*
Briefly transmits: Scene description/mechanism of injury or medical problem		*
Briefly transmits: Chief complaint with brief history of *present* illness		*
Briefly transmits: Associated symptoms (unless able to be deferred to bedside report)		
Briefly transmits: Past medical history (usually deferred to bedside report)		
Briefly transmits: Vital signs		*
Briefly transmits: Level of consciousness/GCS on trauma		*
Briefly transmits: General appearance, distress, cardiac rhythm, blood glucose, and other pertinent findings unable to be deferred to bedside report		
Briefly transmits: Interventions by EMS AND response(s)		*
ETA (the more critical the patient, the earlier you need to notify the receiving facility)		
Does not waste airtime		
Protects privacy of patient		*
Echoes dispatch information and any physician orders		*
Writes down dispatch information or physician orders		
Confirms with facility that message is received		
Demonstrates/verbalizes ability to troubleshoot basic equipment malfunction		
Student exhibits competence with skill		

Any items in the Not Done column that are marked with an * are mandatory for the student to complete. A check mark in the Not Done column of an item with an * indicates that the student was unsuccessful and must attempt the skill again to assure competency. Examiners should use a different-color ink for the second attempt.

☐ Successful   ☐ Unsuccessful   Examiner Initials: _____

Documentation Skills: Patient Care Report (PCR) (EMT Medical—Allergy)

Student: _____   Examiner: _____

Date: _____

	Done ✓	Not Done
Records all pertinent dispatch/scene data, using a consistent format		
Completely identifies all additional resources and personnel		
Documents chief complaint, signs/symptoms, position found, age, sex, and weight		
Identifies and records all pertinent, reportable clinical data for each patient		
Documents SAMPLE and OPQRST if applicable		
Records all pertinent negatives		
Records all pertinent denials		
Records accurate, consistent times and patient information		
Includes relevant oral statements of witnesses, bystanders, and patient in "quotes" when appropriate		
Documents initial assessment findings: airway, breathing, and circulation		
Documents any interventions in initial assessment with patient response		
Documents level of consciousness, GCS (if trauma), and VS		
Documents rapid trauma assessment if applicable		
Documents any interventions in rapid trauma assessment with patient response		
Documents focused history and physical assessment		
Documents any interventions in focused assessment with patient response		
Documents repeat VS (every 5 minutes for critical; every 15 minutes for stable)		
Repeats initial assessment and documents findings		
Records ALL treatments with times and patient response(s) in treatment section		
Documents field impression		
Documents transport to specific facility and transfer of care WITH VERBAL REPORT		
Uses correct grammar, abbreviations, spelling, and terminology		
Writes legibly		
Thoroughly documents refusals, denials of transport, and call cancellations		
Documents patient GCS of 15 PRIOR to signing refusal		
Documents advice given to refusal patient, including "call 9-1-1 for further problems"		
Properly corrects errors and omissions		
Writes cautiously, avoids jargon, opinions, inferences, or any derogatory/libelous remarks		
Signs run report		
Uses EMS supplement form if needed		
Student exhibits competence with skill		

Any items in the Not Done column should be evaluated with student. Check marks in this column do not necessarily mean student was unsuccessful as all lines are not completed on all patients. Evaluation of each PCR should be based on the scenario given.

Student must be able to write an EMS report with consistency and accuracy.

☐ Successful   ☐ Unsuccessful   Examiner Initials: _____

          ©2006 Prentice-Hall Inc.

Overall Scenario Management (EMT Medical—Allergy)

Student: _____   Examiner: _____

Date: _____   Scenario: _____

NOTE: This skill sheet is to be done after the student completes a scenario as the TEAM LEADER. It is to let the student know if he or she is beginning to "put it all together" and use critical thinking skills to manage an EMS call. PLEASE notice that it is graded on a different basis than the basic lab skill sheet.

	Done ✓	Needs to Improve
SCENE MANAGEMENT		
Recognized hazards and controlled scene—safety, crowd, and patient issues		
Recognized hazards, but did not control the scene		
Unsuccessfully attempted to manage the scene	*	
Did not evaluate the scene and took no control of the scene	*	
PATIENT ASSESSMENT		
Performed a timely, organized complete patient assessment		
Performed complete initial, focused, and ongoing assessments, but in a disorganized manner		
Performed an incomplete assessment	*	
Did not perform an initial assessment	*	
PATIENT MANAGEMENT		
Evaluated assessment findings to manage all aspects of patient condition		
Managed the patient's presenting signs and symptoms without considering all of assessment		
Inadequately managed the patient	*	
Did not manage life-threatening conditions	*	
COMMUNICATION		
Communicated well with crew, patient, family, bystanders, and assisting agencies		
Communicated well with patient and crew		
Communicated with patient and crew, but poor communication skills	*	
Unable to communicate effectively	*	
REPORT AND TRANSFER OF CARE		
Identified correct destination for patient transport, gave accurate, brief report over radio, and provided full report at bedside demonstrating thorough understanding of patient condition and pathophysiological processes		
Identified correct destination and gave accurate radio and bedside report, but did not demonstrate understanding of patient condition and pathophysiological processes		
Identified correct destination, but provided inadequate radio and bedside report	*	
Identified inappropriate destination or provided no radio or bedside report	*	
Student exhibits competence with skill		

Any items that are marked with an * indicate the student needs to improve and a check mark should be placed in the right-hand column. A check mark in the right-hand column indicates that the student was unsuccessful and must attempt the skill again to assure competency. Examiners should use a different-color ink for the second attempt.

☐ Successful   ☐ Unsuccessful   Examiner Initials: _____

EMT Patient Assessment: Medical—*Cardiac*

Student: _____   Examiner: _____

Date: _____

	Done ✓	Not Done
Assesses scene safety and utilizes appropriate PPE		*
OVERALL SCENE EVALUATION		
Medical—determines nature of illness/if trauma involved determines MOI		*
Determines the number of patients, location, obstacles, and requests any additional resources as needed		
Verbalizes general impression of the patient as approaches		*
Considers stabilization/spinal motion restriction of spine if trauma involved		*
INITIAL ASSESSMENT		
Determines responsiveness/level of consciousness/AVPU		*
Opens airway with appropriate technique and assesses airway/ventilation		*
Manages airway/ventilation and applies appropriate oxygen therapy in less than 3 minutes		*
Assesses circulation: radial/carotid pulse, skin color, temperature, condition, and turgor		*
Controls any major bleeding		*
Makes rapid transport decision if indicated—calls for ALS		
Obtains BGL, GCS, and complete vital signs		
FOCUSED HISTORY AND PHYSICAL EXAMINATION/RAPID ASSESSMENT		
Obtains SAMPLE history		
Obtains OPQRST for differential diagnosis		
Obtains associated symptoms, pertinent negatives/denials		
Evaluates decision to perform focused exam or completes rapid assessment		*
Vital signs including AVPU (and GCS if trauma)		*
Assesses cardiovascular system including heart sounds, peripheral edema, and peripheral perfusion		*
Assesses pulmonary system including reassessing airway, ventilation, breath sounds, pulse oximetry, chest wall excursion, accessory muscle use, or other signs of distress		*
Assesses neurological system including speech, droop, drift, if applicable, and distal movement and sensation		*
Assesses musculoskeletal and integumentary systems		
Assesses behavioral, psychological, and social aspects of patient and situation		
States field impression of patient—cardiac		*
Verbalizes treatment plan for patient and calls for appropriate intervention(s) including ALS assistance		*
Transfers patient care to ALS with report (if present)		
ONGOING ASSESSMENT		
Repeats initial assessment		*
Repeats vital signs and evaluates trends		*
Evaluates response to treatments		*
Repeats focused assessment regarding patient complaint or injuries		
Gives radio report to receiving facility if no ALS agency present		
Turns over patient care with verbal report		*
Student exhibits competence with skill		

Any items in the Not Done column that are marked with an * are mandatory for the student to complete. A check mark in the Not Done column of an item with an * indicates that the student was unsuccessful and must attempt the skill again to assure competency. Examiners should use a different-color ink for the second attempt.

☐ Successful   ☐ Unsuccessful   Examiner Initials: _____

©2006 Prentice-Hall Inc.

Radio Report (EMT Medical—Cardiac)

Student: _____   **Examiner:** _____

Date: _____

	Done ✓	Not Done
Requests and checks for open channel before speaking		
Presses transmit button 1 second before speaking		
Holds microphone 2–3 in. from mouth		
Speaks slowly and clearly		*
Speaks in a normal voice		
Briefly transmits: Agency, unit designation, identification/name		*
Briefly transmits: Patient's age, sex, weight		*
Briefly transmits: Scene description/mechanism of injury or medical problem		*
Briefly transmits: Chief complaint with brief history of *present* illness		*
Briefly transmits: Associated symptoms (unless able to be deferred to bedside report)		
Briefly transmits: Past medical history (usually deferred to bedside report)		
Briefly transmits: Vital signs		*
Briefly transmits: Level of consciousness/GCS on trauma		*
Briefly transmits: General appearance, distress, cardiac rhythm, blood glucose, and other pertinent findings unable to be deferred to bedside report		
Briefly transmits: Interventions by EMS AND response(s)		*
ETA (the more critical the patient, the earlier you need to notify the receiving facility)		
Does not waste airtime		
Protects privacy of patient		*
Echoes dispatch information and any physician orders		*
Writes down dispatch information or physician orders		
Confirms with facility that message is received		
Demonstrates/verbalizes ability to troubleshoot basic equipment malfunction		
Student exhibits competence with skill		

Any items in the Not Done column that are marked with an * are mandatory for the student to complete. A check mark in the Not Done column of an item with an * indicates that the student was unsuccessful and must attempt the skill again to assure competency. Examiners should use a different-color ink for the second attempt.

☐ Successful   ☐ Unsuccessful   Examiner Initials: _____

©2006 Prentice-Hall Inc.

Documentation Skills: Patient Care Report (PCR) (EMT Medical—Cardiac)

Student: _____   **Examiner:** _____

Date: _____

	Done ✓	Not Done
Records all pertinent dispatch/scene data, using a consistent format		
Completely identifies all additional resources and personnel		
Documents chief complaint, signs/symptoms, position found, age, sex, and weight		
Identifies and records all pertinent, reportable clinical data for each patient		
Documents SAMPLE and OPQRST if applicable		
Records all pertinent negatives		
Records all pertinent denials		
Records accurate, consistent times and patient information		
Includes relevant oral statements of witnesses, bystanders, and patient in "quotes" when appropriate		
Documents initial assessment findings: airway, breathing, and circulation		
Documents any interventions in initial assessment with patient response		
Documents level of consciousness, GCS (if trauma), and VS		
Documents rapid trauma assessment if applicable		
Documents any interventions in rapid trauma assessment with patient response		
Documents focused history and physical assessment		
Documents any interventions in focused assessment with patient response		
Documents repeat VS (every 5 minutes for critical; every 15 minutes for stable)		
Repeats initial assessment and documents findings		
Records ALL treatments with times and patient response(s) in treatment section		
Documents field impression		
Documents transport to specific facility and transfer of care WITH VERBAL REPORT		
Uses correct grammar, abbreviations, spelling, and terminology		
Writes legibly		
Thoroughly documents refusals, denials of transport, and call cancellations		
Documents patient GCS of 15 PRIOR to signing refusal		
Documents advice given to refusal patient, including "call 9-1-1 for further problems"		
Properly corrects errors and omissions		
Writes cautiously, avoids jargon, opinions, inferences, or any derogatory/libelous remarks		
Signs run report		
Uses EMS supplement form if needed		
Student exhibits competence with skill		

Any items in the Not Done column should be evaluated with student. Check marks in this column do not necessarily mean student was unsuccessful as all lines are not completed on all patients. Evaluation of each PCR should be based on the scenario given.

Student must be able to write an EMS report with consistency and accuracy.

☐ Successful   ☐ Unsuccessful   Examiner Initials: _____

©2006 Prentice-Hall Inc.

Overall Scenario Management (EMT Medical—Cardiac)

Student: _____   Examiner: _____

Date: _____   Scenario: _____

NOTE: This skill sheet is to be done after the student completes a scenario as the TEAM LEADER. It is to let the student know if he or she is beginning to "put it all together" and use critical thinking skills to manage an EMS call. PLEASE notice that it is graded on a different basis than the basic lab skill sheet.

	Done ✓	Needs to Improve
SCENE MANAGEMENT		
Recognized hazards and controlled scene—safety, crowd, and patient issues		
Recognized hazards, but did not control the scene		
Unsuccessfully attempted to manage the scene	*	
Did not evaluate the scene and took no control of the scene	*	
PATIENT ASSESSMENT		
Performed a timely, organized complete patient assessment		
Performed complete initial, focused, and ongoing assessments, but in a disorganized manner		
Performed an incomplete assessment	*	
Did not perform an initial assessment	*	
PATIENT MANAGEMENT		
Evaluated assessment findings to manage all aspects of patient condition		
Managed the patient's presenting signs and symptoms without considering all of assessment		
Inadequately managed the patient	*	
Did not manage life-threatening conditions	*	
COMMUNICATION		
Communicated well with crew, patient, family, bystanders, and assisting agencies		
Communicated well with patient and crew		
Communicated with patient and crew, but poor communication skills	*	
Unable to communicate effectively	*	
REPORT AND TRANSFER OF CARE		
Identified correct destination for patient transport, gave accurate, brief report over radio, and provided full report at bedside demonstrating thorough understanding of patient condition and pathophysiological processes		
Identified correct destination and gave accurate radio and bedside report, but did not demonstrate understanding of patient condition and pathophysiological processes		
Identified correct destination, but provided inadequate radio and bedside report	*	
Identified inappropriate destination or provided no radio or bedside report	*	
Student exhibits competence with skill		

Any items that are marked with an * indicate the student needs to improve and a check mark should be placed in the right-hand column. A check mark in the right-hand column indicates that the student was unsuccessful and must attempt the skill again to assure competency. Examiners should use a different-color ink for the second attempt.

☐ Successful   ☐ Unsuccessful   Examiner Initials: _____

©2006 Prentice-Hall Inc.

EMT Patient Assessment: Medical—*Diabetic*

Student: _____   **Examiner:** _____

Date: _____

	Done ✓	Not Done
Assesses scene safety and utilizes appropriate PPE		*
OVERALL SCENE EVALUATION		
Medical—determines nature of illness/if trauma involved determines MOI		*
Determines the number of patients, location, obstacles, and requests any additional resources as needed		
Verbalizes general impression of the patient as approaches		*
Considers stabilization/spinal motion restriction of spine if trauma involved		*
INITIAL ASSESSMENT		
Determines responsiveness/level of consciousness/AVPU		*
Opens airway with appropriate technique and assesses airway/ventilation		*
Manages airway/ventilation and applies appropriate oxygen therapy in less than 3 minutes		*
Assesses circulation: radial/carotid pulse, skin color, temperature, condition, and turgor		*
Controls any major bleeding		*
Makes rapid transport decision if indicated		
Obtains BGL, GCS, and complete vital signs		
FOCUSED HISTORY AND PHYSICAL EXAMINATION/RAPID ASSESSMENT		
Obtains SAMPLE history		
Obtains OPQRST for differential diagnosis		
Obtains associated symptoms, pertinent negatives/denials		
Evaluates decision to perform focused exam or completes rapid assessment		*
Vital signs including AVPU (and GCS if trauma)		*
Assesses cardiovascular system including heart sounds, peripheral edema, and peripheral perfusion		*
Assesses pulmonary system including reassessing airway, ventilation, breath sounds, pulse oximetry, chest wall excursion, accessory muscle use, or other signs of distress		*
Assesses neurological system including speech, droop, drift, if applicable, and distal movement and sensation		*
Assesses musculoskeletal and integumentary systems		
Assesses behavioral, psychological, and social aspects of patient and situation		
States field impression of patient—diabetic emergency (states suspected cause—hypoglycemia or hyperglycemia)		*
Verbalizes treatment plan for patient and calls for appropriate intervention(s)—hypoglycemia, if conscious, gives sugar; if hyperglycemia, calls for ALS		*
Reevaluates transport decision		
ONGOING ASSESSMENT		
Repeats initial assessment		*
Repeats vital signs and evaluates trends		*
Evaluates response to treatments		*
Repeats focused assessment regarding patient complaint or injuries		
Gives radio report to receiving facility		
Turns over patient care with verbal report		*
Student exhibits competence with skill		

Any items in the Not Done column that are marked with an * are mandatory for the student to complete. A check mark in the Not Done column of an item with an * indicates that the student was unsuccessful and must attempt the skill again to assure competency. Examiners should use a different-color ink for the second attempt.

☐ Successful   ☐ Unsuccessful   Examiner Initials: _____

     ©2006 Prentice-Hall Inc.

Radio Report (EMT Medical—Diabetic)

Student: _____   **Examiner:** _____

Date: _____

	Done ✓	Not Done
Requests and checks for open channel before speaking		
Presses transmit button 1 second before speaking		
Holds microphone 2–3 in. from mouth		
Speaks slowly and clearly		*
Speaks in a normal voice		
Briefly transmits: Agency, unit designation, identification/name		*
Briefly transmits: Patient's age, sex, weight		*
Briefly transmits: Scene description/mechanism of injury or medical problem		*
Briefly transmits: Chief complaint with brief history of *present* illness		*
Briefly transmits: Associated symptoms (unless able to be deferred to bedside report)		
Briefly transmits: Past medical history (usually deferred to bedside report)		
Briefly transmits: Vital signs		*
Briefly transmits: Level of consciousness/GCS on trauma		*
Briefly transmits: General appearance, distress, cardiac rhythm, blood glucose, and other pertinent findings unable to be deferred to bedside report		
Briefly transmits: Interventions by EMS AND response(s)		*
ETA (the more critical the patient, the earlier you need to notify the receiving facility)		
Does not waste airtime		
Protects privacy of patient		*
Echoes dispatch information and any physician orders		*
Writes down dispatch information or physician orders		
Confirms with facility that message is received		
Demonstrates/verbalizes ability to troubleshoot basic equipment malfunction		
Student exhibits competence with skill		

Any items in the Not Done column that are marked with an * are mandatory for the student to complete. A check mark in the Not Done column of an item with an * indicates that the student was unsuccessful and must attempt the skill again to assure competency. Examiners should use a different-color ink for the second attempt.

☐ Successful   ☐ Unsuccessful   Examiner Initials: _____

Documentation Skills: Patient Care Report (PCR) (EMT Medical—Diabetic)

Student: _____   Examiner: _____

Date: _____

	Done ✓	Not Done
Records all pertinent dispatch/scene data, using a consistent format		
Completely identifies all additional resources and personnel		
Documents chief complaint, signs/symptoms, position found, age, sex, and weight		
Identifies and records all pertinent, reportable clinical data for each patient		
Documents SAMPLE and OPQRST if applicable		
Records all pertinent negatives		
Records all pertinent denials		
Records accurate, consistent times and patient information		
Includes relevant oral statements of witnesses, bystanders, and patient in "quotes" when appropriate		
Documents initial assessment findings: airway, breathing, and circulation		
Documents any interventions in initial assessment with patient response		
Documents level of consciousness, GCS (if trauma), and VS		
Documents rapid trauma assessment if applicable		
Documents any interventions in rapid trauma assessment with patient response		
Documents focused history and physical assessment		
Documents any interventions in focused assessment with patient response		
Documents repeat VS (every 5 minutes for critical; every 15 minutes for stable)		
Repeats initial assessment and documents findings		
Records ALL treatments with times and patient response(s) in treatment section		
Documents field impression		
Documents transport to specific facility and transfer of care WITH VERBAL REPORT		
Uses correct grammar, abbreviations, spelling, and terminology		
Writes legibly		
Thoroughly documents refusals, denials of transport, and call cancellations		
Documents patient GCS of 15 PRIOR to signing refusal		
Documents advice given to refusal patient, including "call 9-1-1 for further problems"		
Properly corrects errors and omissions		
Writes cautiously, avoids jargon, opinions, inferences, or any derogatory/libelous remarks		
Signs run report		
Uses EMS supplement form if needed		
Student exhibits competence with skill		

Any items in the Not Done column should be evaluated with student. Check marks in this column do not necessarily mean student was unsuccessful as all lines are not completed on all patients. Evaluation of each PCR should be based on the scenario given.

Student must be able to write an EMS report with consistency and accuracy.

☐ Successful   ☐ Unsuccessful   Examiner Initials: _____

   ©2006 Prentice-Hall Inc.

Overall Scenario Management (EMT Medical—Diabetic)

Student: _____   **Examiner:** _____

Date: _____   **Scenario:** _____

NOTE: This skill sheet is to be done after the student completes a scenario as the TEAM LEADER. It is to let the student know if he or she is beginning to "put it all together" and use critical thinking skills to manage an EMS call. PLEASE notice that it is graded on a different basis than the basic lab skill sheet.

	Done ✓	Needs to Improve
SCENE MANAGEMENT		
Recognized hazards and controlled scene—safety, crowd, and patient issues		
Recognized hazards, but did not control the scene		
Unsuccessfully attempted to manage the scene	*	
Did not evaluate the scene and took no control of the scene	*	
PATIENT ASSESSMENT		
Performed a timely, organized complete patient assessment		
Performed complete initial, focused, and ongoing assessments, but in a disorganized manner		
Performed an incomplete assessment	*	
Did not perform an initial assessment	*	
PATIENT MANAGEMENT		
Evaluated assessment findings to manage all aspects of patient condition		
Managed the patient's presenting signs and symptoms without considering all of assessment		
Inadequately managed the patient	*	
Did not manage life-threatening conditions	*	
COMMUNICATION		
Communicated well with crew, patient, family, bystanders, and assisting agencies		
Communicated well with patient and crew		
Communicated with patient and crew, but poor communication skills	*	
Unable to communicate effectively	*	
REPORT AND TRANSFER OF CARE		
Identified correct destination for patient transport, gave accurate, brief report over radio, and provided full report at bedside demonstrating thorough understanding of patient condition and pathophysiological processes		
Identified correct destination and gave accurate radio and bedside report, but did not demonstrate understanding of patient condition and pathophysiological processes		
Identified correct destination, but provided inadequate radio and bedside report	*	
Identified inappropriate destination or provided no radio or bedside report	*	
Student exhibits competence with skill		

Any items that are marked with an * indicate the student needs to improve and a check mark should be placed in the right-hand column. A check mark in the right-hand column indicates that the student was unsuccessful and must attempt the skill again to assure competency. Examiners should use a different-color ink for the second attempt.

☐ Successful   ☐ Unsuccessful   Examiner Initials: _____

EMT Patient Assessment: Medical—*Medical Shock*

Student: _____   Examiner: _____

Date: _____

	Done ✓	Not Done
Assesses scene safety and utilizes appropriate PPE		*
OVERALL SCENE EVALUATION		
Medical—determines nature of illness/if trauma involved determines MOI		*
Determines the number of patients, location, obstacles, and requests any additional resources as needed		
Verbalizes general impression of the patient as approaches		*
Considers stabilization/spinal motion restriction of spine if trauma involved		*
INITIAL ASSESSMENT		
Determines responsiveness/level of consciousness/AVPU		*
Opens airway with appropriate technique and assesses airway/ventilation		*
Manages airway/ventilation and applies appropriate oxygen therapy in less than 3 minutes		*
Assesses circulation: radial/carotid pulse, skin color, temperature, condition, and turgor		*
Controls any major bleeding		*
Makes rapid transport decision if indicated		
Obtains BGL, GCS, and complete vital signs		
FOCUSED HISTORY AND PHYSICAL EXAMINATION/RAPID ASSESSMENT		
Obtains SAMPLE history		
Obtains OPQRST for differential diagnosis		
Obtains associated symptoms, pertinent negatives/denials		
Evaluates decision to perform focused exam or completes rapid assessment		*
Vital signs including AVPU (and GCS if trauma)		*
Assesses cardiovascular system including heart sounds, peripheral edema, and peripheral perfusion		*
Assesses pulmonary system including reassessing airway, ventilation, breath sounds, pulse oximetry, chest wall excursion, accessory muscle use, or other signs of distress		*
Assesses neurological system including speech, droop, drift, if applicable, and distal movement and sensation		*
Assesses musculoskeletal and integumentary systems		
Assesses behavioral, psychological, and social aspects of patient and situation		
States field impression of patient—medical shock (states suspected cause)		*
Verbalizes treatment plan for patient and calls for appropriate intervention(s)—warmth/Trendelenberg/calls ALS		*
Reevaluates transport decision		
ONGOING ASSESSMENT		
Repeats initial assessment		*
Repeats vital signs and evaluates trends		*
Evaluates response to treatments		*
Repeats focused assessment regarding patient complaint or injuries		
Gives radio report to receiving facility		
Turns over patient care with verbal report		*
Student exhibits competence with skill		

Any items in the Not Done column that are marked with an * are mandatory for the student to complete. A check mark in the Not Done column of an item with an * indicates that the student was unsuccessful and must attempt the skill again to assure competency. Examiners should use a different-color ink for the second attempt.

☐ Successful   ☐ Unsuccessful   Examiner Initials: _____

©2006 Prentice-Hall Inc.

Radio Report (EMT Medical—Medical Shock)

Student: _____   **Examiner:** _____

Date: _____

	Done ✓	Not Done
Requests and checks for open channel before speaking		
Presses transmit button 1 second before speaking		
Holds microphone 2–3 in. from mouth		
Speaks slowly and clearly		*
Speaks in a normal voice		
Briefly transmits: Agency, unit designation, identification/name		*
Briefly transmits: Patient's age, sex, weight		*
Briefly transmits: Scene description/mechanism of injury or medical problem		*
Briefly transmits: Chief complaint with brief history of *present* illness		*
Briefly transmits: Associated symptoms (unless able to be deferred to bedside report)		
Briefly transmits: Past medical history (usually deferred to bedside report)		
Briefly transmits: Vital signs		*
Briefly transmits: Level of consciousness/GCS on trauma		*
Briefly transmits: General appearance, distress, cardiac rhythm, blood glucose, and other pertinent findings unable to be deferred to bedside report		
Briefly transmits: Interventions by EMS AND response(s)		*
ETA (the more critical the patient, the earlier you need to notify the receiving facility)		
Does not waste airtime		
Protects privacy of patient		*
Echoes dispatch information and any physician orders		*
Writes down dispatch information or physician orders		
Confirms with facility that message is received		
Demonstrates/verbalizes ability to troubleshoot basic equipment malfunction		
Student exhibits competence with skill		

Any items in the Not Done column that are marked with an * are mandatory for the student to complete. A check mark in the Not Done column of an item with an * indicates that the student was unsuccessful and must attempt the skill again to assure competency. Examiners should use a different-color ink for the second attempt.

☐ Successful   ☐ Unsuccessful   Examiner Initials: _____

Documentation Skills: Patient Care Report (PCR)
(EMT Medical—Medical Shock)

Student: _____   Examiner: _____

Date: _____

	Done ✓	Not Done
Records all pertinent dispatch/scene data, using a consistent format		
Completely identifies all additional resources and personnel		
Documents chief complaint, signs/symptoms, position found, age, sex, and weight		
Identifies and records all pertinent, reportable clinical data for each patient		
Documents SAMPLE and OPQRST if applicable		
Records all pertinent negatives		
Records all pertinent denials		
Records accurate, consistent times and patient information		
Includes relevant oral statements of witnesses, bystanders, and patient in "quotes" when appropriate		
Documents initial assessment findings: airway, breathing, and circulation		
Documents any interventions in initial assessment with patient response		
Documents level of consciousness, GCS (if trauma), and VS		
Documents rapid trauma assessment if applicable		
Documents any interventions in rapid trauma assessment with patient response		
Documents focused history and physical assessment		
Documents any interventions in focused assessment with patient response		
Documents repeat VS (every 5 minutes for critical; every 15 minutes for stable)		
Repeats initial assessment and documents findings		
Records ALL treatments with times and patient response(s) in treatment section		
Documents field impression		
Documents transport to specific facility and transfer of care WITH VERBAL REPORT		
Uses correct grammar, abbreviations, spelling, and terminology		
Writes legibly		
Thoroughly documents refusals, denials of transport, and call cancellations		
Documents patient GCS of 15 PRIOR to signing refusal		
Documents advice given to refusal patient, including "call 9-1-1 for further problems"		
Properly corrects errors and omissions		
Writes cautiously, avoids jargon, opinions, inferences, or any derogatory/libelous remarks		
Signs run report		
Uses EMS supplement form if needed		
Student exhibits competence with skill		

Any items in the Not Done column should be evaluated with student. Check marks in this column do not necessarily mean student was unsuccessful as all lines are not completed on all patients. Evaluation of each PCR should be based on the scenario given.

Student must be able to write an EMS report with consistency and accuracy.

☐ Successful   ☐ Unsuccessful   Examiner Initials: _____

©2006 Prentice-Hall Inc.

Overall Scenario Management (EMT Medical—Medical Shock)

Student: _____   Examiner: _____

Date: _____   Scenario: _____

NOTE: This skill sheet is to be done after the student completes a scenario as the TEAM LEADER. It is to let the student know if he or she is beginning to "put it all together" and use critical thinking skills to manage an EMS call. PLEASE notice that it is graded on a different basis than the basic lab skill sheet.

	Done ✓	Needs to Improve
SCENE MANAGEMENT		
Recognized hazards and controlled scene—safety, crowd, and patient issues		
Recognized hazards, but did not control the scene		
Unsuccessfully attempted to manage the scene	*	
Did not evaluate the scene and took no control of the scene	*	
PATIENT ASSESSMENT		
Performed a timely, organized complete patient assessment		
Performed complete initial, focused, and ongoing assessments, but in a disorganized manner		
Performed an incomplete assessment	*	
Did not perform an initial assessment	*	
PATIENT MANAGEMENT		
Evaluated assessment findings to manage all aspects of patient condition		
Managed the patient's presenting signs and symptoms without considering all of assessment		
Inadequately managed the patient	*	
Did not manage life-threatening conditions	*	
COMMUNICATION		
Communicated well with crew, patient, family, bystanders, and assisting agencies		
Communicated well with patient and crew		
Communicated with patient and crew, but poor communication skills	*	
Unable to communicate effectively	*	
REPORT AND TRANSFER OF CARE		
Identified correct destination for patient transport, gave accurate, brief report over radio and provided full report at bedside demonstrating thorough understanding of patient condition and pathophysiological processes		
Identified correct destination and gave accurate radio and bedside report, but did not demonstrate understanding of patient condition and pathophysiological processes		
Identified correct destination, but provided inadequate radio and bedside report	*	
Identified inappropriate destination or provided no radio or bedside report	*	
Student exhibits competence with skill		

Any items that are marked with an * indicate the student needs to improve and a check mark should be placed in the right-hand column. A check mark in the right-hand column indicates that the student was unsuccessful and must attempt the skill again to assure competency. Examiners should use a different-color ink for the second attempt.

☐ Successful   ☐ Unsuccessful   Examiner Initials: _____

EMT Patient Assessment: Medical—*Respiratory*

Student: _____   **Examiner:** _____

Date: _____

	Done ✓	Not Done
Assesses scene safety and utilizes appropriate PPE		*
OVERALL SCENE EVALUATION		
Medical—determines nature of illness/if trauma involved determines MOI		*
Determines the number of patients, location, obstacles, and requests any additional resources as needed		
Verbalizes general impression of the patient as approaches		*
Considers stabilization/spinal motion restriction of spine if trauma involved		*
INITIAL ASSESSMENT		
Determines responsiveness/level of consciousness/AVPU		*
Opens airway with appropriate technique and assesses airway/ventilation		*
Manages airway/ventilation and applies appropriate oxygen therapy in less than 3 minutes		*
Assesses circulation: radial/carotid pulse, skin color, temperature, condition, and turgor		*
Controls any major bleeding		*
Makes rapid transport decision if indicated		
Obtains BGL, GCS, and complete vital signs		
FOCUSED HISTORY AND PHYSICAL EXAMINATION/RAPID ASSESSMENT		
Obtains SAMPLE history		
Obtains OPQRST for differential diagnosis		
Obtains associated symptoms, pertinent negatives/denials		
Evaluates decision to perform focused exam or completes rapid assessment		*
Vital signs including AVPU (and GCS if trauma)		*
Assesses cardiovascular system including heart sounds, peripheral edema, and peripheral perfusion		*
Assesses pulmonary system including reassessing airway, ventilation, breath sounds, pulse oximetry, chest wall excursion, accessory muscle use, or other signs of distress		*
Assesses neurological system including speech, droop, drift, if applicable, and distal movement and sensation		*
Assesses musculoskeletal and integumentary systems		
Assesses behavioral, psychological, and social aspects of patient and situation		
States field impression of patient—respiratory problem (state suspected cause)		*
Verbalizes treatment plan for patient and calls for appropriate intervention(s)—ALS if needed		*
Reevaluates transport decision		
ONGOING ASSESSMENT		
Repeats initial assessment		*
Repeats vital signs and evaluates trends		*
Evaluates response to treatments		*
Repeats focused assessment regarding patient complaint or injuries		
Gives radio report to receiving facility		
Turns over patient care with verbal report		*
Student exhibits competence with skill		

Any items in the Not Done column that are marked with an * are mandatory for the student to complete. A check mark in the Not Done column of an item with an * indicates that the student was unsuccessful and must attempt the skill again to assure competency. Examiners should use a different-color ink for the second attempt.

☐ Successful   ☐ Unsuccessful   Examiner Initials: _____

        ©2006 Prentice-Hall Inc.

Radio Report (EMT Medical—Respiratory)

Student: _____   Examiner: _____

Date: _____

	Done ✓	Not Done
Requests and checks for open channel before speaking		
Presses transmit button 1 second before speaking		
Holds microphone 2–3 in. from mouth		
Speaks slowly and clearly		*
Speaks in a normal voice		
Briefly transmits: Agency, unit designation, identification/name		*
Briefly transmits: Patient's age, sex, weight		*
Briefly transmits: Scene description/mechanism of injury or medical problem		*
Briefly transmits: Chief complaint with brief history of *present* illness		*
Briefly transmits: Associated symptoms (unless able to be deferred to bedside report)		
Briefly transmits: Past medical history (usually deferred to bedside report)		
Briefly transmits: Vital signs		*
Briefly transmits: Level of consciousness/GCS on trauma		*
Briefly transmits: General appearance, distress, cardiac rhythm, blood glucose, and other pertinent findings unable to be deferred to bedside report		
Briefly transmits: Interventions by EMS AND response(s)		*
ETA (the more critical the patient, the earlier you need to notify the receiving facility)		
Does not waste airtime		
Protects privacy of patient		*
Echoes dispatch information and any physician orders		*
Writes down dispatch information or physician orders		
Confirms with facility that message is received		
Demonstrates/verbalizes ability to troubleshoot basic equipment malfunction		
Student exhibits competence with skill		

Any items in the Not Done column that are marked with an * are mandatory for the student to complete. A check mark in the Not Done column of an item with an * indicates that the student was unsuccessful and must attempt the skill again to assure competency. Examiners should use a different-color ink for the second attempt.

☐ Successful   ☐ Unsuccessful   Examiner Initials: _____

Documentation Skills: Patient Care Report (PCR)
(EMT Medical—Respiratory)

Student: _____   Examiner: _____

Date: _____

	Done ✓	Not Done
Records all pertinent dispatch/scene data, using a consistent format		
Completely identifies all additional resources and personnel		
Documents chief complaint, signs/symptoms, position found, age, sex, and weight		
Identifies and records all pertinent, reportable clinical data for each patient		
Documents SAMPLE and OPQRST if applicable		
Records all pertinent negatives		
Records all pertinent denials		
Records accurate, consistent times and patient information		
Includes relevant oral statements of witnesses, bystanders, and patient in "quotes" when appropriate		
Documents initial assessment findings: airway, breathing, and circulation		
Documents any interventions in initial assessment with patient response		
Documents level of consciousness, GCS (if trauma), and VS		
Documents rapid trauma assessment if applicable		
Documents any interventions in rapid trauma assessment with patient response		
Documents focused history and physical assessment		
Documents any interventions in focused assessment with patient response		
Documents repeat VS (every 5 minutes for critical; every 15 minutes for stable)		
Repeats initial assessment and documents findings		
Records ALL treatments with times and patient response(s) in treatment section		
Documents field impression		
Documents transport to specific facility and transfer of care WITH VERBAL REPORT		
Uses correct grammar, abbreviations, spelling, and terminology		
Writes legibly		
Thoroughly documents refusals, denials of transport, and call cancellations		
Documents patient GCS of 15 PRIOR to signing refusal		
Documents advice given to refusal patient, including "call 9-1-1 for further problems"		
Properly corrects errors and omissions		
Writes cautiously, avoids jargon, opinions, inferences, or any derogatory/libelous remarks		
Signs run report		
Uses EMS supplement form if needed		
Student exhibits competence with skill		

Any items in the Not Done column should be evaluated with student. Check marks in this column do not necessarily mean student was unsuccessful as all lines are not completed on all patients. Evaluation of each PCR should be based on the scenario given.

Student must be able to write an EMS report with consistency and accuracy.

☐ Successful   ☐ Unsuccessful   Examiner Initials: _____

©2006 Prentice-Hall Inc.

Overall Scenario Management (EMT Medical—Respiratory)

Student: _____   Examiner: _____

Date: _____   Scenario: _____

NOTE: This skill sheet is to be done after the student completes a scenario as the TEAM LEADER. It is to let the student know if he or she is beginning to "put it all together" and use critical thinking skills to manage an EMS call. PLEASE notice that it is graded on a different basis than the basic lab skill sheet.

	Done ✓	Needs to Improve
SCENE MANAGEMENT		
Recognized hazards and controlled scene—safety, crowd, and patient issues		
Recognized hazards, but did not control the scene		
Unsuccessfully attempted to manage the scene	*	
Did not evaluate the scene and took no control of the scene	*	
PATIENT ASSESSMENT		
Performed a timely, organized complete patient assessment		
Performed complete initial, focused, and ongoing assessments, but in a disorganized manner		
Performed an incomplete assessment	*	
Did not perform an initial assessment	*	
PATIENT MANAGEMENT		
Evaluated assessment findings to manage all aspects of patient condition		
Managed the patient's presenting signs and symptoms without considering all of assessment		
Inadequately managed the patient	*	
Did not manage life-threatening conditions	*	
COMMUNICATION		
Communicated well with crew, patient, family, bystanders, and assisting agencies		
Communicated well with patient and crew		
Communicated with patient and crew, but poor communication skills	*	
Unable to communicate effectively	*	
REPORT AND TRANSFER OF CARE		
Identified correct destination for patient transport, gave accurate, brief report over radio, and provided full report at bedside demonstrating thorough understanding of patient condition and pathophysiological processes		
Identified correct destination and gave accurate radio and bedside report, but did not demonstrate understanding of patient condition and pathophysiological processes		
Identified correct destination, but provided inadequate radio and bedside report	*	
Identified inappropriate destination or provided no radio or bedside report	*	
Student exhibits competence with skill		

Any items that are marked with an * indicate the student needs to improve and a check mark should be placed in the right-hand column. A check mark in the right-hand column indicates that the student was unsuccessful and must attempt the skill again to assure competency. Examiners should use a different-color ink for the second attempt.

☐ Successful   ☐ Unsuccessful   Examiner Initials: _____

©2006 Prentice-Hall Inc.

EMT Patient Assessment: Medical—*Stroke*

Student: _____   Examiner: _____

Date: _____

	Done ✓	Not Done
Assesses scene safety and utilizes appropriate PPE		*
OVERALL SCENE EVALUATION		
Medical—determines nature of illness/if trauma involved determines MOI		*
Determines the number of patients, location, obstacles, and requests any additional resources as needed		
Verbalizes general impression of the patient as approaches		*
Considers stabilization/spinal motion restriction of spine if trauma involved		*
INITIAL ASSESSMENT		
Determines responsiveness/level of consciousness/AVPU		*
Opens airway with appropriate technique and assesses airway/ventilation		*
Manages airway/ventilation and applies appropriate oxygen therapy in less than 3 minutes		*
Assesses circulation: radial/carotid pulse, skin color, temperature, condition, and turgor		*
Controls any major bleeding		*
Makes rapid transport decision if indicated		
Obtains BGL, GCS, and complete vital signs		
FOCUSED HISTORY AND PHYSICAL EXAMINATION/RAPID ASSESSMENT		
Obtains SAMPLE history—MUST obtain time of ONSET		*
Obtains OPQRST for differential diagnosis		
Obtains associated symptoms, pertinent negatives/denials		
Evaluates decision to perform focused exam or completes rapid assessment		*
Vital signs including AVPU (and GCS if trauma)		*
Assesses cardiovascular system including heart sounds, peripheral edema, and peripheral perfusion		*
Assesses pulmonary system including reassessing airway, ventilation, breath sounds, pulse oximetry, chest wall excursion, accessory muscle use, or other signs of distress		*
Assesses neurological system **including speech, droop, drift** and distal movement and sensation		*
Assesses musculoskeletal and integumentary systems		
Assesses behavioral, psychological, and social aspects of patient and situation		
States field impression of patient—possible stroke		*
Verbalizes treatment plan for patient and calls for appropriate intervention(s)—ALS assistance/ rapid transport		*
Reevaluates transport decision		
ONGOING ASSESSMENT		
Repeats initial assessment		*
Repeats vital signs and evaluates trends		*
Evaluates response to treatments		*
Repeats focused assessment regarding patient complaint or injuries		
Gives radio report to receiving facility		
Turns over patient care with verbal report		*
Student exhibits competence with skill		

Any items in the Not Done column that are marked with an * are mandatory for the student to complete. A check mark in the Not Done column of an item with an * indicates that the student was unsuccessful and must attempt the skill again to assure competency. Examiners should use a different-color ink for the second attempt.

☐ Successful   ☐ Unsuccessful   Examiner Initials: _____

©2006 Prentice-Hall Inc.

Radio Report (EMT Medical—Stroke)

Student: _____   Examiner: _____

Date: _____

	Done ✓	Not Done
Requests and checks for open channel before speaking		
Presses transmit button 1 second before speaking		
Holds microphone 2–3 in. from mouth		
Speaks slowly and clearly		*
Speaks in a normal voice		
Briefly transmits: Agency, unit designation, identification/name		*
Briefly transmits: Patient's age, sex, weight		*
Briefly transmits: Scene description/mechanism of injury or medical problem		*
Briefly transmits: Chief complaint with brief history of *present* illness		*
Briefly transmits: Associated symptoms (unless able to be deferred to bedside report)		
Briefly transmits: Past medical history (usually deferred to bedside report)		
Briefly transmits: Vital signs		*
Briefly transmits: Level of consciousness/GCS on trauma		*
Briefly transmits: General appearance, distress, cardiac rhythm, blood glucose, and other pertinent findings unable to be deferred to bedside report		
Briefly transmits: Interventions by EMS AND response(s)		*
ETA (the more critical the patient, the earlier you need to notify the receiving facility)		
Does not waste airtime		
Protects privacy of patient		*
Echoes dispatch information and any physician orders		*
Writes down dispatch information or physician orders		
Confirms with facility that message is received		
Demonstrates/verbalizes ability to troubleshoot basic equipment malfunction		
Student exhibits competence with skill		

Any items in the Not Done column that are marked with an * are mandatory for the student to complete. A check mark in the Not Done column of an item with an * indicates that the student was unsuccessful and must attempt the skill again to assure competency. Examiners should use a different-color ink for the second attempt.

☐ Successful   ☐ Unsuccessful   Examiner Initials: _____

Documentation Skills: Patient Care Report (PCR) (EMT Medical—Stroke)

Student: _____   Examiner: _____

Date: _____

	Done ✓	Not Done
Records all pertinent dispatch/scene data, using a consistent format		
Completely identifies all additional resources and personnel		
Documents chief complaint, signs/symptoms, position found, age, sex, and weight		
Identifies and records all pertinent, reportable clinical data for each patient		
Documents SAMPLE and OPQRST if applicable		
Records all pertinent negatives		
Records all pertinent denials		
Records accurate, consistent times and patient information		
Includes relevant oral statements of witnesses, bystanders, and patient in "quotes" when appropriate		
Documents initial assessment findings: airway, breathing, and circulation		
Documents any interventions in initial assessment with patient response		
Documents level of consciousness, GCS (if trauma), and VS		
Documents rapid trauma assessment if applicable		
Documents any interventions in rapid trauma assessment with patient response		
Documents focused history and physical assessment		
Documents any interventions in focused assessment with patient response		
Documents repeat VS (every 5 minutes for critical; every 15 minutes for stable)		
Repeats initial assessment and documents findings		
Records ALL treatments with times and patient response(s) in treatment section		
Documents field impression		
Documents transport to specific facility and transfer of care WITH VERBAL REPORT		
Uses correct grammar, abbreviations, spelling, and terminology		
Writes legibly		
Thoroughly documents refusals, denials of transport, and call cancellations		
Documents patient GCS of 15 PRIOR to signing refusal		
Documents advice given to refusal patient, including "call 9-1-1 for further problems"		
Properly corrects errors and omissions		
Writes cautiously, avoids jargon, opinions, inferences, or any derogatory/libelous remarks		
Signs run report		
Uses EMS supplement form if needed		
Student exhibits competence with skill		

Any items in the Not Done column should be evaluated with student. Check marks in this column do not necessarily mean student was unsuccessful as all lines are not completed on all patients. Evaluation of each PCR should be based on the scenario given.

Student must be able to write an EMS report with consistency and accuracy.

☐ Successful   ☐ Unsuccessful   Examiner Initials: _____

          ©2006 Prentice-Hall Inc.

Overall Scenario Management (EMT Medical—Stroke)

Student: _____   Examiner: _____

Date: _____   Scenario: _____

NOTE: This skill sheet is to be done after the student completes a scenario as the TEAM LEADER. It is to let the student know if he or she is beginning to "put it all together" and use critical thinking skills to manage an EMS call. PLEASE notice that it is graded on a different basis than the basic lab skill sheet.

	Done ✓	Needs to Improve
SCENE MANAGEMENT		
Recognized hazards and controlled scene—safety, crowd, and patient issues		
Recognized hazards, but did not control the scene		
Unsuccessfully attempted to manage the scene	*	
Did not evaluate the scene and took no control of the scene	*	
PATIENT ASSESSMENT		
Performed a timely, organized complete patient assessment		
Performed complete initial, focused, and ongoing assessments, but in a disorganized manner		
Performed an incomplete assessment	*	
Did not perform an initial assessment	*	
PATIENT MANAGEMENT		
Evaluated assessment findings to manage all aspects of patient condition		
Managed the patient's presenting signs and symptoms without considering all of assessment		
Inadequately managed the patient	*	
Did not manage life-threatening conditions	*	
COMMUNICATION		
Communicated well with crew, patient, family, bystanders, and assisting agencies		
Communicated well with patient and crew		
Communicated with patient and crew, but poor communication skills	*	
Unable to communicate effectively	*	
REPORT AND TRANSFER OF CARE		
Identified correct destination for patient transport, gave accurate, brief report over radio, and provided full report at bedside demonstrating thorough understanding of patient condition and pathophysiological processes		
Identified correct destination and gave accurate radio and bedside report, but did not demonstrate understanding of patient condition and pathophysiological processes		
Identified correct destination, but provided inadequate radio and bedside report	*	
Identified inappropriate destination or provided no radio or bedside report	*	
Student exhibits competence with skill		

Any items that are marked with an * indicate the student needs to improve and a check mark should be placed in the right-hand column. A check mark in the right-hand column indicates that the student was unsuccessful and must attempt the skill again to assure competency. Examiners should use a different-color ink for the second attempt.

☐ Successful   ☐ Unsuccessful   Examiner Initials: _____

EMT Patient Assessment: Medical—*Examiner's Choice*

Student: _____   **Examiner:** _____

Date: _____

	Done ✓	Not Done
Assesses scene safety and utilizes appropriate PPE		*
OVERALL SCENE EVALUATION		
Medical—determines nature of illness/if trauma involved determines MOI		*
Determines the number of patients, location, obstacles, and requests any additional resources as needed		
Verbalizes general impression of the patient as approaches		*
Considers stabilization/spinal motion restriction of spine if trauma involved		*
INITIAL ASSESSMENT		
Determines responsiveness/level of consciousness/AVPU		*
Opens airway with appropriate technique and assesses airway/ventilation		*
Manages airway/ventilation and applies appropriate oxygen therapy in less than 3 minutes		*
Assesses circulation: radial/carotid pulse, skin color, temperature, condition, and turgor		*
Controls any major bleeding		*
Makes rapid transport decision if indicated		
Obtains BGL, GCS, and complete vital signs		
FOCUSED HISTORY AND PHYSICAL EXAMINATION/RAPID ASSESSMENT		
Obtains SAMPLE history		
Obtains OPQRST for differential diagnosis		
Obtains associated symptoms, pertinent negatives/denials		
Evaluates decision to perform focused exam or completes rapid assessment		*
Vital signs including AVPU (and GCS if trauma)		*
Assesses cardiovascular system including heart sounds, peripheral edema, and peripheral perfusion		*
Assesses pulmonary system including reassessing airway, ventilation, breath sounds, pulse oximetry, chest wall excursion, accessory muscle use, or other signs of distress		*
Assesses neurological system including speech, droop, drift, if applicable, and distal movement and sensation		*
Assesses musculoskeletal and integumentary systems		
Assesses behavioral, psychological, and social aspects of patient and situation		
States field impression of patient—		*
Verbalizes treatment plan for patient and calls for appropriate intervention(s)		*
Reevaluates transport decision		
ONGOING ASSESSMENT		
Repeats initial assessment		*
Repeats vital signs and evaluates trends		*
Evaluates response to treatments		*
Repeats focused assessment regarding patient complaint or injuries		
Gives radio report to receiving facility		
Turns over patient care with verbal report		*
Student exhibits competence with skill		

Any items in the Not Done column that are marked with an * are mandatory for the student to complete. A check mark in the Not Done column of an item with an * indicates that the student was unsuccessful and must attempt the skill again to assure competency. Examiners should use a different-color ink for the second attempt.

☐ Successful   ☐ Unsuccessful   Examiner Initials: _____

    ©2006 Prentice-Hall Inc.

Radio Report (EMT Medical—Examiner's Choice)

Student: _____   **Examiner:** _____

Date: _____

	Done ✓	Not Done
Requests and checks for open channel before speaking		
Presses transmit button 1 second before speaking		
Holds microphone 2–3 in. from mouth		
Speaks slowly and clearly		*
Speaks in a normal voice		
Briefly transmits: Agency, unit designation, identification/name		*
Briefly transmits: Patient's age, sex, weight		*
Briefly transmits: Scene description/mechanism of injury or medical problem		*
Briefly transmits: Chief complaint with brief history of *present* illness		*
Briefly transmits: Associated symptoms (unless able to be deferred to bedside report)		
Briefly transmits: Past medical history (usually deferred to bedside report)		
Briefly transmits: Vital signs		*
Briefly transmits: Level of consciousness/GCS on trauma		*
Briefly transmits: General appearance, distress, cardiac rhythm, blood glucose, and other pertinent findings unable to be deferred to bedside report		
Briefly transmits: Interventions by EMS AND response(s)		*
ETA (the more critical the patient, the earlier you need to notify the receiving facility)		
Does not waste airtime		
Protects privacy of patient		*
Echoes dispatch information and any physician orders		*
Writes down dispatch information or physician orders		
Confirms with facility that message is received		
Demonstrates/verbalizes ability to troubleshoot basic equipment malfunction		
Student exhibits competence with skill		

Any items in the Not Done column that are marked with an * are mandatory for the student to complete. A check mark in the Not Done column of an item with an * indicates that the student was unsuccessful and must attempt the skill again to assure competency. Examiners should use a different-color ink for the second attempt.

☐ Successful   ☐ Unsuccessful   Examiner Initials: _____

©2006 Prentice-Hall Inc.

Documentation Skills: Patient Care Report (PCR)
(EMT Medical—Examiner's Choice)

Student: _____   **Examiner:** _____

Date: _____

	Done ✓	Not Done
Records all pertinent dispatch/scene data, using a consistent format		
Completely identifies all additional resources and personnel		
Documents chief complaint, signs/symptoms, position found, age, sex, and weight		
Identifies and records all pertinent, reportable clinical data for each patient		
Documents SAMPLE and OPQRST if applicable		
Records all pertinent negatives		
Records all pertinent denials		
Records accurate, consistent times and patient information		
Includes relevant oral statements of witnesses, bystanders, and patient in "quotes" when appropriate		
Documents initial assessment findings: airway, breathing, and circulation		
Documents any interventions in initial assessment with patient response		
Documents level of consciousness, GCS (if trauma), and VS		
Documents rapid trauma assessment if applicable		
Documents any interventions in rapid trauma assessment with patient response		
Documents focused history and physical assessment		
Documents any interventions in focused assessment with patient response		
Documents repeat VS (every 5 minutes for critical; every 15 minutes for stable)		
Repeats initial assessment and documents findings		
Records ALL treatments with times and patient response(s) in treatment section		
Documents field impression		
Documents transport to specific facility and transfer of care WITH VERBAL REPORT		
Uses correct grammar, abbreviations, spelling, and terminology		
Writes legibly		
Thoroughly documents refusals, denials of transport, and call cancellations		
Documents patient GCS of 15 PRIOR to signing refusal		
Documents advice given to refusal patient, including "call 9-1-1 for further problems"		
Properly corrects errors and omissions		
Writes cautiously, avoids jargon, opinions, inferences, or any derogatory/libelous remarks		
Signs run report		
Uses EMS supplement form if needed		
Student exhibits competence with skill		

Any items in the Not Done column should be evaluated with student. Check marks in this column do not necessarily mean student was unsuccessful as all lines are not completed on all patients. Evaluation of each PCR should be based on the scenario given.

Student must be able to write an EMS report with consistency and accuracy.

☐ Successful   ☐ Unsuccessful   Examiner Initials: _____

    ©2006 Prentice-Hall Inc.

Overall Scenario Management (EMT Medical—Examiner's Choice)

Student: _____   Examiner: _____

Date: _____   Scenario: _____

NOTE: This skill sheet is to be done after the student completes a scenario as the TEAM LEADER. It is to let the student know if he or she is beginning to "put it all together" and use critical thinking skills to manage an EMS call. PLEASE notice that it is graded on a different basis than the basic lab skill sheet.

	Done ✓	Needs to Improve
SCENE MANAGEMENT		
Recognized hazards and controlled scene—safety, crowd, and patient issues		
Recognized hazards, but did not control the scene		
Unsuccessfully attempted to manage the scene	*	
Did not evaluate the scene and took no control of the scene	*	
PATIENT ASSESSMENT		
Performed a timely, organized complete patient assessment		
Performed complete initial, focused, and ongoing assessments, but in a disorganized manner		
Performed an incomplete assessment	*	
Did not perform an initial assessment	*	
PATIENT MANAGEMENT		
Evaluated assessment findings to manage all aspects of patient condition		
Managed the patient's presenting signs and symptoms without considering all of assessment		
Inadequately managed the patient	*	
Did not manage life-threatening conditions	*	
COMMUNICATION		
Communicated well with crew, patient, family, bystanders, and assisting agencies		
Communicated well with patient and crew		
Communicated with patient and crew, but poor communication skills	*	
Unable to communicate effectively	*	
REPORT AND TRANSFER OF CARE		
Identified correct destination for patient transport, gave accurate, brief report over radio, and provided full report at bedside demonstrating thorough understanding of patient condition and pathophysiological processes		
Identified correct destination and gave accurate radio and bedside report, but did not demonstrate understanding of patient condition and pathophysiological processes		
Identified correct destination, but provided inadequate radio and bedside report	*	
Identified inappropriate destination or provided no radio or bedside report	*	
Student exhibits competence with skill		

Any items that are marked with an * indicate the student needs to improve and a check mark should be placed in the right-hand column. A check mark in the right-hand column indicates that the student was unsuccessful and must attempt the skill again to assure competency. Examiners should use a different-color ink for the second attempt.

☐ Successful   ☐ Unsuccessful   Examiner Initials: _____

©2006 Prentice-Hall Inc.

EMT Patient Assessment: Trauma—*Burn Trauma*

Student: _____   **Examiner:** _____

Date: _____

	Done ✓	Not Done
Assesses scene safety and utilizes appropriate PPE		*
OVERALL SCENE EVALUATION		
Trauma—assesses mechanism of injury/if medical component determines nature of illness		*
Determines the number of patients, location, obstacles, and requests any additional resources as needed		
Verbalizes general impression of the patient as approaches		*
Stabilizes C-spine/spinal motion restriction (SMR) of spine and stops the burning process		*
INITIAL ASSESSMENT/RESUSCITATION		
Determines responsiveness/level of consciousness/AVPU		*
Opens airway with appropriate technique and assesses airway/ventilation		*
Manages airway/ventilation and applies appropriate oxygen therapy in less than 3 minutes		*
Assesses circulation: radial/carotid pulse, skin color, temperature, condition, and turgor		*
Controls any major bleeding		*
Figures BSA of burn (using rule of nines) and makes rapid transport decision		*
Obtains BGL, GCS, and complete vital signs		
RAPID TRAUMA ASSESSMENT (If patient is Trauma Alert or Load and Go)		
Assesses abdomen		
Rapidly palpates each extremity, assessing for obvious injuries and distal PMS		
Provides spinal motion restriction (SMR) on long backboard (LBB), checking posterior torso and legs		
Secures head LAST		
Loads patient/initiates transport (to appropriate LZ, to meet ALS, or to appropriate facility) in less than 10 minutes		
Reassesses ABCs and interventions		
FOCUSED HISTORY AND PHYSICAL ASSESSMENT		
Reassesses interventions and further assesses injuries found		
Obtains vital signs and GCS (Glasgow Coma Score)		
Obtains SAMPLE history		
Inspects and palpates head, facial, and neck regions		
Inspects, palpates, and auscultates chest/thorax		
Inspects and palpates abdomen and pelvis		
Inspects and palpates upper and lower extremities, checking distal PMS		
Inspects and palpates posterior torso		
Manages all injuries/wounds appropriately		
Repeats initial assessment		*
Repeats vital signs and evaluates trends		*
Evaluates response to treatments		*
Performs ongoing assessment		
Gives radio report to receiving facility		
Turns over patient care with verbal report		*
Student exhibits competence with skill		

Any items in the Not Done column that are marked with an * are mandatory for the student to complete. A check mark in the Not Done column of an item with an * indicates that the student was unsuccessful and must attempt the skill again to assure competency. Examiners should use a different-color ink for the second attempt.

☐ Successful   ☐ Unsuccessful   Examiner Initials: _____

©2006 Prentice-Hall Inc.

Radio Report (EMT Trauma—Burn Trauma)

Student: _____   **Examiner:** _____

Date: _____

	Done ✓	Not Done
Requests and checks for open channel before speaking		
Presses transmit button 1 second before speaking		
Holds microphone 2–3 in. from mouth		
Speaks slowly and clearly		*
Speaks in a normal voice		
Briefly transmits: Agency, unit designation, identification/name		*
Briefly transmits: Patient's age, sex, weight		*
Briefly transmits: Scene description/mechanism of injury or medical problem		*
Briefly transmits: Chief complaint with brief history of *present* illness		*
Briefly transmits: Associated symptoms (unless able to be deferred to bedside report)		
Briefly transmits: Past medical history (usually deferred to bedside report)		
Briefly transmits: Vital signs		*
Briefly transmits: Level of consciousness/GCS on trauma		*
Briefly transmits: General appearance, distress, cardiac rhythm, blood glucose, and other pertinent findings unable to be deferred to bedside report		
Briefly transmits: Interventions by EMS AND response(s)		*
ETA (the more critical the patient, the earlier you need to notify the receiving facility)		
Does not waste airtime		
Protects privacy of patient		*
Echoes dispatch information and any physician orders		*
Writes down dispatch information or physician orders		
Confirms with facility that message is received		
Demonstrates/verbalizes ability to troubleshoot basic equipment malfunction		
Student exhibits competence with skill		

Any items in the Not Done column that are marked with an * are mandatory for the student to complete. A check mark in the Not Done column of an item with an * indicates that the student was unsuccessful and must attempt the skill again to assure competency. Examiners should use a different-color ink for the second attempt.

☐ Successful   ☐ Unsuccessful   Examiner Initials: _____

©2006 Prentice-Hall Inc.

Documentation Skills: Patient Care Report (PCR)
(EMT Trauma—Burn Trauma)

Student: _____   Examiner: _____

Date: _____

	Done ✓	Not Done
Records all pertinent dispatch/scene data, using a consistent format		
Completely identifies all additional resources and personnel		
Documents chief complaint, signs/symptoms, position found, age, sex, and weight		
Identifies and records all pertinent, reportable clinical data for each patient		
Documents SAMPLE and OPQRST if applicable		
Records all pertinent negatives		
Records all pertinent denials		
Records accurate, consistent times and patient information		
Includes relevant oral statements of witnesses, bystanders, and patient in "quotes" when appropriate		
Documents initial assessment findings: airway, breathing, and circulation		
Documents any interventions in initial assessment with patient response		
Documents level of consciousness, GCS (if trauma), and VS		
Documents rapid trauma assessment if applicable		
Documents any interventions in rapid trauma assessment with patient response		
Documents focused history and physical assessment		
Documents any interventions in focused assessment with patient response		
Documents repeat VS (every 5 minutes for critical; every 15 minutes for stable)		
Repeats initial assessment and documents findings		
Records ALL treatments with times and patient response(s) in treatment section		
Documents field impression		
Documents transport to specific facility and transfer of care WITH VERBAL REPORT		
Uses correct grammar, abbreviations, spelling, and terminology		
Writes legibly		
Thoroughly documents refusals, denials of transport, and call cancellations		
Documents patient GCS of 15 PRIOR to signing refusal		
Documents advice given to refusal patient, including "call 9-1-1 for further problems"		
Properly corrects errors and omissions		
Writes cautiously, avoids jargon, opinions, inferences, or any derogatory/libelous remarks		
Signs run report		
Uses EMS supplement form if needed		
Student exhibits competence with skill		

Any items in the Not Done column should be evaluated with student. Check marks in this column do not necessarily mean student was unsuccessful as all lines are not completed on all patients. Evaluation of each PCR should be based on the scenario given.

Student must be able to write an EMS report with consistency and accuracy.

☐ Successful   ☐ Unsuccessful   Examiner Initials: _____

©2006 Prentice-Hall Inc.

Overall Scenario Management (EMT Trauma—Burn Trauma)

Student: _____

Examiner: _____

Date: _____

Scenario: _____

NOTE: This skill sheet is to be done after the student completes a scenario as the TEAM LEADER. It is to let the student know if he or she is beginning to "put it all together" and use critical thinking skills to manage an EMS call. PLEASE notice that it is graded on a different basis than the basic lab skill sheet.

	Done ✓	Needs to Improve
SCENE MANAGEMENT		
Recognized hazards and controlled scene—safety, crowd, and patient issues		
Recognized hazards, but did not control the scene		
Unsuccessfully attempted to manage the scene	*	
Did not evaluate the scene and took no control of the scene	*	
PATIENT ASSESSMENT		
Performed a timely, organized complete patient assessment		
Performed complete initial, focused, and ongoing assessments, but in a disorganized manner		
Performed an incomplete assessment	*	
Did not perform an initial assessment	*	
PATIENT MANAGEMENT		
Evaluated assessment findings to manage all aspects of patient condition		
Managed the patient's presenting signs and symptoms without considering all of assessment		
Inadequately managed the patient	*	
Did not manage life-threatening conditions	*	
COMMUNICATION		
Communicated well with crew, patient, family, bystanders, and assisting agencies		
Communicated well with patient and crew		
Communicated with patient and crew, but poor communication skills	*	
Unable to communicate effectively	*	
REPORT AND TRANSFER OF CARE		
Identified correct destination for patient transport, gave accurate, brief report over radio, and provided full report at bedside demonstrating thorough understanding of patient condition and pathophysiological processes		
Identified correct destination and gave accurate radio and bedside report, but did not demonstrate understanding of patient condition and pathophysiological processes		
Identified correct destination, but provided inadequate radio and bedside report	*	
Identified inappropriate destination or provided no radio or bedside report	*	
Student exhibits competence with skill		

Any items that are marked with an * indicate the student needs to improve and a check mark should be placed in the right-hand column. A check mark in the right-hand column indicates that the student was unsuccessful and must attempt the skill again to assure competency. Examiners should use a different-color ink for the second attempt.

☐ Successful   ☐ Unsuccessful   Examiner Initials: _____

EMT Patient Assessment: Trauma—*Chest Trauma*

Student: _____   Examiner: _____

Date: _____

	Done ✓	Not Done
Assesses scene safety and utilizes appropriate PPE		*
OVERALL SCENE EVALUATION		
Trauma—assesses mechanism of injury/if medical component determines nature of illness		*
Determines the number of patients, location, obstacles, and requests any additional resources as needed		
Verbalizes general impression of the patient as approaches		*
Stabilizes C-spine/spinal motion restriction (SMR) of spine		
INITIAL ASSESSMENT/RESUSCITATION		
Determines responsiveness/level of consciousness/AVPU		*
Opens airway with appropriate technique and assesses airway/ventilation		*
Manages airway/ventilation and applies oxygen therapy in less than 3 minutes **(occlusive dsg for open chest)**		*
Assesses circulation: radial/carotid pulse, skin color, temperature, condition, and turgor		*
Controls any major bleeding		*
Makes rapid transport decision		*
Obtains BGL, GCS, and complete vital signs		
RAPID TRAUMA ASSESSMENT (If Patient is Trauma Alert or Load and Go)		
Assesses abdomen		
Rapidly palpates each extremity, assessing for obvious injuries and distal PMS		
Provides spinal motion restriction (SMR) on long backboard (LBB), checking posterior torso and legs		
Secures head LAST		
Loads patient/initiates transport (to appropriate LZ, to meet ALS, or to appropriate facility) in less than 10 minutes		
Reassesses ABCs and interventions		
FOCUSED HISTORY AND PHYSICAL ASSESSMENT		
Reassesses interventions and further assesses injuries found		
Obtains vital signs and GCS (Glasgow Coma Score)		
Obtains SAMPLE history		
Inspects and palpates head, facial, and neck regions		
Inspects, palpates, and auscultates chest/thorax		
Inspects and palpates abdomen and pelvis		
Inspects and palpates upper and lower extremities, checking distal PMS		
Inspects and palpates posterior torso		
Manages all injuries/wounds appropriately		
Repeats initial assessment		*
Repeats vital signs and evaluates trends		*
Evaluates response to treatments		*
Performs ongoing assessment		
Gives radio report to receiving facility		
Turns over patient care with verbal report		*
Student exhibits competence with skill		

Any items in the Not Done column that are marked with an * are mandatory for the student to complete. A check mark in the Not Done column of an item with an * indicates that the student was unsuccessful and must attempt the skill again to assure competency. Examiners should use a different-color ink for the second attempt.

☐ Successful   ☐ Unsuccessful   Examiner Initials: _____

©2006 Prentice-Hall Inc.

Radio Report (EMT Trauma—Chest Trauma)

Student: _____   **Examiner:** _____

Date: _____

	Done ✓	Not Done
Requests and checks for open channel before speaking		
Presses transmit button 1 second before speaking		
Holds microphone 2–3 in. from mouth		
Speaks slowly and clearly		*
Speaks in a normal voice		
Briefly transmits: Agency, unit designation, identification/name		*
Briefly transmits: Patient's age, sex, weight		*
Briefly transmits: Scene description/mechanism of injury or medical problem		*
Briefly transmits: Chief complaint with brief history of *present* illness		*
Briefly transmits: Associated symptoms (unless able to be deferred to bedside report)		
Briefly transmits: Past medical history (usually deferred to bedside report)		
Briefly transmits: Vital signs		*
Briefly transmits: Level of consciousness/GCS on trauma		*
Briefly transmits: General appearance, distress, cardiac rhythm, blood glucose, and other pertinent findings unable to be deferred to bedside report		
Briefly transmits: Interventions by EMS AND response(s)		*
ETA (the more critical the patient, the earlier you need to notify the receiving facility)		
Does not waste airtime		
Protects privacy of patient		*
Echoes dispatch information and any physician orders		*
Writes down dispatch information or physician orders		
Confirms with facility that message is received		
Demonstrates/verbalizes ability to troubleshoot basic equipment malfunction		
Student exhibits competence with skill		

Any items in the Not Done column that are marked with an * are mandatory for the student to complete. A check mark in the Not Done column of an item with an * indicates that the student was unsuccessful and must attempt the skill again to assure competency. Examiners should use a different-color ink for the second attempt.

☐ Successful   ☐ Unsuccessful   Examiner Initials: _____

©2006 Prentice-Hall Inc.

Documentation Skills: Patient Care Report (PCR)
(EMT Trauma—Chest Trauma)

Student: _____   **Examiner:** _____

Date: _____

	Done ✓	Not Done
Records all pertinent dispatch/scene data, using a consistent format		
Completely identifies all additional resources and personnel		
Documents chief complaint, signs/symptoms, position found, age, sex, and weight		
Identifies and records all pertinent, reportable clinical data for each patient		
Documents SAMPLE and OPQRST if applicable		
Records all pertinent negatives		
Records all pertinent denials		
Records accurate, consistent times and patient information		
Includes relevant oral statements of witnesses, bystanders, and patient in "quotes" when appropriate		
Documents initial assessment findings: airway, breathing, and circulation		
Documents any interventions in initial assessment with patient response		
Documents level of consciousness, GCS (if trauma), and VS		
Documents rapid trauma assessment if applicable		
Documents any interventions in rapid trauma assessment with patient response		
Documents focused history and physical assessment		
Documents any interventions in focused assessment with patient response		
Documents repeat VS (every 5 minutes for critical; every 15 minutes for stable)		
Repeats initial assessment and documents findings		
Records ALL treatments with times and patient response(s) in treatment section		
Documents field impression		
Documents transport to specific facility and transfer of care WITH VERBAL REPORT		
Uses correct grammar, abbreviations, spelling, and terminology		
Writes legibly		
Thoroughly documents refusals, denials of transport, and call cancellations		
Documents patient GCS of 15 PRIOR to signing refusal		
Documents advice given to refusal patient, including "call 9-1-1 for further problems"		
Properly corrects errors and omissions		
Writes cautiously, avoids jargon, opinions, inferences, or any derogatory/libelous remarks		
Signs run report		
Uses EMS supplement form if needed		
Student exhibits competence with skill		

Any items in the Not Done column should be evaluated with student. Check marks in this column do not necessarily mean student was unsuccessful as all lines are not completed on all patients. Evaluation of each PCR should be based on the scenario given.

Student must be able to write an EMS report with consistency and accuracy.

☐ Successful   ☐ Unsuccessful   Examiner Initials: _____

©2006 Prentice-Hall Inc.

Overall Scenario Management (EMT Trauma—Chest Trauma)

Student: _____   Examiner: _____

Date: _____   Scenario: _____

NOTE: This skill sheet is to be done after the student completes a scenario as the TEAM LEADER. It is to let the student know if he or she is beginning to "put it all together" and use critical thinking skills to manage an EMS call. PLEASE notice that it is graded on a different basis than the basic lab skill sheet.

	Done ✓	Needs to Improve
SCENE MANAGEMENT		
Recognized hazards and controlled scene—safety, crowd, and patient issues		
Recognized hazards, but did not control the scene		
Unsuccessfully attempted to manage the scene	*	
Did not evaluate the scene and took no control of the scene	*	
PATIENT ASSESSMENT		
Performed a timely, organized complete patient assessment		
Performed complete initial, focused, and ongoing assessments, but in a disorganized manner		
Performed an incomplete assessment	*	
Did not perform an initial assessment	*	
PATIENT MANAGEMENT		
Evaluated assessment findings to manage all aspects of patient condition		
Managed the patient's presenting signs and symptoms without considering all of assessment		
Inadequately managed the patient	*	
Did not manage life-threatening conditions	*	
COMMUNICATION		
Communicated well with crew, patient, family, bystanders, and assisting agencies		
Communicated well with patient and crew		
Communicated with patient and crew, but poor communication skills	*	
Unable to communicate effectively	*	
REPORT AND TRANSFER OF CARE		
Identified correct destination for patient transport, gave accurate, brief report over radio, and provided full report at bedside demonstrating thorough understanding of patient condition and pathophysiological processes		
Identified correct destination and gave accurate radio and bedside report, but did not demonstrate understanding of patient condition and pathophysiological processes		
Identified correct destination, but provided inadequate radio and bedside report	*	
Identified inappropriate destination or provided no radio or bedside report	*	
Student exhibits competence with skill		

Any items that are marked with an * indicate the student needs to improve and a check mark should be placed in the right-hand column. A check mark in the right-hand column indicates that the student was unsuccessful and must attempt the skill again to assure competency. Examiners should use a different-color ink for the second attempt.

☐ Successful   ☐ Unsuccessful   Examiner Initials: _____

EMT Patient Assessment: Trauma—*Extremity Trauma*

Student: _____   Examiner: _____

Date: _____

	Done ✓	Not Done
Assesses scene safety and utilizes appropriate PPE		*
OVERALL SCENE EVALUATION		
Trauma—assesses mechanism of injury/if medical component determines nature of illness		*
Determines the number of patients, location, obstacles, and requests any additional resources as needed		
Verbalizes general impression of the patient as approaches		*
Stabilizes C-spine/spinal motion restriction (SMR) of spine		*
INITIAL ASSESSMENT/RESUSCITATION		
Determines responsiveness/level of consciousness/AVPU		*
Opens airway with appropriate technique and assesses airway/ventilation		*
Manages airway/ventilation and applies appropriate oxygen therapy in less than 3 minutes		*
Assesses circulation: radial/carotid pulse, skin color, temperature, condition, and turgor		*
Controls any major bleeding		*
Makes rapid transport decision		*
Obtains BGL, GCS, and complete vital signs		
RAPID TRAUMA ASSESSMENT (If patient is Trauma Alert or Load and Go)		
Assesses abdomen		
Rapidly palpates each extremity, assessing for obvious injuries and distal PMS		
Provides spinal motion restriction (SMR) on long backboard (LBB), checking posterior torso and legs		
Secures head LAST		
Loads patient/initiates transport (to appropriate LZ, to meet ALS, or to appropriate facility) in less than 10 minutes		
Reassesses ABCs and interventions		
FOCUSED HISTORY AND PHYSICAL ASSESSMENT		
Reassesses interventions and further assesses injuries found		
Obtains vital signs and GCS (Glasgow Coma Score)		
Obtains SAMPLE history		
Inspects and palpates head, facial, and neck regions		
Inspects, palpates, and auscultates chest/thorax		
Inspects and palpates abdomen and pelvis		
Inspects and palpates upper and lower extremities, checking distal PMS		
Inspects and palpates posterior torso		
Manages all injuries/wounds appropriately—SPLINTS—immobilizes joint above and below fracture site		*
Rechecks distal PMS after splint applied		*
Repeats initial assessment		*
Repeats vital signs and evaluates trends		*
Evaluates response to treatments		*
Performs ongoing assessment		
Gives radio report to receiving facility		
Turns over patient care with verbal report		*
Student exhibits competence with skill		

Any items in the Not Done column that are marked with an * are mandatory for the student to complete. A check mark in the Not Done column of an item with an * indicates that the student was unsuccessful and must attempt the skill again to assure competency. Examiners should use a different-color ink for the second attempt.

☐ Successful   ☐ Unsuccessful   Examiner Initials: _____

©2006 Prentice-Hall Inc.

Radio Report (EMT Trauma—Extremity Trauma)

Student: _____   **Examiner:** _____

Date: _____

	Done ✓	Not Done
Requests and checks for open channel before speaking		
Presses transmit button 1 second before speaking		
Holds microphone 2–3 in. from mouth		
Speaks slowly and clearly		*
Speaks in a normal voice		
Briefly transmits: Agency, unit designation, identification/name		*
Briefly transmits: Patient's age, sex, weight		*
Briefly transmits: Scene description/mechanism of injury or medical problem		*
Briefly transmits: Chief complaint with brief history of *present* illness		*
Briefly transmits: Associated symptoms (unless able to be deferred to bedside report)		
Briefly transmits: Past medical history (usually deferred to bedside report)		
Briefly transmits: Vital signs		*
Briefly transmits: Level of consciousness/GCS on trauma		*
Briefly transmits: General appearance, distress, cardiac rhythm, blood glucose, and other pertinent findings unable to be deferred to bedside report		
Briefly transmits: Interventions by EMS AND response(s)		*
ETA (the more critical the patient, the earlier you need to notify the receiving facility)		
Does not waste airtime		
Protects privacy of patient		*
Echoes dispatch information and any physician orders		*
Writes down dispatch information or physician orders		
Confirms with facility that message is received		
Demonstrates/verbalizes ability to troubleshoot basic equipment malfunction		
Student exhibits competence with skill		

Any items in the Not Done column that are marked with an * are mandatory for the student to complete. A check mark in the Not Done column of an item with an * indicates that the student was unsuccessful and must attempt the skill again to assure competency. Examiners should use a different-color ink for the second attempt.

☐ Successful   ☐ Unsuccessful   Examiner Initials: _____

©2006 Prentice-Hall Inc.

Documentation Skills: Patient Care Report (PCR)
(EMT Trauma—Extremity Trauma)

Student: _____   Examiner: _____

Date: _____

	Done ✓	Not Done
Records all pertinent dispatch/scene data, using a consistent format		
Completely identifies all additional resources and personnel		
Documents chief complaint, signs/symptoms, position found, age, sex, and weight		
Identifies and records all pertinent, reportable clinical data for each patient		
Documents SAMPLE and OPQRST if applicable		
Records all pertinent negatives		
Records all pertinent denials		
Records accurate, consistent times and patient information		
Includes relevant oral statements of witnesses, bystanders, and patient in "quotes" when appropriate		
Documents initial assessment findings: airway, breathing, and circulation		
Documents any interventions in initial assessment with patient response		
Documents level of consciousness, GCS (if trauma), and VS		
Documents rapid trauma assessment if applicable		
Documents any interventions in rapid trauma assessment with patient response		
Documents focused history and physical assessment		
Documents any interventions in focused assessment with patient response		
Documents repeat VS (every 5 minutes for critical; every 15 minutes for stable)		
Repeats initial assessment and documents findings		
Records ALL treatments with times and patient response(s) in treatment section		
Documents field impression		
Documents transport to specific facility and transfer of care WITH VERBAL REPORT		
Uses correct grammar, abbreviations, spelling, and terminology		
Writes legibly		
Thoroughly documents refusals, denials of transport, and call cancellations		
Documents patient GCS of 15 PRIOR to signing refusal		
Documents advice given to refusal patient, including "call 9-1-1 for further problems"		
Properly corrects errors and omissions		
Writes cautiously, avoids jargon, opinions, inferences, or any derogatory/libelous remarks		
Signs run report		
Uses EMS supplement form if needed		
Student exhibits competence with skill		

Any items in the Not Done column should be evaluated with student. Check marks in this column do not necessarily mean student was unsuccessful as all lines are not completed on all patients. Evaluation of each PCR should be based on the scenario given.

Student must be able to write an EMS report with consistency and accuracy.

☐ Successful   ☐ Unsuccessful   Examiner Initials: _____

©2006 Prentice-Hall Inc.

Overall Scenario Management (EMT Trauma—Extremity Trauma)

Student: _____   Examiner: _____

Date: _____   Scenario: _____

NOTE: This skill sheet is to be done after the student completes a scenario as the TEAM LEADER. It is to let the student know if he or she is beginning to "put it all together" and use critical thinking skills to manage an EMS call. PLEASE notice that it is graded on a different basis than the basic lab skill sheet.

	Done ✓	Needs to Improve
SCENE MANAGEMENT		
Recognized hazards and controlled scene—safety, crowd, and patient issues		
Recognized hazards, but did not control the scene		
Unsuccessfully attempted to manage the scene	*	
Did not evaluate the scene and took no control of the scene	*	
PATIENT ASSESSMENT		
Performed a timely, organized complete patient assessment		
Performed complete initial, focused, and ongoing assessments, but in a disorganized manner		
Performed an incomplete assessment	*	
Did not perform an initial assessment	*	
PATIENT MANAGEMENT		
Evaluated assessment findings to manage all aspects of patient condition		
Managed the patient's presenting signs and symptoms without considering all of assessment		
Inadequately managed the patient	*	
Did not manage life-threatening conditions	*	
COMMUNICATION		
Communicated well with crew, patient, family, bystanders, and assisting agencies		
Communicated well with patient and crew		
Communicated with patient and crew, but poor communication skills	*	
Unable to communicate effectively	*	
REPORT AND TRANSFER OF CARE		
Identified correct destination for patient transport, gave accurate, brief report over radio, and provided full report at bedside demonstrating thorough understanding of patient condition and pathophysiological processes		
Identified correct destination and gave accurate radio and bedside report, but did not demonstrate understanding of patient condition and pathophysiological processes		
Identified correct destination, but provided inadequate radio and bedside report	*	
Identified inappropriate destination or provided no radio or bedside report	*	
Student exhibits competence with skill		

Any items that are marked with an * indicate the student needs to improve and a check mark should be placed in the right-hand column. A check mark in the right-hand column indicates that the student was unsuccessful and must attempt the skill again to assure competency. Examiners should use a different-color ink for the second attempt.

☐ Successful   ☐ Unsuccessful   Examiner Initials: _____

©2006 Prentice-Hall Inc.

EMT Patient Assessment: Trauma—*Fractured Femur*

Student: _____   **Examiner:** _____

Date: _____

	Done ✓	Not Done
Assesses scene safety and utilizes appropriate PPE		*
OVERALL SCENE EVALUATION		
Trauma—assesses mechanism of injury/if medical component determines nature of illness		*
Determines the number of patients, location, obstacles, and requests any additional resources as needed		
Verbalizes general impression of the patient as approaches		*
Stabilizes C-spine/spinal motion restriction (SMR) of spine		*
INITIAL ASSESSMENT/RESUSCITATION		
Determines responsiveness/level of consciousness/AVPU		*
Opens airway with appropriate technique and assesses airway/ventilation		*
Manages airway/ventilation and applies appropriate oxygen therapy in less than 3 minutes		*
Assesses circulation: radial/carotid pulse, skin color, temperature, condition, and turgor		*
Controls any major bleeding, manually stabilizes fracture site		*
Makes rapid transport decision		*
Obtains BGL, GCS, and complete vital signs		
RAPID TRAUMA ASSESSMENT (If patient is Trauma Alert or Load and Go)		
Assesses abdomen		
Rapidly palpates each extremity, assessing for obvious injuries and distal PMS		
Provides spinal motion restriction (SMR) on long backboard (LBB), checking posterior torso and legs		
Secures head LAST		
Loads patient/initiates transport (to appropriate LZ, to meet ALS, or to appropriate facility) in less than 10 minutes		
Reassesses ABCs and interventions		
FOCUSED HISTORY AND PHYSICAL ASSESSMENT		
Reassesses interventions and further assesses injuries found		
Obtains vital signs and GCS (Glasgow Coma Score)		
Obtains SAMPLE history		
Inspects and palpates head, facial, and neck regions		
Inspects, palpates, and auscultates chest/thorax		
Inspects and palpates abdomen and pelvis		
Inspects and palpates upper and lower extremities, checking distal PMS		
Inspects and palpates posterior torso		
Manages all injuries/wounds appropriately—manually immobilizes or uses traction splint		
Reassesses distal PMS after immobilization or splinting		*
Repeats initial assessment		*
Repeats vital signs and evaluates trends		*
Evaluates response to treatments		*
Performs ongoing assessment		
Gives radio report to receiving facility		
Turns over patient care with verbal report		*
Student exhibits competence with skill		

Any items in the Not Done column that are marked with an * are mandatory for the student to complete. A check mark in the Not Done column of an item with an * indicates that the student was unsuccessful and must attempt the skill again to assure competency. Examiners should use a different-color ink for the second attempt.

☐ Successful   ☐ Unsuccessful   Examiner Initials: _____

©2006 Prentice-Hall Inc.

Radio Report (EMT Trauma—Fractured Femur)

Student: _____   **Examiner:** _____

Date: _____

	Done ✓	Not Done
Requests and checks for open channel before speaking		
Presses transmit button 1 second before speaking		
Holds microphone 2–3 in. from mouth		
Speaks slowly and clearly		*
Speaks in a normal voice		
Briefly transmits: Agency, unit designation, identification/name		*
Briefly transmits: Patient's age, sex, weight		*
Briefly transmits: Scene description/mechanism of injury or medical problem		*
Briefly transmits: Chief complaint with brief history of *present* illness		*
Briefly transmits: Associated symptoms (unless able to be deferred to bedside report)		
Briefly transmits: Past medical history (usually deferred to bedside report)		
Briefly transmits: Vital signs		*
Briefly transmits: Level of consciousness/GCS on trauma		*
Briefly transmits: General appearance, distress, cardiac rhythm, blood glucose, and other pertinent findings unable to be deferred to bedside report		
Briefly transmits: Interventions by EMS AND response(s)		*
ETA (the more critical the patient, the earlier you need to notify the receiving facility)		
Does not waste airtime		
Protects privacy of patient		*
Echoes dispatch information and any physician orders		*
Writes down dispatch information or physician orders		
Confirms with facility that message is received		
Demonstrates/verbalizes ability to troubleshoot basic equipment malfunction		
Student exhibits competence with skill		

Any items in the Not Done column that are marked with an * are mandatory for the student to complete. A check mark in the Not Done column of an item with an * indicates that the student was unsuccessful and must attempt the skill again to assure competency. Examiners should use a different-color ink for the second attempt.

☐ Successful   ☐ Unsuccessful   Examiner Initials: _____

©2006 Prentice-Hall Inc.

Documentation Skills: Patient Care Report (PCR)
(EMT Trauma—Fractured Femur)

Student: _____   Examiner: _____

Date: _____

	Done ✓	Not Done
Records all pertinent dispatch/scene data, using a consistent format		
Completely identifies all additional resources and personnel		
Documents chief complaint, signs/symptoms, position found, age, sex, and weight		
Identifies and records all pertinent, reportable clinical data for each patient		
Documents SAMPLE and OPQRST if applicable		
Records all pertinent negatives		
Records all pertinent denials		
Records accurate, consistent times and patient information		
Includes relevant oral statements of witnesses, bystanders, and patient in "quotes" when appropriate		
Documents initial assessment findings: airway, breathing, and circulation		
Documents any interventions in initial assessment with patient response		
Documents level of consciousness, GCS (if trauma), and VS		
Documents rapid trauma assessment if applicable		
Documents any interventions in rapid trauma assessment with patient response		
Documents focused history and physical assessment		
Documents any interventions in focused assessment with patient response		
Documents repeat VS (every 5 minutes for critical; every 15 minutes for stable)		
Repeats initial assessment and documents findings		
Records ALL treatments with times and patient response(s) in treatment section		
Documents field impression		
Documents transport to specific facility and transfer of care WITH VERBAL REPORT		
Uses correct grammar, abbreviations, spelling, and terminology		
Writes legibly		
Thoroughly documents refusals, denials of transport, and call cancellations		
Documents patient GCS of 15 PRIOR to signing refusal		
Documents advice given to refusal patient, including "call 9-1-1 for further problems"		
Properly corrects errors and omissions		
Writes cautiously, avoids jargon, opinions, inferences, or any derogatory/libelous remarks		
Signs run report		
Uses EMS supplement form if needed		
Student exhibits competence with skill		

Any items in the Not Done column should be evaluated with student. Check marks in this column do not necessarily mean student was unsuccessful as all lines are not completed on all patients. Evaluation of each PCR should be based on the scenario given.

Student must be able to write an EMS report with consistency and accuracy.

☐ Successful   ☐ Unsuccessful   Examiner Initials: _____

©2006 Prentice-Hall Inc.

Overall Scenario Management (EMT Trauma—Fractured Femur)

Student: _____   Examiner: _____

Date: _____   Scenario: _____

NOTE: This skill sheet is to be done after the student completes a scenario as the TEAM LEADER. It is to let the student know if he or she is beginning to "put it all together" and use critical thinking skills to manage an EMS call. PLEASE notice that it is graded on a different basis than the basic lab skill sheet.

	Done ✓	Needs to Improve
SCENE MANAGEMENT		
Recognized hazards and controlled scene—safety, crowd, and patient issues		
Recognized hazards, but did not control the scene		
Unsuccessfully attempted to manage the scene	*	
Did not evaluate the scene and took no control of the scene	*	
PATIENT ASSESSMENT		
Performed a timely, organized complete patient assessment		
Performed complete initial, focused, and ongoing assessments, but in a disorganized manner		
Performed an incomplete assessment	*	
Did not perform an initial assessment	*	
PATIENT MANAGEMENT		
Evaluated assessment findings to manage all aspects of patient condition		
Managed the patient's presenting signs and symptoms without considering all of assessment		
Inadequately managed the patient	*	
Did not manage life-threatening conditions	*	
COMMUNICATION		
Communicated well with crew, patient, family, bystanders, and assisting agencies		
Communicated well with patient and crew		
Communicated with patient and crew, but poor communication skills	*	
Unable to communicate effectively	*	
REPORT AND TRANSFER OF CARE		
Identified correct destination for patient transport, gave accurate, brief report over radio, and provided full report at bedside demonstrating thorough understanding of patient condition and pathophysiological processes		
Identified correct destination and gave accurate radio and bedside report, but did not demonstrate understanding of patient condition and pathophysiological processes		
Identified correct destination, but provided inadequate radio and bedside report	*	
Identified inappropriate destination or provided no radio or bedside report	*	
Student exhibits competence with skill		

Any items that are marked with an * indicate the student needs to improve and a check mark should be placed in the right-hand column. A check mark in the right-hand column indicates that the student was unsuccessful and must attempt the skill again to assure competency. Examiners should use a different-color ink for the second attempt.

☐ Successful   ☐ Unsuccessful   Examiner Initials: _____

EMT Patient Assessment: Trauma—*Head Injury*

Student: _____   **Examiner:** _____

Date: _____

	Done ✓	Not Done
Assesses scene safety and utilizes appropriate PPE		*
OVERALL SCENE EVALUATION		
Trauma—assesses mechanism of injury/if medical component determines nature of illness		*
Determines the number of patients, location, obstacles, and requests any additional resources as needed		
Verbalizes general impression of the patient as approaches		*
Stabilizes C-spine/spinal motion restriction (SMR) of spine		*
INITIAL ASSESSMENT/RESUSCITATION		
Determines responsiveness/level of consciousness/AVPU		*
Opens airway with appropriate technique and assesses airway/ventilation		*
Manages airway/ventilation and applies appropriate oxygen therapy in less than 3 minutes		*
Assesses circulation: radial/carotid pulse, skin color, temperature, condition, and turgor		*
Controls any major bleeding		*
Makes rapid transport decision		*
Obtains BGL, GCS, and complete vital signs		
RAPID TRAUMA ASSESSMENT (If patient is Trauma Alert or Load and Go)		
Assesses abdomen		
Rapidly palpates each extremity, assessing for obvious injuries and distal PMS		
Provides spinal motion restriction (SMR) on long backboard (LBB), checking posterior torso and legs		
Secures head LAST		
Loads patient/initiates transport (to appropriate LZ, to meet ALS, or to appropriate facility) in less than 10 minutes		
Reassesses ABCs and interventions		
FOCUSED HISTORY AND PHYSICAL ASSESSMENT		
Reassesses interventions and further assesses injuries found		
Obtains vital signs and GCS (Glasgow Coma Score)		
Obtains SAMPLE history		
Inspects and palpates head, facial, and neck regions		
Inspects, palpates, and auscultates chest/thorax		
Inspects and palpates abdomen and pelvis		
Inspects and palpates upper and lower extremities, checking distal PMS		
Inspects and palpates posterior torso		
Manages all injuries/wounds appropriately		
Repeats initial assessment		*
Repeats vital signs and evaluates trends		*
Evaluates response to treatments		*
Performs ongoing assessment		
Gives radio report to receiving facility		
Turns over patient care with verbal report		*
Student exhibits competence with skill		

Any items in the Not Done column that are marked with an * are mandatory for the student to complete. A check mark in the Not Done column of an item with an * indicates that the student was unsuccessful and must attempt the skill again to assure competency. Examiners should use a different-color ink for the second attempt.

☐ Successful   ☐ Unsuccessful   Examiner Initials: _____

©2006 Prentice-Hall Inc.

Radio Report (EMT Trauma—Head Injury)

Student: _____   **Examiner:** _____

Date: _____

	Done ✓	Not Done
Requests and checks for open channel before speaking		
Presses transmit button 1 second before speaking		
Holds microphone 2–3 in. from mouth		
Speaks slowly and clearly		*
Speaks in a normal voice		
Briefly transmits: Agency, unit designation, identification/name		*
Briefly transmits: Patient's age, sex, weight		*
Briefly transmits: Scene description/mechanism of injury or medical problem		*
Briefly transmits: Chief complaint with brief history of *present* illness		*
Briefly transmits: Associated symptoms (unless able to be deferred to bedside report)		
Briefly transmits: Past medical history (usually deferred to bedside report)		
Briefly transmits: Vital signs		*
Briefly transmits: Level of consciousness/GCS on trauma		*
Briefly transmits: General appearance, distress, cardiac rhythm, blood glucose, and other pertinent findings unable to be deferred to bedside report		
Briefly transmits: Interventions by EMS AND response(s)		*
ETA (the more critical the patient, the earlier you need to notify the receiving facility)		
Does not waste airtime		
Protects privacy of patient		*
Echoes dispatch information and any physician orders		*
Writes down dispatch information or physician orders		
Confirms with facility that message is received		
Demonstrates/verbalizes ability to troubleshoot basic equipment malfunction		
Student exhibits competence with skill		

Any items in the Not Done column that are marked with an * are mandatory for the student to complete. A check mark in the Not Done column of an item with an * indicates that the student was unsuccessful and must attempt the skill again to assure competency. Examiners should use a different-color ink for the second attempt.

☐ Successful   ☐ Unsuccessful   Examiner Initials: _____

©2006 Prentice-Hall Inc.

Documentation Skills: Patient Care Report (PCR)
(EMT Trauma—Head Injury)

Student: _____   **Examiner:** _____

Date: _____

	Done ✓	Not Done
Records all pertinent dispatch/scene data, using a consistent format		
Completely identifies all additional resources and personnel		
Documents chief complaint, signs/symptoms, position found, age, sex, and weight		
Identifies and records all pertinent, reportable clinical data for each patient		
Documents SAMPLE and OPQRST if applicable		
Records all pertinent negatives		
Records all pertinent denials		
Records accurate, consistent times and patient information		
Includes relevant oral statements of witnesses, bystanders, and patient in "quotes" when appropriate		
Documents initial assessment findings: airway, breathing, and circulation		
Documents any interventions in initial assessment with patient response		
Documents level of consciousness, GCS (if trauma), and VS		
Documents rapid trauma assessment if applicable		
Documents any interventions in rapid trauma assessment with patient response		
Documents focused history and physical assessment		
Documents any interventions in focused assessment with patient response		
Documents repeat VS (every 5 minutes for critical; every 15 minutes for stable)		
Repeats initial assessment and documents findings		
Records ALL treatments with times and patient response(s) in treatment section		
Documents field impression		
Documents transport to specific facility and transfer of care WITH VERBAL REPORT		
Uses correct grammar, abbreviations, spelling, and terminology		
Writes legibly		
Thoroughly documents refusals, denials of transport, and call cancellations		
Documents patient GCS of 15 PRIOR to signing refusal		
Documents advice given to refusal patient, including "call 9-1-1 for further problems"		
Properly corrects errors and omissions		
Writes cautiously, avoids jargon, opinions, inferences, or any derogatory/libelous remarks		
Signs run report		
Uses EMS supplement form if needed		
Student exhibits competence with skill		

Any items in the Not Done column should be evaluated with student. Check marks in this column do not necessarily mean student was unsuccessful as all lines are not completed on all patients. Evaluation of each PCR should be based on the scenario given.

Student must be able to write an EMS report with consistency and accuracy.

☐ Successful   ☐ Unsuccessful   Examiner Initials: _____

©2006 Prentice-Hall Inc.

Overall Scenario Management (EMT Trauma—Head Injury)

Student: _____   **Examiner:** _____

Date: _____   **Scenario:** _____

NOTE: This skill sheet is to be done after the student completes a scenario as the **TEAM LEADER**. It is to let the student know if he or she is beginning to "put it all together" and use critical thinking skills to manage an EMS call. PLEASE notice that it is graded on a different basis than the basic lab skill sheet.

	Done ✓	Needs to Improve
SCENE MANAGEMENT		
Recognized hazards and controlled scene—safety, crowd, and patient issues		
Recognized hazards, but did not control the scene		
Unsuccessfully attempted to manage the scene	*	
Did not evaluate the scene and took no control of the scene	*	
PATIENT ASSESSMENT		
Performed a timely, organized complete patient assessment		
Performed complete initial, focused, and ongoing assessments, but in a disorganized manner		
Performed an incomplete assessment	*	
Did not perform an initial assessment	*	
PATIENT MANAGEMENT		
Evaluated assessment findings to manage all aspects of patient condition		
Managed the patient's presenting signs and symptoms without considering all of assessment		
Inadequately managed the patient	*	
Did not manage life-threatening conditions	*	
COMMUNICATION		
Communicated well with crew, patient, family, bystanders, and assisting agencies		
Communicated well with patient and crew		
Communicated with patient and crew, but poor communication skills	*	
Unable to communicate effectively	*	
REPORT AND TRANSFER OF CARE		
Identified correct destination for patient transport, gave accurate, brief report over radio, and provided full report at bedside demonstrating thorough understanding of patient condition and pathophysiological processes		
Identified correct destination and gave accurate radio and bedside report, but did not demonstrate understanding of patient condition and pathophysiological processes		
Identified correct destination, but provided inadequate radio and bedside report	*	
Identified inappropriate destination or provided no radio or bedside report	*	
Student exhibits competence with skill		

Any items that are marked with an * indicate the student needs to improve and a check mark should be placed in the right-hand column. A check mark in the right-hand column indicates that the student was unsuccessful and must attempt the skill again to assure competency. Examiners should use a different-color ink for the second attempt.

☐ Successful   ☐ Unsuccessful   Examiner Initials: _____

EMT Patient Assessment: Medical—*Pediatric*

Student: _____   Examiner: _____

Date: _____

	Done ✓	Not Done
Assesses scene safety and utilizes appropriate PPE		*
OVERALL SCENE EVALUATION		
Medical—determines nature of illness/if trauma involved determines MOI		*
Determines the number of patients, location, obstacles, and requests any additional resources as needed		
Verbalizes general impression of the patient as approaches		*
Considers stabilization/spinal motion restriction of spine if trauma involved		*
INITIAL ASSESSMENT		
Determines responsiveness/level of consciousness/AVPU		*
Opens airway with appropriate technique and assesses airway/ventilation		*
Manages airway/ventilation and applies appropriate oxygen therapy in less than 3 minutes		*
Assesses circulation: radial/carotid pulse, skin color, temperature, condition, and turgor		*
Controls any major bleeding		*
Makes rapid transport decision if indicated		
Obtains BGL, GCS, and complete vital signs		
FOCUSED HISTORY AND PHYSICAL EXAMINATION/RAPID ASSESSMENT		
Obtains SAMPLE history		
Obtains OPQRST for differential diagnosis		
Obtains associated symptoms, pertinent negatives/denials		
Evaluates decision to perform focused exam or completes rapid assessment		*
Vital signs including AVPU (and GCS if trauma)		*
Assesses cardiovascular system including heart sounds, peripheral edema, and peripheral perfusion		*
Assesses pulmonary system including reassessing airway, ventilation, breath sounds, pulse oximetry, chest wall excursion, accessory muscle use, or other signs of distress		*
Assesses neurological system including distal pulse, movement, and sensation		*
Assesses musculoskeletal and integumentary systems		
Assesses behavioral, psychological, and social aspects of patient and situation		
States field impression of patient—		*
Verbalizes treatment plan for patient and calls for appropriate intervention(s)		*
Reevaluates transport decision		
ONGOING ASSESSMENT		
Repeats initial assessment		*
Repeats vital signs and evaluates trends		*
Evaluates response to treatments		*
Repeats focused assessment regarding patient complaint or injuries		
Gives radio report to receiving facility		
Turns over patient care with verbal report		*
Student exhibits competence with skill		

Any items in the Not Done column that are marked with an * are mandatory for the student to complete. A check mark in the Not Done column of an item with an * indicates that the student was unsuccessful and must attempt the skill again to assure competency. Examiners should use a different-color ink for the second attempt.

☐ Successful   ☐ Unsuccessful   Examiner Initials: _____

©2006 Prentice-Hall Inc.

Radio Report (EMT Medical—Pediatric)

Student: _____   Examiner: _____

Date: _____

	Done ✓	Not Done
Requests and checks for open channel before speaking		
Presses transmit button 1 second before speaking		
Holds microphone 2–3 in. from mouth		
Speaks slowly and clearly		*
Speaks in a normal voice		
Briefly transmits: Agency, unit designation, identification/name		*
Briefly transmits: Patient's age, sex, weight		*
Briefly transmits: Scene description/mechanism of injury or medical problem		*
Briefly transmits: Chief complaint with brief history of *present* illness		*
Briefly transmits: Associated symptoms (unless able to be deferred to bedside report)		
Briefly transmits: Past medical history (usually deferred to bedside report)		
Briefly transmits: Vital signs		*
Briefly transmits: Level of consciousness/GCS on trauma		*
Briefly transmits: General appearance, distress, cardiac rhythm, blood glucose, and other pertinent findings unable to be deferred to bedside report		
Briefly transmits: Interventions by EMS AND response(s)		*
ETA (the more critical the patient, the earlier you need to notify the receiving facility)		
Does not waste airtime		
Protects privacy of patient		*
Echoes dispatch information and any physician orders		*
Writes down dispatch information or physician orders		
Confirms with facility that message is received		
Demonstrates/verbalizes ability to troubleshoot basic equipment malfunction		
Student exhibits competence with skill		

Any items in the Not Done column that are marked with an * are mandatory for the student to complete. A check mark in the Not Done column of an item with an * indicates that the student was unsuccessful and must attempt the skill again to assure competency. Examiners should use a different-color ink for the second attempt.

☐ Successful   ☐ Unsuccessful   Examiner Initials: _____

Documentation Skills: Patient Care Report (PCR)
(EMT Medical—Pediatric)

Student: _____   Examiner: _____

Date: _____

	Done ✓	Not Done
Records all pertinent dispatch/scene data, using a consistent format		
Completely identifies all additional resources and personnel		
Documents chief complaint, signs/symptoms, position found, age, sex, and weight		
Identifies and records all pertinent, reportable clinical data for each patient		
Documents SAMPLE and OPQRST if applicable		
Records all pertinent negatives		
Records all pertinent denials		
Records accurate, consistent times and patient information		
Includes relevant oral statements of witnesses, bystanders, and patient in "quotes" when appropriate		
Documents initial assessment findings: airway, breathing, and circulation		
Documents any interventions in initial assessment with patient response		
Documents level of consciousness, GCS (if trauma), and VS		
Documents rapid trauma assessment if applicable		
Documents any interventions in rapid trauma assessment with patient response		
Documents focused history and physical assessment		
Documents any interventions in focused assessment with patient response		
Documents repeat VS (every 5 minutes for critical; every 15 minutes for stable)		
Repeats initial assessment and documents findings		
Records ALL treatments with times and patient response(s) in treatment section		
Documents field impression		
Documents transport to specific facility and transfer of care WITH VERBAL REPORT		
Uses correct grammar, abbreviations, spelling, and terminology		
Writes legibly		
Thoroughly documents refusals, denials of transport, and call cancellations		
Documents patient GCS of 15 PRIOR to signing refusal		
Documents advice given to refusal patient, including "call 9-1-1 for further problems"		
Properly corrects errors and omissions		
Writes cautiously, avoids jargon, opinions, inferences, or any derogatory/libelous remarks		
Signs run report		
Uses EMS supplement form if needed		
Student exhibits competence with skill		

Any items in the Not Done column should be evaluated with student. Check marks in this column do not necessarily mean student was unsuccessful as all lines are not completed on all patients. Evaluation of each PCR should be based on the scenario given.

Student must be able to write an EMS report with consistency and accuracy.

☐ Successful   ☐ Unsuccessful   Examiner Initials: _____

©2006 Prentice-Hall Inc.

Overall Scenario Management (EMT Medical—Pediatric)

Student: _____   Examiner: _____

Date: _____   Scenario: _____

NOTE: This skill sheet is to be done after the student completes a scenario as the TEAM LEADER. It is to let the student know if he or she is beginning to "put it all together" and use critical thinking skills to manage an EMS call. PLEASE notice that it is graded on a different basis than the basic lab skill sheet.

	Done ✓	Needs to Improve
SCENE MANAGEMENT		
Recognized hazards and controlled scene—safety, crowd, and patient issues		
Recognized hazards, but did not control the scene		
Unsuccessfully attempted to manage the scene	*	
Did not evaluate the scene and took no control of the scene	*	
PATIENT ASSESSMENT		
Performed a timely, organized complete patient assessment		
Performed complete initial, focused, and ongoing assessments, but in a disorganized manner		
Performed an incomplete assessment	*	
Did not perform an initial assessment	*	
PATIENT MANAGEMENT		
Evaluated assessment findings to manage all aspects of patient condition		
Managed the patient's presenting signs and symptoms without considering all of assessment		
Inadequately managed the patient	*	
Did not manage life-threatening conditions	*	
COMMUNICATION		
Communicated well with crew, patient, family, bystanders, and assisting agencies		
Communicated well with patient and crew		
Communicated with patient and crew, but poor communication skills	*	
Unable to communicate effectively	*	
REPORT AND TRANSFER OF CARE		
Identified correct destination for patient transport, gave accurate, brief report over radio, and provided full report at bedside demonstrating thorough understanding of patient condition and pathophysiological processes		
Identified correct destination and gave accurate radio and bedside report, but did not demonstrate understanding of patient condition and pathophysiological processes		
Identified correct destination, but provided inadequate radio and bedside report	*	
Identified inappropriate destination or provided no radio or bedside report	*	
Student exhibits competence with skill		

Any items that are marked with an * indicate the student needs to improve and a check mark should be placed in the right-hand column. A check mark in the right-hand column indicates that the student was unsuccessful and must attempt the skill again to assure competency. Examiners should use a different-color ink for the second attempt.

☐ Successful   ☐ Unsuccessful   Examiner Initials: _____

EMT Patient Assessment: Trauma—*Shock/Hemorrhage*

Student: _____   Examiner: _____

Date: _____

	Done ✓	Not Done
Assesses scene safety and utilizes appropriate PPE		*
OVERALL SCENE EVALUATION		
Trauma—assesses mechanism of injury/if medical component determines nature of illness		*
Determines the number of patients, location, obstacles, and requests any additional resources as needed		
Verbalizes general impression of the patient as approaches		*
Stabilizes C-spine/spinal motion restriction (SMR) of spine		*
INITIAL ASSESSMENT/RESUSCITATION		
Determines responsiveness/level of consciousness/AVPU		*
Opens airway with appropriate technique and assesses airway/ventilation		*
Manages airway/ventilation and applies appropriate oxygen therapy in less than 3 minutes		*
Assesses circulation: radial/carotid pulse, skin color, temperature, condition, and turgor		*
Controls any major bleeding		*
Makes rapid transport decision		*
Obtains BGL, GCS, and complete vital signs		
RAPID TRAUMA ASSESSMENT (If patient is Trauma Alert or Load and Go)		
Assesses abdomen		
Rapidly palpates each extremity, assessing for obvious injuries and distal PMS		
Provides spinal motion restriction (SMR) on long backboard (LBB), checking posterior torso and legs		
Secures head LAST		
Loads patient/initiates transport (to appropriate LZ, to meet ALS, or to appropriate facility) in less than 10 minutes		
Reassesses ABCs and interventions		
FOCUSED HISTORY AND PHYSICAL ASSESSMENT		
Reassesses interventions and further assesses injuries found		
Obtains vital signs and GCS (Glasgow Coma Score)		
Obtains SAMPLE history		
Inspects and palpates head, facial, and neck regions		
Inspects, palpates, and auscultates chest/thorax		
Inspects and palpates abdomen and pelvis		
Inspects and palpates upper and lower extremities, checking distal PMS		
Inspects and palpates posterior torso		
Manages all injuries/wounds appropriately--Trendelenberg, warmth, call for ALS		
Repeats initial assessment		*
Repeats vital signs and evaluates trends		*
Evaluates response to treatments		*
Performs ongoing assessment		
Gives radio report to receiving facility		
Turns over patient care with verbal report		*
Student exhibits competence with skill		

Any items in the Not Done column that are marked with an * are mandatory for the student to complete. A check mark in the Not Done column of an item with an * indicates that the student was unsuccessful and must attempt the skill again to assure competency. Examiners should use a different-color ink for the second attempt.

☐ Successful   ☐ Unsuccessful   Examiner Initials: _____

    ©2006 Prentice-Hall Inc.

Radio Report (EMT Trauma—Shock / Hemorrhage)

Student: _____   **Examiner:** _____

Date: _____

	Done ✓	Not Done
Requests and checks for open channel before speaking		
Presses transmit button 1 second before speaking		
Holds microphone 2–3 in. from mouth		
Speaks slowly and clearly		*
Speaks in a normal voice		
Briefly transmits: Agency, unit designation, identification/name		*
Briefly transmits: Patient's age, sex, weight		*
Briefly transmits: Scene description/mechanism of injury or medical problem		*
Briefly transmits: Chief complaint with brief history of *present* illness		*
Briefly transmits: Associated symptoms (unless able to be deferred to bedside report)		
Briefly transmits: Past medical history (usually deferred to bedside report)		
Briefly transmits: Vital signs		*
Briefly transmits: Level of consciousness/GCS on trauma		*
Briefly transmits: General appearance, distress, cardiac rhythm, blood glucose, and other pertinent findings unable to be deferred to bedside report		
Briefly transmits: Interventions by EMS AND response(s)		*
ETA (the more critical the patient, the earlier you need to notify the receiving facility)		
Does not waste airtime		
Protects privacy of patient		*
Echoes dispatch information and any physician orders		*
Writes down dispatch information or physician orders		
Confirms with facility that message is received		
Demonstrates/verbalizes ability to troubleshoot basic equipment malfunction		
Student exhibits competence with skill		

Any items in the Not Done column that are marked with an * are mandatory for the student to complete. A check mark in the Not Done column of an item with an * indicates that the student was unsuccessful and must attempt the skill again to assure competency. Examiners should use a different-color ink for the second attempt.

☐ Successful   ☐ Unsuccessful   Examiner Initials: _____

Documentation Skills: Patient Care Report (PCR)
(EMT Trauma—Shock/Hemorrhage)

Student: _____   **Examiner:** _____

Date: _____

	Done ✓	Not Done
Records all pertinent dispatch/scene data, using a consistent format		
Completely identifies all additional resources and personnel		
Documents chief complaint, signs/symptoms, position found, age, sex, and weight		
Identifies and records all pertinent, reportable clinical data for each patient		
Documents SAMPLE and OPQRST if applicable		
Records all pertinent negatives		
Records all pertinent denials		
Records accurate, consistent times and patient information		
Includes relevant oral statements of witnesses, bystanders, and patient in "quotes" when appropriate		
Documents initial assessment findings: airway, breathing, and circulation		
Documents any interventions in initial assessment with patient response		
Documents level of consciousness, GCS (if trauma), and VS		
Documents rapid trauma assessment if applicable		
Documents any interventions in rapid trauma assessment with patient response		
Documents focused history and physical assessment		
Documents any interventions in focused assessment with patient response		
Documents repeat VS (every 5 minutes for critical; every 15 minutes for stable)		
Repeats initial assessment and documents findings		
Records ALL treatments with times and patient response(s) in treatment section		
Documents field impression		
Documents transport to specific facility and transfer of care WITH VERBAL REPORT		
Uses correct grammar, abbreviations, spelling, and terminology		
Writes legibly		
Thoroughly documents refusals, denials of transport, and call cancellations		
Documents patient GCS of 15 PRIOR to signing refusal		
Documents advice given to refusal patient, including "call 9-1-1 for further problems"		
Properly corrects errors and omissions		
Writes cautiously, avoids jargon, opinions, inferences, or any derogatory/libelous remarks		
Signs run report		
Uses EMS supplement form if needed		
Student exhibits competence with skill		

Any items in the Not Done column should be evaluated with student. Check marks in this column do not necessarily mean student was unsuccessful as all lines are not completed on all patients. Evaluation of each PCR should be based on the scenario given.

Student must be able to write an EMS report with consistency and accuracy.

☐ Successful   ☐ Unsuccessful   Examiner Initials: _____

©2006 Prentice-Hall Inc.

Overall Scenario Management (EMT Trauma—Shock/Hemorrhage)

Student: _____   Examiner: _____

Date: _____   Scenario: _____

NOTE: This skill sheet is to be done after the student completes a scenario as the TEAM LEADER. It is to let the student know if he or she is beginning to "put it all together" and use critical thinking skills to manage an EMS call. PLEASE notice that it is graded on a different basis than the basic lab skill sheet.

	Done ✓	Needs to Improve
SCENE MANAGEMENT		
Recognized hazards and controlled scene—safety, crowd, and patient issues		
Recognized hazards, but did not control the scene		
Unsuccessfully attempted to manage the scene	*	
Did not evaluate the scene and took no control of the scene	*	
PATIENT ASSESSMENT		
Performed a timely, organized complete patient assessment		
Performed complete initial, focused, and ongoing assessments, but in a disorganized manner		
Performed an incomplete assessment	*	
Did not perform an initial assessment	*	
PATIENT MANAGEMENT		
Evaluated assessment findings to manage all aspects of patient condition		
Managed the patient's presenting signs and symptoms without considering all of assessment		
Inadequately managed the patient	*	
Did not manage life-threatening conditions	*	
COMMUNICATION		
Communicated well with crew, patient, family, bystanders, and assisting agencies		
Communicated well with patient and crew		
Communicated with patient and crew, but poor communication skills	*	
Unable to communicate effectively	*	
REPORT AND TRANSFER OF CARE		
Identified correct destination for patient transport, gave accurate, brief report over radio, and provided full report at bedside demonstrating thorough understanding of patient condition and pathophysiological processes		
Identified correct destination and gave accurate radio and bedside report, but did not demonstrate understanding of patient condition and pathophysiological processes		
Identified correct destination, but provided inadequate radio and bedside report	*	
Identified inappropriate destination or provided no radio or bedside report	*	
Student exhibits competence with skill		

Any items that are marked with an * indicate the student needs to improve and a check mark should be placed in the right-hand column. A check mark in the right-hand column indicates that the student was unsuccessful and must attempt the skill again to assure competency. Examiners should use a different-color ink for the second attempt.

☐ Successful   ☐ Unsuccessful   Examiner Initials: _____

©2006 Prentice-Hall Inc.

Part 4: Special Operations

Fabulous Factoids

Skill Sheets

Daily Discussions and Pertinent Points

FABULOUS FACTOIDS—SPECIAL OPERATIONS

When arriving at a fire scene, try to find out what is burning. In the Cleveland Clinic fire of 1929, 123 deaths were linked to poisoning from oxides of nitrogen released by the burning of nitrocellulose (X-ray films).

Seventy-five percent of all murder victims knew their killer.

Twenty-five percent of them were killed by a relative.

Thomas Edison was afraid of the dark.

Floods cause more death and destruction in the United States than does any other natural disaster.

It takes approximately 720 peanuts to make 1 pound of peanut butter.

The average lightning bolt is 1 inch in diameter.

A strong bolt of lightning can contain as much as 100 million volts of electricity.

Seven times as many men as women are killed by lightning in the United States.

Like an astute detective, the paramedic must use all his or her senses (even taste—for scene safety only) to gather information from the scene.

Julius Caesar was an epileptic.

Twelve thousand Americans are injured by fireworks every year.

©2006 Prentice-Hall Inc.

SKILL SHEETS

Rescue: Phases of a Rescue Operation

Student: _____   **Examiner:** _____

Date: _____

	Done ✓	Not Done
VERBALIZES PHASE I: ARRIVAL AND SIZE-UP		
Identifies TYPE of rescue involved		*
Utilizes appropriate PPE		*
Determines number of patients		*
Calls for appropriate additional resources		*
Implements IMS/ICS as needed		*
VERBALIZES PHASE II: HAZARD CONTROL		
Determines nature of hazards		*
Initiates containment of incident if needed		*
VERBALIZES PHASE III: PATIENT ACCESS		
Formulates access plan		
Briefs and deploys personnel		
Stabilizes patient's location		
VERBALIZES PHASE IV: MEDICAL TREATMENT		
Initiates patient assessment and care		*
Anticipates changing patient condition during remaining phases		*
Calls for any additional resources/equipment that may be needed		*
VERBALIZES PHASE V: DISENTANGLEMENT		
Maintains patient care during disentanglement		*
Continuously evaluates for safety risk to self or patient		*
If increased risk, immediately stops operation and reassesses plan for options		*
Prevents additional injury		*
VERBALIZES PHASE VI: PATIENT PACKAGING		
Maintains patient care during packaging		*
Appropriately packages patient for removal and transport		
Prevents additional injury		
Reassesses plan for transport		
VERBALIZES PHASE VII: REMOVAL AND TRANSPORT		
Maintains patient care during removal and transport		*
Reassesses transport decision based on patient's condition		
Turns over patient care to air transport or hospital with full report		*
Restocks unit and documents incident correctly		
Critiques call with personnel involved with incident		
Student exhibits competence with skill		

This is a knowledge lab. Student attendance is required for successful completion.

☐ Successful   ☐ Unsuccessful   Examiner Initials: _____

Rescue: Highway Operations Strategies

Student: _____   Examiner: _____

Date: _____

	Done ✓	Not Done
INITIAL SCENE SIZE-UP		
Establishes command		*
Calls for additional resources		*
Locates and triages all patients		*
HAZARD CONTROL		
Checks for electrical wires/hazardous materials		*
Sets out flares		
Parks vehicle between traffic and patient care		*
Directs incoming units in a manner that permits optimal traffic flow, but provides protection for rescuers		
Verbalizes awareness of fuel/fire dangers		*
Checks for energy-absorbing bumpers/air bags		
Checks for unstable vehicles		*
ASSESSES DEGREE OF ENTRAPMENT AND IDENTIFIES MOST EFFICIENT MEANS OF EXTRICATION		
Tries all doors		*
Checks for window/windshield access		
ESTABLISHES CIRCLE OF OPERATIONS		
Sets up inner circle for rescue		
Sets up outer circle for staging/LZ		
PERFORMS TREATMENT, PACKAGING, AND REMOVAL		
Performs appropriate treatment, packaging, and removal		
Student exhibits competence with skill		

This is a knowledge acquisition lab. Student participation is required for successful completion.

☐ Successful   ☐ Unsuccessful   Examiner Initials: _____

©2006 Prentice-Hall Inc.

Extrication: Determining Mechanism of Injury (MOI)

Student: _____   Examiner: _____

Date: _____

NOTE: Lead extrication lab instructor chooses several vehicles with different areas of damage (or shows pictures) and assigns each student or group of students a different "patient location" (driver, passenger behind driver, etc.). Student(s) must identify mechanism(s) of injury, types of forces exerted, and possible injuries of patient. Student(s) should write directly on this lab sheet.

	Done ✓	Not Done
Vehicle 1: Type of vehicle— Area(s) of damage— Patient position in vehicle— MOI/forces involved— Anticipated injuries—		
Vehicle 2: Type of vehicle— Area(s) of damage— Patient position in vehicle— MOI/forces involved— Anticipated injuries—		
Vehicle 3: Type of vehicle— Area(s) of damage— Patient position in vehicle— MOI/forces involved— Anticipated injuries—		
Student exhibits competence with skill		

This is a knowledge acquisition lab. Student participation is required for successful completion.

☐ Successful   ☐ Unsuccessful   Examiner Initials: _____

Extrication: Vehicle Stabilization

Student: _____   **Examiner:** _____

Date: _____

	Done ✓	Not Done
Assesses scene safety and utilizes appropriate PPE		*
Using cribbing, stabilizes a vehicle on:		
All four wheels		
Side		
Roof		
An embankment/incline		
Using ropes, stabilizes a vehicle on:		
All four wheels		
Side		
Roof		
An embankment/incline		
Using lifting devices (such as air bags), stabilizes a vehicle on:		
All four wheels		
Side		
Roof		
An embankment/incline		
Using spare tires, stabilizes a vehicle on:		
All four wheels		
Side		
Roof		
An embankment/incline		
Using chains, stabilizes a vehicle on:		
All four wheels		
Side		
Roof		
An embankment/incline		
Using hand winches, stabilizes a vehicle on:		
All four wheels		
Side		
Roof		
An embankment/incline		
Student exhibits competence with skill		

This is a knowledge acquisition lab. Student participation is required for successful completion.

☐ Successful   ☐ Unsuccessful   Examiner Initials: _____

©2006 Prentice-Hall Inc.

Extrication: Using Basic Hand Tools

Student: _____   Examiner: _____

Date: _____

	Done ✓	Not Done
Assesses scene safety and utilizes appropriate PPE		*
Using basic hand tools, gains patient access through a stuck door		
Using basic hand tools, gains patient access through tempered glass		
Using basic hand tools, gains patient access through safety glass		
Using basic hand tools, gains patient access through the trunk		
Using basic hand tools, gains patient access through the floor		
Using basic hand tools, removes the roof		
Using basic hand tools, demonstrates dash displacement/roll-up		
Using basic hand tools, demonstrates steering wheel and steering column displacement		
Using basic hand tools, gains access through the roof		
Student exhibits competence with skill		

This is a knowledge acquisition lab. Student participation is required for successful completion.

☐ Successful   ☐ Unsuccessful   Examiner Initials: _____

High-Angle Rescue: Stokes for Lift/Rough Terrain

Student: _____   **Examiner:** _____

Date: _____

	Done ✓	Not Done
Assesses scene safety and utilizes appropriate PPE		*
Provides spinal motion restriction (SMR) on long backboard (LBB)		*
For rough terrain, shields patient from dirt, dust, debris, falling objects, or low branches		*
Secures LBB to Stokes basket, then "laces" strapping across top of Stokes, securing patient and shielding material		*
Safely removes patient from area with 6–8 man carry		
Verbalizes that high-angle and low-angle rescues require advanced training to perform and skilled rescuers with specialized equipment		*
HIGH ANGLE		
If asked to assist, maintains SMR, explains rescue plan, and in reverse procedure of helmet removal, maintains manual C-spine and places helmet on patient		
Assists with application of safety harness and leg stirrups to patient, reassuring patient		
Secures patient to LBB, keeping straps of safety harness and leg stirrups available		
Secures LBB to Stokes basket		
Depending on anticipated removal and transport time, initiates IV therapy		
Places monitoring equipment (BP cuff, monitor, pulse ox, etc.) on patient		*
Thoroughly pads patient in Stokes, leaving equipment access, airway access, and access to patient for distal PMS checks		*
Places blanket(s), if needed, and shielding material over patient, leaving access to straps of safety harness and leg stirrups, medical equipment, and patient		
Introduces patient to special rescue team members if not done previously		
Special rescue team will tie litter line to patient harness, belay line to Stokes, and gravity "tip line" in case patient vomits and needs airway management		
Rechecks padding and "laces" patient into Stokes basket, preparing for removal		
Maintains communication with patient, reassures patient, and provides report to team		
Student exhibits competence with skill		

Any items in the Not Done column that are marked with an * are mandatory for the student to complete. A check mark in the Not Done column of an item with an * indicates that the student was unsuccessful and must attempt the skill again to assure competency. Examiners should use a different-color ink for the second attempt.

☐ Successful   ☐ Unsuccessful   Examiner Initials: _____

                    ©2006 Prentice-Hall Inc.

High-Angle Rescue: Vertical Lift without a Stokes

Student: _____   Examiner: _____

Date: _____

	Done ✓	Not Done *
Assesses scene safety and utilizes appropriate PPE		*
Calls for additional resources		*
Recognizes need for short distance vertical lift		*
Maintains C-spine SMR and applies helmet to patient, then C-collar		*
Maintains manual C-spine and secures chest to LBB, explaining rescue plan to patient		*
Applies leg straps or seat harness (padding wherever necessary) and secures to LBB to prevent patient slipping as LBB is lifted		
Straps torso and legs to LBB, then secures head		
Pads all voids well		*
Checks condition of all straps (or ropes) to be used for lift for signs of fraying		
Threads lift straps through top and sides of board for team at top to lift patient		
Applies straps through bottom of board for team members at feet to stabilize LBB during lift		
With assistance of team members at patient (ground) level to avoid dragging patient on ground, team members at top slowly begin lift		
When patient is perpendicular to ground (upright), ground level team members recheck all straps and padding—prior to lifting bottom of LBB into air		
When verified that patient is secured, ground team members take stabilizing straps, and lifting team slowly raises patient upward		
After lift accomplished, removes lift and stabilizing straps, leaving patient in SMR, and initiates transport		*
Continues patient care during transport		*
Student exhibits competence with skill		

Any items in the Not Done column that are marked with an * are mandatory for the student to complete. A check mark in the Not Done column of an item with an * indicates that the student was unsuccessful and must attempt the skill again to assure competency. Examiners should use a different-color ink for the second attempt.

☐ Successful   ☐ Unsuccessful   Examiner Initials: _____

©2006 Prentice-Hall Inc.

High-Angle Rescue: Litter-Carrying Techniques

Student: _____   Examiner: _____

Date: _____

NOTE: Instructor advises that patient must be evacuated over rough terrain using techniques of lift straps, passing over obstructions, and "leapfrogging."

	Done ✓	Not Done
Assesses scene safety and utilizes appropriate PPE		*
Packages patient in Stokes basket—pads WELL		*
Stretcher lift straps: "Laces" webbing straps through and over top rails on each side, making three loops (for three litter bearers on each side)		*
Each litter bearer faces head end of Stokes, ducks under his or her "loop," and places loop strap on OUTSIDE shoulder using hand next to Stokes (inside hand) to lift and steady Stokes		*
Litter bearers distribute lift straps to equalize weight—easier if bearers close in height		*
On command of predesignated person at head, bearers lift Stokes and begin removal		*
Passing patient over obstruction: If using lift straps, bearers must remove themselves from straps		
Two rescuers/bearers move forward/beyond obstruction (such as rock) and other four rescuers/bearers pass head of Stokes forward over obstacle/obstruction		
Two rescuers at head and two of rear rescuers balance Stokes on obstruction while other two rescuers at rear move around obstruction to head of Stokes		
With four rescuers at head, Stokes is eased across/over obstruction until patient's weight is able to be balanced by four rescuers at head		
Two rear rescuers now move forward past obstruction and removal can continue		
If obstruction too wide to safely pass Stokes forward, lift straps may be removed and utilized as a pulling strap for rescuers at head and a stabilizing strap for rescuers at rear		
Verbalizes that leapfrogging can be used for rapid removal situations with 12–18 available rescuers moving patient over flat, rough terrain		
Packages patient in Stokes and first team of six lifts Stokes for carry while other team or teams of six move forward to await pass-off		
Verbalizes that when lifting team reaches fresh team, Stokes is transferred and carried by new team while team just relieved moves forward, has time to rest, and awaits another pass-off		
Student exhibits competence with skill		

Any items in the Not Done column that are marked with an * are mandatory for the student to complete. A check mark in the Not Done column of an item with an * indicates that the student was unsuccessful and must attempt the skill again to assure competency. Examiners should use a different-color ink for the second attempt.

☐ Successful   ☐ Unsuccessful   Examiner Initials: _____

©2006 Prentice-Hall Inc.

High-Angle Rescue: Packaging for Aerial Evacuation

Student: _____   **Examiner:** _____

Date: _____

	Done ✓	Not Done
Assesses scene safety and utilizes appropriate PPE		*
Requests additional resources—advises Control/Dispatch that aerial evacuation necessary		*
Verbalizes awareness that cannot call for "helicopter" without advising of need for aerial rescue as all helicopters are not equipped for this specialized rescue technique		*
Packages patient in Stokes in same manner as for vertical lift and explains rescue plan		*
Upon arrival of helicopter, assists with securing aerial lift harness/apparatus to Stokes basket		
Gives report to helicopter rescuer and introduces to patient		*
Assists helicopter rescuer who will be accompanying patient during lift with harness, and checks all straps being used on Stokes and helicopter rescuer for fraying		
Assists with belay line attachment (to prevent twisting of Stokes and rescuer during lift)		
Student exhibits competence with skill		

Any items in the Not Done column that are marked with an * are mandatory for the student to complete. A check mark in the Not Done column of an item with an * indicates that the student was unsuccessful and must attempt the skill again to assure competency. Examiners should use a different-color ink for the second attempt.

☐ Successful   ☐ Unsuccessful   Examiner Initials: _____

Water Rescue: H-E-L-P/Self-Rescue

Student: _____   Examiner: _____

Date: _____

NOTE: At beginning of water rescue, examiner starts in shallow end of pool and verifies ALL participants able to swim!

	Done ✓	Not Done
Verbalizes H-E-L-P is Heat Escape Lessening Position		*
Verbalizes position can reduce heat loss up to 60%		
Performs "jellyfish" or fetal position in pool (face in water, curls and holds legs against body)—when needs breath, opens curl slightly and raises head		
Performs head-up tuck position in pool		
Examiner gently "pushes" student into deep end of pool to perform self-rescue techniques.		
Covers mouth and nose during entry		
Protects head and keeps face out of water if possible (if able to adjust balance, enters water with legs in "striding position")		
Verbalizes NOT attempting to stand if moving/swift water		
Removes boots/shoes and long pants		
Floats on back with head toward nearest shore/side of pool at 45° angle		
Continues to float, frequently raising head to get position or look for obstacles (in swift water float feet first with head up to watch for obstacles or eddies—possible point of exit)		
Verbalizes that if river curves, needs to try steering to inside of curve		
Student exhibits competence with skill		

This is a knowledge acquisition lab. Student attendance is required for successful completion.

☐ Successful   ☐ Unsuccessful   Examiner Initials: _____

©2006 Prentice-Hall Inc.

Water Rescue: Donning a Personal Flotation Device (PFD)

Student: _____   **Examiner:** _____

Date: _____

	Done ✓	Not Done
Selects appropriately sized PFD (chest pads must be able to reach across chest and be approximated with enough leeway in strap length to be able to adjust)		
Fastens leg straps and steps in, putting jacket portion on last, OR puts jacket portion on and reaches through legs to rear straps, pulls through legs, and fastens to front of PFD		
Adjusts chest straps to approximate chest pads, allow good respiratory excursion, and allow freedom of arm movement		
Adjusts leg straps to firmly (but comfortably) fit and securely maintain jacket position		
Readjusts chest straps (as jacket has moved down slightly with leg strap adjustments)		
Verbalizes that "water wings" and jackets or vests put on leaving leg straps unsecured are inadequate PFDs for rescue operations		*
Student exhibits competence with skill		

This is a knowledge acquisition lab. Student attendance is required for successful completion.

☐ Successful   ☐ Unsuccessful   Examiner Initials: _____

Water Rescue: Reach-Throw-Row-Go

Student: _____   Examiner: _____

Date: _____

	Done ✓	Not Done

Identifies water rescue incident
   Surface water
   Submerged
   Flat water
   Moving water
   Scene hazards complicating rescue
		*

Determines number of patients, type of rescue, and calls for additional resources		*
Utilizes appropriate PPE, INCLUDING personal flotation device (PFD)		*
Assures that ALL personnel on shore have on PFDs		*
Attempts to "talk in" victim/assists in victim self-rescue		*
Attempts to REACH victim with pole or long rescue device as team member(s) "anchor" rescuer to prevent loss of balance		*
If victim beyond reach, attempts to THROW flotation device with line or rescue buoy to victim, pulling victim in to shore (have team members "anchor" rescuer before pulling)		*
If victim unable to be pulled to shore due to swift water, distance, or injuries, calls for boat rescue to ROW out to victim		*
Verbalizes that water entry—GO—is a last resort		*
If rescue circumstances appropriate for GO—utilizes dual safety lines with minimum of two team members manning each line (ideally from opposite sides of water, if possible)		
Obtains PFD to apply to victim, and attaches PFD for victim to a shore line manned with two team members as anchors to pull victim to shore		
In swift water, enters upstream and angles in toward victim, moving with current		
Upon reaching victim, properly applies PFD to victim		
If situation permits, stays close to victim, providing any care possible—IF NO RISK TO RESCUER		
Team members on shore initiate care as soon as victim is pulled safely on shore		
Student exhibits competence with skill		

Any items that are marked with an * indicate the student needs to improve and a check mark should be placed in the right-hand column. A check mark in the right-hand column indicates that the student was unsuccessful and must attempt the skill again to assure competency. Examiners should use a different-color ink for the second attempt.

☐ Successful   ☐ Unsuccessful   Examiner Initials: _____

          ©2006 Prentice-Hall Inc.

Water Rescue: Throw-Bag/Rescue Buoy/Noodle

Student: _____   Examiner: _____

Date: _____

	Done ✓	Not Done
Attempts to use REACH rescue method first		*
Obtains water rescue throw-bag, inflates if needed, and checks line connection at bag end		*
Anchors throw-bag line to sturdy, stationary, immovable object on shore (or has two team members anchor—line will be shortened as team members must wrap line around waist)		
If moving water or victim, checks current direction		
Loosely coils line and underhand throws bag slightly up current and PAST victim		*
If victim unable to reach due to distance, adjusts length of line; if unable to reach due to throw, adjusts throw and repeats		
Verbalizes goal is to get throw-bag line to up-current side of victim		
Verbalizes that rescue buoy can be utilized in the same manner, but may also be utilized to assist rescuer as a flotation device if water entry necessary, especially through surf		
Verbalizes that in pool/flat-water rescue, the child toy "noodle" can be utilized as a reach device OR rescuer can swim to within "noodle" reach of victim (NOT close enough for victim to grab rescuer) and pass end of noodle to victim to use as flotation device		
Student exhibits competence with skill		

Any items in the Not Done column that are marked with an * are mandatory for the student to complete. A check mark in the Not Done column of an item with an * indicates that the student was unsuccessful and must attempt the skill again to assure competency. Examiners should use a different-color ink for the second attempt.

☐ Successful   ☐ Unsuccessful   Examiner Initials: _____

Water Rescue: In-Water Spinal Motion Restriction (SMR)

Student: _____   Examiner: _____

Date: _____

NOTE: Examiner should have students perform in-water SMR in SHALLOW end of pool first (where they can stand), then in the deep end. Have students rescue an unresponsive patient (face down in water).

	Done ✓	Not Done
Assures all rescue team members have on PFDs		*
Verbalizes knowledge that in-water SMR is done ONLY in flat water—in moving/swift water, patient needs to be removed to shore/calm water first, for rescuer/patient safety		*
Initial rescuer approaches patient from front, continually watching patient, for rescuer safety		*
Performs arm grab (reaches for both arms, which will be underwater, and moves them up to "splint" head) swivel with axial rotation to place patient on his or her back, face out of water		
Applies manual C-spine motion restriction with trauma jaw-thrust and maintains airway		*
Has second rescuer come in from side of patient and apply C-collar		
Maintaining airway and C-spine, patient can now be ventilated until LBB arrives		
In-water rescuers submerge LBB at an angle to "cut" through the water and allow LBB to "float" up under victim, controlling speed of ascent		
If rescuers able to stand, may secure victim to LBB at this time, if in deep water, maintains manual C-spine and rescue team swims patient on LBB in to shore/side of pool		
Directs securing patient to LBB (head LAST)		*
Has in-water rescuers remain in water to assist poolside/shoreline team in extrication		
Assures that patient is removed HEAD first to maintain airway and avoid axial compression of spine by patient's body weight		*
Assures that rescue team members present and safe at all times		*
Verbalizes that if packaging patient for extrication by boat, patient needs to be secured to LBB, if possible, and placed in Stokes basket for safe removal from water		
Student exhibits competence with skill		

Any items in the Not Done column that are marked with an * are mandatory for the student to complete. A check mark in the Not Done column of an item with an * indicates that the student was unsuccessful and must attempt the skill again to assure competency. Examiners should use a different-color ink for the second attempt.

☐ Successful   ☐ Unsuccessful   Examiner Initials: _____

Hazardous Materials: Research and Risk Determination

Student: _____   Examiner: _____

Date: _____

NOTE: Examiner will collect lab sheets and write down a different hazardous substance for each student. Give sheets back to students to research material and answer the following questions/write down the following information. Students will turn sheets back in and grading will be on a pass/fail basis.

Books that should be available to students are *North American Emergency Response Guidebook,* MSDS sheets, any other reference books preferred by instructor(s).

SUBSTANCE/MATERIAL: _____

	Pass	*Fail*
What are the substance's physical and chemical characteristics?		
What are the hazards?		
What are the appropriate actions to be taken?		
What is the appropriate medical response?		
Determine the risk of secondary contamination.		
What is CAMEO®?		
What is CHEMTREC?		
What is CHEMTEL, Inc.?		

☐ Successful   ☐ Unsuccessful   Examiner Initials: _____

Hazardous Materials: Two-Step Decontamination Method

Student: _____   Examiner: _____

Date: _____

	Done ✓	Not Done
Assesses scene safety and utilizes appropriate PPE		*
Sizes up incident and assesses toxicological risk		*
Activates IMS/ICS and initiates containment		*
Establishes command/turns over command when IMS/ICS personnel arrive		*
Examiner advises that this is a fast-breaking incident and a patient is walking up to you right now.		
Removes all patient clothing, personal effects, shoes, socks, etc.		*
Directs partner to prepare for two-step decon (obtain "kiddie" pool, soap, and hose)		
Brushes patient off to remove any dry particles		*
Washes and rinses patient with soap and water, making sure he or she does not stay in runoff		*
Empties pool into large container		*
Washes and rinses patient again with soap and water		*
Wraps and prepares for transfer to triage/treatment area(s)		*
Student exhibits competence with skill		

Any items in the Not Done column that are marked with an * are mandatory for the student to complete. A check mark in the Not Done column of an item with an * indicates that the student was unsuccessful and must attempt the skill again to assure competency. Examiners should use a different-color ink for the second attempt.

☐ Successful   ☐ Unsuccessful   Examiner Initials: _____

   ©2006 Prentice-Hall Inc.

Hazardous Materials: Eight-Step Decontamination Method

Student: _____   Examiner: _____

Date: _____

	Done ✓	Not Done
Assesses scene safety and utilizes appropriate PPE		*
Sizes up incident and assesses toxicological risk		*
Activates IMS/ICS and initiates containment		*
Establishes command/turns over command when IMS/ICS personnel arrive		*
Examiner advises that student is now in complete decontamination corridor and must remove patient from the hot zone using the eight-step decontamination process.		
1. Enters the decon area in hot zone and mechanically removes contaminants from victim		
2. Drops equipment in a tool-drop area and removes outer gloves		
3. Meets decon personnel and, along with victim, is showered and scrubbed to remove gross contamination, with surface decon dilution being removed and conducted into a contained area—victim may be moved ahead to step 6 or 7		
4. Removes and isolates SCBA (if reentry necessary, dons new SCBA from noncontaminated area)		
5. Removes all protective clothing, articles being isolated, labeled for disposal, and placed on contaminated side		
6. Removes all personal clothing (victims who have not had clothing removed will have it removed here), with all items isolated in plastic bags and labeled for storage or disposal		
7. Receives full-body washing (along with victim), using soft scrub brushes or sponges, water, and mild soap or detergent—cleaning tools are bagged for later disposal		
8. Is evaluated by EMS, completes exposure record, and is transported (if needed), while victim receives rapid assessment and stabilization before being transported		
Student exhibits competence with skill		

The above steps are an example of a relatively thorough decontamination process. Local protocols will vary. Students in lab can use lab sheets to read from during this lab—the simulated decon should involve students playing the roles of rescuer, victim, decon personnel, and EMS providers who receive victim and rescuer at end of decontamination process. Have fun with it! This is probably the ONLY haz-mat decon you CAN have fun with.

This is a knowledge acquisition lab. Student participation is required for successful completion.

☐ Successful   ☐ Unsuccessful   Examiner Initials: _____

MCI: Start Triage System

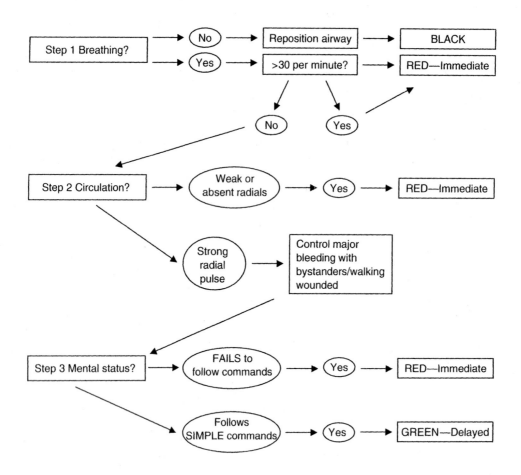

30—2—"Can Do": Once you arrive on scene with a mass casualty incident (MCI), you announce on the PA that all the people who were involved in the incident are to go to a location of your designation. With the "walking wounded" out of the way, you can begin tagging the injured according to the START algorithm here: "30"—Breathing; "2"—Capillary refill; "Can Do"—Simple commands. You can use walking wounded and bystanders to help maintain airways or hold pressure on wounds. It is the mission of triage personnel to categorize patients, not to start treatment. Attempt to spend as little time as possible on any one victim.

©2006 Prentice-Hall Inc.

MCI: Triage of MCI Patients Using Start System—Tabletop Exercise

Student: _____   **Examiner:** _____

Date: _____

	Done ✓	Not Done
Assesses scene safety and utilizes appropriate PPE (multiple gloves on each hand and in belt)		*
Assesses the need to use the START triage system		*
Asks all patients who can walk to go to a predetermined area		*
Properly classes patient 1		
Properly classes patient 2		
Properly classes patient 3		
Properly classes patient 4		
Properly classes patient 5		
Properly classes patient 6		
Properly classes patient 7		
Properly classes patient 8		
Properly classes patient 9		
Properly classes patient 10		
Properly classes patient 11		
Finished classification of all patients within 11 minutes		*
Student exhibits competence with skill		

Any items in the Not Done column that are marked with an * are mandatory for the student to complete. A check mark in the Not Done column of an item with an * indicates that the student was unsuccessful and must attempt the skill again to assure competency. Examiners should use a different-color ink for the second attempt.

☐ Successful   ☐ Unsuccessful   Examiner Initials: _____

Special Operations: Contact and Cover

Student: _____   **Examiner:** _____

Date: _____

	Done ✓	Not Done
Assesses scene safety and utilizes appropriate PPE		*
Verbalizes that even with presence of law enforcement, scenes may become unsafe—especially abuse, assault, behavioral emergencies, and domestic violence scenes		*
Verbalizes that in cases of potential escalation, EMS personnel need to use the "contact and cover" technique		
Recognizes situation calls for contact and cover		*
Designates team member/partner as "cover" and proceeds to "contact" patient		*
Contact person initiates assessment and emergency treatment while cover person observes scene (optimally stands at 90° angle to partner) for dangers		*
Cover person remains in observational role and keeps clear pathway to door for rapid exit		*
Expeditiously removes patient from scene and performs further treatment in unit		*
Student exhibits competence with skill		

Any items in the Not Done column that are marked with an * are mandatory for the student to complete. A check mark in the Not Done column of an item with an * indicates that the student was unsuccessful and must attempt the skill again to assure competency. Examiners should use a different-color ink for the second attempt.

☐ Successful   ☐ Unsuccessful   Examiner Initials: _____

©2006 Prentice-Hall Inc.

Special Operations: Cover and Conceal

Student: _____   Examiner: _____

Date: _____

	Done ✓	Not Done
Assesses scene safety and utilizes appropriate PPE		*
Recognizes scene has become unsafe and rescuer must take cover/concealment		*
Verbalizes that **concealment** hides body (bushes, doors, curtains, etc.) but does not stop bullets		*
Verbalizes that **cover** hides body AND protects from bullets/projectiles (solid, impenetrable objects such as brick walls, rocks, trees, car engines, etc.)		*
In case of cover, checks surroundings for possibility that bullets might ricochet		
Student exhibits competence with skill		

Any items in the Not Done column that are marked with an * are mandatory for the student to complete. A check mark in the Not Done column of an item with an * indicates that the student was unsuccessful and must attempt the skill again to assure competency. Examiners should use a different-color ink for the second attempt.

☐ Successful   ☐ Unsuccessful   Examiner Initials: _____

Special Operations: Evasive Tactics

Student: _____   **Examiner:** _____

Date: _____

	Done ✓	Not Done
Assesses scene safety and utilizes appropriate PPE		*
Recognizes scene has become unsafe and identifies need to use evasive tactics		*
Calls for help/pushes alarm button on radio		*
Uses distraction of throwing piece of equipment or household furnishing such as trash can/garbage can (at attacker if present)		
Makes rapid retreat from scene, wedging stretcher in doorway if inside residence		*
Overturns objects, the larger the better, in path of attacker		
After exiting residence, anticipates moves of attacker and splits from partner, making counter moves and watching moves of attacker for protection of self and partner		
Uses unconventional path while retreating and concealment techniques as needed		
If attacker is armed, uses solid objects (trees, houses, etc.) between self and attacker—advises incoming law enforcement of situation		*
If attacker is armed, does NOT retreat to rescue unit as attacker will anticipate—verbalizes safety of self and partner primary concern		
Student exhibits competence with skill		

Any items in the Not Done column that are marked with an * are mandatory for the student to complete. A check mark in the Not Done column of an item with an * indicates that the student was unsuccessful and must attempt the skill again to assure competency. Examiners should use a different-color ink for the second attempt.

☐ Successful   ☐ Unsuccessful   Examiner Initials: _____

©2006 Prentice-Hall Inc.

DAILY DISCUSSIONS AND PERTINENT POINTS— SPECIAL OPERATIONS

Student: _____   Date: _____

Instructor: _____

	Instructor Initials
Describe the common hazards found at the scene of a trauma and a medical patient.	
Describe methods of making an unsafe scene safe.	
Explain the rationale for crew members to evaluate scene safety prior to entering.	
Describe the incidence, morbidity, and mortality of unintentional and alleged unintentional events.	
Identify the human, environmental, and socioeconomic impacts of unintentional and alleged unintentional events.	
Discuss common mechanisms of injury/nature of illness.	
Discuss the reason for identifying the total number of patients at the scene.	
Explain the reasons for identifying the need for additional help or assistance.	
Explain the reason for prioritizing a patient for care and transport.	
Identify patients who may require expeditious transport.	
Discuss the reasons for reconsidering the mechanism of injury.	
Describe the criteria and procedure for air medical transport.	
Value the need to serve as the patient advocate to ensure appropriate patient transportation via ground or air.	
Explain the need for the incident management system (IMS)/incident command system (ICS) in managing EMS incidents.	
Define the term *multiple casualty incident (MCI)*.	
Define the term *disaster management*.	
Describe essential elements of scene size-up when arriving at a potential MCI.	
Describe the role of the paramedics and EMS systems in planning for MCIs and disasters.	

Describe the functional components of the IMS in terms of the following:
  a. Command
  b. Finance
  c. Logistics
  d. Operations
  e. Planning	

Define the following types of incidents and how they affect medical management:
  a. Open or uncontained incident
  b. Closed or contained incident	

Differentiate between singular and unified command and when each is most applicable.	
Describe the role of command.	
Describe the need for transfer of command and procedures for transferring it.	
Differentiate between command procedures used at small-, medium-, and large-scale medical incidents.	
Explain the local/regional threshold for establishing command and implementation of the IMS, including threshold MCI declaration.	

List and describe the functions of the following groups and leaders in ICS as each pertains to EMS incidents:
  a. Safety
  b. Logistics
  c. Rehabilitation
  d. Staging
  e. Treatment
  f. Triage
  g. Transportation
  h. Extrication/rescue
  i. Disposition of deceased (morgue)
  j. Communications	

(continued)

DAILY DISCUSSIONS AND PERTINENT POINTS—
SPECIAL OPERATIONS (*continued*)

Student: _____   **Date:** _____

Instructor: _____

	Instructor Initials
Describe the methods and rationale for identifying specific functions and leaders for those functions.	
Describe the role of both command posts and emergency operations centers in MCI and disaster management.	
Describe the role of the physician at MCIs.	
Define triage and describe the principles of triage.	
Describe the START method of initial triage.	
Given a list of 20 patients with various multiple injuries, determine the appropriate triage priority with 90% accuracy.	
Given color-coded tags and numerical priorities, assign the following terms to each: a. Immediate b. Delayed c. Hold d. Deceased	
Define *primary* and *secondary* triage.	
Describe when primary and secondary triage techniques should be implemented.	
Describe the need for, and techniques used in, tracking patients during MCIs.	
Describe techniques used to allocate patients to hospitals and track them.	
Describe modifications of telecommunications procedures during MCIs.	
List and describe the essential equipment to provide logistical support to MCI operations to include: a. Airway, respiratory, and hemorrhage control b. Burn management c. Patient packaging/immobilization	
List the physical and psychological signs of critical incident stress (CIS).	
Describe the role of CIS management sessions in MCIs.	
Describe the role of the following exercises in preparation for MCIs: a. Tabletop exercises b. Small and large MCI drills	
Understand the rationale for initiating incident command even at a small MCI event.	
Explain the rationale for having efficient and effective communications as part of an incident command/management system.	
Explain why common problems of an MCI can have an adverse effect on an entire incident.	
Define the term *rescue*.	
Explain the medical and mechanical aspects of rescue situations.	
Explain the role of the paramedic in delivering care at the site of the injury, continuing through the rescue process and to definitive care.	
Describe the phases of a rescue operation.	
List and describe the types of PPE needed to safely operate in the rescue environment to include: a. Head protection b. Eye protection c. Hand protection d. Personal flotation device (PFD) e. Thermal protection/layering systems f. High-visibility clothing g. Specialized footwear	
Explain the differences in risk between moving water and flat-water rescue.	
Explain the effects of immersion hypothermia on the ability to survive sudden immersion and self-rescue.	
Explain the phenomenon of the cold protective response in cold water drowning situations.	

©2006 Prentice-Hall Inc.

Identify the poisonous gases commonly found in confined spaces to include:
  a. Hydrogen sulfide (H_2S)
  b. Carbon dioxide (CO_2)
  c. Carbon monoxide (CO)
  d. Low/high oxygen concentrations (FiO_2)
  e. Methane (CH_4)
  f. Ammonia (NH_3)
  g. Nitrogen dioxide (NO_2)

Explain the hazard of cave-in during trench rescue operations.

Describe the effects of traffic flow on the highway rescue incident, including limited access superhighways and regular access highways.

List and describe the following techniques to reduce scene risk at highway incidents:
  a. Apparatus placement
  b. Headlights and emergency vehicle lighting
  c. Cones, flares
  d. Reflective and high-visibility clothing

List and describe the hazards associated with the following auto/truck components:
  a. Energy absorbing bumpers
  b. Air bag/supplemental restraint systems
  c. Catalytic converters and conventional fuel systems
  d. Stored energy
  e. Alternate fuel systems

Given a diagram of a passenger auto, identify the following structures:
  a. A, B, C, D posts
  b. Fire wall
  c. Unibody versus frame designs

Describe methods for emergency stabilization using rope, cribbing, jacks, spare tire, and come-alongs for vehicles found on their:
  a. Wheels
  b. Side
  c. Roof
  d. Inclines

Describe the electrical hazards commonly found at highway incidents (above and below ground).

Explain the difference between tempered and safety glass: identify their locations on a vehicle and how to break them safely.

Explain typical door anatomy and methods to access through stuck doors.

Explain SRS or air bag systems and methods to neutralize them.

Define the following terms:
  a. Low angle
  b. High angle
  c. Belay
  d. Rappel
  e. Scrambling
  f. Hasty rope slide

Explain techniques to be used in nontechnical litter carries over rough terrain.

Explain the procedures for low-angle litter evacuation to include:
  a. Anchoring
  b. Litter/rope attachment
  c. Lowering and raising procedures

Explain nontechnical high-angle rescue procedures using aerial apparatus.

Develop specific skill in emergency stabilization of vehicles and access procedures and an awareness of specific extrication strategies.

Explain assessment procedures and modifications necessary when caring for entrapped patients.

List the equipment necessary for an off-road medical pack.

Explain specific methods of improvisation for assessment, spinal motion restriction, and extremity splinting.

Explain the indications, contraindications, and methods of pain control for entrapped patients.

Explain the need for, and techniques of, thermal control for entrapped patients.

Explain the pathophysiology of crush trauma syndrome.

Develop an understanding of the medical issues involved in providing care for a patient in a rescue environment.

Develop proficiency in patient packaging and evacuation techniques that pertain to hazardous or rescue environments.

(continued)

DAILY DISCUSSIONS AND PERTINENT POINTS—
SPECIAL OPERATIONS (*continued*)

Student: _____   **Date:** _____

Instructor: _____

	Instructor Initials
Explain the different types of "Stokes" or basket stretchers and the advantages and disadvantages associated with each.	
Explain the role of the paramedic/EMS responder in terms of the following: a. Incident size-up b. Assessment of toxicologic risk c. Appropriate decontamination methods d. Treatment of semidecontaminated patients e. Transportation of semidecontaminated patients	
Size up a simulated hazardous materials (haz-mat) incident and determine the following: a. Potential hazards to the rescuers, public, and environment b. Potential risk of primary contamination to patients c. Potential risk of secondary contamination to rescuers	
Identify resources for substance identification, decontamination, and treatment information including the following: a. Poison control center b. Medical control c. Material safety data sheets (MSDS) d. Reference textbooks e. Computer databases (CAMEO) f. CHEMTREC g. Technical specialists h. Agency for toxic substances and disease registry	
Explain the following terms/concepts: a. Primary contamination risk b. Secondary contamination risk	
List and describe the following routes of exposure: a. Topical b. Respiratory c. Gastrointestinal d. Parenteral	
Explain the following toxicologic principles: a. Acute and delayed toxicity b. Route of exposure c. Local versus systemic effects d. Dose response e. Synergistic effects	
Explain how the substance and route of contamination alters triage and decontamination methods.	
Explain the limitations of field decontamination procedures.	
Explain the use and limitations of PPE in hazardous material situations.	
List and explain the common signs, symptoms, and treatment for the following substances: a. Corrosives (acids/alkalis) b. Pulmonary irritants (ammonia/chlorine) c. Pesticides (carbamates/organophosphates) d. Chemical asphyxiants (cyanide/carbon monoxide) e. Hydrocarbon solvents (xylene/methylene chloride)	
Explain the potential risk associated with invasive procedures performed on contaminated patients.	
Given a contaminated patient, determine the level of decontamination necessary and: a. Level of rescuer PPE b. Decontamination methods c. Treatment d. Transportation and patient isolation techniques	

©2006 Prentice-Hall Inc.

Identify local facilities and resources capable of treating patients exposed to hazardous materials.	
Given an incident involving hazardous materials, determine the hazards present to the patient and paramedic.	

Define the following and explain their importance to the risk assessment process:
  a. Boiling point
  b. Flammable/explosive limits
  c. Flash point
  d. Ignition temperature
  e. Specific gravity
  f. Vapor density
  g. Vapor pressure
  h. Water solubility
  i. Alpha radiation
  j. Beta radiation
  k. Gamma radiation	

Define the toxicologic terms and their use in the risk assessment process:
  a. Threshold limit value (TLV)
  b. Lethal concentration and doses (LD)
  c. Parts per million/billion (ppm/ppb)
  d. Immediately dangerous to life and health (IDLH)
  e. Permissible exposure limit (PEL)
  f. Short-term exposure limit (TLV-STEL)
  g. Ceiling level (TLV-C)	

Determine the factors that determine where and when to treat a patient, to include:
  a. Substance toxicity
  b. Patient condition
  c. Availability of decontamination	

Determine the appropriate level of PPE to include:
  a. Types, applications, use, and limitations
  b. Use of chemical compatibility chart	

Explain decontamination procedures when functioning in the following modes:
  a. Critical patient rapid two-step decontamination process
  b. Noncritical patient eight-step decontamination process	

Explain specific decontamination procedures.	

Explain the four most common decontamination solutions used to include:
  a. Water
  b. Water and tincture of green soap
  c. Isopropyl alcohol
  d. Vegetable oil	

Identify the areas of the body difficult to decontaminate to include:
  a. Scalp/hair
  b. Ears/ear canals/nostrils
  c. Axilla
  d. Fingernails
  e. Navel
  f. Groin/buttocks/genitalia
  g. Behind knees
  h. Between toes, toenails	

Explain the medical monitoring procedures of hazardous material team members to be used both pre- and postentry, to include:
  a. Vital signs
  b. Body weight
  c. General health
  d. Neurologic status
  e. ECG	

Explain the factors that influence the heat stress of hazardous material team personnel to include:
  a. Hydration
  b. Physical fitness
  c. Ambient temperature
  d. Activity
  e. Level of PPE
  f. Duration of activity	

(continued)

DAILY DISCUSSIONS AND PERTINENT POINTS—
SPECIAL OPERATIONS (*continued*)

Student: _____   Date: _____

Instructor: _____

	Instructor Initials
Explain the documentation necessary for haz-mat medical monitoring and rehabilitation operations: a. The substance b. The toxicity and danger of secondary contamination c. Appropriate PPE and suit breakthrough time d. Appropriate level of decontamination e. Appropriate antidote and medical treatment f. Transportation method	
Integrate the principles and practices of hazardous materials response in an effective manner to prevent and limit contamination, morbidity, and mortality.	
Explain the organizational benefits of having standard operating procedures (SOPs), for using the incident management system, or for using the incident command system.	
Demonstrate the use of local/regional triage tagging system used for primary and secondary triage in a simulated lab exercise.	
Given a simulated tabletop MCI with 5–10 patients: a. Establish unified or singular command b. Conduct a scene assessment c. Determine scene objectives d. Formulate an incident plan e. Request appropriate resources f. Determine need for ICS expansion and groups g. Coordinate communications and group leaders h. Coordinate outside agencies	
Given a classroom simulation of an MCI with 5–10 patients, fulfill the role of triage group leader.	
Given a classroom simulation of an MCI with 5–10 patients, fulfill the role of treatment group leader.	
Given a classroom simulation of an MCI with 5–10 patients, fulfill the role of transportation group leader.	
Explain how EMS providers are often mistaken for the police.	
Explain specific techniques for risk reduction when approaching the following types of routine EMS scenes: a. Highway encounters b. Violent street incidents c. Residences and "dark houses"	
Describe warning signs of potentially violent situations.	
Explain emergency evasive techniques for potentially violent situations including: a. Threats of physical violence b. Firearms encounters c. Edged weapon encounters	
Explain EMS considerations for the following types of violent or potentially violent situations: a. Gangs and gang violence b. Hostage/sniper situations c. Clandestine drug labs d. Domestic violence e. Emotionally disturbed people	
Explain the following techniques: a. Field "contact and cover" procedures during assessment and care b. Evasive tactics c. Concealment techniques	
Describe police evidence considerations and techniques to assist in evidence preservation.	

©2006 Prentice-Hall Inc.

SECTION 2
Advanced Airway Management

Fabulous Factoids
Skill Sheets
Daily Discussions and Pertinent Points

FABULOUS FACTOIDS—ADVANCED AIRWAY MANAGEMENT

NEVER use the technique of placing Miller blade "all the way in" and "pulling back until you see the epiglottis drop."

Esophageal intubation is lethal if you do not recognize it immediately.

The only indication for a surgical airway is the inability to establish an airway by any other method.

Never withhold oxygen from any patient for whom it is indicated.

Sometimes a physical exam won't help in diagnosing respiratory burns. Sooty sputum is present in only 50% of cases, hoarseness in less than 25%, and singed nasal hairs in only 13%. MOI is a better indicator in most cases.

Pay attention to anything in the patient's mouth that may become an airway obstruction.

Children are NOT little adults. Don't treat them as if they were.

Size for size, the strongest muscle in your body is the masseter. One masseter is located on each side of the mouth. Working together, the masseters give the biting force of about 150 pounds—not a good thing for a paramedic's fingers.

Believe it or not—you CAN intubate a patient without RSI!!

Discuss respiratory failure and intubating a conscious patient WITHOUT RSI.

Twenty-first century paramedics are prehospital practitioners of emergency medicine—not field technicians.

Why are there interstate highways in Hawaii?

You would have been a scholar in the Middle Ages—barely 5% of the people were literate.

The two lines that connect the bottom of your nose to your lip are called the philtrum.

The world's first recorded tonsillectomy was performed in 1000 B.C.

It takes 3 minutes for a fresh mosquito bite to begin to itch.

The life span of a taste bud is 10 days.

Drugs of the Section (see Emergency Drug Quiz Key, p. xxxi):

Versed
Amidate
Anectine
Norcuron

Pathophysiologies of the Section: 2.01–2.04 (see Checklist, p. 595)

©2006 Prentice-Hall Inc.

SKILL SHEETS

Bag-Valve-Mask Ventilation

Student: _____   Examiner: _____

Date: _____

	Done ✓	Not Done
Determines scene safety and utilizes appropriate PPE		*
Manually opens the airway using appropriate technique for patient condition		*
Checks mouth for foreign bodies, blood, loose teeth, or other potential airway obstruction		*
Suctions or clears airway as indicated		
Inserts simple airway adjunct		
Fits appropriately sized mask to bag-valve device		*
Creates tight mask-to-face seal		*
Ventilates patient for 30 seconds/8–10 breaths with adequate tidal volume for patient condition		*
Observes chest rise and fall, chest wall excursion and evaluates compliance		*
Connects oxygen reservoir and adjusts flow rate to fill reservoir		*
Turns ventilation over to assistant and bilaterally auscultates breath sounds for baseline		*
Creates tight mask-to-face seal with two hands		
Instructs assistant to resume ventilation		
Provides adequate ventilation for at least 1 minute		
Evaluates patient response		*
Student exhibits competence with skill		

Any items in the Not Done column that are marked with an * are mandatory for the student to complete. A check mark in the Not Done column of an item with an * indicates that the student was unsuccessful and must attempt the skill again to assure competency. Examiners should use a different-color ink for the second attempt.

☐ Successful   ☐ Unsuccessful   Examiner Initials: _____

Adult Ventilatory Management

Student: _____   **Examiner:** _____

Date: _____

	Done ✓	Not Done
Assesses scene safety and utilizes appropriate PPE		*
Manually opens the airway with technique appropriate for patient condition		*
Checks mouth for blood or potential airway obstruction		*
Suctions or removes loose teeth or foreign materials as needed		
Inserts simple adjunct (oropharyngeal or nasopharyngeal airway)		
Directs assistant to ventilate patient with bag-valve-mask device (room air)		*
Observes chest rise/fall and auscultates bilaterally over lungs for baseline		*
Obtains effective ventilation in less than 30 seconds		*
Attaches oxygen reservoir to bag-valve-mask device and connects to high-flow oxygen		
Ventilates patient and evaluates chest wall/lung compliance		*
Directs assistant to preoxygenate patient		*
Identifies/selects proper equipment for intubation		
Checks laryngoscope light and cuff of ET tube		
Removes all air from cuff and properly inserts stylet if used		
Removes airway adjunct		
Positions patient's head properly and has assistant perform Sellick's maneuver		*
Opens mouth and gently inserts blade while sweeping tongue to side		*
Has assistant maintain Sellick's pressure		
Gently elevates mandible with laryngoscope and visualizes cords		*
Introduces ET tube to side of blade and visualizes tube passing through cords		*
"Threads" ET tube off stylet (if used) maintaining hold on ET tube as stylet removed		
Inflates cuff to proper pressure and disconnects syringe		*
Disconnects mask from bag-valve device and attaches to ET tube without releasing ET tube		
Directs ventilation of patient while maintaining Sellick's maneuver and holding ET tube in place		
Confirms proper placement by auscultation over epigastrium and bilaterally over each lung		*
Directs assistant to release cricoid pressure		*
Secures ET tube		*
Reassesses bilateral lung sounds and compliance		*
Uses secondary device to confirm tube placement		*
Assesses patient's response to intervention		*
Student exhibits competence with skill		

Any items in the Not Done column that are marked with an * are mandatory for the student to complete. A check mark in the Not Done column of an item with an * indicates that the student was unsuccessful and must attempt the skill again to assure competency. Examiners should use a different-color ink for the second attempt.

☐ Successful   ☐ Unsuccessful   Examiner Initials: _____

                    ©2006 Prentice-Hall Inc.

Endotracheal Intubation with Suspected Cervical Spine

Student: _____   **Examiner:** _____

Date: _____

	Done ✓	Not Done
Determines scene safety and utilizes appropriate PPE		*
Opens the airway manually with trauma jaw-thrust while assistant maintains C-spine SMR		*
Checks mouth for blood or potential airway obstruction		*
Suctions or removes loose teeth or foreign materials as needed		
Inserts simple airway adjunct (oropharyngeal airway)		
Directs assistant to ventilate patient with bag-valve-mask device (room air)		*
Observes chest rise/fall and auscultates bilaterally over lungs for baseline		*
Obtains effective ventilation in less than 30 seconds		*
Attaches oxygen reservoir to bag-valve-mask device and connects to high-flow oxygen		
Ventilates patient and evaluates chest wall/lung compliance		*
Directs assistant to preoxygenate patient with assistant maintaining C-spine SMR		*
Identifies/selects proper equipment for intubation		
Checks laryngoscope light and cuff of ET tube		
Removes all air from cuff and properly inserts stylet if used		
Directs assistant to face patient and establish cervical spine SMR from front		
Intubating paramedic sits behind patient on ground with legs straddling patient's shoulders		
Moves up until patient's head is secured		
Removes OPA and directs assistant to perform Sellick's maneuver		*
Opens mouth and gently inserts blade while sweeping tongue to side		*
Gently elevates mandible with laryngoscope and leans backward to visualize cords		*
Inserts ET tube and visualizes as tube is advanced through cords		*
"Threads" ET tube off stylet (if used), maintaining hold on ET tube as stylet removed		
Inflates cuff to proper pressure and disconnects syringe		*
Disconnects mask from bag-valve device and attaches to ET tube without releasing ET tube		
Directs ventilation of patient while maintaining Sellick's maneuver and holding ET tube in place		
Confirms proper placement by auscultation over epigastrium and bilaterally over each lung		*
Directs assistant to release cricoid pressure		*
Secures ET tube		*
Reassesses bilateral lung sounds and compliance		*
Uses secondary device to confirm tube placement		*
Assesses patient's response to intervention		*
Student exhibits competence with skill		

Any items in the Not Done column that are marked with an * are mandatory for the student to complete. A check mark in the Not Done column of an item with an * indicates that the student was unsuccessful and must attempt the skill again to assure competency. Examiners should use a different-color ink for the second attempt.

☐ Successful   ☐ Unsuccessful   Examiner Initials: _____

©2006 Prentice-Hall Inc.

Dual Lumen (Biluminal) Airway Insertion

Student: _____   Examiner: _____

Date: _____

	Done ✓	Not Done
Utilizes appropriate PPE		*
Opens the airway manually—assures unresponsiveness		*
Opens mouth and checks for blood, loose teeth, or foreign matter		
Suctions or removes potential airway debris as needed		
Inserts simple airway adjunct (oropharyngeal or nasopharyngeal airway)		
Ventilates patient immediately (with room air)		
Obtains effective patient ventilation in less than 30 seconds		*
Attaches oxygen to bag-valve-mask at high flow and uses reservoir if available		
Effectively ventilates patient for 30 seconds		*
Auscultates over bilateral lung fields for baseline lung sounds		*
Directs assistant to take over preoxygenation		*
Checks/prepares airway device		*
Lubricates distal tip of the device (may be verbalized)		
Positions head properly and removes airway adjunct if inserted		
Assures unresponsiveness and performs a tongue-jaw lift		
Inserts dual lumen airway according to manufacturer's instructions		*
Inflates cuffs and secures airway device in sequence recommended for device		*
Removes syringes		*
Attaches bag-valve device to first lumen (esophageal) and ventilates		*
Auscultates over epigastrium to confirm placement		*
If hears gurgling over epigastrium, verbalizes that tube is in trachea		
Changes bag-valve device to second (tracheal) lumen and ventilates		
Auscultates over epigastrium and bilateral lungs to verify effective ventilations		*
Observes for rise and fall of chest, patient color change, and improvement		*
Secures device or confirms that the device remains properly secured		*
Student exhibits competence with skill		

Any items in the Not Done column that are marked with an * are mandatory for the student to complete. A check mark in the Not Done column of an item with an * indicates that the student was unsuccessful and must attempt the skill again to assure competency. Examiners should use a different-color ink for the second attempt.

☐ Successful   ☐ Unsuccessful   Examiner Initials: _____

©2006 Prentice-Hall Inc.

Nasotracheal Intubation

Student: _____   **Examiner:** _____

Date: _____

	Done ✓	Not Done
Utilizes appropriate PPE		*
Preoxygenates with 100% oxygen		*
Prepares ET tube with syringe and lubricant, checks cuff		
Inspects nose and selects larger nostril, evaluating septum		
Inserts tube into nostril with bevel along the floor of the nostril or facing nasal septum		
As tube drops into posterior pharynx, listens closely at tube end for respirations		
With patient's next inhalation, advances ET tube quickly into trachea past cords		*
Watches for condensation, feels for exhaled air, and observes for cough		
Holding ET tube with one hand, inflates cuff with 5–10 cc air using other hand		*
Removes syringe, maintaining hold on ET tube for placement		*
Verifies tube placement by observing chest rise and auscultating breath sounds with synchronized breath from BVM		*
Uses secondary device to confirm placement		*
Secures tube with tape or commercial device and rechecks breath sounds		*
Assesses patient's response to intervention		*
Periodically rechecks tube placement		
Student exhibits competence with skill		

Any items in the Not Done column that are marked with an * are mandatory for the student to complete. A check mark in the Not Done column of an item with an * indicates that the student was unsuccessful and must attempt the skill again to assure competency. Examiners should use a different-color ink for the second attempt.

☐ Successful   ☐ Unsuccessful   Examiner Initials: _____

Lighted Stylet

Student: _____   **Examiner:** _____

Date: _____

	Done ✓	Not Done
Utilizes appropriate PPE		*
Manually opens airway and ventilates patient with 100% oxygen		*
Inserts simple airway adjunct		
Directs assistant to assume BVM ventilations and assesses bilateral baseline lung sounds		*
Assembles and checks equipment		
Uses 7.5–8.5 mm ET tube		*
Places stylet in ET tube, bending it proximal to cuff		*
With patient supine and head in neutral position, kneels to face patient and turns on stylet		
Removes adjunct and places bite block to rear molars of one side of patient's mouth		*
Verifies unresponsiveness and inserts index and middle fingers deeply into patient's mouth and with thumb under bony part of chin, lifts tongue and jaw forward		*
Inserts ET tube/stylet into patient's mouth, advancing into hypopharynx		*
Uses "hooking" action with ET tube/stylet to lift epiglottis out of the way		*
Holds stylet stationary when circle of light visible at level of Adam's apple		*
Gently "threads" ET tube off stylet approximately 1–2 cm while withdrawing stylet		*
Inflates cuff with 5–10 cc of air and removes syringe, never releasing ET tube		*
Attaches bag-valve device and delivers breath while holding ET tube		
Auscultates over epigastrium and bilaterally over each lung		*
Secures ET tube		*
Uses secondary device to confirm tube placement		*
Reassesses bilateral breath sounds and compliance		*
Assesses patient's response to intervention		*
Reconfirms tube placement		
Student exhibits competence with skill		

Any items in the Not Done column that are marked with an * are mandatory for the student to complete. A check mark in the Not Done column of an item with an * indicates that the student was unsuccessful and must attempt the skill again to assure competency. Examiners should use a different-color ink for the second attempt.

☐ Successful   ☐ Unsuccessful   Examiner Initials: _____

©2006 Prentice-Hall Inc.

Digital Intubation

Student: _____   **Examiner:** _____

Date: _____

	Done ✓	Not Done
Utilizes PPE and assures unresponsiveness		*
Directs assistant to preoxygenate the patient with 100% oxygen		
Auscultates bilateral lung sounds for baseline		*
Prepares ET tube with syringe and lubrication if indicated—checks cuff		
Instructs team member to stabilize the head and neck as needed		
Positions self at left shoulder facing the patient		
Places a bite block between the patient's molars to prevent biting		*
Inserts the middle and index fingers of the left hand into the patient's mouth and "walks" down the midline tugging forward on the tongue		
Palpates the epiglottis with the middle finger		*
Presses the epiglottis forward and inserts the endotracheal tube anterior to the fingers		*
Advances the tube, pushing it with the right hand, using the index finger to maintain the tip of the tube against the middle finger, directing it to the epiglottis		
Using the middle and index fingers, directs the tube tip between the epiglottis and the fingers, advancing the tube through the cords		*
Holds the tube in place and inflates the distal cuff with 10 cc of air, immediately removing syringe		*
Effectively ventilates patient with 100% oxygen in less than 30 seconds from last breath given		*
Verifies proper placement by watching for chest rise, auscultating for bilateral breath sounds, and watching for condensation in the tube on exhalation		*
Secures the tube with tape or commercial device		*
Uses secondary device to confirm tube placement		*
Assesses patient's response to intervention		*
Periodically rechecks tube placement		
Student exhibits competence with skill		

Any items in the Not Done column that are marked with an * are mandatory for the student to complete. A check mark in the Not Done column of an item with an * indicates that the student was unsuccessful and must attempt the skill again to assure competency. Examiners should use a different-color ink for the second attempt.

☐ Successful   ☐ Unsuccessful   Examiner Initials: _____

EGTA/EOA Insertion

Student: _____   **Examiner:** _____

Date: _____

NOTE: EOA (esophageal obturator airway) is inserted with same technique except for placement of the nasogastric tube.

	Done ✓	Not Done
Utilizes appropriate PPE and assures unresponsiveness		*
Preoxygenates with 100% oxygen and assesses compliance		*
Turns over ventilation to assistant and prepares EGTA with syringe and lubricant, checks cuffs		
Assembles airway, seating mask with "click"		*
Auscultates bilateral lung sounds for baseline		
Places patient supine and kneels at the top of his or her head		
Inserts EGTA at midline through oropharynx using a tongue-jaw lift maneuver, advancing it past the hypopharynx to the depth indicated by markings on tube so black rings are between patient's teeth and mask is sealed against face		*
Inflates pharyngeal cuff with 100 ml of air		*
Removes syringe		*
Ventilates with BVM device attached to high-flow oxygen		*
Auscultates over epigastrium and bilaterally over lungs		*
Applies pulse oximeter		
Secures tube with tape or commercial device, continues ventilations, and rechecks lung sounds		*
Periodically rechecks tube placement		
Inserts nasogastric tube through port and advances into stomach		
Checks gastric tube placement using 30–50 ml air, then hooks to suction to empty stomach		
Disconnects from suction or places to intermittent suction after stomach contents evacuated		
Assesses patient's response to intervention		*
Student exhibits competence with skill		

Any items in the Not Done column that are marked with an * are mandatory for the student to complete. A check mark in the Not Done column of an item with an * indicates that the student was unsuccessful and must attempt the skill again to assure competency. Examiners should use a different-color ink for the second attempt.

☐ Successful   ☐ Unsuccessful   Examiner Initials: _____

©2006 Prentice-Hall Inc.

Orogastric Tube Insertion—Unresponsive

Student: _____   Examiner: _____

Date: _____

	Done ✓	Not Done
Utilizes appropriate PPE		*
Obtains equipment (suction, NG tube, lubricant, tape, irrigating syringe, water)		
Verifies secure airway in unresponsive patient		*
Positions patient supine		
Measures tube from hypogastric region to earlobe to mouth and tapes depth marking		*
Lubricates tube		*
Passes tip through oral cavity to posterior pharynx (along tongue side of ET tube)		*
Passes tube slowly and posteriorly, checking mouth for curling		*
Determines proper tube placement by auscultation over epigastrium of injected AIR		*
Aspirates stomach contents for secondary verification		*
Secures tube in place		*
Places to suction (continuous only for emptying initial contents, then intermittent)		
Saves gastric contents		
Documents procedure correctly		
Assesses patient's response to intervention		*
Student exhibits competence with skill		

Any items in the Not Done column that are marked with an * are mandatory for the student to complete. A check mark in the Not Done column of an item with an * indicates that the student was unsuccessful and must attempt the skill again to assure competency. Examiners should use a different-color ink for the second attempt.

☐ Successful   ☐ Unsuccessful   Examiner Initials: _____

Nasogastric Tube Insertion

Student: _____   **Examiner:** _____

Date: _____

	Done ✓	Not Done
Utilizes appropriate PPE		*
Obtains equipment (suction, NG tube, lubricant, tape, irrigating syringe, water, straw, basin)		
Explains procedure to conscious patient or verifies secure airway in unresponsive patient		*
Positions patient (supine for unresponsive, high Fowler's for conscious)		
Measures tube from hypogastric region to earlobe to nose and tapes depth marking		*
Checks for larger nostril and palpates with little finger to assess patency		*
Lubricates tube		
Passes tip through nostril anterior to posterior along floor of nasal passage (straight back)		*
Guides tube to nasopharynx		
Advises conscious patient to continue drinking as tube is passed to measured depth		
Passes tube slowly and posteriorly in unresponsive patient, checking mouth for curling		
Determines proper tube placement by auscultation over epigastrium of injected AIR		*
Secures tube in place		*
Places to suction (continuous only for emptying initial contents, then intermittent)		
Saves gastric contents		
Documents procedure correctly		
Assesses patient's response to intervention		*
Student exhibits competence with skill		

Any items in the Not Done column that are marked with an * are mandatory for the student to complete. A check mark in the Not Done column of an item with an * indicates that the student was unsuccessful and must attempt the skill again to assure competency. Examiners should use a different-color ink for the second attempt.

☐ Successful   ☐ Unsuccessful   Examiner Initials: _____

©2006 Prentice-Hall Inc.

Automatic Transport Ventilator (ATV)

Student: _____

Date: _____

Examiner: _____

	Done ✓	Not Done
Utilizes appropriate PPE		*
Hooks disposable patient circuit to ventilator		*
Checks connections of oxygen hoses and tubings		*
Turns oxygen supply on and checks cylinder contents		*
Verifies controls are set to desired parameters		*
Sets frequency to 12 BPM		
Sets tidal volume to 10 ml/kg, then backs down slightly		
Sets pressure relief at 40 cmH$_2$O		
Sets air mix to 100%		
Auscultates lung sounds to verify tube placement and ventilation of both lungs		*
Turns switch on and briefly occludes patient connection port with thumb to check that peak inflation pressure reading on manometer is appropriate for patient condition		*
Applies patient port to ET tube or face mask to patient (with manually maintained airway)		*
Monitors rise and fall of chest, breath sounds, pressure manometer, and EtCO$_2$		*
If spontaneous breathing, sets to SMMV (synchronized minimum mandatory ventilation)		
Adjusts as indicated by patient condition and readings		
Able to verbalize actions to be taken for alarm signal (DOPE) Check lung sounds for tube placement (Dislodged) Check for obstructed airway (Obstructed) Check lung sounds for equality (Pneumothorax) Check hose for kink and pressure relief setting (Equipment)		*
Adjusts tidal volume		
Assesses patient's response to intervention		*
Student exhibits competence with skill		

Any items in the Not Done column that are marked with an * are mandatory for the student to complete. A check mark in the Not Done column of an item with an * indicates that the student was unsuccessful and must attempt the skill again to assure competency. Examiners should use a different-color ink for the second attempt.

☐ Successful   ☐ Unsuccessful   Examiner Initials: _____

Pleural Decompression

Student: _____   **Examiner:** _____

Date: _____

	Done ✓	Not Done
Utilizes appropriate PPE		*
Evaluates patient for indications and obtains baseline lung sounds and assessment		*
Prepares equipment (14 gauge 2¼-in. catheter-over-needle) and explains procedure to patient		
Palpates at 2nd intercostal space/midclavicular line		*
Cleanses site appropriately		
Inserts needle at superior border of 3rd rib, avoiding artery, vein, and nerve		*
Advances until feels "pop" and rush of air released		*
Checks patient for improvement in clinical status		*
Removes needle from catheter, disposes of needle properly, and applies flutter valve		*
Secures in place		
Reassesses patient for improvement		*
Documents procedure and response correctly		
Student exhibits competence with skill		

Any items in the Not Done column that are marked with an * are mandatory for the student to complete. A check mark in the Not Done column of an item with an * indicates that the student was unsuccessful and must attempt the skill again to assure competency. Examiners should use a different-color ink for the second attempt.

☐ Successful   ☐ Unsuccessful   Examiner Initials: _____

©2006 Prentice-Hall Inc.

Ventilation of an Obstructed Trach

Student: _____   Examiner: _____

Date: _____

	Done ✓	Not Done
Utilizes appropriate PPE		*
Attempts ventilation by bag-valve device to trach tube		*
Attempts BVM ventilation via mask over mouth and nose while setting up for suction		*
Suctions through tracheostomy tube using sterile technique		*
If still unable to ventilate and trach tube has inner cannula, deflates cuff if present and removes inner cannula		
Attempts to suction through outer cannula		
If no spontaneous breathing and inner cannula not patent, inserts appropriately sized ET tube through outer cannula until cuff just past end of outer cannula (1–2 cm)		
Inflates cuff with 5–10 cc of air and immediately removes syringe		
Ventilates and confirms chest rise and fall in less than 3 minutes		*
Auscultates bilateral lung sounds		*
Confirms placement with secondary device		*
Assesses patient's response to intervention		*
Student exhibits competence with skill		

Any items in the Not Done column that are marked with an * are mandatory for the student to complete. A check mark in the Not Done column of an item with an * indicates that the student was unsuccessful and must attempt the skill again to assure competency. Examiners should use a different-color ink for the second attempt.

☐ Successful   ☐ Unsuccessful   Examiner Initials: _____

CPAP/BiPAP

Student: _____   Examiner: _____

Date: _____

	Done ✓	Not Done
Utilizes appropriate PPE		*
Explains procedure to patient and obtains full set of vitals		*
Hooks disposable patient circuit to ventilator		*
Checks connections of oxygen hoses and tubing		*
Turns oxygen supply on and checks cylinder contents		*
Verifies controls are set to desired parameters		*
Sets frequency to 12 BPM		
Sets tidal volume to 10 ml/kg, then backs down slightly		
Sets pressure relief at 40 cmH$_2$O		
Sets air mix to 100%		
Auscultates lung sounds to verify ventilation of both lungs and obtain baseline		*
Turns switch on and briefly occludes patient connection port with thumb to check that peak inflation pressure reading on manometer is appropriate for patient condition		*
Applies patient port to face mask to patient (with manually maintained airway) and checks for proper seal		*
Monitors rise and fall of chest, breath sounds, and pressure manometer		*
If spontaneous breathing, sets to SMMV (synchronized minimum mandatory ventilation)		
Adjusts as indicated by patient condition and readings		
Able to verbalize actions to be taken for alarm signal (DOPE) Check lung sounds for tube placement (Dislodged) Check for obstructed airway (Obstructed) Check lung sounds for equality (Pneumothorax) Check hose for kink and pressure relief setting (Equipment)		*
Adjusts tidal volume		
Assesses patient's response to intervention		*
Student exhibits competence with skill		

Any items in the Not Done column that are marked with an * are mandatory for the student to complete. A check mark in the Not Done column of an item with an * indicates that the student was unsuccessful and must attempt the skill again to assure competency. Examiners should use a different-color ink for the second attempt.

☐ Successful   ☐ Unsuccessful   Examiner Initials: _____

©2006 Prentice-Hall Inc.

Rapid Sequence Induction with Neuromuscular Blockade

Student: _____   Examiner: _____

Date: _____

	Done ✓	Not Done
Utilizes appropriate PPE		*
Verifies allergies and recognizes contraindication of succinylcholine with hyperkalemia		
Assembles and checks required equipment		
Ensures IV in place and patent		*
Auscultates bilateral lung sounds for baseline		*
Places patient on cardiac monitor and pulse oximeter		*
Preoxygenates with 100% oxygen		
Considers premedicating with Versed, Etomidate, Atropine, Lidocaine per protocols		*
SEDATES before administers paralytic if patient VS allow		*
Has assistant apply Sellick's maneuver until proper ET tube placement confirmed		*
Administers Succinylcholine 1–2 mg/kg IVP and continues oxygenation		*
Watches for apnea and jaw relaxation		*
Performs endotracheal intubation, inflates cuff, and removes syringe		*
Confirms proper ET tube placement by auscultating over epigastrium and each lung		*
Directs assistant to release Sellick's maneuver		*
Secures ET tube		*
Auscultates bilateral lung sounds to reconfirm tube placement		*
Reconfirms tube placement with secondary device		*
Assesses patient's response to intervention		*
Student exhibits competence with skill		

Any items in the Not Done column that are marked with an * are mandatory for the student to complete. A check mark in the Not Done column of an item with an * indicates that the student was unsuccessful and must attempt the skill again to assure competency. Examiners should use a different-color ink for the second attempt.

☐ Successful   ☐ Unsuccessful   Examiner Initials: _____

Needle Cricothyrotomy

Student: _____   Examiner: _____

Date: _____

	Done ✓	Not Done
Utilizes appropriate PPE		*
Places patient supine and hyperextends neck if no cervical trauma suspected		
Positions at patient's side and directs assistant to attempt ventilations with 100% oxygen		
Prepares equipment, attaches large-bore needle with catheter to 10–20 ml syringe		
Palpates thyroid cartilage and cricoid cartilage		*
Identifies and places finger on cricothyroid membrane (CTM)		*
Maintaining placement, cleanses site appropriately		
Firmly grasps laryngeal cartilages and reconfirms CTM		*
Inserts needle into CTM at midline, directed 45° caudally		*
Advances needle no more than 1 cm and aspirates with syringe		*
Confirms placement and advances catheter while withdrawing needle and syringe unit		*
Reconfirms placement and secures catheter in place (does not release catheter)		*
Checks adequacy of ventilations; chest rise, bilateral breath sounds		
If spontaneous ventilations are absent or inadequate, begins transtracheal jet ventilation		
Connects one end of oxygen tubing to catheter, other end to jet ventilator or using "whistle-tip" and oxygen tank, covers hole for inspiration (allows adequate lung expansion)		*
Watches chest carefully, turning off release valve or opening whistle-tip as soon as chest rises		*
Verbalizes problem of carbon dioxide retention with this ventilation method		*
Continues ventilatory support, assessing for adequacy of ventilations and complications		
Assesses patient's response to intervention		*
Student exhibits competence with skill		

Any items in the Not Done column that are marked with an * are mandatory for the student to complete. A check mark in the Not Done column of an item with an * indicates that the student was unsuccessful and must attempt the skill again to assure competency. Examiners should use a different-color ink for the second attempt.

☐ Successful   ☐ Unsuccessful   Examiner Initials: _____

©2006 Prentice-Hall Inc.

Surgical Cricothyrotomy

Student: _____   Examiner: _____

Date: _____

	Done ✓	Not Done
Utilizes appropriate PPE		*
Determines necessity for surgical cricothyrotomy (unable to ventilate, FBAO, etc.)		*
Prepares equipment		
Assures maintenance of cervical spine motion restriction if appropriate		*
Locates thyroid cartilage and cricoid cartilage		
Finds cricothyroid membrane (CTM)		*
Cleanses site appropriately		
Stabilizes cartilages with one hand		*
Uses scalpel to make 1–2 cm vertical or horizontal (per protocol) skin incision over membrane		*
Makes 1 cm incision in horizontal plane through CTM		*
Inserts safety cover of catheter or a hemostat into incision to hold incision open		
Removes scalpel and disposes in appropriate container		
Inserts either cuffed ET tube or Shiley trach tube through incision into trachea		*
Inflates cuff and ventilates		*
Confirms placement with auscultation, chest rise and fall, and $EtCO_2$ monitoring		*
Uses secondary confirmation device		*
Secures tube in place		*
Assesses patient's response to intervention		*
Student exhibits competence with skill		

Any items in the Not Done column that are marked with an * are mandatory for the student to complete. A check mark in the Not Done column of an item with an * indicates that the student was unsuccessful and must attempt the skill again to assure competency. Examiners should use a different-color ink for the second attempt.

☐ Successful   ☐ Unsuccessful   Examiner Initials: _____

Pediatric Ventilatory Management

Student: _____   Examiner: _____

Date: _____

	Done ✓	Not Done
Assesses scene safety and utilizes appropriate PPE		*
Manually opens the airway with technique appropriate to patient condition		*
Checks mouth for blood or potential airway compromising matter		*
Suctions or removes foreign body IF VISUALIZED		
Properly inserts simple adjunct (oropharyngeal or nasopharyngeal airway)		
Ventilates patient with BVM device in less than 20 seconds, assessing chest wall compliance		*
Directs assistant to ventilate		
Observes chest movement and auscultates for baseline bilateral lung sounds		
Attaches oxygen reservoir to bag-valve-mask device and connects to high-flow oxygen		
Directs assistant to preoxygenate patient		*
Identifies/selects proper equipment for intubation—uncuffed tube		
Checks laryngoscope to assure operational with good light source		
Places patient on cardiac monitor to continuously hear heart rate during intubation		*
Positions patient in neutral or sniffing position and removes airway adjunct if inserted		*
Gently inserts blade while displacing tongue (holds laryngoscope gently with two fingers and thumb)		*
Gently elevates mandible with laryngoscope and visualizes cords		*
Gently inserts ET tube to side of blade and visualizes tube passing through cords		*
Verbalizes smallest portion of pediatric airway is at the cricothyroid ring		
Disconnects mask from bag-valve device and attaches to ET tube without releasing ET tube		*
Directs ventilation of patient while holding ET tube in place		*
Confirms proper placement by auscultation over epigastrium and bilaterally over each lung		*
Uses secondary confirmation device		*
Secures ET tube and restricts cervical spine motion to maintain proper ET tube placement		*
Reassesses ET tube placement and heart rate		*
Considers OGT to decrease any abdominal distension compromising ventilation		
Assesses patient's response to intervention		*
Student exhibits competence with skill		

Any items in the Not Done column that are marked with an * are mandatory for the student to complete. A check mark in the Not Done column of an item with an * indicates that the student was unsuccessful and must attempt the skill again to assure competency. Examiners should use a different-color ink for the second attempt.

☐ Successful   ☐ Unsuccessful   Examiner Initials: _____

©2006 Prentice-Hall Inc.

End Tidal Carbon Dioxide Monitoring

Student: _____   Examiner: _____

Date: _____

	Done ✓	Not Done
Utilizes appropriate PPE		*
Explains procedure to patient		
Prepares disposable sensor and hooks tubing to device		
Turns on device and calibrates		*
Grasps ET tube to stabilize and removes bag-valve device		*
Inserts EtCO$_2$ sensor to end of ET tube and reattaches bag-valve device		*
Monitors reading for trends and adjusts ventilations accordingly		*
Evaluates patient condition/correlation to reading and treats appropriately		*
Documents results and actions		
Student exhibits competence with skill		

Any items in the Not Done column that are marked with an * are mandatory for the student to complete. A check mark in the Not Done column of an item with an * indicates that the student was unsuccessful and must attempt the skill again to assure competency. Examiners should use a different-color ink for the second attempt.

☐ Successful   ☐ Unsuccessful   Examiner Initials: _____

Extubation

Student: _____   **Examiner:** _____

Date: _____

	Done ✓	Not Done
Utilizes appropriate PPE		*
Assesses patient level of consciousness and respiratory parameters		*
Verifies patient respiratory effort and tidal volumes adequate for extubation		*
Verifies suction equipment set up and working		*
Explains procedure to patient		*
Removes tape or tube holder		
Has patient take a few deep breaths while still on oxygen		*
Removes air from balloon and detaches syringe when empty (pilot balloon flat)		*
Removes oxygen and has patient exhale forcefully or cough		*
Rapidly removes ET tube during exhalation or cough		*
Suctions as needed and places on supplemental oxygen until patient calms		*
Reassesses patient and documents correctly		*
Student exhibits competence with skill		

Any items in the Not Done column that are marked with an * are mandatory for the student to complete. A check mark in the Not Done column of an item with an * indicates that the student was unsuccessful and must attempt the skill again to assure competency. Examiners should use a different-color ink for the second attempt.

☐ Successful   ☐ Unsuccessful   Examiner Initials: _____

©2006 Prentice-Hall Inc.

Documentation Skills: Patient Care Report (PCR)

Student: _____   Examiner: _____

Date: _____

	Done ✓	Not Done
Records all pertinent dispatch/scene data, using a consistent format		
Completely identifies all additional resources and personnel		
Documents chief complaint, signs/symptoms, position found, age, sex, and weight		
Identifies and records all pertinent, reportable clinical data for each patient		
Documents SAMPLE and OPQRST if applicable		
Records all pertinent negatives		
Records all pertinent denials		
Records accurate, consistent times and patient information		
Includes relevant oral statements of witnesses, bystanders, and patient in "quotes" when appropriate		
Documents initial assessment findings: airway, breathing, and circulation		
Documents any interventions in initial assessment with patient response		
Documents level of consciousness, GCS (if trauma), and VS		
Documents rapid trauma assessment if applicable		
Documents any interventions in rapid trauma assessment with patient response		
Documents focused history and physical assessment		
Documents any interventions in focused assessment with patient response		
Documents repeat VS (every 5 minutes for critical; every 15 minutes for stable)		
Repeats initial assessment and documents findings		
Records ALL treatments with times and patient response(s) in treatment section		
Documents field impression		
Documents transport to specific facility and transfer of care WITH VERBAL REPORT		
Uses correct grammar, abbreviations, spelling, and terminology		
Writes legibly		
Thoroughly documents refusals, denials of transport, and call cancellations		
Documents patient GCS of 15 PRIOR to signing refusal		
Documents advice given to refusal patient, including "call 9-1-1 for further problems"		
Properly corrects errors and omissions		
Writes cautiously, avoids jargon, opinions, inferences, or any derogatory/libelous remarks		
Signs run report		
Uses EMS supplement form if needed		
Student exhibits competence with skill		

Any items in the Not Done column should be evaluated with student. Check marks in this column do not necessarily mean student was unsuccessful as all lines are not completed on all patients. Evaluation of each PCR should be based on the scenario given.

Student must be able to write an EMS report with consistency and accuracy.

☐ Successful   ☐ Unsuccessful   Examiner Initials: _____

DAILY DISCUSSIONS AND PERTINENT POINTS— ADVANCED AIRWAY MANAGEMENT SKILLS LAB

Student: _____   **Examiner:** _____

Date: _____

	Instructor Initials
Assess personal practices relative to the responsibility for personal safety, the safety of the crew, the patient, and bystanders.	
Identify health hazards and potential crime areas within the community served.	
Explain the primary objective of airway maintenance.	
Identify commonly neglected prehospital skills related to airway.	
Explain the risk of infection to EMS providers associated with ventilation.	
Describe the indications, contraindications, advantages, disadvantages, complications, equipment, and technique for tracheobronchial suctioning in the intubated patient.	
Identify special considerations of tracheobronchial suctioning in the intubated patient.	
Describe the indications, contraindications, advantages, disadvantages, complications, and techniques for inserting an oropharyngeal and nasopharyngeal airway.	
Explain the advantage of the two-person method when ventilating with the bag-valve-mask.	
Describe the indications, contraindications, advantages, disadvantages, complications, liter flow range, and concentration of delivered oxygen for supplemental oxygen delivery devices.	
Describe laryngoscopy for the removal of a foreign body airway obstruction (FBAO).	
Describe the indications, contraindications, advantages, disadvantages, complications, and techniques for direct laryngoscopy.	
Describe visual landmarks for direct laryngoscopy.	
Describe use of cricoid pressure during intubation.	
Defend the need to oxygenate and ventilate a patient.	
Defend the necessity of establishing and/or maintaining patency of a patient's airway.	
Comply with standard precautions to defend against infectious and communicable diseases in classroom, labs, and clinical areas.	

©2006 Prentice-Hall Inc.

SECTION 3

Patient Assessment and Respiratory

Fabulous Factoids

Skill Sheets

Overall Scenario Management—Allergy
Patient Assessment: Respiratory—Anaphylaxis
Scenario Intubation—Anaphylaxis
Scenario IV Insertion—Anaphylaxis
Scenario Radio Report—Anaphylaxis
Scenario Patient Care Report (PCR)—Anaphylaxis
Overall Scenario Management—Anaphylaxis

Daily Discussions and Pertinent Points

©2006 Prentice-Hall Inc.

FABULOUS FACTOIDS—PATIENT ASSESSMENT AND RESPIRATORY

Probably 80–95% of your field diagnosis will come from patient history. For medical cases history is the most vital component of the assessment.

Common errors in lung auscultation include trying to listen through clothing (rales), listening in a noisy environment, and misinterpreting stethoscope tubing rubbing against objects and chest hairs as adventitious sounds.

In some people anisocoria (unequal pupils) is normal.

Repeat VS often and look for trends.

The index finger is the most sensitive finger on your hand.

Abnormal respirations require rapid interventions.

The decisions you make as a paramedic will be only as good as the information you gather.

The smallest bones in your body are in your ear—the stirrup is smaller than an ant.

Respiratory emergencies are among the most common emergencies EMS personnel are called upon to treat.

PPOPPA (P4OA)—major causes of dyspnea
> Pulmonary embolism
> Pulmonary edema
> Obstruction
> Pneumothorax
> Pneumonia
> Asthma (COPD)

As acid increases, bodily function decreases.

Patients with COPD who experience a sudden onset of increased dyspnea often have spontaneous pneumothorax. Why? (blebs)

The immune system is responsible for the 3 Rs:
> Recognize
> React
> Remove

Mark Twain gave the following medical advice: "Be careful about reading health books. You may die of a misprint."

Drugs of the Section (see Emergency Drug Quiz Key, pp. xxxi–xxxii):

Ventolin
Epinephrine
Benadryl
Narcan

Pathophysiologies of the Section: 3.01–3.09 (see Checklist, p. 595)

Stethoscope Placement

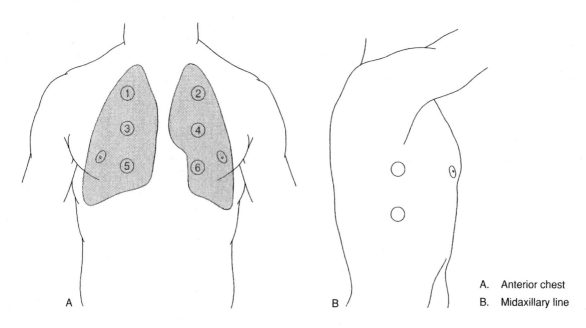

A. Anterior chest
B. Midaxillary line

Student: _____   Examiner: _____

Date: _____

	Done ✓	Not Done
Utilizes appropriate PPE		*
Explains procedure to the patient		
Instructs the patient to open his or her mouth and take slow, deep breaths after each placement of the stethoscope		
Identifies all 16 points of auscultation		*
Identifies where each type of lung sound is normally auscultated (tracheal, bronchial, bronchovesicular, vesicular)		*
Assesses patient's response to intervention		*
Student exhibits competence with skill		

Any items in the Not Done column that are marked with an * are mandatory for the student to complete. A check mark in the Not Done column of an item with an * indicates that the student was unsuccessful and must attempt the skill again to assure competency. Examiners should use a different-color ink for the second attempt.

☐ Successful   ☐ Unsuccessful   Examiner Initials: _____

     ©2006 Prentice-Hall Inc.

Breath Sounds Identification

Student: _____   Examiner: _____

Date: _____

NOTE: Lung sounds to be identified by use of generator, video, or audiotape for consistency.

	Done ✓	Not Done
Identifies rhonchi		*
Identifies wheezes		*
Identifies friction rub		*
Identifies stridor		*
Identifies rales (also known as crackles)		*
Identifies absent lung sounds		*
Assesses patient's response to intervention		*
Student exhibits competence with skill		

Any items in the Not Done column that are marked with an * are mandatory for the student to complete. A check mark in the Not Done column of an item with an * indicates that the student was unsuccessful and must attempt the skill again to assure competency. Examiners should use a different-color ink for the second attempt.

☐ Successful   ☐ Unsuccessful   Examiner Initials: _____

Complete Physical Examination

Student: _____   Examiner: _____

Date: _____

NOTE: Students may use textbook and classmates may "coach" during this skill.

	Done ✓	Not Done
Utilizes appropriate PPE		
Demonstrates examination of the skin, hair, and nails		
Demonstrates examination of the head and neck		
Demonstrates examination of the eyes		
Demonstrates examination of the ears		
Demonstrates assessment of visual acuity		
Demonstrates examination of the nose		
Demonstrates examination of the mouth and pharynx		
Demonstrates examination of the thorax and ventilation		
Demonstrates examination of the posterior chest		
Demonstrates auscultation of the chest		
Demonstrates percussion of the chest		
Demonstrates examination of the anterior chest		
Demonstrates special examination techniques related to the assessment of the chest		
Demonstrates examination of the arterial pulse (location, rate, rhythm, and amplitude)		
Demonstrates examination of the jugular venous pressure and pulsations		
Demonstrates examination of the heart and blood vessels		
Demonstrates special examination techniques of the cardiovascular assessment		
Demonstrates examination of the abdomen		
Demonstrates auscultation of the abdomen		
Verbalizes external visual examination of the female genitalia		
Verbalizes examination of the male genitalia		
Demonstrates examination of the peripheral vascular system		
Demonstrates examination of the musculoskeletal system		
Demonstrates examination of the nervous system		
Student exhibits competence with skill		

This is a knowledge acquisition lab. Student participation is required for successful completion.

☐ Successful   ☐ Unsuccessful   Examiner Initials: _____

©2006 Prentice-Hall Inc.

Glasgow Coma Score (GCS) Evaluation

Student: _____   Examiner: _____

Date: _____

	Done ✓	Not Done
Utilizes appropriate PPE		*
Properly demonstrates and scores EYE OPENING: Spontaneous (4)		
Properly demonstrates and scores EYE OPENING: To speech (3)		
Properly demonstrates and scores EYE OPENING: To pain (2)		
Properly demonstrates and scores EYE OPENING: No response (1)		
Properly demonstrates and scores VERBAL: Oriented (5)		
Properly demonstrates and scores VERBAL: Confused (4)		
Properly demonstrates and scores VERBAL: Inappropriate (3)		
Properly demonstrates and scores VERBAL: Garbled (2)		
Properly demonstrates and scores VERBAL: No verbal response (1)		
Properly demonstrates and scores MOTOR: Obeys command (6)		
Properly demonstrates and scores MOTOR: Localizes pain (5)		
Properly demonstrates and scores MOTOR: Withdraws from pain (4)		
Properly demonstrates and scores MOTOR: Flexion to pain (3)		
Properly demonstrates and scores MOTOR: Extension to pain (2)		
Properly demonstrates and scores MOTOR: No response to pain (1)		
Correctly scores at least four patients with 100% accuracy		*
Student exhibits competence with skill		

Any items in the Not Done column that are marked with an * are mandatory for the student to complete. A check mark in the Not Done column of an item with an * indicates that the student was unsuccessful and must attempt the skill again to assure competency. Examiners should use a different-color ink for the second attempt.

☐ Successful   ☐ Unsuccessful   Examiner Initials: _____

One-Minute Cranial Exam

Student: _____   **Examiner:** _____

Date: _____

	Done ✓	Not Done
Utilizes appropriate PPE		*
Checks CN II and III by direct pupillary response to light		*
Checks CN III, IV, and VI by "H" test for extraocular movements		
Checks CN V by having patient clench teeth, palpates masseter and temporal muscles, and tests sensory to forehead, cheek, and tongue		
Checks CN VII by having patient show teeth		
Checks CN IX and X by having patient say "aaaahhhh" and watching uvula movement and checking gag reflex if not contraindicated		
Checks CN XII by having patient stick out tongue		
Checks CN VIII by Romberg test (balance) and hearing		
Checks CN XI by having patient shrug shoulders and turn head		
Student exhibits competence with skill		

Any items in the Not Done column that are marked with an * are mandatory for the student to complete. A check mark in the Not Done column of an item with an * indicates that the student was unsuccessful and must attempt the skill again to assure competency. Examiners should use a different-color ink for the second attempt.

☐ Successful   ☐ Unsuccessful   Examiner Initials: _____

                    ©2006 Prentice-Hall Inc.

Peak Expiratory Flow Testing

Student: _____   **Examiner:** _____

Date: _____

	Done ✓	Not Done
Utilizes appropriate PPE		*
Obtains patient history for "zone" (green, yellow, red)		
Verifies meter calibrated and zeroed		
Explains procedure to patient		*
Places disposable mouthpiece onto flow meter		*
Has patient take 2–3 deep breaths and exhale fully		*
Has patient breathe in, place mouthpiece, and exhale forcefully		*
Takes reading and repeats process		*
Uses best of the two readings, notes "zone" comparison		*
Approximates patient's norm (10 ml/kg with adjustment for respiratory history)		*
Administers breathing treatment		
Performs peak flow testing again to evaluate treatment efficacy		
Reassesses patient		
Documents procedures and treatment with response		
Student exhibits competence with skill		

Any items in the Not Done column that are marked with an * are mandatory for the student to complete. A check mark in the Not Done column of an item with an * indicates that the student was unsuccessful and must attempt the skill again to assure competency. Examiners should use a different-color ink for the second attempt.

☐ Successful   ☐ Unsuccessful   Examiner Initials: _____

Clinical Decision-Making

Student: _____   **Examiner:** _____

Date: _____

	Done ✓	Not Done
Assesses for scene safety and utilizes appropriate PPE		*
READS the scene:		
Observes general environmental conditions		
Observes immediate surroundings		
Observes interaction among or between family members		
Observes mechanism of injury		*
READS the patient:		
Observes level of consciousness		
Observes skin color		
Observes patient's position and location		
Observes any obvious deformity, asymmetry, or obvious hemorrhage		
Determines chief complaint		
Initiates physical contact to develop rapport and reassurance		
Evaluates patient to assess skin temp and condition		
Evaluates patient to assess radial and carotid pulse rate and quality		
Auscultates for problems with upper and lower airways		
Identifies life threats with ABCs		
Takes full set of vital signs		*
REACTS:		
Manages life threats as found		
Determines most common and serious existing conditions		
Initiates treatment of patient accordingly		*
REEVALUATES:		
Conducts focused and detailed physical assessment		
Assesses response to initial management interventions		
Discovers other less obvious problems		
REVISES:		
Changes or stops interventions that are not working		
Tries new interventions as appropriate		*
REVIEWS:		
Conducts run critique that is honest and critical		
Looks for ways to improve patient management		
Student exhibits competence with skill		

Any items in the Not Done column that are marked with an * are mandatory for the student to complete. A check mark in the Not Done column of an item with an * indicates that the student was unsuccessful and must attempt the skill again to assure competency. Examiners should use a different-color ink for the second attempt.

☐ Successful   ☐ Unsuccessful   Examiner Initials: _____

©2006 Prentice-Hall Inc.

Documentation Skills: Advanced Patient Care Report (PCR)

Student: _____   **Examiner:** _____

Date: _____

	Done ✓	Not Done
Records all pertinent dispatch/scene data, using a consistent format		
Completely identifies all additional resources and personnel		
Documents chief complaint, signs/symptoms, position found, age, sex, and weight		
Identifies and records all pertinent, reportable clinical data for each patient		
Documents SAMPLE and OPQRST if applicable		
Records all pertinent negatives		
Records all pertinent denials		
Records accurate, consistent times and patient information		
Includes relevant oral statements of witnesses, bystanders, and patient in "quotes" when appropriate		
Documents initial assessment findings: airway, breathing, and circulation		
Documents any interventions in initial assessment with patient response		
Documents level of consciousness, GCS (if trauma), and VS		
Documents rapid trauma assessment if applicable		
Documents any interventions in rapid trauma assessment with patient response		
Documents focused history and physical assessment		
Documents any interventions in focused assessment with patient response		
Documents repeat VS (every 5 minutes for critical; every 15 minutes for stable)		
Repeats initial assessment and documents findings		
Records ALL treatments with times and patient response(s) in treatment section		
Documents field impression		
Documents transport to specific facility and transfer of care WITH VERBAL REPORT		
Uses correct grammar, abbreviations, spelling, and terminology		
Writes legibly		
Thoroughly documents refusals, denials of transport, and call cancellations		
Documents patient GCS of 15 PRIOR to signing refusal		
Documents advice given to refusal patient, including "call 9-1-1 for further problems"		
Properly corrects errors and omissions		
Writes cautiously, avoids jargon, opinions, inferences, or any derogatory/libelous remarks		
Signs run report		
Uses EMS supplement form if needed		
Student exhibits competence with skill		

Any items in the Not Done column should be evaluated with student. Check marks in this column do not necessarily mean student was unsuccessful as all lines are not completed on all patients. Evaluation of each PCR should be based on the scenario given.

Student must be able to write an EMS report with consistency and accuracy.

☐ Successful   ☐ Unsuccessful   Examiner Initials: _____

©2006 Prentice-Hall Inc.

Patient Assessment: Respiratory—Dyspnea

Student: _____   Examiner: _____

Date: _____   Scenario: _____

	Done ✓	Not Done
Assesses scene safety and utilizes appropriate PPE		*
OVERALL SCENE EVALUATION		
Medical—determines nature of illness/if trauma involved determines MOI		*
Determines the number of patients, location, obstacles, and requests any additional resources as needed		
Verbalizes general impression of the patient as approaches		*
Considers stabilization/spinal motion restriction of spine if trauma involved		*
INITIAL ASSESSMENT		
Determines responsiveness/level of consciousness/AVPU		*
Opens airway with appropriate technique and assesses airway/ventilation		*
Manages airway/ventilation and applies appropriate oxygen therapy in less than 3 minutes		*
Assesses circulation: radial/carotid pulse, skin color, temperature, condition, and turgor		*
Controls any major bleeding		*
Makes rapid transport decision if indicated		
Initiates IV, obtains BGL, GCS, and complete vital signs		
FOCUSED HISTORY AND PHYSICAL EXAMINATION/RAPID ASSESSMENT		
Obtains SAMPLE history		
Obtains OPQRST for differential diagnosis		
Obtains associated symptoms, pertinent negatives/denials		
Evaluates decision to perform focused exam or completes rapid assessment		*
Vital signs including AVPU (and GCS if trauma)		*
Assesses cardiovascular system including heart sounds, peripheral edema, and peripheral perfusion		*
Assesses pulmonary system including reassessing airway, ventilation, breath sounds, pulse oximetry, chest wall excursion, accessory muscle use, or other signs of distress		*
Assesses neurological system including speech, droop, drift, if applicable, and distal movement and sensation		*
Assesses musculoskeletal and integumentary systems		
Assesses behavioral, psychological, and social aspects of patient and situation		
States field impression of patient—dyspnea (states suspected cause)		*
Verbalizes treatment plan for patient and calls for appropriate intervention(s)—cardiac monitor, meds		*
Reevaluates transport decision		
ONGOING ASSESSMENT		
Repeats initial assessment		*
Repeats vital signs and evaluates trends		*
Evaluates response to treatments		*
Repeats focused assessment regarding patient complaint or injuries		
Gives radio report to receiving facility		
Turns over patient care with verbal report		*
Student exhibits competence with skill		

Any items in the Not Done column that are marked with an * are mandatory for the student to complete. A check mark in the Not Done column of an item with an * indicates that the student was unsuccessful and must attempt the skill again to assure competency. Examiners should use a different-color ink for the second attempt.

☐ Successful   ☐ Unsuccessful   Examiner Initials: _____

    ©2006 Prentice-Hall Inc.

Scenario Intubation—Dyspnea

Student: _____   Examiner: _____

Date: _____

	Done ✓	Not Done
Assesses scene safety and utilizes appropriate PPE		*
Manually opens the airway with technique appropriate for patient condition		*
Checks mouth for blood or potential airway obstruction		*
Suctions or removes loose teeth or foreign materials as needed		
Inserts simple adjunct (oropharyngeal or nasopharyngeal airway)		
Directs assistant to ventilate patient with bag-valve-mask device (room air)		*
Observes chest rise/fall and auscultates bilaterally over lungs for baseline		*
Obtains effective ventilation in less than 30 seconds		*
Attaches oxygen reservoir to bag-valve-mask device and connects to high-flow oxygen		
Ventilates patient and evaluates chest wall/lung compliance		*
Directs assistant to preoxygenate patient		*
Identifies/selects proper equipment for intubation		
Checks laryngoscope light and cuff of ET tube		
Removes all air from cuff and properly inserts stylet if used		
Removes airway adjunct		
Positions patient's head properly and has assistant perform Sellick's maneuver		*
Opens mouth and gently inserts blade while sweeping tongue to side		*
Has assistant maintain Sellick's pressure		
Gently elevates mandible with laryngoscope and visualizes cords		*
Introduces ET tube to side of blade and visualizes tube passing through cords		*
"Threads" ET tube off stylet (if used), maintaining hold on ET tube as stylet removed		
Inflates cuff to proper pressure and disconnects syringe		*
Disconnects mask from bag-valve device and attaches to ET tube without releasing ET tube		
Directs ventilation of patient while maintaining Sellick's maneuver and holding ET tube in place		
Confirms proper placement by auscultation over epigastrium and bilaterally over each lung		*
Directs assistant to release cricoid pressure		*
Secures ET tube		*
Reassesses bilateral lung sounds and compliance		*
Uses secondary device to confirm tube placement		*
Assesses patient's response to intervention		*
Student exhibits competence with skill		

Any items in the Not Done column that are marked with an * are mandatory for the student to complete. A check mark in the Not Done column of an item with an * indicates that the student was unsuccessful and must attempt the skill again to assure competency. Examiners should use a different-color ink for the second attempt.

☐ Successful   ☐ Unsuccessful   Examiner Initials: _____

Scenario IV Insertion—Dyspnea

Student: _____   Examiner: _____

Date: _____

	Done ✓	Not Done
Selects appropriate IV fluid, checking clarity, color, and expiration date		*
Selects appropriate catheter		
Selects appropriate administration set		
Properly inserts IV tubing into the IV bag		*
Prepares administration set (fills drip chamber and flushes tubing)		*
Cuts or tears tape (at any time before venipuncture)		*
Applies constricting band (checks distal pulse to assure NOT a tourniquet)		*
Palpates suitable vein		*
Cleanses site appropriately		*
Utilizes appropriate PPE		*
Inserts catheter with sterile technique		*
Verbalizes flash/blood return and advances catheter slightly farther		*
Occludes vein with finger at distal end of catheter and removes stylet		
Immediately disposes (or verbalizes disposal) of needle/sharp in proper container		
Obtains blood sample or connects IV tubing to catheter		
Obtains BGL (blood glucose level)		*
Releases constricting band		*
Runs IV for a brief period to ensure patency and adjusts flow rate as appropriate		*
Checks IV site for signs of infiltration		*
Secures catheter (tapes securely or verbalizes)		*
Attaches label with size of catheter, date, time, and "prehospital"		*
Assesses patient's response to intervention		*
Student exhibits competence with skill		

Any items in the Not Done column that are marked with an * are mandatory for the student to complete. A check mark in the Not Done column of an item with an * indicates that the student was unsuccessful and must attempt the skill again to assure competency. Examiners should use a different-color ink for the second attempt.

☐ Successful   ☐ Unsuccessful   Examiner Initials: _____

©2006 Prentice-Hall Inc.

Scenario Radio Report—Dyspnea

Student: _____   Examiner: _____

Date: _____

	Done ✓	Not Done
Requests and checks for open channel before speaking		
Presses transmit button 1 second before speaking		
Holds microphone 2–3 in. from mouth		
Speaks slowly and clearly		*
Speaks in a normal voice		
Briefly transmits: Agency, unit designation, identification/name		*
Briefly transmits: Patient's age, sex, weight		*
Briefly transmits: Scene description/mechanism of injury or medical problem		*
Briefly transmits: Chief complaint with brief history of *present* illness		*
Briefly transmits: Associated symptoms (unless able to be deferred to bedside report)		
Briefly transmits: Past medical history (usually deferred to bedside report)		
Briefly transmits: Vital signs		*
Briefly transmits: Level of consciousness/GCS on trauma		*
Briefly transmits: General appearance, distress, cardiac rhythm, blood glucose, and other pertinent findings unable to be deferred to bedside report		
Briefly transmits: Interventions by EMS AND response(s)		*
ETA (the more critical the patient, the earlier you need to notify the receiving facility)		
Does not waste airtime		
Protects privacy of patient		*
Echoes dispatch information and any physician orders		*
Writes down dispatch information or physician orders		
Confirms with facility that message is received		
Demonstrates/verbalizes ability to troubleshoot basic equipment malfunction		
Student exhibits competence with skill		

Any items in the Not Done column that are marked with an * are mandatory for the student to complete. A check mark in the Not Done column of an item with an * indicates that the student was unsuccessful and must attempt the skill again to assure competency. Examiners should use a different-color ink for the second attempt.

☐ Successful   ☐ Unsuccessful   Examiner Initials: _____

Scenario Patient Care Report (PCR)—Dyspnea

Student: _____   Examiner: _____

Date: _____

	Done ✓	Not Done
Records all pertinent dispatch/scene data, using a consistent format		
Completely identifies all additional resources and personnel		
Documents chief complaint, signs/symptoms, position found, age, sex, and weight		
Identifies and records all pertinent, reportable clinical data for each patient		
Documents SAMPLE and OPQRST if applicable		
Records all pertinent negatives		
Records all pertinent denials		
Records accurate, consistent times and patient information		
Includes relevant oral statements of witnesses, bystanders, and patient in "quotes" when appropriate		
Documents initial assessment findings: airway, breathing, and circulation		
Documents any interventions in initial assessment with patient response		
Documents level of consciousness, GCS (if trauma), and VS		
Documents rapid trauma assessment if applicable		
Documents any interventions in rapid trauma assessment with patient response		
Documents focused history and physical assessment		
Documents any interventions in focused assessment with patient response		
Documents repeat VS (every 5 minutes for critical; every 15 minutes for stable)		
Repeats initial assessment and documents findings		
Records ALL treatments with times and patient response(s) in treatment section		
Documents field impression		
Documents transport to specific facility and transfer of care WITH VERBAL REPORT		
Uses correct grammar, abbreviations, spelling, and terminology		
Writes legibly		
Thoroughly documents refusals, denials of transport, and call cancellations		
Documents patient GCS of 15 PRIOR to signing refusal		
Documents advice given to refusal patient, including "call 9-1-1 for further problems"		
Properly corrects errors and omissions		
Writes cautiously, avoids jargon, opinions, inferences, or any derogatory/libelous remarks		
Signs run report		
Uses EMS supplement form if needed		
Student exhibits competence with skill		

Any items in the Not Done column should be evaluated with student. Check marks in this column do not necessarily mean student was unsuccessful as all lines are not completed on all patients. Evaluation of each PCR should be based on the scenario given.

Student must be able to write an EMS report with consistency and accuracy.

☐ Successful   ☐ Unsuccessful   Examiner Initials: _____

©2006 Prentice-Hall Inc.

Overall Scenario Management—Dyspnea

Student: _____   Examiner: _____

Date: _____   Scenario: _____

NOTE: This skill sheet is to be done after the student completes a scenario as the TEAM LEADER. It is to let the student know if he or she is beginning to "put it all together" and use critical thinking skills to manage an EMS call. PLEASE notice that it is graded on a different basis than the basic lab skill sheet.

	Done ✓	Needs to Improve
SCENE MANAGEMENT		
Recognized hazards and controlled scene—safety, crowd, and patient issues		
Recognized hazards, but did not control the scene		
Unsuccessfully attempted to manage the scene	*	
Did not evaluate the scene and took no control of the scene	*	
PATIENT ASSESSMENT		
Performed a timely, organized complete patient assessment		
Performed complete initial, focused, and ongoing assessments, but in a disorganized manner		
Performed an incomplete assessment	*	
Did not perform an initial assessment	*	
PATIENT MANAGEMENT		
Evaluated assessment findings to manage all aspects of patient condition		
Managed the patient's presenting signs and symptoms without considering all of assessment		
Inadequately managed the patient	*	
Did not manage life-threatening conditions	*	
COMMUNICATION		
Communicated well with crew, patient, family, bystanders, and assisting agencies		
Communicated well with patient and crew		
Communicated with patient and crew, but poor communication skills	*	
Unable to communicate effectively	*	
REPORT AND TRANSFER OF CARE		
Identified correct destination for patient transport, gave accurate, brief report over radio, and provided full report at bedside demonstrating thorough understanding of patient condition and pathophysiological processes		
Identified correct destination and gave accurate radio and bedside report, but did not demonstrate understanding of patient condition and pathophysiological processes		
Identified correct destination, but provided inadequate radio and bedside report	*	
Identified inappropriate destination or provided no radio or bedside report	*	
Student exhibits competence with skill		

Any items that are marked with an * indicate the student needs to improve and a check mark should be placed in the right-hand column. A check mark in the right-hand column indicates that the student was unsuccessful and must attempt the skill again to assure competency. Examiners should use a different-color ink for the second attempt.

☐ Successful   ☐ Unsuccessful   Examiner Initials: _____

Patient Assessment: Respiratory—Dyspnea

Student: _____   Examiner: _____

Date: _____   Scenario: _____

	Done ✓	Not Done
Assesses scene safety and utilizes appropriate PPE		*
OVERALL SCENE EVALUATION		
Medical—determines nature of illness/if trauma involved determines MOI		*
Determines the number of patients, location, obstacles, and requests any additional resources as needed		
Verbalizes general impression of the patient as approaches		*
Considers stabilization/spinal motion restriction of spine if trauma involved		*
INITIAL ASSESSMENT		
Determines responsiveness/level of consciousness/AVPU		*
Opens airway with appropriate technique and assesses airway/ventilation		*
Manages airway/ventilation and applies appropriate oxygen therapy in less than 3 minutes		*
Assesses circulation: radial/carotid pulse, skin color, temperature, condition, and turgor		*
Controls any major bleeding		*
Makes rapid transport decision if indicated		
Initiates IV, obtains BGL, GCS, and complete vital signs		
FOCUSED HISTORY AND PHYSICAL EXAMINATION/RAPID ASSESSMENT		
Obtains SAMPLE history		
Obtains OPQRST for differential diagnosis		
Obtains associated symptoms, pertinent negatives/denials		
Evaluates decision to perform focused exam or completes rapid assessment		*
Vital signs including AVPU (and GCS if trauma)		*
Assesses cardiovascular system including heart sounds, peripheral edema, and peripheral perfusion		*
Assesses pulmonary system including reassessing airway, ventilation, breath sounds, pulse oximetry, chest wall excursion, accessory muscle use, or other signs of distress		*
Assesses neurological system including speech, droop, drift, if applicable, and distal movement and sensation		*
Assesses musculoskeletal and integumentary systems		
Assesses behavioral, psychological, and social aspects of patient and situation		
States field impression of patient—dyspnea (states suspected cause)		*
Verbalizes treatment plan for patient and calls for appropriate intervention(s)—cardiac monitor, meds		*
Reevaluates transport decision		
ONGOING ASSESSMENT		
Repeats initial assessment		*
Repeats vital signs and evaluates trends		*
Evaluates response to treatments		*
Repeats focused assessment regarding patient complaint or injuries		
Gives radio report to receiving facility		
Turns over patient care with verbal report		*
Student exhibits competence with skill		

Any items in the Not Done column that are marked with an * are mandatory for the student to complete. A check mark in the Not Done column of an item with an * indicates that the student was unsuccessful and must attempt the skill again to assure competency. Examiners should use a different-color ink for the second attempt.

☐ Successful   ☐ Unsuccessful   Examiner Initials: _____

©2006 Prentice-Hall Inc.

Scenario Intubation—Dyspnea

Student: _____   Examiner: _____

Date: _____

	Done ✓	Not Done
Assesses scene safety and utilizes appropriate PPE		*
Manually opens the airway with technique appropriate for patient condition		*
Checks mouth for blood or potential airway obstruction		*
Suctions or removes loose teeth or foreign materials as needed		
Inserts simple adjunct (oropharyngeal or nasopharyngeal airway)		
Directs assistant to ventilate patient with bag-valve-mask device (room air)		*
Observes chest rise/fall and auscultates bilaterally over lungs for baseline		*
Obtains effective ventilation in less than 30 seconds		*
Attaches oxygen reservoir to bag-valve-mask device and connects to high-flow oxygen		
Ventilates patient and evaluates chest wall/lung compliance		*
Directs assistant to preoxygenate patient		*
Identifies/selects proper equipment for intubation		
Checks laryngoscope light and cuff of ET tube		
Removes all air from cuff and properly inserts stylet if used		
Removes airway adjunct		
Positions patient's head properly and has assistant perform Sellick's maneuver		*
Opens mouth and gently inserts blade while sweeping tongue to side		*
Has assistant maintain Sellick's pressure		
Gently elevates mandible with laryngoscope and visualizes cords		*
Introduces ET tube to side of blade and visualizes tube passing through cords		*
"Threads" ET tube off stylet (if used), maintaining hold on ET tube as stylet removed		
Inflates cuff to proper pressure and disconnects syringe		*
Disconnects mask from bag-valve device and attaches to ET tube without releasing ET tube		
Directs ventilation of patient while maintaining Sellick's maneuver and holding ET tube in place		
Confirms proper placement by auscultation over epigastrium and bilaterally over each lung		*
Directs assistant to release cricoid pressure		*
Secures ET tube		*
Reassesses bilateral lung sounds and compliance		*
Uses secondary device to confirm tube placement		*
Assesses patient's response to intervention		*
Student exhibits competence with skill		

Any items in the Not Done column that are marked with an * are mandatory for the student to complete. A check mark in the Not Done column of an item with an * indicates that the student was unsuccessful and must attempt the skill again to assure competency. Examiners should use a different-color ink for the second attempt.

☐ Successful   ☐ Unsuccessful   Examiner Initials: _____

Scenario IV Insertion—Dyspnea

Student: _____   Examiner: _____

Date: _____

	Done ✓	Not Done
Selects appropriate IV fluid, checking clarity, color, and expiration date		*
Selects appropriate catheter		
Selects appropriate administration set		
Properly inserts IV tubing into the IV bag		*
Prepares administration set (fills drip chamber and flushes tubing)		*
Cuts or tears tape (at any time before venipuncture)		*
Applies constricting band (checks distal pulse to assure NOT a tourniquet)		*
Palpates suitable vein		*
Cleanses site appropriately		*
Utilizes appropriate PPE		*
Inserts catheter with sterile technique		*
Verbalizes flash/blood return and advances catheter slightly farther		*
Occludes vein with finger at distal end of catheter and removes stylet		
Immediately disposes (or verbalizes disposal) of needle/sharp in proper container		
Obtains blood sample or connects IV tubing to catheter		
Obtains BGL (blood glucose level)		*
Releases constricting band		*
Runs IV for a brief period to ensure patency and adjusts flow rate as appropriate		*
Checks IV site for signs of infiltration		*
Secures catheter (tapes securely or verbalizes)		*
Attaches label with size of catheter, date, time, and "prehospital"		*
Assesses patient's response to intervention		*
Student exhibits competence with skill		

Any items in the Not Done column that are marked with an * are mandatory for the student to complete. A check mark in the Not Done column of an item with an * indicates that the student was unsuccessful and must attempt the skill again to assure competency. Examiners should use a different-color ink for the second attempt.

☐ Successful   ☐ Unsuccessful   Examiner Initials: _____

©2006 Prentice-Hall Inc.

Scenario Radio Report—Dyspnea

Student: _____   **Examiner:** _____

Date: _____

	Done ✓	Not Done
Requests and checks for open channel before speaking		
Presses transmit button 1 second before speaking		
Holds microphone 2–3 in. from mouth		
Speaks slowly and clearly		*
Speaks in a normal voice		
Briefly transmits: Agency, unit designation, identification/name		*
Briefly transmits: Patient's age, sex, weight		*
Briefly transmits: Scene description/mechanism of injury or medical problem		*
Briefly transmits: Chief complaint with brief history of *present* illness		*
Briefly transmits: Associated symptoms (unless able to be deferred to bedside report)		
Briefly transmits: Past medical history (usually deferred to bedside report)		
Briefly transmits: Vital signs		*
Briefly transmits: Level of consciousness/GCS on trauma		*
Briefly transmits: General appearance, distress, cardiac rhythm, blood glucose, and other pertinent findings unable to be deferred to bedside report		
Briefly transmits: Interventions by EMS AND response(s)		*
ETA (the more critical the patient, the earlier you need to notify the receiving facility)		
Does not waste airtime		
Protects privacy of patient		*
Echoes dispatch information and any physician orders		*
Writes down dispatch information or physician orders		
Confirms with facility that message is received		
Demonstrates/verbalizes ability to troubleshoot basic equipment malfunction		
Student exhibits competence with skill		

Any items in the Not Done column that are marked with an * are mandatory for the student to complete. A check mark in the Not Done column of an item with an * indicates that the student was unsuccessful and must attempt the skill again to assure competency. Examiners should use a different-color ink for the second attempt.

☐ Successful   ☐ Unsuccessful   Examiner Initials: _____

Scenario Patient Care Report (PCR)—Dyspnea

Student: _____   Examiner: _____

Date: _____

	Done ✓	Not Done
Records all pertinent dispatch/scene data, using a consistent format		
Completely identifies all additional resources and personnel		
Documents chief complaint, signs/symptoms, position found, age, sex, and weight		
Identifies and records all pertinent, reportable clinical data for each patient		
Documents SAMPLE and OPQRST if applicable		
Records all pertinent negatives		
Records all pertinent denials		
Records accurate, consistent times and patient information		
Includes relevant oral statements of witnesses, bystanders, and patient in "quotes" when appropriate		
Documents initial assessment findings: airway, breathing, and circulation		
Documents any interventions in initial assessment with patient response		
Documents level of consciousness, GCS (if trauma), and VS		
Documents rapid trauma assessment if applicable		
Documents any interventions in rapid trauma assessment with patient response		
Documents focused history and physical assessment		
Documents any interventions in focused assessment with patient response		
Documents repeat VS (every 5 minutes for critical; every 15 minutes for stable)		
Repeats initial assessment and documents findings		
Records ALL treatments with times and patient response(s) in treatment section		
Documents field impression		
Documents transport to specific facility and transfer of care WITH VERBAL REPORT		
Uses correct grammar, abbreviations, spelling, and terminology		
Writes legibly		
Thoroughly documents refusals, denials of transport, and call cancellations		
Documents patient GCS of 15 PRIOR to signing refusal		
Documents advice given to refusal patient, including "call 9-1-1 for further problems"		
Properly corrects errors and omissions		
Writes cautiously, avoids jargon, opinions, inferences, or any derogatory/libelous remarks		
Signs run report		
Uses EMS supplement form if needed		
Student exhibits competence with skill		

Any items in the Not Done column should be evaluated with student. Check marks in this column do not necessarily mean student was unsuccessful as all lines are not completed on all patients. Evaluation of each PCR should be based on the scenario given.

Student must be able to write an EMS report with consistency and accuracy.

☐ Successful   ☐ Unsuccessful   Examiner Initials: _____

     ©2006 Prentice-Hall Inc.

Overall Scenario Management—Dyspnea

Student: _____   Examiner: _____

Date: _____   Scenario: _____

NOTE: This skill sheet is to be done after the student completes a scenario as the TEAM LEADER. It is to let the student know if he or she is beginning to "put it all together" and use critical thinking skills to manage an EMS call. PLEASE notice that it is graded on a different basis than the basic lab skill sheet.

	Done	Needs to Improve
SCENE MANAGEMENT		
Recognized hazards and controlled scene—safety, crowd, and patient issues		
Recognized hazards, but did not control the scene		
Unsuccessfully attempted to manage the scene	*	
Did not evaluate the scene and took no control of the scene	*	
PATIENT ASSESSMENT		
Performed a timely, organized complete patient assessment		
Performed complete initial, focused, and ongoing assessments, but in a disorganized manner		
Performed an incomplete assessment	*	
Did not perform an initial assessment	*	
PATIENT MANAGEMENT		
Evaluated assessment findings to manage all aspects of patient condition		
Managed the patient's presenting signs and symptoms without considering all of assessment		
Inadequately managed the patient	*	
Did not manage life-threatening conditions	*	
COMMUNICATION		
Communicated well with crew, patient, family, bystanders, and assisting agencies		
Communicated well with patient and crew		
Communicated with patient and crew, but poor communication skills	*	
Unable to communicate effectively	*	
REPORT AND TRANSFER OF CARE		
Identified correct destination for patient transport, gave accurate, brief report over radio, and provided full report at bedside demonstrating thorough understanding of patient condition and pathophysiological processes		
Identified correct destination and gave accurate radio and bedside report, but did not demonstrate understanding of patient condition and pathophysiological processes		
Identified correct destination, but provided inadequate radio and bedside report	*	
Identified inappropriate destination or provided no radio or bedside report	*	
Student exhibits competence with skill		

Any items that are marked with an * indicate the student needs to improve and a check mark should be placed in the right-hand column. A check mark in the right-hand column indicates that the student was unsuccessful and must attempt the skill again to assure competency. Examiners should use a different-color ink for the second attempt.

☐ Successful   ☐ Unsuccessful   Examiner Initials: _____

Patient Assessment: Respiratory—Allergy

Student: _____   Examiner: _____

Date: _____   Scenario: _____

	Done ✓	Not Done
Assesses scene safety and utilizes appropriate PPE		*
OVERALL SCENE EVALUATION		
Medical—determines nature of illness/if trauma involved determines MOI		*
Determines the number of patients, location, obstacles, and requests any additional resources as needed		
Verbalizes general impression of the patient as approaches		*
Considers stabilization/spinal motion restriction of spine if trauma involved		*
INITIAL ASSESSMENT		
Determines responsiveness/level of consciousness/AVPU		*
Opens airway with appropriate technique and assesses airway/ventilation		*
Manages airway/ventilation and applies appropriate oxygen therapy in less than 3 minutes		*
Assesses circulation: radial/carotid pulse, skin color, temperature, condition, and turgor		*
Controls any major bleeding		*
Makes rapid transport decision if indicated		
Initiates IV, obtains BGL, GCS, and complete vital signs		
FOCUSED HISTORY AND PHYSICAL EXAMINATION/RAPID ASSESSMENT		
Obtains SAMPLE history		
Obtains OPQRST for differential diagnosis		
Obtains associated symptoms, pertinent negatives/denials		
Evaluates decision to perform focused exam or completes rapid assessment		*
Vital signs including AVPU (and GCS if trauma)		*
Assesses cardiovascular system including heart sounds, peripheral edema, and peripheral perfusion		*
Assesses pulmonary system including reassessing airway, ventilation, breath sounds, pulse oximetry, chest wall excursion, accessory muscle use, or other signs of distress		*
Assesses neurological system including speech, droop, drift, if applicable, and distal movement and sensation		*
Assesses musculoskeletal and integumentary systems		
Assesses behavioral, psychological, and social aspects of patient and situation		
States field impression of patient—possible allergic reaction		*
Verbalizes treatment plan for patient and calls for appropriate intervention(s)—Albuterol, Benadryl, Epinephrine prn		*
Reevaluates transport decision		
ONGOING ASSESSMENT		
Repeats initial assessment		*
Repeats vital signs and evaluates trends		*
Evaluates response to treatments		*
Repeats focused assessment regarding patient complaint or injuries		
Gives radio report to receiving facility		
Turns over patient care with verbal report		*
Student exhibits competence with skill		

Any items in the Not Done column that are marked with an * are mandatory for the student to complete. A check mark in the Not Done column of an item with an * indicates that the student was unsuccessful and must attempt the skill again to assure competency. Examiners should use a different-color ink for the second attempt.

☐ Successful   ☐ Unsuccessful   Examiner Initials: _____

     ©2006 Prentice-Hall Inc.

Scenario Intubation—Allergy

Student: _____   Examiner: _____

Date: _____

	Done ✓	Not Done
Assesses scene safety and utilizes appropriate PPE		*
Manually opens the airway with technique appropriate for patient condition		*
Checks mouth for blood or potential airway obstruction		*
Suctions or removes loose teeth or foreign materials as needed		
Inserts simple adjunct (oropharyngeal or nasopharyngeal airway)		
Directs assistant to ventilate patient with bag-valve-mask device (room air)		*
Observes chest rise/fall and auscultates bilaterally over lungs for baseline		*
Obtains effective ventilation in less than 30 seconds		*
Attaches oxygen reservoir to bag-valve-mask device and connects to high-flow oxygen		
Ventilates patient and evaluates chest wall/lung compliance		*
Directs assistant to preoxygenate patient		*
Identifies/selects proper equipment for intubation		
Checks laryngoscope light and cuff of ET tube		
Removes all air from cuff and properly inserts stylet if used		
Removes airway adjunct		
Positions patient's head properly and has assistant perform Sellick's maneuver		*
Opens mouth and gently inserts blade while sweeping tongue to side		*
Has assistant maintain Sellick's pressure		
Gently elevates mandible with laryngoscope and visualizes cords		*
Introduces ET tube to side of blade and visualizes tube passing through cords		*
"Threads" ET tube off stylet (if used), maintaining hold on ET tube as stylet removed		
Inflates cuff to proper pressure and disconnects syringe		*
Disconnects mask from bag-valve device and attaches to ET tube without releasing ET tube		
Directs ventilation of patient while maintaining Sellick's maneuver and holding ET tube in place		
Confirms proper placement by auscultation over epigastrium and bilaterally over each lung		*
Directs assistant to release cricoid pressure		*
Secures ET tube		*
Reassesses bilateral lung sounds and compliance		*
Uses secondary device to confirm tube placement		*
Assesses patient's response to intervention		*
Student exhibits competence with skill		

Any items in the Not Done column that are marked with an * are mandatory for the student to complete. A check mark in the Not Done column of an item with an * indicates that the student was unsuccessful and must attempt the skill again to assure competency. Examiners should use a different-color ink for the second attempt.

☐ Successful   ☐ Unsuccessful   Examiner Initials: _____

Scenario IV Insertion—Allergy

Student: _____   **Examiner:** _____

Date: _____

	Done ✓	Not Done
Selects appropriate IV fluid, checking clarity, color, and expiration date		*
Selects appropriate catheter		
Selects appropriate administration set		
Properly inserts IV tubing into the IV bag		*
Prepares administration set (fills drip chamber and flushes tubing)		*
Cuts or tears tape (at any time before venipuncture)		*
Applies constricting band (checks distal pulse to assure NOT a tourniquet)		*
Palpates suitable vein		*
Cleanses site appropriately		*
Utilizes appropriate PPE		*
Inserts catheter with sterile technique		*
Verbalizes flash/blood return and advances catheter slightly farther		*
Occludes vein with finger at distal end of catheter and removes stylet		
Immediately disposes (or verbalizes disposal) of needle/sharp in proper container		
Obtains blood sample or connects IV tubing to catheter		
Obtains BGL (blood glucose level)		*
Releases constricting band		*
Runs IV for a brief period to ensure patency and adjusts flow rate as appropriate		*
Checks IV site for signs of infiltration		*
Secures catheter (tapes securely or verbalizes)		*
Attaches label with size of catheter, date, time, and "prehospital"		*
Assesses patient's response to intervention		*
Student exhibits competence with skill		

Any items in the Not Done column that are marked with an * are mandatory for the student to complete. A check mark in the Not Done column of an item with an * indicates that the student was unsuccessful and must attempt the skill again to assure competency. Examiners should use a different-color ink for the second attempt.

☐ Successful   ☐ Unsuccessful   Examiner Initials: _____

©2006 Prentice-Hall Inc.

Scenario Radio Report—Allergy

Student: _____   Examiner: _____

Date: _____

	Done ✓	Not Done
Requests and checks for open channel before speaking		
Presses transmit button 1 second before speaking		
Holds microphone 2–3 in. from mouth		
Speaks slowly and clearly		*
Speaks in a normal voice		
Briefly transmits: Agency, unit designation, identification/name		*
Briefly transmits: Patient's age, sex, weight		*
Briefly transmits: Scene description/mechanism of injury or medical problem		*
Briefly transmits: Chief complaint with brief history of *present* illness		*
Briefly transmits: Associated symptoms (unless able to be deferred to bedside report)		
Briefly transmits: Past medical history (usually deferred to bedside report)		
Briefly transmits: Vital signs		*
Briefly transmits: Level of consciousness/GCS on trauma		*
Briefly transmits: General appearance, distress, cardiac rhythm, blood glucose, and other pertinent findings unable to be deferred to bedside report		
Briefly transmits: Interventions by EMS AND response(s)		*
ETA (the more critical the patient, the earlier you need to notify the receiving facility)		
Does not waste airtime		
Protects privacy of patient		*
Echoes dispatch information and any physician orders		*
Writes down dispatch information or physician orders		
Confirms with facility that message is received		
Demonstrates/verbalizes ability to troubleshoot basic equipment malfunction		
Student exhibits competence with skill		

Any items in the Not Done column that are marked with an * are mandatory for the student to complete. A check mark in the Not Done column of an item with an * indicates that the student was unsuccessful and must attempt the skill again to assure competency. Examiners should use a different-color ink for the second attempt.

☐ Successful   ☐ Unsuccessful   Examiner Initials: _____

©2006 Prentice-Hall Inc.

Scenario Patient Care Report (PCR)—Allergy

Student: _____   **Examiner:** _____

Date: _____

	Done ✓	Not Done
Records all pertinent dispatch/scene data, using a consistent format		
Completely identifies all additional resources and personnel		
Documents chief complaint, signs/symptoms, position found, age, sex, and weight		
Identifies and records all pertinent, reportable clinical data for each patient		
Documents SAMPLE and OPQRST if applicable		
Records all pertinent negatives		
Records all pertinent denials		
Records accurate, consistent times and patient information		
Includes relevant oral statements of witnesses, bystanders, and patient in "quotes" when appropriate		
Documents initial assessment findings: airway, breathing, and circulation		
Documents any interventions in initial assessment with patient response		
Documents level of consciousness, GCS (if trauma), and VS		
Documents rapid trauma assessment if applicable		
Documents any interventions in rapid trauma assessment with patient response		
Documents focused history and physical assessment		
Documents any interventions in focused assessment with patient response		
Documents repeat VS (every 5 minutes for critical; every 15 minutes for stable)		
Repeats initial assessment and documents findings		
Records ALL treatments with times and patient response(s) in treatment section		
Documents field impression		
Documents transport to specific facility and transfer of care WITH VERBAL REPORT		
Uses correct grammar, abbreviations, spelling, and terminology		
Writes legibly		
Thoroughly documents refusals, denials of transport, and call cancellations		
Documents patient GCS of 15 PRIOR to signing refusal		
Documents advice given to refusal patient, including "call 9-1-1 for further problems"		
Properly corrects errors and omissions		
Writes cautiously, avoids jargon, opinions, inferences, or any derogatory/libelous remarks		
Signs run report		
Uses EMS supplement form if needed		
Student exhibits competence with skill		

Any items in the Not Done column should be evaluated with student. Check marks in this column do not necessarily mean student was unsuccessful as all lines are not completed on all patients. Evaluation of each PCR should be based on the scenario given.

Student must be able to write an EMS report with consistency and accuracy.

☐ Successful   ☐ Unsuccessful   Examiner Initials: _____

©2006 Prentice-Hall Inc.

Overall Scenario Management—Allergy

Student: _____   Examiner: _____

Date: _____   Scenario: _____

NOTE: This skill sheet is to be done after the student completes a scenario as the TEAM LEADER. It is to let the student know if he or she is beginning to "put it all together" and use critical thinking skills to manage an EMS call. PLEASE notice that it is graded on a different basis than the basic lab skill sheet.

	Done ✓	Needs to Improve
SCENE MANAGEMENT		
Recognized hazards and controlled scene—safety, crowd, and patient issues		
Recognized hazards, but did not control the scene		
Unsuccessfully attempted to manage the scene	*	
Did not evaluate the scene and took no control of the scene	*	
PATIENT ASSESSMENT		
Performed a timely, organized complete patient assessment		
Performed complete initial, focused, and ongoing assessments, but in a disorganized manner		
Performed an incomplete assessment	*	
Did not perform an initial assessment	*	
PATIENT MANAGEMENT		
Evaluated assessment findings to manage all aspects of patient condition		
Managed the patient's presenting signs and symptoms without considering all of assessment		
Inadequately managed the patient	*	
Did not manage life-threatening conditions	*	
COMMUNICATION		
Communicated well with crew, patient, family, bystanders, and assisting agencies		
Communicated well with patient and crew		
Communicated with patient and crew, but poor communication skills	*	
Unable to communicate effectively	*	
REPORT AND TRANSFER OF CARE		
Identified correct destination for patient transport, gave accurate, brief report over radio, and provided full report at bedside demonstrating thorough understanding of patient condition and pathophysiological processes		
Identified correct destination and gave accurate radio and bedside report, but did not demonstrate understanding of patient condition and pathophysiological processes		
Identified correct destination, but provided inadequate radio and bedside report	*	
Identified inappropriate destination or provided no radio or bedside report	*	
Student exhibits competence with skill		

Any items that are marked with an * indicate the student needs to improve and a check mark should be placed in the right-hand column. A check mark in the right-hand column indicates that the student was unsuccessful and must attempt the skill again to assure competency. Examiners should use a different-color ink for the second attempt.

☐ Successful   ☐ Unsuccessful   Examiner Initials: _____

Patient Assessment: Respiratory—Allergy

Student: _____   Examiner: _____

Date: _____   Scenario: _____

	Done ✓	Not Done
Assesses scene safety and utilizes appropriate PPE		*
OVERALL SCENE EVALUATION		
Medical—determines nature of illness/if trauma involved determines MOI		*
Determines the number of patients, location, obstacles, and requests any additional resources as needed		
Verbalizes general impression of the patient as approaches		*
Considers stabilization/spinal motion restriction of spine if trauma involved		*
INITIAL ASSESSMENT		
Determines responsiveness/level of consciousness/AVPU		*
Opens airway with appropriate technique and assesses airway/ventilation		*
Manages airway/ventilation and applies appropriate oxygen therapy in less than 3 minutes		*
Assesses circulation: radial/carotid pulse, skin color, temperature, condition, and turgor		*
Controls any major bleeding		*
Makes rapid transport decision if indicated		
Initiates IV, obtains BGL, GCS, and complete vital signs		
FOCUSED HISTORY AND PHYSICAL EXAMINATION/RAPID ASSESSMENT		
Obtains SAMPLE history		
Obtains OPQRST for differential diagnosis		
Obtains associated symptoms, pertinent negatives/denials		
Evaluates decision to perform focused exam or completes rapid assessment		*
Vital signs including AVPU (and GCS if trauma)		*
Assesses cardiovascular system including heart sounds, peripheral edema, and peripheral perfusion		*
Assesses pulmonary system including reassessing airway, ventilation, breath sounds, pulse oximetry, chest wall excursion, accessory muscle use, or other signs of distress		*
Assesses neurological system including speech, droop, drift, if applicable, and distal movement and sensation		*
Assesses musculoskeletal and integumentary systems		
Assesses behavioral, psychological, and social aspects of patient and situation		
States field impression of patient—possible allergic reaction		*
Verbalizes treatment plan for patient and calls for appropriate intervention(s)—Albuterol, Benadryl, Epinephrine prn		*
Reevaluates transport decision		
ONGOING ASSESSMENT		
Repeats initial assessment		*
Repeats vital signs and evaluates trends		*
Evaluates response to treatments		*
Repeats focused assessment regarding patient complaint or injuries		
Gives radio report to receiving facility		
Turns over patient care with verbal report		*
Student exhibits competence with skill		

Any items in the Not Done column that are marked with an * are mandatory for the student to complete. A check mark in the Not Done column of an item with an * indicates that the student was unsuccessful and must attempt the skill again to assure competency. Examiners should use a different-color ink for the second attempt.

☐ Successful   ☐ Unsuccessful   Examiner Initials: _____

     ©2006 Prentice-Hall Inc.

Scenario Intubation—Allergy

Student: _____   **Examiner:** _____

Date: _____

	Done ✓	Not Done
Assesses scene safety and utilizes appropriate PPE		*
Manually opens the airway with technique appropriate for patient condition		*
Checks mouth for blood or potential airway obstruction		*
Suctions or removes loose teeth or foreign materials as needed		
Inserts simple adjunct (oropharyngeal or nasopharyngeal airway)		
Directs assistant to ventilate patient with bag-valve-mask device (room air)		*
Observes chest rise/fall and auscultates bilaterally over lungs for baseline		*
Obtains effective ventilation in less than 30 seconds		*
Attaches oxygen reservoir to bag-valve-mask device and connects to high-flow oxygen		
Ventilates patient and evaluates chest wall/lung compliance		*
Directs assistant to preoxygenate patient		*
Identifies/selects proper equipment for intubation		
Checks laryngoscope light and cuff of ET tube		
Removes all air from cuff and properly inserts stylet if used		
Removes airway adjunct		
Positions patient's head properly and has assistant perform Sellick's maneuver		*
Opens mouth and gently inserts blade while sweeping tongue to side		*
Has assistant maintain Sellick's pressure		
Gently elevates mandible with laryngoscope and visualizes cords		*
Introduces ET tube to side of blade and visualizes tube passing through cords		*
"Threads" ET tube off stylet (if used), maintaining hold on ET tube as stylet removed		
Inflates cuff to proper pressure and disconnects syringe		*
Disconnects mask from bag-valve device and attaches to ET tube without releasing ET tube		
Directs ventilation of patient while maintaining Sellick's maneuver and holding ET tube in place		
Confirms proper placement by auscultation over epigastrium and bilaterally over each lung		*
Directs assistant to release cricoid pressure		*
Secures ET tube		*
Reassesses bilateral lung sounds and compliance		*
Uses secondary device to confirm tube placement		*
Assesses patient's response to intervention		*
Student exhibits competence with skill		

Any items in the Not Done column that are marked with an * are mandatory for the student to complete. A check mark in the Not Done column of an item with an * indicates that the student was unsuccessful and must attempt the skill again to assure competency. Examiners should use a different-color ink for the second attempt.

☐ Successful   ☐ Unsuccessful   Examiner Initials: _____

Scenario IV Insertion—Allergy

Student: _____   Examiner: _____

Date: _____

	Done ✓	Not Done
Selects appropriate IV fluid, checking clarity, color, and expiration date		*
Selects appropriate catheter		
Selects appropriate administration set		
Properly inserts IV tubing into the IV bag		*
Prepares administration set (fills drip chamber and flushes tubing)		*
Cuts or tears tape (at any time before venipuncture)		*
Applies constricting band (checks distal pulse to assure NOT a tourniquet)		*
Palpates suitable vein		*
Cleanses site appropriately		*
Utilizes appropriate PPE		*
Inserts catheter with sterile technique		*
Verbalizes flash/blood return and advances catheter slightly farther		*
Occludes vein with finger at distal end of catheter and removes stylet		
Immediately disposes (or verbalizes disposal) of needle/sharp in proper container		
Obtains blood sample or connects IV tubing to catheter		
Obtains BGL (blood glucose level)		*
Releases constricting band		*
Runs IV for a brief period to ensure patency and adjusts flow rate as appropriate		*
Checks IV site for signs of infiltration		*
Secures catheter (tapes securely or verbalizes)		*
Attaches label with size of catheter, date, time, and "prehospital"		*
Assesses patient's response to intervention		*
Student exhibits competence with skill		

Any items in the Not Done column that are marked with an * are mandatory for the student to complete. A check mark in the Not Done column of an item with an * indicates that the student was unsuccessful and must attempt the skill again to assure competency. Examiners should use a different-color ink for the second attempt.

☐ Successful   ☐ Unsuccessful   Examiner Initials: _____

©2006 Prentice-Hall Inc.

Scenario Radio Report—Allergy

Student: _____   **Examiner:** _____

Date: _____

	Done ✓	Not Done
Requests and checks for open channel before speaking		
Presses transmit button 1 second before speaking		
Holds microphone 2–3 in. from mouth		
Speaks slowly and clearly		*
Speaks in a normal voice		
Briefly transmits: Agency, unit designation, identification/name		*
Briefly transmits: Patient's age, sex, weight		*
Briefly transmits: Scene description/mechanism of injury or medical problem		*
Briefly transmits: Chief complaint with brief history of *present* illness		*
Briefly transmits: Associated symptoms (unless able to be deferred to bedside report)		
Briefly transmits: Past medical history (usually deferred to bedside report)		
Briefly transmits: Vital signs		*
Briefly transmits: Level of consciousness/GCS on trauma		*
Briefly transmits: General appearance, distress, cardiac rhythm, blood glucose, and other pertinent findings unable to be deferred to bedside report		
Briefly transmits: Interventions by EMS AND response(s)		*
ETA (the more critical the patient, the earlier you need to notify the receiving facility)		
Does not waste airtime		
Protects privacy of patient		*
Echoes dispatch information and any physician orders		*
Writes down dispatch information or physician orders		
Confirms with facility that message is received		
Demonstrates/verbalizes ability to troubleshoot basic equipment malfunction		
Student exhibits competence with skill		

Any items in the Not Done column that are marked with an * are mandatory for the student to complete. A check mark in the Not Done column of an item with an * indicates that the student was unsuccessful and must attempt the skill again to assure competency. Examiners should use a different-color ink for the second attempt.

☐ Successful   ☐ Unsuccessful   Examiner Initials: _____

Scenario Patient Care Report (PCR)—Allergy

Student: _____   Examiner: _____

Date: _____

	Done ✓	Not Done
Records all pertinent dispatch/scene data, using a consistent format		
Completely identifies all additional resources and personnel		
Documents chief complaint, signs/symptoms, position found, age, sex, and weight		
Identifies and records all pertinent, reportable clinical data for each patient		
Documents SAMPLE and OPQRST if applicable		
Records all pertinent negatives		
Records all pertinent denials		
Records accurate, consistent times and patient information		
Includes relevant oral statements of witnesses, bystanders, and patient in "quotes" when appropriate		
Documents initial assessment findings: airway, breathing, and circulation		
Documents any interventions in initial assessment with patient response		
Documents level of consciousness, GCS (if trauma), and VS		
Documents rapid trauma assessment if applicable		
Documents any interventions in rapid trauma assessment with patient response		
Documents focused history and physical assessment		
Documents any interventions in focused assessment with patient response		
Documents repeat VS (every 5 minutes for critical; every 15 minutes for stable)		
Repeats initial assessment and documents findings		
Records ALL treatments with times and patient response(s) in treatment section		
Documents field impression		
Documents transport to specific facility and transfer of care WITH VERBAL REPORT		
Uses correct grammar, abbreviations, spelling, and terminology		
Writes legibly		
Thoroughly documents refusals, denials of transport, and call cancellations		
Documents patient GCS of 15 PRIOR to signing refusal		
Documents advice given to refusal patient, including "call 9-1-1 for further problems"		
Properly corrects errors and omissions		
Writes cautiously, avoids jargon, opinions, inferences, or any derogatory/libelous remarks		
Signs run report		
Uses EMS supplement form if needed		
Student exhibits competence with skill		

Any items in the Not Done column should be evaluated with student. Check marks in this column do not necessarily mean student was unsuccessful as all lines are not completed on all patients. Evaluation of each PCR should be based on the scenario given.

Student must be able to write an EMS report with consistency and accuracy.

☐ Successful   ☐ Unsuccessful   Examiner Initials: _____

©2006 Prentice-Hall Inc.

Overall Scenario Management—Allergy

Student: _____   Examiner: _____

Date: _____   Scenario: _____

NOTE: This skill sheet is to be done after the student completes a scenario as the TEAM LEADER. It is to let the student know if he or she is beginning to "put it all together" and use critical thinking skills to manage an EMS call. PLEASE notice that it is graded on a different basis than the basic lab skill sheet.

	Done ✓	Needs to Improve
SCENE MANAGEMENT		
Recognized hazards and controlled scene—safety, crowd, and patient issues		
Recognized hazards, but did not control the scene		
Unsuccessfully attempted to manage the scene	*	
Did not evaluate the scene and took no control of the scene	*	
PATIENT ASSESSMENT		
Performed a timely, organized complete patient assessment		
Performed complete initial, focused, and ongoing assessments, but in a disorganized manner		
Performed an incomplete assessment	*	
Did not perform an initial assessment	*	
PATIENT MANAGEMENT		
Evaluated assessment findings to manage all aspects of patient condition		
Managed the patient's presenting signs and symptoms without considering all of assessment		
Inadequately managed the patient	*	
Did not manage life-threatening conditions	*	
COMMUNICATION		
Communicated well with crew, patient, family, bystanders, and assisting agencies		
Communicated well with patient and crew		
Communicated with patient and crew, but poor communication skills	*	
Unable to communicate effectively	*	
REPORT AND TRANSFER OF CARE		
Identified correct destination for patient transport, gave accurate, brief report over radio, and provided full report at bedside demonstrating thorough understanding of patient condition and pathophysiological processes		
Identified correct destination and gave accurate radio and bedside report, but did not demonstrate understanding of patient condition and pathophysiological processes		
Identified correct destination, but provided inadequate radio and bedside report	*	
Identified inappropriate destination or provided no radio or bedside report	*	
Student exhibits competence with skill		

Any items that are marked with an * indicate the student needs to improve and a check mark should be placed in the right-hand column. A check mark in the right-hand column indicates that the student was unsuccessful and must attempt the skill again to assure competency. Examiners should use a different-color ink for the second attempt.

☐ Successful   ☐ Unsuccessful   Examiner Initials: _____

Patient Assessment: Respiratory—Anaphylaxis

Student: _____   Examiner: _____

Date: _____   Scenario: _____

	Done ✓	Not Done
Assesses scene safety and utilizes appropriate PPE		*
OVERALL SCENE EVALUATION		
Medical—determines nature of illness/if trauma involved determines MOI		*
Determines the number of patients, location, obstacles, and requests any additional resources as needed		
Verbalizes general impression of the patient as approaches		*
Considers stabilization/spinal motion restriction of spine if trauma involved		*
INITIAL ASSESSMENT		
Determines responsiveness/level of consciousness/AVPU		*
Opens airway with appropriate technique and assesses airway/ventilation		*
Manages airway/ventilation and applies appropriate oxygen therapy in less than 3 minutes		*
Assesses circulation: radial/carotid pulse, skin color, temperature, condition, and turgor		*
Controls any major bleeding		*
Makes rapid transport decision—recognizes anaphylaxis as critical patient		
Initiates IV, obtains BGL, GCS, and complete vital signs		
FOCUSED HISTORY AND PHYSICAL EXAMINATION/RAPID ASSESSMENT		
Obtains SAMPLE history		
Obtains OPQRST for differential diagnosis		
Obtains associated symptoms, pertinent negatives/denials		
Evaluates decision to perform focused exam or completes rapid assessment		*
Vital signs including AVPU (and GCS if trauma)		*
Assesses cardiovascular system including heart sounds, peripheral edema, and peripheral perfusion		*
Assesses pulmonary system including reassessing airway, ventilation, breath sounds, pulse oximetry, chest wall excursion, accessory muscle use, or other signs of distress		*
Assesses neurological system including speech, droop, drift, if applicable, and distal movement and sensation		*
Assesses musculoskeletal and integumentary systems		
Assesses behavioral, psychological, and social aspects of patient and situation		
States field impression of patient—anaphylaxis		*
Verbalizes treatment plan for patient and calls for appropriate intervention(s)—Epinephrine intubation as needed		*
Reevaluates transport decision		
ONGOING ASSESSMENT		
Repeats initial assessment		*
Repeats vital signs and evaluates trends		*
Evaluates response to treatments		*
Repeats focused assessment regarding patient complaint or injuries		
Gives radio report to receiving facility		
Turns over patient care with verbal report		*
Student exhibits competence with skill		

Any items in the Not Done column that are marked with an * are mandatory for the student to complete. A check mark in the Not Done column of an item with an * indicates that the student was unsuccessful and must attempt the skill again to assure competency. Examiners should use a different-color ink for the second attempt.

☐ Successful   ☐ Unsuccessful   Examiner Initials: _____

©2006 Prentice-Hall Inc.

Scenario Intubation—Anaphylaxis

Student: _____   Examiner: _____

Date: _____

	Done ✓	Not Done
Assesses scene safety and utilizes appropriate PPE		*
Manually opens the airway with technique appropriate for patient condition		*
Checks mouth for blood or potential airway obstruction		*
Suctions or removes loose teeth or foreign materials as needed		
Inserts simple adjunct (oropharyngeal or nasopharyngeal airway)		
Directs assistant to ventilate patient with bag-valve-mask device (room air)		*
Observes chest rise/fall and auscultates bilaterally over lungs for baseline		*
Obtains effective ventilation in less than 30 seconds		*
Attaches oxygen reservoir to bag-valve-mask device and connects to high-flow oxygen		
Ventilates patient and evaluates chest wall/lung compliance		*
Directs assistant to preoxygenate patient		*
Identifies/selects proper equipment for intubation		
Checks laryngoscope light and cuff of ET tube		
Removes all air from cuff and properly inserts stylet if used		
Removes airway adjunct		
Positions patient's head properly and has assistant perform Sellick's maneuver		*
Opens mouth and gently inserts blade while sweeping tongue to side		*
Has assistant maintain Sellick's pressure		
Gently elevates mandible with laryngoscope and visualizes cords		*
Introduces ET tube to side of blade and visualizes tube passing through cords		*
"Threads" ET tube off stylet (if used) maintaining hold on ET tube as stylet removed		
Inflates cuff to proper pressure and disconnects syringe		*
Disconnects mask from bag-valve device and attaches to ET tube without releasing ET tube		
Directs ventilation of patient while maintaining Sellick's maneuver and holding ET tube in place		
Confirms proper placement by auscultation over epigastrium and bilaterally over each lung		*
Directs assistant to release cricoid pressure		*
Secures ET tube		*
Reassesses bilateral lung sounds and compliance		*
Uses secondary device to confirm tube placement		*
Assesses patient's response to intervention		*
Student exhibits competence with skill		

Any items in the Not Done column that are marked with an * are mandatory for the student to complete. A check mark in the Not Done column of an item with an * indicates that the student was unsuccessful and must attempt the skill again to assure competency. Examiners should use a different-color ink for the second attempt.

☐ Successful   ☐ Unsuccessful   Examiner Initials: _____

Scenario IV Insertion—Anaphylaxis

Student: _____   Examiner: _____

Date: _____

	Done ✓	Not Done
Selects appropriate IV fluid, checking clarity, color, and expiration date		*
Selects appropriate catheter		
Selects appropriate administration set		
Properly inserts IV tubing into the IV bag		*
Prepares administration set (fills drip chamber and flushes tubing)		*
Cuts or tears tape (at any time before venipuncture)		*
Applies constricting band (checks distal pulse to assure NOT a tourniquet)		*
Palpates suitable vein		*
Cleanses site appropriately		*
Utilizes appropriate PPE		*
Inserts catheter with sterile technique		*
Verbalizes flash/blood return and advances catheter slightly farther		*
Occludes vein with finger at distal end of catheter and removes stylet		
Immediately disposes (or verbalizes disposal) of needle/sharp in proper container		
Obtains blood sample or connects IV tubing to catheter		
Obtains BGL (blood glucose level)		*
Releases constricting band		*
Runs IV for a brief period to ensure patency and adjusts flow rate as appropriate		*
Checks IV site for signs of infiltration		*
Secures catheter (tapes securely or verbalizes)		*
Attaches label with size of catheter, date, time, and "prehospital"		*
Assesses patient's response to intervention		*
Student exhibits competence with skill		

Any items in the Not Done column that are marked with an * are mandatory for the student to complete. A check mark in the Not Done column of an item with an * indicates that the student was unsuccessful and must attempt the skill again to assure competency. Examiners should use a different-color ink for the second attempt.

☐ Successful   ☐ Unsuccessful   Examiner Initials: _____

©2006 Prentice-Hall Inc.

Scenario Radio Report—Anaphylaxis

Student: _____   **Examiner:** _____

Date: _____

	Done ✓	Not Done
Requests and checks for open channel before speaking		
Presses transmit button 1 second before speaking		
Holds microphone 2–3 in. from mouth		
Speaks slowly and clearly		*
Speaks in a normal voice		
Briefly transmits: Agency, unit designation, identification/name		*
Briefly transmits: Patient's age, sex, weight		*
Briefly transmits: Scene description/mechanism of injury or medical problem		*
Briefly transmits: Chief complaint with brief history of *present* illness		*
Briefly transmits: Associated symptoms (unless able to be deferred to bedside report)		
Briefly transmits: Past medical history (usually deferred to bedside report)		
Briefly transmits: Vital signs		*
Briefly transmits: Level of consciousness/GCS on trauma		*
Briefly transmits: General appearance, distress, cardiac rhythm, blood glucose, and other pertinent findings unable to be deferred to bedside report		
Briefly transmits: Interventions by EMS AND response(s)		*
ETA (the more critical the patient, the earlier you need to notify the receiving facility)		
Does not waste airtime		
Protects privacy of patient		*
Echoes dispatch information and any physician orders		*
Writes down dispatch information or physician orders		
Confirms with facility that message is received		
Demonstrates/verbalizes ability to troubleshoot basic equipment malfunction		
Student exhibits competence with skill		

Any items in the Not Done column that are marked with an * are mandatory for the student to complete. A check mark in the Not Done column of an item with an * indicates that the student was unsuccessful and must attempt the skill again to assure competency. Examiners should use a different-color ink for the second attempt.

☐ Successful   ☐ Unsuccessful   Examiner Initials: _____

Scenario Patient Care Report (PCR)—Anaphylaxis

Student: _____   Examiner: _____

Date: _____

	Done ✓	Not Done
Records all pertinent dispatch/scene data, using a consistent format		
Completely identifies all additional resources and personnel		
Documents chief complaint, signs/symptoms, position found, age, sex, and weight		
Identifies and records all pertinent, reportable clinical data for each patient		
Documents SAMPLE and OPQRST if applicable		
Records all pertinent negatives		
Records all pertinent denials		
Records accurate, consistent times and patient information		
Includes relevant oral statements of witnesses, bystanders, and patient in "quotes" when appropriate		
Documents initial assessment findings: airway, breathing, and circulation		
Documents any interventions in initial assessment with patient response		
Documents level of consciousness, GCS (if trauma), and VS		
Documents rapid trauma assessment if applicable		
Documents any interventions in rapid trauma assessment with patient response		
Documents focused history and physical assessment		
Documents any interventions in focused assessment with patient response		
Documents repeat VS (every 5 minutes for critical; every 15 minutes for stable)		
Repeats initial assessment and documents findings		
Records ALL treatments with times and patient response(s) in treatment section		
Documents field impression		
Documents transport to specific facility and transfer of care WITH VERBAL REPORT		
Uses correct grammar, abbreviations, spelling, and terminology		
Writes legibly		
Thoroughly documents refusals, denials of transport, and call cancellations		
Documents patient GCS of 15 PRIOR to signing refusal		
Documents advice given to refusal patient, including "call 9-1-1 for further problems"		
Properly corrects errors and omissions		
Writes cautiously, avoids jargon, opinions, inferences, or any derogatory/libelous remarks		
Signs run report		
Uses EMS supplement form if needed		
Student exhibits competence with skill		

Any items in the Not Done column should be evaluated with student. Check marks in this column do not necessarily mean student was unsuccessful as all lines are not completed on all patients. Evaluation of each PCR should be based on the scenario given.

Student must be able to write an EMS report with consistency and accuracy.

☐ Successful   ☐ Unsuccessful   Examiner Initials: _____

©2006 Prentice-Hall Inc.

Overall Scenario Management—Anaphylaxis

Student: _____   Examiner: _____

Date: _____   Scenario: _____

NOTE: This skill sheet is to be done after the student completes a scenario as the **TEAM LEADER.** It is to let the student know if he or she is beginning to "put it all together" and use critical thinking skills to manage an EMS call. PLEASE notice that it is graded on a different basis than the basic lab skill sheet.

	Done ✓	Needs to Improve
SCENE MANAGEMENT		
Recognized hazards and controlled scene—safety, crowd, and patient issues		
Recognized hazards, but did not control the scene		
Unsuccessfully attempted to manage the scene	*	
Did not evaluate the scene and took no control of the scene	*	
PATIENT ASSESSMENT		
Performed a timely, organized complete patient assessment		
Performed complete initial, focused, and ongoing assessments, but in a disorganized manner		
Performed an incomplete assessment	*	
Did not perform an initial assessment	*	
PATIENT MANAGEMENT		
Evaluated assessment findings to manage all aspects of patient condition		
Managed the patient's presenting signs and symptoms without considering all of assessment		
Inadequately managed the patient	*	
Did not manage life-threatening conditions	*	
COMMUNICATION		
Communicated well with crew, patient, family, bystanders, and assisting agencies		
Communicated well with patient and crew		
Communicated with patient and crew, but poor communication skills	*	
Unable to communicate effectively	*	
REPORT AND TRANSFER OF CARE		
Identified correct destination for patient transport, gave accurate, brief report over radio, and provided full report at bedside demonstrating thorough understanding of patient condition and pathophysiological processes		
Identified correct destination and gave accurate radio and bedside report, but did not demonstrate understanding of patient condition and pathophysiological processes		
Identified correct destination, but provided inadequate radio and bedside report	*	
Identified inappropriate destination or provided no radio or bedside report	*	
Student exhibits competence with skill		

Any items that are marked with an * indicate the student needs to improve and a check mark should be placed in the right-hand column. A check mark in the right-hand column indicates that the student was unsuccessful and must attempt the skill again to assure competency. Examiners should use a different-color ink for the second attempt.

☐ Successful   ☐ Unsuccessful   Examiner Initials: _____

DAILY DISCUSSIONS AND PERTINENT POINTS— PATIENT ASSESSMENT AND RESPIRATORY

Student: _____   **Date:** _____

Instructor: _____

	Instructor Initials
Summarize developmental considerations of various age groups that influence patient interviewing.	
Discuss interviewing considerations used by paramedics in cross-cultural communications.	
Discuss the importance of empathy when obtaining a health history and demonstrate empathy in both lab and clinical areas.	
Discuss the importance of confidentiality when obtaining a health history and demonstrate maintaining confidentiality in both lab and clinical areas.	
Describe the techniques of inspection, palpation, percussion, and auscultation.	
Discuss the need to demonstrate a caring attitude when performing physical examination skills.	
Discuss the importance of a professional appearance and demeanor when performing physical examination skills.	
Appreciate the limitations of conducting a physical exam in the out-of-hospital environment.	
Explain the importance of forming a general impression of the patient.	
Serve as a role model for others, explaining how patient situations affect your evaluation of mechanism of illness or injury.	
Explain the importance of performing an initial assessment.	
Discuss the need to demonstrate a caring attitude when performing an initial assessment.	
Attend to the feelings that patients with medical conditions may be experiencing.	
Value the need for maintaining a professional caring attitude when performing a focused history and physical exam.	
Explain the rationale for the feelings that these patients might be experiencing.	
Discuss the need to demonstrate a caring attitude when performing a detailed physical examination.	
Explain the value of performing an ongoing assessment.	
Recognize and respect the feelings that patients might experience during assessment.	
Explain the value of trending assessment components to other health care professionals who assume care of the patient.	
Appreciate the use of scenarios to develop high-level clinical decision-making skills.	
Defend the importance of considering differentials in patient care.	
Advocate and practice the process of complete patient assessment on all patients.	
Identify internal and external factors that affect a patient/bystander interview conducted by a paramedic.	
Define *communication*.	
Restate the strategies for developing patient rapport.	
Summarize the methods to assess mental status based on interviewing techniques.	
Evaluate the importance of a general survey.	
Describe the examination of skin, hair, and nails.	
Describe the examination of the peripheral vascular system.	
Differentiate normal and abnormal findings of the peripheral vascular system.	
Describe the examination of the musculoskeletal system.	
Differentiate normal and abnormal findings of the musculoskeletal system.	
Describe the examination of the nervous system.	
Differentiate normal and abnormal findings of the nervous system.	
Describe the examination of the cranial nerves.	
Differentiate normal and abnormal findings of the cranial nerves.	
Describe the general guidelines of recording examination information.	
Discuss the considerations of examination of an infant or child.	
Summarize the reasons for forming a general impression of the patient.	

©2006 Prentice-Hall Inc.

Discuss the reasons for repeating the initial assessment as part of the ongoing assessment.	
Describe the components of the ongoing assessment and trending of assessment components.	
Discuss medical identification devices/systems.	
Defend the position that clinical decision-making is the cornerstone of effective paramedic practice.	
Practice facilitating behaviors when thinking under pressure, in both lab and clinical areas.	
Recognize and value the assessment and treatment of patients with respiratory diseases.	
Indicate appreciation for the critical nature of accurate field impressions of patients with respiratory diseases and conditions.	
Explain how effective assessment is critical to clinical decision-making.	
Explain how the paramedic's attitude affects assessment and decision-making.	
Explain how uncooperative patients affect assessment and decision-making.	
Restate the strategies to obtain information from the patient.	
Practice integrating patient history and medications with assessment, diagnostics, and treatment plan, in classroom, lab, and clinical areas.	
Restate the strategies for developing patient rapport.	
Review techniques for a complete physical examination.	
Provide examples of open-ended and closed or direct questions.	
Discuss common errors made by paramedics when interviewing patients.	
Identify the nonverbal skills that are used in patient interviewing.	
List and explain the rationale for carrying the essential patient care items.	
Discuss the reasons for doing a thorough rig checkout whenever you come on duty.	

SECTION 4

✳

IV Therapy and Medication Administration

Fabulous Factoids

Skill Sheets

Medication Administration via Gastric Tube
Guidelines for Parenteral Medications
Subcutaneous Injection
Intramuscular Injection
Cannulation of the External Jugular Vein
Daily Discussions and Pertinent Points

FABULOUS FACTOIDS—IV THERAPY AND MEDICATION ADMINISTRATION

Don't "slap up" a vein—it can cause vasospasm rather than vasodilation. Use warm compresses.

The goal of drug dosing is to achieve the minimum therapeutic effect by the lowest dose possible and avoid toxic effects of higher doses. Start with lower doses of emergency meds. You can always give more.

The fetus does not have a functioning blood–brain barrier. Consider all drugs given to Mom as going to the baby's brain.

Why do you need to know all this information about pharmacology? Example: Because Lidocaine is metabolized in the liver, you might give lower doses to people with liver disease (alcoholics, hepatitis). Because insulin is eliminated by the kidneys, diabetics with renal failure may have higher levels of insulin and become hypoglycemic faster. This information is crucial and relates directly to street medicine.

When discussing drug receptors, think of a "lock and key" analogy.

IV drip rates:

$$\frac{\text{Volume} \times \text{Tubing}}{\text{Time in minutes}} = \text{Drops/minute}$$

Drug dosages:

$$\frac{\text{Desired}}{\text{Have}} \times \text{Solution} = \text{Dose}$$

Drugs of the Section (see Emergency Drug Quiz Key, p. xxxi):

Pitressin
Cardizem
Levophed
50% dextrose
Glucagon
Atropine
Intropin
Lasix

Pathophysiologies of the Section: 4.01–4.05 (see Checklist, p. 595)

SKILL SHEETS

Blood Draw Using a Syringe (1) and Vacutainer (2)

Student: _____   Examiner: _____

Date: _____

	Done ✓	Not Done
Utilizes appropriate PPE		*
Attaches needle to syringe (1) or vacutainer needle to vacutainer (2), obtains all tubes		*
Positions patient with arm extended and palm supine		
Secures constricting band above site, checks presence of distal PMS after application		*
Instructs patient to open and clench fist several times		
Selects appropriate vein		*
Cleanses site with proper technique		*
Anchors vein distal to puncture site and warns patient to expect puncture		*
Inserts needle, bevel up, at 30° angle into vessel, noting vein entry "popping sensation"		*
(1) Slowly draws plunger back, filling syringe (avoids hemolysis) (2) Places vacutainer tube and, holding base of vacutainer SECURELY anchored, presses vacutainer tube onto interior needle, puncturing top of tube		*
Observes blood fill syringe/tubes and gently removes last tube		*
Releases constricting band		*
Places DSD over insertion site and rapidly withdraws needle, placing pressure over site		*
Elevates arm while maintaining pressure (or having patient hold)		
(1) Empties syringe into appropriate tubes		
Properly disposes of sharps		*
Rechecks puncture site for hemostasis and applies dressing		*
Labels all tubes correctly (patient name, date, time, your initials)		*
Student exhibits competence with skill		

Any items in the Not Done column that are marked with an * are mandatory for the student to complete. A check mark in the Not Done column of an item with an * indicates that the student was unsuccessful and must attempt the skill again to assure competency. Examiners should use a different-color ink for the second attempt.

☐ Successful   ☐ Unsuccessful   Examiner Initials: _____

   ©2006 Prentice-Hall Inc.

IV Solution Setup

Student: _____   **Examiner:** _____

Date: _____

	Done ✓	Not Done
Washes hands		*
Selects appropriate IV fluid		*
Removes protective cover and checks fluid, clarity, and expiration date		*
Selects appropriate tubing for IV administration rate		*
Removes safety cover from IV bag port		
Removes safety cover from IV tubing "spike" keeping spike sterile		*
Inverts fluid bag and inserts spike so it pierces membrane		*
Clamps off tubing and pinches drip chamber PRIOR to turning upright		
Flips IV bag and tubing upright, releasing drip chamber only		*
Fills drip chamber to appropriate level		*
Opens clamp and runs IV fluid through to end of tubing		*
Checks IV line for presence of bubbles		*
Student exhibits competence with skill		

Any items in the Not Done column that are marked with an * are mandatory for the student to complete. A check mark in the Not Done column of an item with an * indicates that the student was unsuccessful and must attempt the skill again to assure competency. Examiners should use a different-color ink for the second attempt.

☐ Successful   ☐ Unsuccessful   Examiner Initials: _____

Changing IV Solution Bag

Student: _____   **Examiner:** _____

Date: _____

	Done ✓	Not Done
Utilizes appropriate PPE		*
Checks for correct solution and amount/container size		*
Removes protective cover and checks color, clarity, and expiration date		*
Removes used container from IV pole, clamps tubing, inverts container, and removes tubing		
Removes plug of new container, keeping area sterile		*
Inserts spike through opening of new container, piercing membrane		*
Hangs new container		
Verifies drip chamber still has fluid in it		*
Opens clamp and regulates drip rate		*
Documents correctly		
Assesses patient's response to intervention		*
Student exhibits competence with skill		

Any items in the Not Done column that are marked with an * are mandatory for the student to complete. A check mark in the Not Done column of an item with an * indicates that the student was unsuccessful and must attempt the skill again to assure competency. Examiners should use a different-color ink for the second attempt.

☐ Successful   ☐ Unsuccessful   Examiner Initials: _____

©2006 Prentice-Hall Inc.

Changing IV Bag and Tubing

Student: _____   **Examiner:** _____

Date: _____

	Done ✓	Not Done
Utilizes appropriate PPE		*
Checks for correct solution and amount (size of container)		*
Removes protective cover and checks color, clarity, and expiration date		*
Attaches new administration set to new bag and primes tubing, maintaining sterility		*
Clamps IV now hanging (old one) and loosens tape securing catheter hub		*
Places antiseptic swab under connecting hub of IV catheter and loosens connection		
Observes site for redness/infiltration, tourniquets tip of catheter with finger		*
Removes safety tip of new tubing, keeping area sterile, and exchanges for old tubing		*
Hangs new container		
Verifies drip chamber still has fluid in it		*
Opens clamp and regulates drip rate		*
Cleanses venipuncture site		*
Reapplies sterile dressing and updates label		*
Documents correctly		
Assesses patient's response to intervention		*
Student exhibits competence with skill		

Any items in the Not Done column that are marked with an * are mandatory for the student to complete. A check mark in the Not Done column of an item with an * indicates that the student was unsuccessful and must attempt the skill again to assure competency. Examiners should use a different-color ink for the second attempt.

☐ Successful   ☐ Unsuccessful   Examiner Initials: _____

IV Drip Rate Calculations

Student: _____   **Examiner:** _____

Date: _____

	Done ✓	Not Done
Identifies volume to be infused in 1 hour		
Identifies proper drop factor of tubing to be used		
Calculates number of drops per minute IV is to flow		*
Adjusts drip rate appropriately, timing drops with watch		*
Monitors frequently for rate change		
_____ cc to run over _____ hours (Instructor record problem given)		*
Student uses _____ tubing (Instructor choice)		
Student runs at _____ drops per minute (Instructor counts actual drip rate)		
_____ cc to run over _____ hours (Instructor record problem given)		
Student uses _____ tubing (Instructor choice)		
Student runs at _____ drops per minute (Instructor counts actual drip rate)		
_____ cc to run over _____ hours (Instructor record problem given)		*
Student uses _____ tubing (Instructor choice)		
Student runs at _____ drops per minute (Instructor counts actual drip rate)		
_____ cc to run over _____ hours (Instructor record problem given)		
Student uses _____ tubing (Instructor choice)		
Students runs at _____ drops per minute (Instructor counts actual drip rate)		
<u>100</u> cc to run over <u>20</u> minutes		*
Student uses _____ tubing (Instructor choice)		
Student runs at _____ drops per minute (Instructor counts actual drip rate)		
Student exhibits competence with skill		

Any items in the Not Done column that are marked with an * are mandatory for the student to complete. A check mark in the Not Done column of an item with an * indicates that the student was unsuccessful and must attempt the skill again to assure competency. Examiners should use a different-color ink for the second attempt.

☐ Successful   ☐ Unsuccessful   Examiner Initials: _____

©2006 Prentice-Hall Inc.

Peripheral IV Insertion

Student: _____   Examiner: _____

Date: _____   Scenario: _____

	Done ✓	Not Done
Selects appropriate IV fluid, checking clarity, color, and expiration date		*
Selects appropriate catheter		
Selects appropriate administration set		
Properly inserts IV tubing into the IV bag		*
Prepares administration set (fills drip chamber and flushes tubing)		*
Cuts or tears tape (at any time before venipuncture)		*
Applies constricting band (checks distal pulse to assure NOT a tourniquet)		*
Palpates suitable vein		*
Cleanses site appropriately		*
Utilizes appropriate PPE		*
Inserts catheter with sterile technique		*
Verbalizes flash/blood return and advances catheter slightly farther		*
Occludes vein with finger at distal end of catheter and removes stylet		
Immediately disposes (or verbalizes disposal) of needle/sharp in proper container		
Obtains blood sample or connects IV tubing to catheter		
Obtains BGL (blood glucose level)		*
Releases constricting band		*
Runs IV for a brief period to ensure patency and adjusts flow rate as appropriate		*
Checks IV site for signs of infiltration		*
Secures catheter (tapes securely or verbalizes)		*
Attaches label with size of catheter, date, time, and "prehospital"		*
Assesses patient's response to intervention		*
Student exhibits competence with skill		

Any items in the Not Done column that are marked with an * are mandatory for the student to complete. A check mark in the Not Done column of an item with an * indicates that the student was unsuccessful and must attempt the skill again to assure competency. Examiners should use a different-color ink for the second attempt.

☐ Successful   ☐ Unsuccessful   Examiner Initials: _____

IV Push/Bolus (IVP)

Student: _____   **Examiner:** _____

Date: _____

NOTE: This skill is to be done after student successfully starts IV.
     Check here (_____) if student did not establish a patent IV and do not evaluate IV bolus medication.

Intravenous Bolus Medication	Done ✓	Not Done
Asks patient for known allergies		*
Selects correct medication and checks color, clarity, and expiration date		*
Assures correct concentration of the drug		*
Assembles prefilled syringe correctly and dispels air		
Continues to utilize appropriate PPE		*
Cleanses injection site (Y-port or hub) and inserts syringe		*
Reaffirms medication **and patient allergies**		*
Stops IV flow (pinches tubing)		*
Administers correct dose at proper push rate		*
Disposes/verbalizes disposal of syringe (and needle if used) in proper container		*
Flushes tubing (runs wide open for brief period)		*
Adjusts drip rate to TKO/KVO or previous rate of flow		*
Verbalizes need to observe patient for desired effect/adverse side effects		*
Student exhibits competence with skill		

Any items in the Not Done column that are marked with an * are mandatory for the student to complete. A check mark in the Not Done column of an item with an * indicates that the student was unsuccessful and must attempt the skill again to assure competency. Examiners should use a different-color ink for the second attempt.

☐ Successful   ☐ Unsuccessful   Examiner Initials: _____

©2006 Prentice-Hall Inc.

IV PIGGYBACK (IVPB)

Student: _____   **Examiner:** _____

Date: _____

	Done ✓	Not Done
Utilizes appropriate PPE		*
Obtains patient allergies and explains procedure		*
Checks patency of IV and evaluates site		*
Selects correct IV fluid		*
Checks IV fluid for clarity, expiration date		*
Selects correct medication		*
Checks label for correct drug, concentration, and expiration date		*
Checks medication for cloudiness or discoloration		*
Prepares correct amount of medication		*
Cleanses IV bag injection port and injects medication into bag and mixes thoroughly		*
Labels IV bag with medication added, amount, time, date, and initials		*
Connects administration set and flushes through line		*
Attaches needle or needleless device to line		*
Cleanses medication port on IV line and inserts needle/needleless device		*
Places piggyback bag higher than primary IV bag		*
Stops flow of primary IV line and adjusts IVPB infusion to desired rate		*
Secures needle to IV port (not necessary if needleless device)		
Monitors patient for desired effects and potential complications		*
Correctly records IV piggyback administration and patient response		*
Student exhibits competence with skill		

Any items in the Not Done column that are marked with an * are mandatory for the student to complete. A check mark in the Not Done column of an item with an * indicates that the student was unsuccessful and must attempt the skill again to assure competency. Examiners should use a different-color ink for the second attempt.

☐ Successful   ☐ Unsuccessful   Examiner Initials: _____

IV Pump

Student: _____   **Examiner:** _____

Date: _____

	Done ✓	Not Done
Utilizes appropriate PPE		*
Confirms patency of IV		*
Evaluates IV insertion site		*
Ensures that infusion pump has power source (electric or battery)		
Prepares solution container and pump administration set		*
Primes tubing, if indicated, per manufacturer's recommendations		*
Threads tubing through pump per manufacturer's recommendations		*
Primes tubing at this time if not done previously		
Calculates drip rate for pump infusion (usually in cc/hr)		*
If new IV necessary, performs venipuncture and attaches PRIMED tubing		
Opens tubing clamp and turns on pump		*
Sets IV pump to correct infusion rate and volume per manufacturer's recommendations		*
Sets alarm		*
Assesses patient's response to intervention		*
Monitors at regular intervals		*
Student exhibits competence with skill		

Any items in the Not Done column that are marked with an * are mandatory for the student to complete. A check mark in the Not Done column of an item with an * indicates that the student was unsuccessful and must attempt the skill again to assure competency. Examiners should use a different-color ink for the second attempt.

☐ Successful   ☐ Unsuccessful   Examiner Initials: _____

©2006 Prentice-Hall Inc.

Adjusting IV Pump Rate

Student: _____   **Examiner:** _____

Date: _____

	Done ✓	Not Done
Utilizes appropriate PPE		*
Ensures that infusion pump has power source (electric or battery)		*
Assures patency of IV line and checks insertion site for redness or pain		*
Checks fluid hanging and tubing line		*
Calculates new rate for fluid infusion		*
Checks settings on pump for amount of fluid infused at present rate		*
Checks amount of fluid remaining		*
Pauses IV pump and clamps off tubing leading to patient on patient's side of pump		*
Changes rate on pump according to manufacturer's recommendations		*
Presses start and unclamps tubing to patient		*
Checks IV site as fluid infuses at new rate		*
Checks that pump alarms are on		*
Assesses patient's response to intervention		*
Monitors at regular intervals		
Student exhibits competence with skill		

Any items in the Not Done column that are marked with an * are mandatory for the student to complete. A check mark in the Not Done column of an item with an * indicates that the student was unsuccessful and must attempt the skill again to assure competency. Examiners should use a different-color ink for the second attempt.

☐ Successful   ☐ Unsuccessful   Examiner Initials: _____

Discontinuing an IV

Student: _____   **Examiner:** _____

Date: _____

	Done ✓	Not Done
Utilizes appropriate PPE		*
Explains procedure to patient		
Clamps the infusion tubing		*
Holds catheter firmly and loosens tape or transparent dressing from venipuncture site		*
Places a DSD over insertion site		
Pulls catheter gently in reverse direction of insertion until removed		*
Holds pressure to site firmly until good hemostasis (elevates arm if needed)		*
Applies dressing to puncture site		*
Disposes of used catheter in proper container		*
Assesses patient's response to intervention		*
Student exhibits competence with skill		

Any items in the Not Done column that are marked with an * are mandatory for the student to complete. A check mark in the Not Done column of an item with an * indicates that the student was unsuccessful and must attempt the skill again to assure competency. Examiners should use a different-color ink for the second attempt.

☐ Successful   ☐ Unsuccessful   Examiner Initials: _____

©2006 Prentice-Hall Inc.

Preparing a Medication from an Ampule

Student: _____   Examiner: _____

Date: _____

	Done ✓	Not Done
Checks patient allergies and physician order		*
Selects FILTER needle and appropriately sized syringe for the type of administration/medication		
Secures the hub of the needle to the tip of the syringe		
Selects the correct medication ampule, checks clarity, color, and expiration date		*
Holds ampule with gauze pad and flicks ampule with fingertip to get fluid into base		*
Holds ampule with gauze or alcohol swab on top and base sections		
Breaks ampule open by holding upright and breaking away from self		*
Removes needle cap		
Inserts FILTER needle into ampule so fluid covers bevel		*
Pulls back on plunger and withdraws correct amount of medication		*
Rechecks medication and amount		*
Changes filter needle to proper needle for medication administration		*
Disposes of filter needle in proper container		*
Examines barrel of syringe for air and expels any extra fluid, rechecking amount		*
Prepares to administer medication to patient		*
Student exhibits competence with skill		

Any items in the Not Done column that are marked with an * are mandatory for the student to complete. A check mark in the Not Done column of an item with an * indicates that the student was unsuccessful and must attempt the skill again to assure competency. Examiners should use a different-color ink for the second attempt.

☐ Successful   ☐ Unsuccessful   Examiner Initials: _____

Preparing a Medication from a Vial

Student: _____   Examiner: _____

Date: _____

	Done ✓	Not Done
Checks patient allergies and physician order		*
Selects appropriate needle and syringe for the type of medication and administration route		
Secures the hub of the needle to the tip of the syringe		
Selects the correct medication vial, checks clarity, color, and expiration date		*
Removes protective cap from vial if present		
Cleanses stopper		*
Removes protective cap from needle		
Pulls plunger back to same volume to be withdrawn from vial		*
Inserts needle through center of stopper		*
Injects air from syringe into vial		*
Inverts vial so fluid covers bevel of needle and withdraws correct amount of medication		*
Withdraws needle from stopper and rechecks medication and amount		*
Examines barrel of syringe for air and expels any extra fluid, rechecking amount		*
Prepares to administer medication to patient		
Student exhibits competence with skill		

Any items in the Not Done column that are marked with an * are mandatory for the student to complete. A check mark in the Not Done column of an item with an * indicates that the student was unsuccessful and must attempt the skill again to assure competency. Examiners should use a different-color ink for the second attempt.

☐ Successful   ☐ Unsuccessful   Examiner Initials: _____

©2006 Prentice-Hall Inc.

Preparing a Medication from Two Vials in One Syringe

Student: _____   Examiner: _____

Date: _____

	Done ✓	Not Done
Checks patient allergies and physician order		*
Verifies compatibility of medications to be administered		*
Selects appropriate needle and syringe for amount and type of medication and administration route	.	
Secures the hub of the needle to the tip of the syringe		
Selects the correct medication vials, checks clarity, color, and expiration date of both		*
Removes protective caps from vials if present		
Cleanses stoppers		*
Removes protective cap from needle		
Pulls plunger back to same volume to be withdrawn from vial 1		*
Inserts needle through center of stopper of vial 1, being careful NOT to touch solution		*
Injects air from syringe into vial, being careful NOT to touch solution, and withdraws needle		*
Pulls plunger back to same volume to be withdrawn from vial 2		*
Inserts needle through center of stopper of vial 2		*
Injects air into vial		*
Inverts vial so fluid covers bevel of needle and withdraws correct amount of medication		*
Examines barrel of syringe for air and expels any extra fluid, rechecking amount		*
Withdraws needle from stopper and rechecks medication and amount		*
Inverts vial 1 and inserts needle through center of stopper so fluid covers bevel of needle		*
Pulls plunger back to withdraw correct amount of medication from vial		*
Disposes of vial 1 as it is now contaminated		*
Examines barrel of syringe for air and rechecks total amount		*
Prepares to administer medication to patient		
Student exhibits competence with skill		

Any items in the Not Done column that are marked with an * are mandatory for the student to complete. A check mark in the Not Done column of an item with an * indicates that the student was unsuccessful and must attempt the skill again to assure competency. Examiners should use a different-color ink for the second attempt.

☐ Successful   ☐ Unsuccessful   Examiner Initials: _____

Preparing a Medication from an Ampule and a Vial in One Syringe

Student: _____   Examiner: _____

Date: _____

	Done ✓	Not Done
Checks patient allergies and physician order		*
Verifies compatibility of medications to be administered		*
Selects appropriate needle and syringe for amount and type of medication and administration route		
Secures the hub of the needle to the tip of the syringe		
Selects the correct medication vial, checks clarity, color, and expiration date		*
Removes protective cap from vial if present		
Cleanses stopper		*
Selects the correct medication ampule, checks clarity, color, and expiration date		*
Safely flicks medication into base of ampule		*
Safely breaks open ampule		*
Removes protective cap from needle		
Pulls plunger back to same volume to be withdrawn from vial		*
Inserts needle through center of stopper of vial		*
Injects air into vial		*
Inverts vial so fluid covers bevel of needle and withdraws correct amount of medication		*
Withdraws needle from stopper and rechecks medication and amount		*
Changes needle to FILTER needle, disposing of original needle in proper container		*
Inserts needle into ampule so fluid covers bevel of needle		*
Pulls plunger back to withdraw correct amount of medication from ampule		*
Examines barrel of syringe for air and rechecks total amount of medication		*
Changes needle to appropriate needle for administration, disposing of filter needle in proper container		*
Prepares to administer medication to patient		
Student exhibits competence with skill		

Any items in the Not Done column that are marked with an * are mandatory for the student to complete. A check mark in the Not Done column of an item with an * indicates that the student was unsuccessful and must attempt the skill again to assure competency. Examiners should use a different-color ink for the second attempt.

☐ Successful   ☐ Unsuccessful   Examiner Initials: _____

©2006 Prentice-Hall Inc.

Six Rights of Medication Administration

Student: _____   Examiner: _____

Date: _____

	Done ✓	Not Done
Verbalizes—Right patient		*
Verbalizes—Right medication		*
Verbalizes—Right dosage		*
Verbalizes—Right time		*
Verbalizes—Right route		*
Verbalizes—Right documentation		*
Student exhibits competence with skill		

Any items in the Not Done column that are marked with an * are mandatory for the student to complete. A check mark in the Not Done column of an item with an * indicates that the student was unsuccessful and must attempt the skill again to assure competency. Examiners should use a different-color ink for the second attempt.

☐ Successful   ☐ Unsuccessful   Examiner Initials: _____

Oral (PO) Medication Administration

Student: _____   **Examiner:** _____

Date: _____

	Done ✓	Not Done
Utilizes appropriate PPE		*
Elicits patient allergies and explains procedure		*
Selects correct medication and checks physician order		*
Checks label for correct name, concentration/strength, and expiration date		*
Inspects medication for discoloration, particles, or humidity damage		*
Prepares correct amount of medication and gets something for patient to drink		*
Obtains baseline level of pain or other signs/symptoms medication is to help		*
Gives patient sip of water and verifies patient can swallow		*
Administers medication to patient		*
Checks patient's mouth for absence of medication		*
Monitors patient for desired effects of medication or potential complications		*
Reasesses and documents effects of medication		*
Student exhibits competence with skill		

Any items in the Not Done column that are marked with an * are mandatory for the student to complete. A check mark in the Not Done column of an item with an * indicates that the student was unsuccessful and must attempt the skill again to assure competency. Examiners should use a different-color ink for the second attempt.

☐ Successful   ☐ Unsuccessful   Examiner Initials: _____

©2006 Prentice-Hall Inc.

Sublingual (SL) Medication Administration

Student: _____   Examiner: _____

Date: _____

	Done ✓	Not Done
Utilizes appropriate PPE		*
Checks physician order, elicits patient allergies, and explains procedure		*
Selects correct medication (if NTG asks patient re: performance enhancer use within 24–72 hr)		*
Checks label for correct name, concentration, and expiration date		*
Inspects medication for discoloration, particles, or humidity damage		
Prepares correct amount of medication		*
Obtains baseline level of pain or other signs/symptoms medication is to help		*
Asks patient to open his or her mouth and lift his or her tongue		*
Administers medication under tongue		*
Instructs patient to close mouth		
Monitors patient for desired effects of medication or potential complications		*
Reassesses and documents effects of medication		*
Student exhibits competence with skill		

Any items in the Not Done column that are marked with an * are mandatory for the student to complete. A check mark in the Not Done column of an item with an * indicates that the student was unsuccessful and must attempt the skill again to assure competency. Examiners should use a different-color ink for the second attempt.

☐ Successful   ☐ Unsuccessful   Examiner Initials: _____

Rectal Medication Administration

Student: _____   Examiner: _____

Date: _____

	Done ✓	Not Done
Utilizes appropriate PPE		*
Checks physician order, elicits patient allergies, and explains procedure		*
Selects correct medication		*
Checks label for correct name, concentration/strength, and expiration date		*
Inspects medication for discoloration, particles, or humidity damage		*
Prepares correct amount of medication and removes needle, disposes of needle properly		*
Places hub of 14 gauge catheter (or ET tube) on end of syringe (catheter WITHOUT needle)		*
Obtains baseline level of pain or other signs/symptoms medication is to help		*
Inserts catheter into patient's rectum and injects medication		*
Withdraws catheter and holds patient's buttocks together for minimum 5 minutes		*
Monitors patient for desired effects of medication or potential complications		*
Reassesses and documents effects of medication		*
Student exhibits competence with skill		

Any items in the Not Done column that are marked with an * are mandatory for the student to complete. A check mark in the Not Done column of an item with an * indicates that the student was unsuccessful and must attempt the skill again to assure competency. Examiners should use a different-color ink for the second attempt.

☐ Successful   ☐ Unsuccessful   Examiner Initials: _____

     ©2006 Prentice-Hall Inc.

Metered Dose Inhaler (MDI) Medication Administration

Student: _____   Examiner: _____

Date: _____

	Done ✓	Not Done
Utilizes appropriate PPE		*
Checks physician order (or verifies protocol)		
Obtains proper equipment and medication (checks concentration and expiration date)		*
Checks patient allergies and 6 Rs of medication administration		*
Explains procedure to patient		*
Assembles inhaler, shakes well, and removes mouthpiece cover		*
Blocks patient's nose		
Has patient forcefully exhale, close lips on mouthpiece, then inhale deeply through mouth		*
As patient inhales, presses metered dose inhaler		*
Unblocks nose and holds mouth partially shut (if possible) because patient may cough/sneeze		
Assists patient until he or she can tolerate medication		
Observes for effects and documents administration		
Student exhibits competence with skill		

Any items in the Not Done column that are marked with an * are mandatory for the student to complete. A check mark in the Not Done column of an item with an * indicates that the student was unsuccessful and must attempt the skill again to assure competency. Examiners should use a different-color ink for the second attempt.

☐ Successful   ☐ Unsuccessful   Examiner Initials: _____

Handheld Nebulizer Medication Administration

Student: _____   Examiner: _____

Date: _____

	Done ✓	Not Done
Utilizes appropriate PPE		*
Ensures that patient has adequate tidal volume for procedure		*
Elicits allergy history and explains procedure		*
Checks physician order and selects correct medication		*
Inspects medication for clarity, discoloration, and expiration date		*
Obtains baseline lung sounds		*
Places patient on cardiac monitor		*
Places medication into nebulizer reservoir and tightly closes		*
Hooks appropriate end of nebulizer tubing to oxygen source		*
Secures mouthpiece or mask to reservoir end		
Turns on oxygen until mist flows from mouthpiece of nebulizer		
Places mask on patient or assists patient in holding mouthpiece and closing off nose		
Encourages patient to breathe slowly with adequate tidal volume		
Adjusts oxygen flow so medicated mist is inhaled with each breath, not flowing throughout		*
Monitors patient throughout administration		*
Reassesses patient for change in condition—both desired and undesired effects		*
Correctly documents administration and patient response		
Student exhibits competence with skill		

Any items in the Not Done column that are marked with an * are mandatory for the student to complete. A check mark in the Not Done column of an item with an * indicates that the student was unsuccessful and must attempt the skill again to assure competency. Examiners should use a different-color ink for the second attempt.

☐ Successful   ☐ Unsuccessful   Examiner Initials: _____

©2006 Prentice-Hall Inc.

In-line Nebulizer Medication Administration

Student: _____ **Examiner:** _____

Date: _____

	Done ✓	Not Done
Utilizes appropriate PPE		*
Ensures that patient has adequate tidal volume for procedure		*
Elicits allergy history and explains procedure		
Checks physician order and selects correct medication		*
Inspects medication for clarity, discoloration, and expiration date		*
Obtains baseline lung sounds		*
Places patient on cardiac monitor		*
Places medication into nebulizer reservoir and tightly closes		
Hooks appropriate end of nebulizer tubing to oxygen source		
Hooks up patient circuit to nebulizer reservoir		
Turns on oxygen until mist flows from patient end of nebulizer		*
Places nebulizer circuit to endotracheal tube or CPAP/BiPAP mask		*
Encourages breathing patient to breathe slowly with adequate tidal volume		
Adjusts oxygen flow so medicated mist is inhaled with each breath		*
Ventilates patient without spontaneous respirations, using PPV device		*
Monitors patient throughout administration		*
Reassesses patient for change in condition—both desired and undesired effects		*
Correctly documents administration and patient response		
Student exhibits competence with skill		

Any items in the Not Done column that are marked with an * are mandatory for the student to complete. A check mark in the Not Done column of an item with an * indicates that the student was unsuccessful and must attempt the skill again to assure competency. Examiners should use a different-color ink for the second attempt.

☐ Successful   ☐ Unsuccessful   Examiner Initials: _____

Endotracheal Medication Administration*

Student: _____   Examiner: _____

Date: _____

	Done ✓	Not Done
Utilizes appropriate PPE (including goggles if not a closed administration system)		*
Attempts to obtain patient allergies and explains procedure		*
Checks physician order and selects correct medication		*
Checks label for correct drug, concentration, and expiration date		*
Checks medication for cloudiness or discoloration		*
Prepares correct amount of medication		*
Hyperventilates patient		
Rechecks medication and dosage		*
Removes the ventilation device		
Administers the medication down the ET tube (follows by NS if necessary)		*
Replaces ventilation device and hyperventilates patient		*
Monitors patient for desired effects and potential complications		*
Correctly records medication and patient response		
Student exhibits competence with skill		

Any items in the Not Done column that are marked with an * are mandatory for the student to complete. A check mark in the Not Done column of an item with an * indicates that the student was unsuccessful and must attempt the skill again to assure competency. Examiners should use a different-color ink for the second attempt.

☐ Successful   ☐ Unsuccessful   Examiner Initials: _____

*Endotracheal administration is an alternate route for SELECTED medications (LEAN—Lidocaine, Epinephrine, Atropine, Narcan) when unable to obtain other routes. Vasopressin is also considered as potentially able to be administered via the endotracheal route; however there is no research on the appropriate dosage for administration. (Some like to remember NAVEL for the ET administration of drugs due to vasopressin)

©2006 Prentice-Hall Inc.

Nasal Spray Medication Administration

Student: _____ Examiner: _____

Date: _____

	Done ✓	Not Done
Utilizes appropriate PPE		*
Obtains medication and 4 × 4		*
Checks physician order (or protocol), medication, concentration, and expiration date		*
Checks patient allergies and 6 Rs of medication administration		*
Explains procedure to conscious patient		*
Places nasal spray or nasal administration device to larger nostril		*
Has patient forcefully exhale then inhale deeply		
As patient inhales, presses open nostril closed and squeezes nasal spray into other nostril		
Unblocks closed nostril and holds medicated nostril shut because patient may cough/sneeze		
Holds medicated nostril shut until patient can tolerate medication or has patient "sniff"		
Observes for effects and documents administration		*
Student exhibits competence with skill		

Any items in the Not Done column that are marked with an * are mandatory for the student to complete. A check mark in the Not Done column of an item with an * indicates that the student was unsuccessful and must attempt the skill again to assure competency. Examiners should use a different-color ink for the second attempt.

☐ Successful   ☐ Unsuccessful   Examiner Initials: _____

Eye Medication Administration

Student: _____   **Examiner:** _____

Date: _____

	Done ✓	Not Done
Utilizes appropriate PPE		*
Obtains medication and 4 × 4		*
Checks physician order (or protocol), medication, concentration, and expiration date		*
Checks patient allergies and 6 Rs of medication administration		*
Explains procedure to conscious patient		
Tilts patient's head so that eye receiving medication is down and perpendicular to floor (allowing medication to flow away from inner canthus)		*
Uses 4 × 4 to indirectly pull down lower lid of proper eye, exposing conjunctival membrane		*
Applies proper number of drops to conjunctiva at inner canthus or thin line of ointment along conjunctival sac		*
Has patient close eye to limit tears washing medication out		*
Cleanses around eye		
Observes for effects and documents administration		*
Student exhibits competence with skill		

Any items in the Not Done column that are marked with an * are mandatory for the student to complete. A check mark in the Not Done column of an item with an * indicates that the student was unsuccessful and must attempt the skill again to assure competency. Examiners should use a different-color ink for the second attempt.

☐ Successful   ☐ Unsuccessful   Examiner Initials: _____

©2006 Prentice-Hall Inc.

Medication Administration via Nasogastric Tube

Student: _____   **Examiner:** _____

Date: _____

	Done ✓	Not Done
Utilizes appropriate PPE		*
Obtains equipment: irrigating syringe, water		*
Checks physician order (or protocol), medication, concentration, and expiration date		*
Checks patient allergies and 6 Rs of medication administration		*
Explains procedure to conscious patient or verifies secure airway in unresponsive patient		*
Determines proper tube placement by auscultation over epigastrium of injected AIR		*
Aspirates for stomach contents if present		
Instills medication into NG tube		*
Flushes NG tube with 20–30 cc water or saline		*
Clamps NG tube for 20–30 minutes for medication absorption to take place		*
Observes for effects and documents administration		*
Student exhibits competence with skill		

Any items in the Not Done column that are marked with an * are mandatory for the student to complete. A check mark in the Not Done column of an item with an * indicates that the student was unsuccessful and must attempt the skill again to assure competency. Examiners should use a different-color ink for the second attempt.

☐ Successful   ☐ Unsuccessful   Examiner Initials: _____

Medication Administration via Gastric Tube

Student: _____   Examiner: _____

Date: _____

	Done ✓	Not Done
Checks physician order and utilizes appropriate PPE		*
Obtains equipment: irrigating syringe, water		*
Checks medication, concentration, and expiration date		*
Checks patient allergies and the 6 Rs of medication administration		*
Prepares medication in cone-tipped syringe		*
Explains procedure to conscious patient		
Determines proper tube placement by auscultation over epigastrium of injected AIR		*
Aspirates for stomach contents, if present, irrigates gastric tube		*
Instills medication into gastric tube		*
Flushes gastric tube with 30–50 cc of warm water or saline		*
Clamps gastric tube for 20–30 minutes for medication absorption to take place		*
Observes for effects and documents administration		*
Student exhibits competence with skill		

Any items in the Not Done column that are marked with an * are mandatory for the student to complete. A check mark in the Not Done column of an item with an * indicates that the student was unsuccessful and must attempt the skill again to assure competency. Examiners should use a different-color ink for the second attempt.

☐ Successful   ☐ Unsuccessful   Examiner Initials: _____

©2006 Prentice-Hall Inc.

Guidelines for Parenteral Medications

1. Hold the aseptic swab between the fingers of your nondominant hand.
2. Cleanse site with an antiseptic swab by applying at the center of the site and gently rotating outward in a circular fashion.
3. Grasp the syringe between the forefinger and thumb of your dominant hand. If the angle of insertion is 15° or 45°, rotate the needle so that the bevel is facing up.
4. For a 15° angle insertion: Stretch the skin taut between the thumb and forefinger of the nondominant hand. For a 45° angle insertion: Pinch the skin and subQ tissue between the thumb and forefinger of the nondominant hand. For a 90° angle insertion: Stretch the skin taut between the thumb and forefinger of the nondominant hand.
5. For subQ or IM: Inject the needle firmly and swiftly into the center of the prepared site until needle shaft is fully inserted. For the intradermal: Inject the needle slowly and gently just under the skin surface, with the bevel facing upward.
6. Positioning the patient for the injection:
   - Subcutaneous: position of comfort that exposes the selected site
   - Intramuscular
     Ventrogluteal: supine, lateral, or prone, with knee and hip flexed on the side of the injection site
     Dorsogluteal: prone, with feet turned inward, or lateral, with upper knee and hip flexed and placed over lower leg
     Vastus lateralis: supine with knee slightly flexed
     Deltoid: lower arm flexed but relaxed (i.e., hand on hip)
7. After insertion, gently pull back on the plunger and aspirate to check that needle is NOT in a vein. If blood appears, withdraw and discard the entire syringe. Prepare a new dose of the medication and begin again.

Exceptions to Guidelines

- Heparin is not aspirated.
- Injected heparin is not massaged.

Subcutaneous Injection

Student: _____   **Examiner:** _____

Date: _____

	Done ✓	Not Done
Checks physician order or protocol		*
Obtains patient allergies and explains procedure		*
Selects correct medication		*
Checks label for correct drug, concentration, and expiration date		*
Checks medication for cloudiness or discoloration		*
Obtains baseline level of pain or other signs/symptoms medication is to help		*
Prepares correct amount of medication		*
Utilizes appropriate PPE		*
Chooses and cleanses injection site appropriately		*
Rechecks allergies, correct drug, and correct dose		*
Inserts needle at 45° angle and aspirates for blood return		*
If no blood return, injects medication at appropriate rate		*
Places DSD over insertion site and holds while quickly removing needle		
Massages site, if appropriate, while disposing of needle and syringe in proper container		*
Checks site for hemostasis and applies dressing		*
Monitors patient for desired effects and potential complications		*
Correctly records injection and patient response		
Student exhibits competence with skill		

Any items in the Not Done column that are marked with an * are mandatory for the student to complete. A check mark in the Not Done column of an item with an * indicates that the student was unsuccessful and must attempt the skill again to assure competency. Examiners should use a different-color ink for the second attempt.

☐ Successful   ☐ Unsuccessful   Examiner Initials: _____

©2006 Prentice-Hall Inc.

Intramuscular Injection

Student: _____

Examiner: _____

Date: _____

	Done ✓	Not Done
Checks physician order or protocol		*
Obtains patient allergies and explains procedure		*
Selects correct medication		*
Checks label for correct drug, concentration, and expiration date		*
Checks medication for cloudiness or discoloration		*
Prepares correct amount of medication		*
Obtains baseline level of pain or other signs/symptoms medication is to help		*
Utilizes appropriate PPE		*
Chooses and cleanses injection site appropriately		*
Rechecks allergies, correct drug, and correct dose		*
Inserts needle at 90° angle and aspirates for blood return		*
If no blood return, injects medication at appropriate rate		*
Places DSD over insertion site and holds while quickly removing needle		
Massages site, if appropriate, while disposing of needle and syringe in proper container		*
Checks site for hemostasis and applies dressing		*
Monitors patient for desired effects and potential complications		*
Correctly records injection site and patient response		
Student exhibits competence with skill		

Any items in the Not Done column that are marked with an * are mandatory for the student to complete. A check mark in the Not Done column of an item with an * indicates that the student was unsuccessful and must attempt the skill again to assure competency. Examiners should use a different-color ink for the second attempt.

☐ Successful   ☐ Unsuccessful   Examiner Initials: _____

Cannulation of the External Jugular Vein

Student: _____   Examiner: _____

Date: _____

	Done ✓	Not Done
Utilizes appropriate PPE		*
Checks selected IV fluid to ensure proper fluid and setup		*
Selects appropriate catheter		*
Prepares equipment		
Places patient in Trendelenberg position with head turned to opposite side—DO NOT TURN HEAD IF CERVICAL SPINE TRAUMA SUSPECTED		
Palpates vein and cleanses site appropriately		*
Aligns catheter in caudal direction		*
"Tourniquets" vein with one finger		
Inserts catheter midway between angle of jaw and midclavicular line		*
Notes or verbalizes flashback		
Releases tourniquet finger and occludes catheter tip and vein while removing stylet		*
Obtains BGL and disposes of needle in appropriate container		*
Connects tubing and runs IV to check placement and assure patency		*
Checks site and secures catheter		*
Adjusts flow rate		
Assesses patient's response to intervention		*
Student exhibits competence with skill		

Any items in the Not Done column that are marked with an * are mandatory for the student to complete. A check mark in the Not Done column of an item with an * indicates that the student was unsuccessful and must attempt the skill again to assure competency. Examiners should use a different-color ink for the second attempt.

☐ Successful   ☐ Unsuccessful   Examiner Initials: _____

©2006 Prentice-Hall Inc.

DAILY DISCUSSIONS AND PERTINENT POINTS— IV THERAPY AND MEDICATION ADMINISTRATION

Student: _____   Date: _____

Instructor: _____

	Instructor Initials
Serve as a role model for obtaining a history and identifying classifications of drugs in both lab and clinical areas.	
Defend the administration of drugs by a paramedic to affect positive therapeutic effect.	
Advocate drug education through identification of drug classifications.	
Comply with paramedic standards of medication administration.	
Comply with universal precautions and body substance isolation by utilizing the appropriate PPE in both lab and clinical areas.	
Defend a pharmacologic management plan for medication administration.	
Serve as a role model for medical asepsis in both lab and clinical areas.	
Serve as a role model for advocacy while performing medication administration in both lab and clinical areas.	
Discuss legal aspects affecting medication administration.	
Describe the use of universal precautions and BSI procedures (appropriate PPE) when administering a medication.	
Differentiate among the different dosage forms of oral medications.	
In both lab and clinical areas, serve as a role model for disposing of contaminated items and sharps.	

SECTION 5

*

Trauma

Fabulous Factoids
  MVC Charting

Skill Sheets
  Rapid Extrication
  Rapid Trauma Assessment
  Glasgow Coma Score (GCS) Evaluation
  Rule of Nines
  Helmet Removal
  Infant/Child Car Seat Spinal Motion Restriction (SMR)
  Critical Trauma "Load and Go"
  Pleural Decompression
  Patient Assessment: Trauma—Abdominal Trauma
  Endotracheal Intubation with Suspected Cervical Spine—Abdominal Trauma
  Scenario IV Insertion—Abdominal Trauma
  Scenario Radio Report—Abdominal Trauma
  Scenario Patient Care Report (PCR)—Abdominal Trauma
  Overall Scenario Management—Abdominal Trauma
  Patient Assessment: Trauma—Abuse/Assault
  Endotracheal Intubation with Suspected Cervical Spine—Abuse/Assault
  Scenario IV Insertion—Abuse/Assault
  Scenario Radio Report—Abuse/Assault
  Scenario Patient Care Report (PCR)—Abuse/Assault
  Overall Scenario Management—Abuse/Assault
  Patient Assessment: Trauma—Burn Trauma
  Endotracheal Intubation with Suspected Cervical Spine—Burn Trauma
  Scenario IV Insertion—Burn Trauma
  Scenario Radio Report—Burn Trauma
  Scenario Patient Care Report (PCR)—Burn Trauma
  Overall Scenario Management—Burn Trauma
  Patient Assessment: Trauma—Geriatric Trauma
  Endotracheal Intubation with Suspected Cervical Spine—Geriatric Trauma
  Scenario IV Insertion—Geriatric Trauma
  Scenario Radio Report—Geriatric Trauma
  Scenario Patient Care Report (PCR)—Geriatric Trauma
  Overall Scenario Management—Geriatric Trauma
  Patient Assessment: Trauma—Head/Facial/Neck Trauma
  Endotracheal Intubation with Suspected Cervical Spine—Head/Facial/Neck Trauma
  Scenario IV Insertion—Head/Facial/Neck Trauma

Daily Discussions and Pertinent Points

FABULOUS FACTOIDS—TRAUMA

Patients experiencing loss of consciousness resulting from blunt trauma should be seen by a physician, no matter how stable their condition seems.

In adult vehicle versus pedestrian collisions, there are actually three collisions. The bumper hits the patient, the patient hits the windshield or hood, and the patient hits the ground.

Know the indicators for decision to transport rapidly. Always err on the side of caution. Look for subtle signs of serious injury or deterioration and expect the worst.

Everything and everyone in a moving ambulance should be secured in some way. In a deceleration collision, anything not secured to the vehicle becomes a rapidly moving projectile.

Twenty-five percent of abdominal knife wounds involve the diaphragm and chest.

Primary injuries are most often overlooked while secondary and tertiary are most often treated.

In some people anisocoria (unequal pupils) is normal.

The classic elements in a traffic fatality with head injury include a single-car, high-speed, head-on collision on a dark rural road, and a young intoxicated driver.

The greatest number of spinal cord injuries occurs among males ages 16–20.

The classic case of epidural hematoma is a blow to the side of the head with a brief loss of consciousness, followed by a lucid interval, followed by a decreasing level of consciousness.

If the patient with a subdural hematoma is comatose, mortality is 60–90%.

Often the patient with CSF in the mouth complains of a "salty" taste.

During the French Revolution, Antoine Lavoisier (1743–1794), a French chemist, was beheaded. He told a friend that he would continue blinking for as long as possible to see how long he remained conscious after the guillotine. It was 15 seconds!!

C-spine injuries are present in approximately 1–2% of all blunt trauma patients and in 5–10% of patients with head trauma.

Recreational road bicycling is increasing in popularity, particularly among adults 40–60 years old. During an accident, recreational bicyclists can and do suffer head and brain injuries, even when wearing ANSI- or SNELL-approved helmets. Look on the outside of the victim's helmet for a medical symbol. If there is a symbol, the victim's ID, medical, and insurance information may be found in a folded packet stuck between the helmet's vent holes or inside the helmet.

The decision to immobilize can be made from MOI alone. Absence of clinical findings (pain) does not rule out significant spinal injuries, even in the ambulatory patient.

Most tension pneumos are caused by overuse of positive pressure ventilation with PEEP valves.

Four things can happen with a flail chest: decreased vital lung capacity, increased labored breathing, decreased tidal volume from pain, and lung contusions. All four are bad.

D_5W rapidly diffuses into tissues, with up to two-thirds NS and LR lost to interstitial space within the first hour (3:1 replacement).

The classic Beck's Triad includes muffled heart sounds, decreasing pulse pressure, and JVD.

Look for a classic "hood sign" with traumatic asphyxia—caused by bursting of capillary beds from extreme pressure. It appears from nipple line up.

Severe force is required to fracture ribs 1, 2, and 3 because they are so well protected by surrounding structures. If they are fractured, expect severe underlying injuries and a high mortality rate (up to 30%). There is no such thing prehospital as a simple rib fracture. Any person with a fractured rib should be suspected of having associated lung tissue damage.

Aortic rupture is the most common cause of sudden death from MVC or long fall.

High mortality from blunt abdominal trauma is due to the widespread energy transfer and injury pattern.

Some 90% of hip dislocations are posterior, usually from "down and under" MVC.

Your elderly stroke patient cannot speak and cannot complain. She is lying on the floor. What should you check for? (wrists for Colles' fracture from trying to break fall)

©2006 Prentice-Hall Inc.

Whether you are immobilizing the finger or the entire body, the principles are the same: Align the bone ends with a rigid splint; immobilize the adjacent joints; perform distal PMS on all extremities before and after splinting.

You're born with 300 bones, but have only 206 as an adult—some fuse.

Some 40% of knee dislocations have associated vascular damage, whereas 25–35% have associated nerve damage.

Never test the depth of a river with both feet.

Emergency departments treat twice as many left-handed people for accidents as right-handed people.

Drugs of the Section (see Emergency Drug Quiz Key, p. xxxi):

Lidocaine
Morphine

Pathophysiologies of the Section: 5.01–5.41 (see Checklist, pp. 595–596)

MVC Charting

Many calls for an MVC (motor vehicle collision) result in multiple patients and multiple patient refusals. There is no time in the middle of the call to document each patient, all the patients' information, MOI (mechanism of injury), where they were sitting, whether or not they were restrained, and do a fully complete narrative. The following diagram will provide much of this information at a glance. On the sheet on which you record the patient information and vitals, just draw this diagram to use later for your documentation.

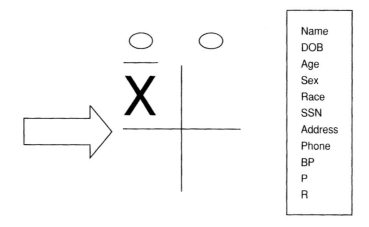

The two circles at the top are the headlights; therefore, the X (patient) indicates that *this* patient was the DRIVER of the vehicle with damage to the driver's side, but slightly behind the driver (as indicated by the arrow). The LINE in front of the driver (a seat belt) means the patient WAS restrained; NO line means NOT restrained, and a line with a ? means it is unknown whether restrained. You should always be consistent in documentation of restraints, no matter the "system" you use. This diagram also works with multiple patients who are injured and transported; just put the suspected injuries or findings in a note to the left of the diagram.

©2006 Prentice-Hall Inc.

SKILL SHEETS

Rapid Extrication

Student: _____   **Examiner:** _____

Date: _____

	Done ✓	Not Done
Utilizes appropriate PPE		*
Directs assistant to place/maintain head in a neutral in-line position from behind		*
Directs same assistant to maintain manual SMR of the head/cervical spine		*
Does a rapid survey, then applies the appropriately sized cervical collar		*
Assesses distal PMS prior to movement		*
Slides LBB slightly beneath patient's buttocks with 2nd assistant/PD supporting end of LBB		*
Directs 3rd assistant to enter vehicle from opposite side to support legs during swivel		
Maintaining right arm down axial spine and left arm laterally angled across chest, swivels patient approximately 45° until C-spine motion restriction can be taken by either 2nd or 3rd assistant (after moving around), then transferred back after C-spine person moves out from behind patient		*
Swivels patient (as a unit) remainder of distance and, still supporting axial spine, lowers to LBB		*
Directs team to carefully slide the patient completely onto the LBB with axial movement only		*
Reassesses distal PMS		*
Directs/assists with careful movement of LBB to stretcher		*
Secures patient to LBB, then LBB to stretcher		*
Assesses patient's response to intervention		*
Student exhibits competence with skill		

Any items in the Not Done column that are marked with an * are mandatory for the student to complete. A check mark in the Not Done column of an item with an * indicates that the student was unsuccessful and must attempt the skill again to assure competency. Examiners should use a different-color ink for the second attempt.

☐ Successful   ☐ Unsuccessful   Examiner Initials: _____

©2006 Prentice-Hall Inc.

Rapid Trauma Assessment

Student: _____   **Examiner:** _____

Date: _____

	Done ✓	Not Done
Utilizes appropriate PPE		*
Assures C-spine motion restriction is being maintained		*
In assessing areas students may use DCAP-BTLS* or DCAP-BLS-TIC*		
HEAD: Palpates the head and facial bones		*
Periodically examines gloves for blood		
NECK: Inspects and palpates anterior neck		*
Checks for tracheal deviation		
Checks for subcutaneous emphysema		
Checks for jugular vein distention		
Inspects and palpates posterior neck for tenderness, irregularity, or edema		
CHEST: Inspects and palpates the chest		*
Checks for subcutaneous emphysema		
Auscultates both lungs		
ABDOMEN: Inspects and palpates abdomen		*
PELVIS: Evaluates the pelvic ring		*
EXTREMITIES: Inspects and palpates all four extremities		
Evaluates distal neurovascular function—PMS (pulse, movement, sensation)		*
POSTERIOR: Inspects and palpates posterior trunk, buttocks		*
Student exhibits competence with skill		

Any items in the Not Done column that are marked with an * are mandatory for the student to complete. A check mark in the Not Done column of an item with an * indicates that the student was unsuccessful and must attempt the skill again to assure competency. Examiners should use a different-color ink for the second attempt.

☐ Successful   ☐ Unsuccessful   Examiner Initials: _____

- DCAP-BTLS: Deformities, Contusions, Abrasions, Penetrations, Burns, Tenderness, Lacerations, Swelling
- DCAP-BLS-TIC: Deformities, Contusions, Abrasions, Penetrations, Burns, Lacerations, Swelling, Tenderness, Instability, Crepitus

Glasgow Coma Score (GCS) Evaluation

Student: _____   **Examiner:** _____

Date: _____

	Done ✓	Not Done
Utilizes appropriate PPE		*
Properly demonstrates and scores EYE OPENING: Spontaneous (4)		
Properly demonstrates and scores EYE OPENING: To speech (3)		
Properly demonstrates and scores EYE OPENING: To pain (2)		
Properly demonstrates and scores EYE OPENING: No response (1)		
Properly demonstrates and scores VERBAL: Oriented (5)		
Properly demonstrates and scores VERBAL: Confused (4)		
Properly demonstrates and scores VERBAL: Inappropriate (3)		
Properly demonstrates and scores VERBAL: Garbled (2)		
Properly demonstrates and scores VERBAL: No verbal response (1)		
Properly demonstrates and scores MOTOR: Obeys command (6)		
Properly demonstrates and scores MOTOR: Localizes pain (5)		
Properly demonstrates and scores MOTOR: Withdraws from pain (4)		
Properly demonstrates and scores MOTOR: Flexion to pain (3)		
Properly demonstrates and scores MOTOR: Extension to pain (2)		
Properly demonstrates and scores MOTOR: No response to pain (1)		
Correctly scores four patients with 100% accuracy		*
Student exhibits competence with skill		

Any items in the Not Done column that are marked with an * are mandatory for the student to complete. A check mark in the Not Done column of an item with an * indicates that the student was unsuccessful and must attempt the skill again to assure competency. Examiners should use a different-color ink for the second attempt.

☐ Successful   ☐ Unsuccessful   Examiner Initials: _____

©2006 Prentice-Hall Inc.

Rule of Nines

Student: _____   **Examiner:** _____

Date: _____

	Done ✓	Not Done
Properly scores an infant's arm (9%)		
Properly scores an adult's back (18%)		
Properly scores an infant's leg (14%)		
Properly scores an adult's chest and abdomen (18%)		
Properly scores an infant's head (18%)		
Properly scores an adult's head (9%)		
Properly scores an infant's back (18%)		
Properly scores an adult's leg (18%)		
Properly scores an infant's genitalia (1%)		
Properly scores an adult's arm (9%)		
Properly scores an infant's chest and abdomen (18%)		
Properly scores an adult's genitalia (1%)		
Properly scores three simulated patients with 100% accuracy		*
Student exhibits competence with skill		

Any items in the Not Done column that are marked with an * are mandatory for the student to complete. A check mark in the Not Done column of an item with an * indicates that the student was unsuccessful and must attempt the skill again to assure competency. Examiners should use a different-color ink for the second attempt.

☐ Successful   ☐ Unsuccessful   Examiner Initials: _____

Helmet Removal

Student: _____   **Examiner:** _____

Date: _____

	Done ✓	Not Done
Utilizes appropriate PPE		*
Positions self above or behind the victim, stabilizes the head and neck by holding the helmet and the patient's neck		*
Directs assistant to remove the chin strap		
Directs assistant to assume stabilization by placing one hand under neck and occiput, the other on anterior neck with thumb on one angle of the mandible, index and middle fingers on other angle of mandible		*
Removes the helmet by pulling out laterally on each side to clear the ears and then up to remove. Tilts full-face helmet back to clear the nose		*
After removal of helmet, assumes motion restriction of neck by grasping head on either side with fingers holding one angle of jaw and occiput		
Directs placement of properly sized cervical collar		
Assesses patient's response to intervention		*
Student exhibits competence with skill		

Any items in the Not Done column that are marked with an * are mandatory for the student to complete. A check mark in the Not Done column of an item with an * indicates that the student was unsuccessful and must attempt the skill again to assure competency. Examiners should use a different-color ink for the second attempt.

☐ Successful   ☐ Unsuccessful   Examiner Initials: _____

©2006 Prentice-Hall Inc.

Infant/Child Car Seat Spinal Motion Restriction (SMR)

Student: _____   Examiner: _____

Date: _____

	Done ✓	Not Done
Assesses scene safety and utilizes appropriate PPE		*
Takes or directs manual cervical SMR		*
Performs ABCD, including distal PMS		*
Checks car seat integrity		*
Performs visual and palpation body survey for glass and DCAP-BLS-TIC/DCAP-BTLS		*
Resecures restraining straps		
Restricts motion of head and shoulders with towel roll or blanket roll as appropriate		*
Reassesses ABCD and distal PMS		*
Secures car seat to rescue unit		*
Monitors infant/child at all times		*
Student exhibits competence with skill		

Any items in the Not Done column that are marked with an * are mandatory for the student to complete. A check mark in the Not Done column of an item with an * indicates that the student was unsuccessful and must attempt the skill again to assure competency. Examiners should use a different-color ink for the second attempt.

☐ Successful   ☐ Unsuccessful   Examiner Initials: _____

©2006 Prentice-Hall Inc.

Critical Trauma "Load and Go"

Student: _____   **Examiner:** _____

Date: _____

	Done ✓	Not Done
Airway obstruction that cannot be quickly relieved by mechanical methods such as suction, forceps, or intubation		
Traumatic cardiopulmonary arrest		

Conditions resulting in possible inadequate breathing:
    Large open chest wound (sucking chest wound)
    Large flail chest
    Tension pneumothorax
    Major blunt chest injury		

Shock		
Head injury with unconsciousness, unequal pupils, or decreasing level of consciousness		
Tender or rigid abdomen		
Unstable pelvis		
Bilateral femur fractures		
Able to verbalize 9 out of 11 criteria		*
Student exhibits competence with skill		

Any items in the Not Done column that are marked with an * are mandatory for the student to complete. A check mark in the Not Done column of an item with an * indicates that the student was unsuccessful and must attempt the skill again to assure competency. Examiners should use a different-color ink for the second attempt.

☐ Successful   ☐ Unsuccessful   Examiner Initials: _____

©2006 Prentice-Hall Inc.

Pleural Decompression

Student: _____   **Examiner:** _____

Date: _____

	Done ✓	Not Done
Utilizes appropriate PPE		
Evaluates patient for indications and obtains baseline lung sounds and assessment		
Prepares equipment (14 gauge 2¼-in. catheter-over-needle) and explains procedure to patient		
Palpates at 2nd intercostal space/midclavicular line		
Cleanses site appropriately		
Inserts needle at superior border of 3rd rib, avoiding artery, vein, and nerve		
Advances until feels "pop" and rush of air released		
Checks patient for improvement in clinical status		
Removes needle from catheter, disposes of needle properly, and applies flutter valve		
Secures in place		
Reassesses patient for improvement		
Documents procedure and response correctly		
Student exhibits competence with skill		

Any items in the Not Done column that are marked with an * are mandatory for the student to complete. A check mark in the Not Done column of an item with an * indicates that the student was unsuccessful and must attempt the skill again to assure competency. Examiners should use a different-color ink for the second attempt.

☐ Successful   ☐ Unsuccessful   Examiner Initials: _____

Patient Assessment: Trauma—Abdominal Trauma

Student: _____   Examiner: _____

Date: _____   Scenario: _____

	Done ✓	Not Done
Assesses scene safety and utilizes appropriate PPE		*
OVERALL SCENE EVALUATION		
Trauma—assesses mechanism of injury/if medical component determines nature of illness		*
Determines the number of patients, location, obstacles, and requests any additional resources as needed		
Verbalizes general impression of the patient as approaches		*
Stabilizes C-spine/spinal motion restriction (SMR) of spine		*
INITIAL ASSESSMENT/RESUSCITATION		
Determines responsiveness/level of consciousness/AVPU		*
Opens airway with appropriate technique and assesses airway/ventilation		*
Manages airway/ventilation and applies appropriate oxygen therapy in less than 3 minutes		*
Assesses circulation: radial/carotid pulse, skin color, temperature, condition, and turgor		*
Controls any major bleeding		*
Makes rapid transport decision		*
Obtains IV (2 if indicated), BGL, GCS, and complete vital signs		
RAPID TRAUMA ASSESSMENT (If patient is Trauma Alert or Load and Go)		
Assesses abdomen		
Rapidly palpates each extremity, assessing for obvious injuries and distal PMS		
Provides spinal motion restriction (SMR) on long backboard (LBB), checking posterior torso and legs		
Secures head LAST		
Identifies patient problem: abdominal trauma		*
Loads patient/initiates transport (to appropriate LZ or to appropriate facility) in less than 10 minutes		*
Reassesses ABCs and interventions		*
FOCUSED HISTORY AND PHYSICAL ASSESSMENT		
Reassesses interventions and further assesses injuries found		
Obtains vital signs and GCS (Glasgow Coma Score)		
Obtains SAMPLE history		
Inspects and palpates head, facial, and neck regions		
Inspects, palpates, and auscultates chest/thorax		
Inspects and palpates abdomen and pelvis		
Inspects and palpates upper and lower extremities, checking distal PMS		
Inspects and palpates posterior torso		
Manages all injuries/wounds appropriately—moist dressing for evisceration, stabilize impaled object, etc.		
Repeats initial assessment, vital signs, and evaluates trends		*
Evaluates response to interventions/treatments		*
Performs ongoing assessment (VS every 5 minutes for critical patient/every 15 minutes for stable patient)		
Gives radio report to receiving facility		
Turns over patient care with verbal report		*
Student exhibits competence with skill		

Any items in the Not Done column that are marked with an * are mandatory for the student to complete. A check mark in the Not Done column of an item with an * indicates that the student was unsuccessful and must attempt the skill again to assure competency. Examiners should use a different-color ink for the second attempt.

☐ Successful   ☐ Unsuccessful   Examiner Initials: _____

©2006 Prentice-Hall Inc.

Endotracheal Intubation with Suspected Cervical Spine— Abdominal Trauma

Student: _____   **Examiner:** _____

Date: _____

	Done ✓	Not Done
Determines scene safety and utilizes appropriate PPE		*
Opens the airway manually with trauma jaw-thrust while assistant maintains C-spine SMR		*
Checks mouth for blood or potential airway obstruction		*
Suctions or removes loose teeth or foreign materials as needed		
Inserts simple airway adjunct (oropharyngeal airway)		
Directs assistant to ventilate patient with bag-valve-mask device (room air)		*
Observes chest rise/fall and auscultates bilaterally over lungs for baseline		*
Obtains effective ventilation in less than 30 seconds		*
Attaches oxygen reservoir to bag-valve-mask device and connects to high-flow oxygen		
Ventilates patient and evaluates chest wall/lung compliance		*
Directs assistant to preoxygenate patient with assistant maintaining C-spine SMR		*
Identifies/selects proper equipment for intubation		
Checks laryngoscope light and cuff of ET tube		
Removes all air from cuff and properly inserts stylet if used		
Directs assistant to face patient and establish cervical spine SMR from front		
Intubating paramedic sits behind patient on ground with legs straddling patient's shoulders		
Moves up until patient's head is secured		
Removes OPA and directs assistant to perform Sellick's maneuver		*
Opens mouth and gently inserts blade while sweeping tongue to side		*
Gently elevates mandible with laryngoscope and leans backward to visualize cords		*
Inserts ET tube and visualizes as tube is advanced through cords		*
"Threads" ET tube off stylet (if used), maintaining hold on ET tube as stylet removed		
Inflates cuff to proper pressure and disconnects syringe		*
Disconnects mask from bag-valve device and attaches to ET tube without releasing ET tube		
Directs ventilation of patient while maintaining Sellick's maneuver and holding ET tube in place		
Confirms proper placement by auscultation over epigastrium and bilaterally over each lung		*
Directs assistant to release cricoid pressure		*
Secures ET tube		*
Reassesses bilateral lung sounds and compliance		*
Uses secondary device to confirm tube placement		*
Assesses patient's response to intervention		*
Student exhibits competence with skill		

Any items in the Not Done column that are marked with an * are mandatory for the student to complete. A check mark in the Not Done column of an item with an * indicates that the student was unsuccessful and must attempt the skill again to assure competency. Examiners should use a different-color ink for the second attempt.

☐ Successful   ☐ Unsuccessful   Examiner Initials: _____

©2006 Prentice-Hall Inc.

Scenario IV Insertion—Abdominal Trauma

Student: _____   Examiner: _____

Date: _____

	Done ✓	Not Done
Selects appropriate IV fluid, checking clarity, color, and expiration date		*
Selects appropriate catheter		
Selects appropriate administration set		
Properly inserts IV tubing into the IV bag		*
Prepares administration set (fills drip chamber and flushes tubing)		*
Cuts or tears tape (at any time before venipuncture)		*
Applies constricting band (checks distal pulse to assure NOT a tourniquet)		*
Palpates suitable vein		*
Cleanses site appropriately		*
Utilizes appropriate PPE		*
Inserts catheter with sterile technique		*
Verbalizes flash/blood return and advances catheter slightly farther		*
Occludes vein with finger at distal end of catheter and removes stylet		
Immediately disposes (or verbalizes disposal) of needle/sharp in proper container		
Obtains blood sample or connects IV tubing to catheter		
Obtains BGL (blood glucose level)		*
Releases constricting band		*
Runs IV for a brief period to ensure patency and adjusts flow rate as appropriate		*
Checks IV site for signs of infiltration		*
Secures catheter (tapes securely or verbalizes)		*
Attaches label with size of catheter, date, time, and "prehospital"		*
Assesses patient's response to intervention		*
Student exhibits competence with skill		

Any items in the Not Done column that are marked with an * are mandatory for the student to complete. A check mark in the Not Done column of an item with an * indicates that the student was unsuccessful and must attempt the skill again to assure competency. Examiners should use a different-color ink for the second attempt.

☐ Successful   ☐ Unsuccessful   Examiner Initials: _____

©2006 Prentice-Hall Inc.

Scenario Radio Report—Abdominal Trauma

Student: _____   **Examiner:** _____

Date: _____

	Done ✓	Not Done
Requests and checks for open channel before speaking		
Presses transmit button 1 second before speaking		
Holds microphone 2–3 in. from mouth		
Speaks slowly and clearly		*
Speaks in a normal voice		
Briefly transmits: Agency, unit designation, identification/name		*
Briefly transmits: Patient's age, sex, weight		*
Briefly transmits: Scene description/mechanism of injury or medical problem		*
Briefly transmits: Chief complaint with brief history of *present* illness		*
Briefly transmits: Associated symptoms (unless able to be deferred to bedside report)		
Briefly transmits: Past medical history (usually deferred to bedside report)		
Briefly transmits: Vital signs		*
Briefly transmits: Level of consciousness/GCS on trauma		*
Briefly transmits: General appearance, distress, cardiac rhythm, blood glucose, and other pertinent findings unable to be deferred to bedside report		
Briefly transmits: Interventions by EMS AND response(s)		*
ETA (the more critical the patient, the earlier you need to notify the receiving facility)		
Does not waste airtime		
Protects privacy of patient		*
Echoes dispatch information and any physician orders		*
Writes down dispatch information or physician orders		
Confirms with facility that message is received		
Demonstrates/verbalizes ability to troubleshoot basic equipment malfunction		
Student exhibits competence with skill		

Any items in the Not Done column that are marked with an * are mandatory for the student to complete. A check mark in the Not Done column of an item with an * indicates that the student was unsuccessful and must attempt the skill again to assure competency. Examiners should use a different-color ink for the second attempt.

☐ Successful   ☐ Unsuccessful   Examiner Initials: _____

Scenario Patient Care Report (PCR)—Abdominal Trauma

Student: _____   Examiner: _____

Date: _____

	Done ✓	Not Done
Records all pertinent dispatch/scene data, using a consistent format		
Completely identifies all additional resources and personnel		
Documents chief complaint, signs/symptoms, position found, age, sex, and weight		
Identifies and records all pertinent, reportable clinical data for each patient		
Documents SAMPLE and OPQRST if applicable		
Records all pertinent negatives		
Records all pertinent denials		
Records accurate, consistent times and patient information		
Includes relevant oral statements of witnesses, bystanders, and patient in "quotes" when appropriate		
Documents initial assessment findings: airway, breathing, and circulation		
Documents any interventions in initial assessment with patient response		
Documents level of consciousness, GCS (if trauma), and VS		
Documents rapid trauma assessment if applicable		
Documents any interventions in rapid trauma assessment with patient response		
Documents focused history and physical assessment		
Documents any interventions in focused assessment with patient response		
Documents repeat VS (every 5 minutes for critical; every 15 minutes for stable)		
Repeats initial assessment and documents findings		
Records ALL treatments with times and patient response(s) in treatment section		
Documents field impression		
Documents transport to specific facility and transfer of care WITH VERBAL REPORT		
Uses correct grammar, abbreviations, spelling, and terminology		
Writes legibly		
Thoroughly documents refusals, denials of transport, and call cancellations		
Documents patient GCS of 15 PRIOR to signing refusal		
Documents advice given to refusal patient, including "call 9-1-1 for further problems"		
Properly corrects errors and omissions		
Writes cautiously, avoids jargon, opinions, inferences, or any derogatory/libelous remarks		
Signs run report		
Uses EMS supplement form if needed		
Student exhibits competence with skill		

Any items in the Not Done column should be evaluated with student. Check marks in this column do not necessarily mean student was unsuccessful as all lines are not completed on all patients. Evaluation of each PCR should be based on the scenario given.

Student must be able to write an EMS report with consistency and accuracy.

☐ Successful   ☐ Unsuccessful   Examiner Initials: _____

    ©2006 Prentice-Hall Inc.

Overall Scenario Management—Abdominal Trauma

Student: _____   Examiner: _____

Date: _____   Scenario: _____

NOTE: This skill sheet is to be done after the student completes a scenario as the TEAM LEADER. It is to let the student know if he or she is beginning to "put it all together" and use critical thinking skills to manage an EMS call. PLEASE notice that it is graded on a different basis than the basic lab skill sheet.

	Done ✓	Needs to Improve
SCENE MANAGEMENT		
Recognized hazards and controlled scene—safety, crowd, and patient issues		
Recognized hazards, but did not control the scene		
Unsuccessfully attempted to manage the scene	*	
Did not evaluate the scene and took no control of the scene	*	
PATIENT ASSESSMENT		
Performed a timely, organized complete patient assessment		
Performed complete initial, focused, and ongoing assessments, but in a disorganized manner		
Performed an incomplete assessment	*	
Did not perform an initial assessment	*	
PATIENT MANAGEMENT		
Evaluated assessment findings to manage all aspects of patient condition		
Managed the patient's presenting signs and symptoms without considering all of assessment		
Inadequately managed the patient	*	
Did not manage life-threatening conditions	*	
COMMUNICATION		
Communicated well with crew, patient, family, bystanders, and assisting agencies		
Communicated well with patient and crew		
Communicated with patient and crew, but poor communication skills	*	
Unable to communicate effectively	*	
REPORT AND TRANSFER OF CARE		
Identified correct destination for patient transport, gave accurate, brief report over radio, and provided full report at bedside demonstrating thorough understanding of patient condition and pathophysiological processes		
Identified correct destination and gave accurate radio and bedside report, but did not demonstrate understanding of patient condition and pathophysiological processes		
Identified correct destination, but provided inadequate radio and bedside report	*	
Identified inappropriate destination or provided no radio or bedside report	*	
Student exhibits competence with skill		

Any items that are marked with an * indicate the student needs to improve and a check mark should be placed in the right-hand column. A check mark in the right-hand column indicates that the student was unsuccessful and must attempt the skill again to assure competency. Examiners should use a different-color ink for the second attempt.

☐ Successful   ☐ Unsuccessful   Examiner Initials: _____

Patient Assessment: Trauma—Abuse/Assault

Student: _____   Examiner: _____

Date: _____   Scenario: _____

	Done ✓	Not Done
Assesses scene safety and utilizes appropriate PPE		*
OVERALL SCENE EVALUATION		
Trauma—assesses mechanism of injury/if medical component determines nature of illness		*
Determines the number of patients, location, obstacles, and requests any additional resources as needed		
Verbalizes general impression of the patient as approaches		*
Stabilizes C-spine/spinal motion restriction (SMR) of spine		*
INITIAL ASSESSMENT/RESUSCITATION		
Determines responsiveness/level of consciousness/AVPU		*
Opens airway with appropriate technique and assesses airway/ventilation		*
Manages airway/ventilation and applies appropriate oxygen therapy in less than 3 minutes		*
Assesses circulation: radial/carotid pulse, skin color, temperature, condition, and turgor		*
Controls any major bleeding		*
Makes rapid transport decision		*
Obtains IV (2 if indicated), BGL, GCS, and complete vital signs		
RAPID TRAUMA ASSESSMENT (If patient is Trauma Alert or Load and Go)		
Assesses abdomen		
Rapidly palpates each extremity, assessing for obvious injuries and distal PMS		
Provides spinal motion restriction (SMR) on long backboard (LBB), checking posterior torso and legs		
Secures head LAST		
Identifies patient problem: assault/suspected abuse (specify injuries)		*
Loads patient/initiates transport (to appropriate LZ or to appropriate facility) in less than 10 minutes		*
Reassesses ABCs and interventions		*
FOCUSED HISTORY AND PHYSICAL ASSESSMENT		
Reassesses interventions and further assesses injuries found		
Obtains vital signs and GCS (Glasgow Coma Score)		
Obtains SAMPLE history		
Inspects and palpates head, facial, and neck regions		
Inspects, palpates, and auscultates chest/thorax		
Inspects and palpates abdomen and pelvis		
Inspects and palpates upper and lower extremities, checking distal PMS		
Inspects and palpates posterior torso		
Manages all injuries/wounds appropriately—verbalize possible need to notify ABUSE HOTLINE or PD		
Repeats initial assessment, vital signs, and evaluates trends		*
Evaluates response to interventions/treatments		*
Performs ongoing assessment (VS every 5 minutes for critical patient/every 15 minutes for stable patient)		
Gives radio report to receiving facility		
Turns over patient care with verbal report—OBTAINS NAME OF PERSON NOTIFIED OF SUSPECTED ABUSE		*
Student exhibits competence with skill		

Any items in the Not Done column that are marked with an * are mandatory for the student to complete. A check mark in the Not Done column of an item with an * indicates that the student was unsuccessful and must attempt the skill again to assure competency. Examiners should use a different-color ink for the second attempt.

☐ Successful   ☐ Unsuccessful   Examiner Initials: _____

©2006 Prentice-Hall Inc.

Endotracheal Intubation with Suspected Cervical Spine—Abuse/Assault

Student: _____   Examiner: _____

Date: _____

	Done ✓	Not Done
Determines scene safety and utilizes appropriate PPE		*
Opens the airway manually with trauma jaw-thrust while assistant maintains C-spine SMR		*
Checks mouth for blood or potential airway obstruction		*
Suctions or removes loose teeth or foreign materials as needed		
Inserts simple airway adjunct (oropharyngeal airway)		
Directs assistant to ventilate patient with bag-valve-mask device (room air)		*
Observes chest rise/fall and auscultates bilaterally over lungs for baseline		*
Obtains effective ventilation in less than 30 seconds		*
Attaches oxygen reservoir to bag-valve-mask device and connects to high-flow oxygen		
Ventilates patient and evaluates chest wall/lung compliance		*
Directs assistant to preoxygenate patient with assistant maintaining C-spine SMR		*
Identifies/selects proper equipment for intubation		
Checks laryngoscope light and cuff of ET tube		
Removes all air from cuff and properly inserts stylet if used		
Directs assistant to face patient and establish cervical spine SMR from front		
Intubating paramedic sits behind patient on ground with legs straddling patient's shoulders		
Moves up until patient's head is secured		
Removes OPA and directs assistant to perform Sellick's maneuver		*
Opens mouth and gently inserts blade while sweeping tongue to side		*
Gently elevates mandible with laryngoscope and leans backward to visualize cords		*
Inserts ET tube and visualizes as tube is advanced through cords		*
"Threads" ET tube off stylet (if used), maintaining hold on ET tube as stylet removed		
Inflates cuff to proper pressure and disconnects syringe		*
Disconnects mask from bag-valve device and attaches to ET tube without releasing ET tube		
Directs ventilation of patient while maintaining Sellick's maneuver and holding ET tube in place		
Confirms proper placement by auscultation over epigastrium and bilaterally over each lung		*
Directs assistant to release cricoid pressure		*
Secures ET tube		*
Reassesses bilateral lung sounds and compliance		*
Uses secondary device to confirm tube placement		*
Assesses patient's response to intervention		*
Student exhibits competence with skill		

Any items in the Not Done column that are marked with an * are mandatory for the student to complete. A check mark in the Not Done column of an item with an * indicates that the student was unsuccessful and must attempt the skill again to assure competency. Examiners should use a different-color ink for the second attempt.

☐ Successful   ☐ Unsuccessful   Examiner Initials: _____

Scenario IV Insertion—Abuse/Assault

Student: _____   Examiner: _____

Date: _____

	Done ✓	Not Done
Selects appropriate IV fluid, checking clarity, color, and expiration date		*
Selects appropriate catheter		
Selects appropriate administration set		
Properly inserts IV tubing into the IV bag		*
Prepares administration set (fills drip chamber and flushes tubing)		*
Cuts or tears tape (at any time before venipuncture)		*
Applies constricting band (checks distal pulse to assure NOT a tourniquet)		*
Palpates suitable vein		*
Cleanses site appropriately		*
Utilizes appropriate PPE		*
Inserts catheter with sterile technique		*
Verbalizes flash/blood return and advances catheter slightly farther		*
Occludes vein with finger at distal end of catheter and removes stylet		
Immediately disposes (or verbalizes disposal) of needle/sharp in proper container		
Obtains blood sample or connects IV tubing to catheter		
Obtains BGL (blood glucose level)		*
Releases constricting band		*
Runs IV for a brief period to ensure patency and adjusts flow rate as appropriate		*
Checks IV site for signs of infiltration		*
Secures catheter (tapes securely or verbalizes)		*
Attaches label with size of catheter, date, time, and "prehospital"		*
Assesses patient's response to intervention		*
Student exhibits competence with skill		

Any items in the Not Done column that are marked with an * are mandatory for the student to complete. A check mark in the Not Done column of an item with an * indicates that the student was unsuccessful and must attempt the skill again to assure competency. Examiners should use a different-color ink for the second attempt.

☐ Successful   ☐ Unsuccessful   Examiner Initials: _____

©2006 Prentice-Hall Inc.

Scenario Radio Report—Abuse/Assault

Student: _____   **Examiner:** _____

Date: _____

	Done ✓	Not Done
Requests and checks for open channel before speaking		
Presses transmit button 1 second before speaking		
Holds microphone 2–3 in. from mouth		
Speaks slowly and clearly		*
Speaks in a normal voice		
Briefly transmits: Agency, unit designation, identification/name		*
Briefly transmits: Patient's age, sex, weight		*
Briefly transmits: Scene description/mechanism of injury or medical problem		*
Briefly transmits: Chief complaint with brief history of *present* illness		*
Briefly transmits: Associated symptoms (unless able to be deferred to bedside report)		
Briefly transmits: Past medical history (usually deferred to bedside report)		
Briefly transmits: Vital signs		*
Briefly transmits: Level of consciousness/GCS on trauma		*
Briefly transmits: General appearance, distress, cardiac rhythm, blood glucose, and other pertinent findings unable to be deferred to bedside report		
Briefly transmits: Interventions by EMS AND response(s)		*
ETA (the more critical the patient, the earlier you need to notify the receiving facility)		
Does not waste airtime		
Protects privacy of patient		*
Echoes dispatch information and any physician orders		*
Writes down dispatch information or physician orders		
Confirms with facility that message is received		
Demonstrates/verbalizes ability to troubleshoot basic equipment malfunction		
Student exhibits competence with skill		

Any items in the Not Done column that are marked with an * are mandatory for the student to complete. A check mark in the Not Done column of an item with an * indicates that the student was unsuccessful and must attempt the skill again to assure competency. Examiners should use a different-color ink for the second attempt.

☐ Successful   ☐ Unsuccessful   Examiner Initials: _____

Scenario Patient Care Report (PCR)—Abuse/Assault

Student: _____   **Examiner:** _____

Date: _____

	Done ✓	Not Done
Records all pertinent dispatch/scene data, using a consistent format		
Completely identifies all additional resources and personnel		
Documents chief complaint, signs/symptoms, position found, age, sex, and weight		
Identifies and records all pertinent, reportable clinical data for each patient		
Documents SAMPLE and OPQRST if applicable		
Records all pertinent negatives		
Records all pertinent denials		
Records accurate, consistent times and patient information		
Includes relevant oral statements of witnesses, bystanders, and patient in "quotes" when appropriate		
Documents initial assessment findings: airway, breathing, and circulation		
Documents any interventions in initial assessment with patient response		
Documents level of consciousness, GCS (if trauma), and VS		
Documents rapid trauma assessment if applicable		
Documents any interventions in rapid trauma assessment with patient response		
Documents focused history and physical assessment		
Documents any interventions in focused assessment with patient response		
Documents repeat VS (every 5 minutes for critical; every 15 minutes for stable)		
Repeats initial assessment and documents findings		
Records ALL treatments with times and patient response(s) in treatment section		
Documents field impression		
Documents transport to specific facility and transfer of care WITH VERBAL REPORT		
DOCUMENTS NAME OF PERSON GIVEN THE REPORT OF SUSPECTED ABUSE		*
Uses correct grammar, abbreviations, spelling, and terminology		
Writes legibly		
Thoroughly documents refusals, denials of transport, and call cancellations		
Documents patient GCS of 15 PRIOR to signing refusal		
Documents advice given to refusal patient, including "call 9-1-1 for further problems"		
Properly corrects errors and omissions		
Writes cautiously, avoids jargon, opinions, inferences, or any derogatory/libelous remarks		
Signs run report		
Uses EMS supplement form if needed		
Student exhibits competence with skill		

Any items in the Not Done column should be evaluated with student. Check marks in this column do not necessarily mean student was unsuccessful as all lines are not completed on all patients. Evaluation of each PCR should be based on the scenario given.

Student must be able to write an EMS report with consistency and accuracy.

☐ Successful   ☐ Unsuccessful   Examiner Initials: _____

©2006 Prentice-Hall Inc.

Overall Scenario Management—Abuse/Assault

Student: _____   Examiner: _____

Date: _____   Scenario: _____

NOTE: This skill sheet is to be done after the student completes a scenario as the TEAM LEADER. It is to let the student know if he or she is beginning to "put it all together" and use critical thinking skills to manage an EMS call. PLEASE notice that it is graded on a different basis than the basic lab skill sheet.

	Done ✓	Needs to Improve
SCENE MANAGEMENT		
Recognized hazards and controlled scene—safety, crowd, and patient issues		
Recognized hazards, but did not control the scene		
Unsuccessfully attempted to manage the scene	*	
Did not evaluate the scene and took no control of the scene	*	
PATIENT ASSESSMENT		
Performed a timely, organized complete patient assessment		
Performed complete initial, focused, and ongoing assessments, but in a disorganized manner		
Performed an incomplete assessment	*	
Did not perform an initial assessment	*	
PATIENT MANAGEMENT		
Evaluated assessment findings to manage all aspects of patient condition		
Managed the patient's presenting signs and symptoms without considering all of assessment		
Inadequately managed the patient	*	
Did not manage life-threatening conditions	*	
COMMUNICATION		
Communicated well with crew, patient, family, bystanders, and assisting agencies		
Communicated well with patient and crew		
Communicated with patient and crew, but poor communication skills	*	
Unable to communicate effectively	*	
REPORT AND TRANSFER OF CARE		
Identified correct destination for patient transport, gave accurate, brief report over radio, and provided full report at bedside demonstrating thorough understanding of patient condition and pathophysiological processes		
Identified correct destination and gave accurate radio and bedside report, but did not demonstrate understanding of patient condition and pathophysiological processes		
Identified correct destination, but provided inadequate radio and bedside report	*	
Identified inappropriate destination or provided no radio or bedside report	*	
Student exhibits competence with skill		

Any items that are marked with an * indicate the student needs to improve and a check mark should be placed in the right-hand column. A check mark in the right-hand column indicates that the student was unsuccessful and must attempt the skill again to assure competency. Examiners should use a different-color ink for the second attempt.

☐ Successful   ☐ Unsuccessful   Examiner Initials: _____

Patient Assessment: Trauma—Burn Trauma

Student: _____   Examiner: _____

Date: _____   Scenario: _____

	Done ✓	Not Done
Assesses scene safety and utilizes appropriate PPE		*
OVERALL SCENE EVALUATION		
Trauma—assesses mechanism of injury/if medical component determines nature of illness		*
Determines the number of patients, location, obstacles, and requests any additional resources as needed		
Verbalizes general impression of the patient as approaches		*
Stabilizes C-spine/spinal motion restriction (SMR) of spine and stops the burning process		*
INITIAL ASSESSMENT/RESUSCITATION		
Determines responsiveness/level of consciousness/AVPU		*
Opens airway with appropriate technique and assesses airway/ventilation		*
Manages airway/ventilation and applies appropriate oxygen therapy in less than 3 minutes		*
Assesses circulation: radial/carotid pulse, skin color, temperature, condition, and turgor		*
Controls any major bleeding and covers burned areas with clean or sterile DRY sheet or dressing		*
Calculates BSA burned using rule of nines and makes rapid transport decision		*
Obtains IV (2 if indicated), BGL, GCS, and complete vital signs		
RAPID TRAUMA ASSESSMENT (If patient is Trauma Alert or Load and Go)		
Assesses abdomen		
Rapidly palpates each extremity, assessing for obvious injuries and distal PMS		
Provides spinal motion restriction (SMR) on long backboard (LBB), checking posterior torso and legs		
Secures head LAST		
Identifies patient problem: burn trauma		*
Loads patient/initiates transport (to appropriate LZ or to appropriate facility) in less than 10 minutes		*
Reassesses ABCs and interventions		*
FOCUSED HISTORY AND PHYSICAL ASSESSMENT		
Reassesses interventions and further assesses injuries found		
Obtains vital signs and GCS (Glasgow Coma Score)		
Obtains SAMPLE history		
Inspects and palpates head, facial, and neck regions		
Inspects, palpates, and auscultates chest/thorax		
Inspects and palpates abdomen and pelvis		
Inspects and palpates upper and lower extremities, checking distal PMS		
Inspects and palpates posterior torso		
Manages all injuries/wounds appropriately—calculates IV fluid therapy using Parkland Formula		
Repeats initial assessment, vital signs, and evaluates trends		*
Evaluates response to interventions/treatments		*
Performs ongoing assessment (VS every 5 minutes for critical patient/every 15 minutes for stable patient)		
Gives radio report to receiving facility		
Turns over patient care with verbal report		*
Student exhibits competence with skill		

Any items in the Not Done column that are marked with an * are mandatory for the student to complete. A check mark in the Not Done column of an item with an * indicates that the student was unsuccessful and must attempt the skill again to assure competency. Examiners should use a different-color ink for the second attempt.

☐ Successful   ☐ Unsuccessful   Examiner Initials: _____

    ©2006 Prentice-Hall Inc.

Endotracheal Intubation with Suspected Cervical Spine—Burn Trauma

Student: _____   **Examiner:** _____

Date: _____

	Done ✓	Not Done
Determines scene safety and utilizes appropriate PPE		*
Opens the airway manually with trauma jaw-thrust while assistant maintains C-spine SMR		*
Checks mouth for blood or potential airway obstruction		*
Suctions or removes loose teeth or foreign materials as needed		
Inserts simple airway adjunct (oropharyngeal airway)		
Directs assistant to ventilate patient with bag-valve-mask device (room air)		*
Observes chest rise/fall and auscultates bilaterally over lungs for baseline		*
Obtains effective ventilation in less than 30 seconds		*
Attaches oxygen reservoir to bag-valve-mask device and connects to high-flow oxygen		
Ventilates patient and evaluates chest wall/lung compliance		*
Directs assistant to preoxygenate patient with assistant maintaining C-spine SMR		*
Identifies/selects proper equipment for intubation		
Checks laryngoscope light and cuff of ET tube		
Removes all air from cuff and properly inserts stylet if used		
Directs assistant to face patient and establish cervical spine SMR from front		
Intubating paramedic sits behind patient on ground with legs straddling patient's shoulders		
Moves up until patient's head is secured		
Removes OPA and directs assistant to perform Sellick's maneuver		*
Opens mouth and gently inserts blade while sweeping tongue to side		*
Gently elevates mandible with laryngoscope and leans backward to visualize cords		*
Inserts ET tube and visualizes as tube is advanced through cords		*
"Threads" ET tube off stylet (if used), maintaining hold on ET tube as stylet removed		
Inflates cuff to proper pressure and disconnects syringe		*
Disconnects mask from bag-valve device and attaches to ET tube without releasing ET tube		
Directs ventilation of patient while maintaining Sellick's maneuver and holding ET tube in place		
Confirms proper placement by auscultation over epigastrium and bilaterally over each lung		*
Directs assistant to release cricoid pressure		*
Secures ET tube		*
Reassesses bilateral lung sounds and compliance		*
Uses secondary device to confirm tube placement		*
Assesses patient's response to intervention		*
Student exhibits competence with skill		

Any items in the Not Done column that are marked with an * are mandatory for the student to complete. A check mark in the Not Done column of an item with an * indicates that the student was unsuccessful and must attempt the skill again to assure competency. Examiners should use a different-color ink for the second attempt.

☐ Successful   ☐ Unsuccessful   Examiner Initials: _____

Scenario IV Insertion—Burn Trauma

Student: _____   Examiner: _____

Date: _____

	Done ✓	Not Done
Selects appropriate IV fluid, checking clarity, color, and expiration date		*
Selects appropriate catheter		
Selects appropriate administration set		
Properly inserts IV tubing into the IV bag		*
Prepares administration set (fills drip chamber and flushes tubing)		*
Cuts or tears tape (at any time before venipuncture)		*
Applies constricting band (checks distal pulse to assure NOT a tourniquet)		*
Palpates suitable vein		*
Cleanses site appropriately		*
Utilizes appropriate PPE		*
Inserts catheter with sterile technique		*
Verbalizes flash/blood return and advances catheter slightly farther		*
Occludes vein with finger at distal end of catheter and removes stylet		
Immediately disposes (or verbalizes disposal) of needle/sharp in proper container		
Obtains blood sample or connects IV tubing to catheter		
Obtains BGL (blood glucose level)		*
Releases constricting band		*
Runs IV for a brief period to ensure patency and adjusts flow rate as appropriate		*
Checks IV site for signs of infiltration		*
Secures catheter (tapes securely or verbalizes)		*
Attaches label with size of catheter, date, time, and "prehospital"		*
Assesses patient's response to intervention		*
Student exhibits competence with skill		

Any items in the Not Done column that are marked with an * are mandatory for the student to complete. A check mark in the Not Done column of an item with an * indicates that the student was unsuccessful and must attempt the skill again to assure competency. Examiners should use a different-color ink for the second attempt.

☐ Successful   ☐ Unsuccessful   Examiner Initials: _____

©2006 Prentice-Hall Inc.

Scenario Radio Report—Burn Trauma

Student: _____   **Examiner:** _____

Date: _____

	Done ✓	Not Done
Requests and checks for open channel before speaking		
Presses transmit button 1 second before speaking		
Holds microphone 2–3 in. from mouth		
Speaks slowly and clearly		*
Speaks in a normal voice		
Briefly transmits: Agency, unit designation, identification/name		*
Briefly transmits: Patient's age, sex, weight		*
Briefly transmits: Scene description/mechanism of injury or medical problem		*
Briefly transmits: Chief complaint with brief history of *present* illness		*
Briefly transmits: Associated symptoms (unless able to be deferred to bedside report)		
Briefly transmits: Past medical history (usually deferred to bedside report)		
Briefly transmits: Vital signs		*
Briefly transmits: Level of consciousness/GCS on trauma		*
Briefly transmits: General appearance, distress, cardiac rhythm, blood glucose, and other pertinent findings unable to be deferred to bedside report		
Briefly transmits: Interventions by EMS AND response(s)		*
ETA (the more critical the patient, the earlier you need to notify the receiving facility)		
Does not waste airtime		
Protects privacy of patient		*
Echoes dispatch information and any physician orders		*
Writes down dispatch information or physician orders		
Confirms with facility that message is received		
Demonstrates/verbalizes ability to troubleshoot basic equipment malfunction		
Student exhibits competence with skill		

Any items in the Not Done column that are marked with an * are mandatory for the student to complete. A check mark in the Not Done column of an item with an * indicates that the student was unsuccessful and must attempt the skill again to assure competency. Examiners should use a different-color ink for the second attempt.

☐ Successful   ☐ Unsuccessful   Examiner Initials: _____

Scenario Patient Care Report (PCR)—Burn Trauma

Student: _____   Examiner: _____

Date: _____

	Done ✓	Not Done
Records all pertinent dispatch/scene data, using a consistent format		
Completely identifies all additional resources and personnel		
Documents chief complaint, signs/symptoms, position found, age, sex, and weight		
Identifies and records all pertinent, reportable clinical data for each patient		
Documents SAMPLE and OPQRST if applicable		
Records all pertinent negatives		
Records all pertinent denials		
Records accurate, consistent times and patient information		
Includes relevant oral statements of witnesses, bystanders, and patient in "quotes" when appropriate		
Documents initial assessment findings: airway, breathing, and circulation		
Documents any interventions in initial assessment with patient response		
Documents level of consciousness, GCS (if trauma), and VS		
Documents rapid trauma assessment if applicable		
Documents any interventions in rapid trauma assessment with patient response		
Documents focused history and physical assessment		
Documents any interventions in focused assessment with patient response		
Documents repeat VS (every 5 minutes for critical; every 15 minutes for stable)		
Repeats initial assessment and documents findings		
Records ALL treatments with times and patient response(s) in treatment section		
Documents field impression		
Documents transport to specific facility and transfer of care WITH VERBAL REPORT		
Uses correct grammar, abbreviations, spelling, and terminology		
Writes legibly		
Thoroughly documents refusals, denials of transport, and call cancellations		
Documents patient GCS of 15 PRIOR to signing refusal		
Documents advice given to refusal patient, including "call 9-1-1 for further problems"		
Properly corrects errors and omissions		
Writes cautiously, avoids jargon, opinions, inferences, or any derogatory/libelous remarks		
Signs run report		
Uses EMS supplement form if needed		
Student exhibits competence with skill		

Any items in the Not Done column should be evaluated with student. Check marks in this column do not necessarily mean student was unsuccessful as all lines are not completed on all patients. Evaluation of each PCR should be based on the scenario given.

Student must be able to write an EMS report with consistency and accuracy.

☐ Successful   ☐ Unsuccessful   Examiner Initials: _____

©2006 Prentice-Hall Inc.

Overall Scenario Management—Burn Trauma

Student: _____   Examiner: _____

Date: _____   Scenario: _____

NOTE: This skill sheet is to be done after the student completes a scenario as the **TEAM LEADER.** It is to let the student know if he or she is beginning to "put it all together" and use critical thinking skills to manage an EMS call. PLEASE notice that it is graded on a different basis than the basic lab skill sheet.

	Done ✓	Needs to Improve
SCENE MANAGEMENT		
Recognized hazards and controlled scene—safety, crowd, and patient issues		
Recognized hazards, but did not control the scene		
Unsuccessfully attempted to manage the scene	*	
Did not evaluate the scene and took no control of the scene	*	
PATIENT ASSESSMENT		
Performed a timely, organized complete patient assessment		
Performed complete initial, focused, and ongoing assessments, but in a disorganized manner		
Performed an incomplete assessment	*	
Did not perform an initial assessment	*	
PATIENT MANAGEMENT		
Evaluated assessment findings to manage all aspects of patient condition		
Managed the patient's presenting signs and symptoms without considering all of assessment		
Inadequately managed the patient	*	
Did not manage life-threatening conditions	*	
COMMUNICATION		
Communicated well with crew, patient, family, bystanders, and assisting agencies		
Communicated well with patient and crew		
Communicated with patient and crew, but poor communication skills	*	
Unable to communicate effectively	*	
REPORT AND TRANSFER OF CARE		
Identified correct destination for patient transport, gave accurate, brief report over radio, and provided full report at bedside demonstrating thorough understanding of patient condition and pathophysiological processes		
Identified correct destination and gave accurate radio and bedside report, but did not demonstrate understanding of patient condition and pathophysiological processes		
Identified correct destination, but provided inadequate radio and bedside report	*	
Identified inappropriate destination or provided no radio or bedside report	*	
Student exhibits competence with skill		

Any items that are marked with an * indicate the student needs to improve and a check mark should be placed in the right-hand column. A check mark in the right-hand column indicates that the student was unsuccessful and must attempt the skill again to assure competency. Examiners should use a different-color ink for the second attempt.

☐ Successful   ☐ Unsuccessful   Examiner Initials: _____

©2006 Prentice-Hall Inc.

Patient Assessment: Trauma—Geriatric Trauma

Student: _____   Examiner: _____

Date: _____   Scenario: _____

	Done ✓	Not Done
Assesses scene safety and utilizes appropriate PPE		*
OVERALL SCENE EVALUATION		
Trauma—assesses mechanism of injury/if medical component determines nature of illness		*
Determines the number of patients, location, obstacles, and requests any additional resources as needed		
Verbalizes general impression of the patient as approaches		*
Stabilizes C-spine/spinal motion restriction (SMR) of spine		*
INITIAL ASSESSMENT/RESUSCITATION		
Determines responsiveness/level of consciousness/AVPU		*
Opens airway with appropriate technique and assesses airway/ventilation		*
Manages airway/ventilation and applies appropriate oxygen therapy in less than 3 minutes		*
Assesses circulation: radial/carotid pulse, skin color, temperature, condition, and turgor		*
Controls any major bleeding		*
Makes rapid transport decision		*
Obtains IV (2 if indicated), BGL, GCS, and complete vital signs		
RAPID TRAUMA ASSESSMENT (If patient is Trauma Alert or Load and Go)		
Assesses abdomen		
Rapidly palpates each extremity, assessing for obvious injuries and distal PMS		
Provides spinal motion restriction (SMR) on long backboard (LBB), checking posterior torso and legs		
Secures head LAST		
Identifies patient problem: geriatric trauma (identify specific injuries and considerations due to age)		*
Loads patient/initiates transport (to appropriate LZ or to appropriate facility) in less than 10 minutes		*
Reassesses ABCs and interventions		*
FOCUSED HISTORY AND PHYSICAL ASSESSMENT		
Reassesses interventions and further assesses injuries found		
Obtains vital signs and GCS (Glasgow Coma Score)		
Obtains SAMPLE history		
Inspects and palpates head, facial, and neck regions		
Inspects, palpates, and auscultates chest/thorax		
Inspects and palpates abdomen and pelvis		
Inspects and palpates upper and lower extremities, checking distal PMS		
Inspects and palpates posterior torso		
Manages all injuries/wounds appropriately, with consideration for age-related problems, skin integrity, etc.		
Repeats initial assessment, vital signs, and evaluates trends		*
Evaluates response to interventions/treatments		*
Performs ongoing assessment (VS every 5 minutes for critical patient/every 15 minutes for stable patient)		
Gives radio report to receiving facility		
Turns over patient care with verbal report		*
Student exhibits competence with skill		

Any items in the Not Done column that are marked with an * are mandatory for the student to complete. A check mark in the Not Done column of an item with an * indicates that the student was unsuccessful and must attempt the skill again to assure competency. Examiners should use a different-color ink for the second attempt.

☐ Successful   ☐ Unsuccessful   Examiner Initials: _____

          ©2006 Prentice-Hall Inc.

Endotracheal Intubation with Suspected Cervical Spine— Geriatric Trauma

Student: _____ Examiner: _____

Date: _____

	Done ✓	Not Done
Determines scene safety and utilizes appropriate PPE		*
Opens the airway manually with trauma jaw-thrust while assistant maintains C-spine SMR		*
Checks mouth for blood or potential airway obstruction		*
Suctions or removes loose teeth or foreign materials as needed		
Inserts simple airway adjunct (oropharyngeal airway)		
Directs assistant to ventilate patient with bag-valve-mask device (room air)		*
Observes chest rise/fall and auscultates bilaterally over lungs for baseline		*
Obtains effective ventilation in less than 30 seconds		*
Attaches oxygen reservoir to bag-valve-mask device and connects to high-flow oxygen		
Ventilates patient and evaluates chest wall/lung compliance		*
Directs assistant to preoxygenate patient with assistant maintaining C-spine SMR		*
Identifies/selects proper equipment for intubation		
Checks laryngoscope light and cuff of ET tube		
Removes all air from cuff and properly inserts stylet if used		
Directs assistant to face patient and establish cervical spine SMR from front		
Intubating paramedic sits behind patient on ground with legs straddling patient's shoulders		
Moves up until patient's head is secured		
Removes OPA and directs assistant to perform Sellick's maneuver		*
Opens mouth and gently inserts blade while sweeping tongue to side		*
Gently elevates mandible with laryngoscope and leans backward to visualize cords		*
Inserts ET tube and visualizes as tube is advanced through cords		*
"Threads" ET tube off stylet (if used), maintaining hold on ET tube as stylet removed		
Inflates cuff to proper pressure and disconnects syringe		*
Disconnects mask from bag-valve device and attaches to ET tube without releasing ET tube		
Directs ventilation of patient while maintaining Sellick's maneuver and holding ET tube in place		
Confirms proper placement by auscultation over epigastrium and bilaterally over each lung		*
Directs assistant to release cricoid pressure		*
Secures ET tube		*
Reassesses bilateral lung sounds and compliance		*
Uses secondary device to confirm tube placement		*
Assesses patient's response to intervention		*
Student exhibits competence with skill		

Any items in the Not Done column that are marked with an * are mandatory for the student to complete. A check mark in the Not Done column of an item with an * indicates that the student was unsuccessful and must attempt the skill again to assure competency. Examiners should use a different-color ink for the second attempt.

☐ Successful   ☐ Unsuccessful   Examiner Initials: _____

Scenario IV Insertion—Geriatric Trauma

Student: _____   Examiner: _____

Date: _____

	Done ✓	Not Done
Selects appropriate IV fluid, checking clarity, color, and expiration date		*
Selects appropriate catheter		
Selects appropriate administration set		
Properly inserts IV tubing into the IV bag		*
Prepares administration set (fills drip chamber and flushes tubing)		*
Cuts or tears tape (at any time before venipuncture)		*
Applies constricting band (checks distal pulse to assure NOT a tourniquet)		*
Palpates suitable vein		*
Cleanses site appropriately		*
Utilizes appropriate PPE		*
Inserts catheter with sterile technique		*
Verbalizes flash/blood return and advances catheter slightly farther		*
Occludes vein with finger at distal end of catheter and removes stylet		
Immediately disposes (or verbalizes disposal) of needle/sharp in proper container		
Obtains blood sample or connects IV tubing to catheter		
Obtains BGL (blood glucose level)		*
Releases constricting band		*
Runs IV for a brief period to ensure patency and adjusts flow rate as appropriate		*
Checks IV site for signs of infiltration		*
Secures catheter (tapes securely or verbalizes)		*
Attaches label with size of catheter, date, time, and "prehospital"		*
Assesses patient's response to intervention		*
Student exhibits competence with skill		

Any items in the Not Done column that are marked with an * are mandatory for the student to complete. A check mark in the Not Done column of an item with an * indicates that the student was unsuccessful and must attempt the skill again to assure competency. Examiners should use a different-color ink for the second attempt.

☐ Successful   ☐ Unsuccessful   Examiner Initials: _____

©2006 Prentice-Hall Inc.

Scenario Radio Report—Geriatric Trauma

Student: _____   **Examiner:** _____

Date: _____

	Done ✓	Not Done
Requests and checks for open channel before speaking		
Presses transmit button 1 second before speaking		
Holds microphone 2–3 in. from mouth		
Speaks slowly and clearly		*
Speaks in a normal voice		
Briefly transmits: Agency, unit designation, identification/name		*
Briefly transmits: Patient's age, sex, weight		*
Briefly transmits: Scene description/mechanism of injury or medical problem		*
Briefly transmits: Chief complaint with brief history of *present* illness		*
Briefly transmits: Associated symptoms (unless able to be deferred to bedside report)		
Briefly transmits: Past medical history (usually deferred to bedside report)		
Briefly transmits: Vital signs		*
Briefly transmits: Level of consciousness/GCS on trauma		*
Briefly transmits: General appearance, distress, cardiac rhythm, blood glucose, and other pertinent findings unable to be deferred to bedside report		
Briefly transmits: Interventions by EMS AND response(s)		*
ETA (the more critical the patient, the earlier you need to notify the receiving facility)		
Does not waste airtime		
Protects privacy of patient		*
Echoes dispatch information and any physician orders		*
Writes down dispatch information or physician orders		
Confirms with facility that message is received		
Demonstrates/verbalizes ability to troubleshoot basic equipment malfunction		
Student exhibits competence with skill		

Any items in the Not Done column that are marked with an * are mandatory for the student to complete. A check mark in the Not Done column of an item with an * indicates that the student was unsuccessful and must attempt the skill again to assure competency. Examiners should use a different-color ink for the second attempt.

☐ Successful   ☐ Unsuccessful   Examiner Initials: _____

©2006 Prentice-Hall Inc.

Scenario Patient Care Report (PCR)—Geriatric Trauma

Student: _____   Examiner: _____

Date: _____

	Done ✓	Not Done
Records all pertinent dispatch/scene data, using a consistent format		
Completely identifies all additional resources and personnel		
Documents chief complaint, signs/symptoms, position found, age, sex, and weight		
Identifies and records all pertinent, reportable clinical data for each patient		
Documents SAMPLE and OPQRST if applicable		
Records all pertinent negatives		
Records all pertinent denials		
Records accurate, consistent times and patient information		
Includes relevant oral statements of witnesses, bystanders, and patient in "quotes" when appropriate		
Documents initial assessment findings: airway, breathing, and circulation		
Documents any interventions in initial assessment with patient response		
Documents level of consciousness, GCS (if trauma), and VS		
Documents rapid trauma assessment if applicable		
Documents any interventions in rapid trauma assessment with patient response		
Documents focused history and physical assessment		
Documents any interventions in focused assessment with patient response		
Documents repeat VS (every 5 minutes for critical; every 15 minutes for stable)		
Repeats initial assessment and documents findings		
Records ALL treatments with times and patient response(s) in treatment section		
Documents field impression		
Documents transport to specific facility and transfer of care WITH VERBAL REPORT		
Uses correct grammar, abbreviations, spelling, and terminology		
Writes legibly		
Thoroughly documents refusals, denials of transport, and call cancellations		
Documents patient GCS of 15 PRIOR to signing refusal		
Documents advice given to refusal patient, including "call 9-1-1 for further problems"		
Properly corrects errors and omissions		
Writes cautiously, avoids jargon, opinions, inferences, or any derogatory/libelous remarks		
Signs run report		
Uses EMS supplement form if needed		
Student exhibits competence with skill		

Any items in the Not Done column should be evaluated with student. Check marks in this column do not necessarily mean student was unsuccessful as all lines are not completed on all patients. Evaluation of each PCR should be based on the scenario given.

Student must be able to write an EMS report with consistency and accuracy.

☐ Successful   ☐ Unsuccessful   Examiner Initials: _____

©2006 Prentice-Hall Inc.

Overall Scenario Management—Geriatric Trauma

Student: _____   Examiner: _____

Date: _____   Scenario: _____

NOTE: This skill sheet is to be done after the student completes a scenario as the **TEAM LEADER**. It is to let the student know if he or she is beginning to "put it all together" and use critical thinking skills to manage an EMS call. PLEASE notice that it is graded on a different basis than the basic lab skill sheet.

	Done ✓	Needs to Improve
SCENE MANAGEMENT		
Recognized hazards and controlled scene—safety, crowd, and patient issues		
Recognized hazards, but did not control the scene		
Unsuccessfully attempted to manage the scene	*	
Did not evaluate the scene and took no control of the scene	*	
PATIENT ASSESSMENT		
Performed a timely, organized complete patient assessment		
Performed complete initial, focused, and ongoing assessments, but in a disorganized manner		
Performed an incomplete assessment	*	
Did not perform an initial assessment	*	
PATIENT MANAGEMENT		
Evaluated assessment findings to manage all aspects of patient condition		
Managed the patient's presenting signs and symptoms without considering all of assessment		
Inadequately managed the patient	*	
Did not manage life-threatening conditions	*	
COMMUNICATION		
Communicated well with crew, patient, family, bystanders, and assisting agencies		
Communicated well with patient and crew		
Communicated with patient and crew, but poor communication skills	*	
Unable to communicate effectively	*	
REPORT AND TRANSFER OF CARE		
Identified correct destination for patient transport, gave accurate, brief report over radio, and provided full report at bedside demonstrating thorough understanding of patient condition and pathophysiological processes		
Identified correct destination and gave accurate radio and bedside report, but did not demonstrate understanding of patient condition and pathophysiological processes		
Identified correct destination, but provided inadequate radio and bedside report	*	
Identified inappropriate destination or provided no radio or bedside report	*	
Student exhibits competence with skill		

Any items that are marked with an * indicate the student needs to improve and a check mark should be placed in the right-hand column. A check mark in the right-hand column indicates that the student was unsuccessful and must attempt the skill again to assure competency. Examiners should use a different-color ink for the second attempt.

☐ Successful   ☐ Unsuccessful   Examiner Initials: _____

Patient Assessment: Trauma—Head/Facial/Neck Trauma

Student: _____   Examiner: _____

Date: _____   Scenario: _____

	Done ✓	Not Done
Assesses scene safety and utilizes appropriate PPE		*
OVERALL SCENE EVALUATION		
Trauma—assesses mechanism of injury/if medical component determines nature of illness		*
Determines the number of patients, location, obstacles, and requests any additional resources as needed		
Verbalizes general impression of the patient as approaches		*
Stabilizes C-spine/spinal motion restriction (SMR) of spine		*
INITIAL ASSESSMENT/RESUSCITATION		
Determines responsiveness/level of consciousness/AVPU		*
Opens airway with appropriate technique and assesses airway/ventilation		*
Manages airway/ventilation and applies appropriate oxygen therapy in less than 3 minutes		*
Assesses circulation: radial/carotid pulse, skin color, temperature, condition, and turgor		*
Controls any major bleeding—occlusive dressing if vascular neck trauma		*
Makes rapid transport decision		*
Obtains IV (2 if indicated), BGL, GCS, and complete vital signs		
RAPID TRAUMA ASSESSMENT (If patient is Trauma Alert or Load and Go)		
Assesses abdomen		
Rapidly palpates each extremity, assessing for obvious injuries and distal PMS		
Provides spinal motion restriction (SMR) on long backboard (LBB), checking posterior torso and legs		
Secures head LAST		
Identifies patient problem: head/facial/neck trauma (specify injuries)		*
Loads patient/initiates transport (to appropriate LZ or to appropriate facility) in less than 10 minutes		*
Reassesses ABCs and interventions		*
FOCUSED HISTORY AND PHYSICAL ASSESSMENT		
Reassesses interventions and further assesses injuries found		
Obtains vital signs and GCS (Glasgow Coma Score)		
Obtains SAMPLE history		
Inspects and palpates head, facial, and neck regions		
Inspects, palpates, and auscultates chest/thorax		
Inspects and palpates abdomen and pelvis		
Inspects and palpates upper and lower extremities, checking distal PMS		
Inspects and palpates posterior torso		
Manages all injuries/wounds appropriately—intensive monitoring for potential airway compromise; does NOT hyperventilate traumatic brain injury unless signs of herniation present		
Repeats initial assessment, vital signs, and evaluates trends		*
Evaluates response to interventions/treatments		*
Performs ongoing assessment (VS every 5 minutes for critical patient/every 15 minutes for stable patient)		
Gives radio report to receiving facility		
Turns over patient care with verbal report		*
Student exhibits competence with skill		

Any items in the Not Done column that are marked with an * are mandatory for the student to complete. A check mark in the Not Done column of an item with an * indicates that the student was unsuccessful and must attempt the skill again to assure competency. Examiners should use a different-color ink for the second attempt.

☐ Successful   ☐ Unsuccessful   Examiner Initials: _____

©2006 Prentice-Hall Inc.

Endotracheal Intubation with Suspected Cervical Spine—Head/Facial/Neck Trauma

Student: _____   **Examiner:** _____

Date: _____

	Done ✓	Not Done
Determines scene safety and utilizes appropriate PPE		*
Opens the airway manually with trauma jaw-thrust while assistant maintains C-spine SMR		*
Checks mouth for blood or potential airway obstruction		*
Suctions or removes loose teeth or foreign materials as needed		
Inserts simple airway adjunct (oropharyngeal airway)		
Directs assistant to ventilate patient with bag-valve-mask device (room air)		*
Observes chest rise/fall and auscultates bilaterally over lungs for baseline		*
Obtains effective ventilation in less than 30 seconds		*
Attaches oxygen reservoir to bag-valve-mask device and connects to high-flow oxygen		
Ventilates patient and evaluates chest wall/lung compliance		*
Directs assistant to preoxygenate patient with assistant maintaining C-spine SMR		*
Identifies/selects proper equipment for intubation		
Checks laryngoscope light and cuff of ET tube		
Removes all air from cuff and properly inserts stylet if used		
Directs assistant to face patient and establish cervical spine SMR from front		
Intubating paramedic sits behind patient on ground with legs straddling patient's shoulders		
Moves up until patient's head is secured		
Removes OPA and directs assistant to perform Sellick's maneuver		*
Opens mouth and gently inserts blade while sweeping tongue to side		*
Gently elevates mandible with laryngoscope and leans backward to visualize cords		*
Inserts ET tube and visualizes as tube is advanced through cords		*
"Threads" ET tube off stylet (if used), maintaining hold on ET tube as stylet removed		
Inflates cuff to proper pressure and disconnects syringe		*
Disconnects mask from bag-valve device and attaches to ET tube without releasing ET tube		
Directs ventilation of patient while maintaining Sellick's maneuver and holding ET tube in place		
Confirms proper placement by auscultation over epigastrium and bilaterally over each lung		*
Directs assistant to release cricoid pressure		*
Secures ET tube		*
Reassesses bilateral lung sounds and compliance		*
Uses secondary device to confirm tube placement		*
Assesses patient's response to intervention		*
Student exhibits competence with skill		

Any items in the Not Done column that are marked with an * are mandatory for the student to complete. A check mark in the Not Done column of an item with an * indicates that the student was unsuccessful and must attempt the skill again to assure competency. Examiners should use a different-color ink for the second attempt.

☐ Successful   ☐ Unsuccessful   Examiner Initials: _____

©2006 Prentice-Hall Inc.

Scenario IV Insertion—Head/Facial/Neck Trauma

Student: _____   **Examiner:** _____

Date: _____

	Done ✓	Not Done
Selects appropriate IV fluid, checking clarity, color, and expiration date		*
Selects appropriate catheter		
Selects appropriate administration set		
Properly inserts IV tubing into the IV bag		*
Prepares administration set (fills drip chamber and flushes tubing)		*
Cuts or tears tape (at any time before venipuncture)		*
Applies constricting band (checks distal pulse to assure NOT a tourniquet)		*
Palpates suitable vein		*
Cleanses site appropriately		*
Utilizes appropriate PPE		*
Inserts catheter with sterile technique		*
Verbalizes flash/blood return and advances catheter slightly farther		*
Occludes vein with finger at distal end of catheter and removes stylet		
Immediately disposes (or verbalizes disposal) of needle/sharp in proper container		
Obtains blood sample or connects IV tubing to catheter		
Obtains BGL (blood glucose level)		*
Releases constricting band		*
Runs IV for a brief period to ensure patency and adjusts flow rate as appropriate		*
Checks IV site for signs of infiltration		*
Secures catheter (tapes securely or verbalizes)		*
Attaches label with size of catheter, date, time, and "prehospital"		*
Assesses patient's response to intervention		*
Student exhibits competence with skill		

Any items in the Not Done column that are marked with an * are mandatory for the student to complete. A check mark in the Not Done column of an item with an * indicates that the student was unsuccessful and must attempt the skill again to assure competency. Examiners should use a different-color ink for the second attempt.

☐ Successful   ☐ Unsuccessful   Examiner Initials: _____

©2006 Prentice-Hall Inc.

Scenario Radio Report—Head/Facial/Neck Trauma

Student: _____

Examiner: _____

Date: _____

	Done ✓	Not Done
Requests and checks for open channel before speaking		
Presses transmit button 1 second before speaking		
Holds microphone 2–3 in. from mouth		
Speaks slowly and clearly		*
Speaks in a normal voice		
Briefly transmits: Agency, unit designation, identification/name		*
Briefly transmits: Patient's age, sex, weight		*
Briefly transmits: Scene description/mechanism of injury or medical problem		*
Briefly transmits: Chief complaint with brief history of *present* illness		*
Briefly transmits: Associated symptoms (unless able to be deferred to bedside report)		
Briefly transmits: Past medical history (usually deferred to bedside report)		
Briefly transmits: Vital signs		*
Briefly transmits: Level of consciousness/GCS on trauma		*
Briefly transmits: General appearance, distress, cardiac rhythm, blood glucose, and other pertinent findings unable to be deferred to bedside report		
Briefly transmits: Interventions by EMS AND response(s)		*
ETA (the more critical the patient, the earlier you need to notify the receiving facility)		
Does not waste airtime		
Protects privacy of patient		*
Echoes dispatch information and any physician orders		*
Writes down dispatch information or physician orders		
Confirms with facility that message is received		
Demonstrates/verbalizes ability to troubleshoot basic equipment malfunction		
Student exhibits competence with skill		

Any items in the Not Done column that are marked with an * are mandatory for the student to complete. A check mark in the Not Done column of an item with an * indicates that the student was unsuccessful and must attempt the skill again to assure competency. Examiners should use a different-color ink for the second attempt.

☐ Successful   ☐ Unsuccessful   Examiner Initials: _____

©2006 Prentice-Hall Inc.

Scenario Patient Care Report (PCR)—Head/Facial/Neck Trauma

Student: _____   **Examiner:** _____

Date: _____

	Done ✓	Not Done
Records all pertinent dispatch/scene data, using a consistent format		
Completely identifies all additional resources and personnel		
Documents chief complaint, signs/symptoms, position found, age, sex, and weight		
Identifies and records all pertinent, reportable clinical data for each patient		
Documents SAMPLE and OPQRST if applicable		
Records all pertinent negatives		
Records all pertinent denials		
Records accurate, consistent times and patient information		
Includes relevant oral statements of witnesses, bystanders, and patient in "quotes" when appropriate		
Documents initial assessment findings: airway, breathing, and circulation		
Documents any interventions in initial assessment with patient response		
Documents level of consciousness, GCS (if trauma), and VS		
Documents rapid trauma assessment if applicable		
Documents any interventions in rapid trauma assessment with patient response		
Documents focused history and physical assessment		
Documents any interventions in focused assessment with patient response		
Documents repeat VS (every 5 minutes for critical; every 15 minutes for stable)		
Repeats initial assessment and documents findings		
Records ALL treatments with times and patient response(s) in treatment section		
Documents field impression		
Documents transport to specific facility and transfer of care WITH VERBAL REPORT		
Uses correct grammar, abbreviations, spelling, and terminology		
Writes legibly		
Thoroughly documents refusals, denials of transport, and call cancellations		
Documents patient GCS of 15 PRIOR to signing refusal		
Documents advice given to refusal patient, including "call 9-1-1 for further problems"		
Properly corrects errors and omissions		
Writes cautiously, avoids jargon, opinions, inferences, or any derogatory/libelous remarks		
Signs run report		
Uses EMS supplement form if needed		
Student exhibits competence with skill		

Any items in the Not Done column should be evaluated with student. Check marks in this column do not necessarily mean student was unsuccessful as all lines are not completed on all patients. Evaluation of each PCR should be based on the scenario given.

Student must be able to write an EMS report with consistency and accuracy.

☐ Successful   ☐ Unsuccessful   Examiner Initials: _____

©2006 Prentice-Hall Inc.

Overall Scenario Management—Head/Facial/Neck Trauma

Student: _____   Examiner: _____

Date: _____   Scenario: _____

NOTE: This skill sheet is to be done after the student completes a scenario as the TEAM LEADER. It is to let the student know if he or she is beginning to "put it all together" and use critical thinking skills to manage an EMS call. PLEASE notice that it is graded on a different basis than the basic lab skill sheet.

	Done ✓	Needs to Improve
SCENE MANAGEMENT		
Recognized hazards and controlled scene—safety, crowd, and patient issues		
Recognized hazards, but did not control the scene		
Unsuccessfully attempted to manage the scene	*	
Did not evaluate the scene and took no control of the scene	*	
PATIENT ASSESSMENT		
Performed a timely, organized complete patient assessment		
Performed complete initial, focused, and ongoing assessments, but in a disorganized manner		
Performed an incomplete assessment	*	
Did not perform an initial assessment	*	
PATIENT MANAGEMENT		
Evaluated assessment findings to manage all aspects of patient condition		
Managed the patient's presenting signs and symptoms without considering all of assessment		
Inadequately managed the patient	*	
Did not manage life-threatening conditions	*	
COMMUNICATION		
Communicated well with crew, patient, family, bystanders, and assisting agencies		
Communicated well with patient and crew		
Communicated with patient and crew, but poor communication skills	*	
Unable to communicate effectively	*	
REPORT AND TRANSFER OF CARE		
Identified correct destination for patient transport, gave accurate, brief report over radio, and provided full report at bedside demonstrating thorough understanding of patient condition and pathophysiological processes		
Identified correct destination and gave accurate radio and bedside report, but did not demonstrate understanding of patient condition and pathophysiological processes		
Identified correct destination, but provided inadequate radio and bedside report	*	
Identified inappropriate destination or provided no radio or bedside report	*	
Student exhibits competence with skill		

Any items that are marked with an * indicate the student needs to improve and a check mark should be placed in the right-hand column. A check mark in the right-hand column indicates that the student was unsuccessful and must attempt the skill again to assure competency. Examiners should use a different-color ink for the second attempt.

☐ Successful   ☐ Unsuccessful   Examiner Initials: _____

Patient Assessment: Trauma—Musculoskeletal Trauma

Student: _____   **Examiner:** _____

Date: _____   **Scenario:** _____

	Done ✓	Not Done
Assesses scene safety and utilizes appropriate PPE		*
OVERALL SCENE EVALUATION		
Trauma—assesses mechanism of injury/if medical component determines nature of illness		*
Determines the number of patients, location, obstacles, and requests any additional resources as needed		
Verbalizes general impression of the patient as approaches		*
Stabilizes C-spine/spinal motion restriction (SMR) of spine		*
INITIAL ASSESSMENT/RESUSCITATION		
Determines responsiveness/level of consciousness/AVPU		*
Opens airway with appropriate technique and assesses airway/ventilation		*
Manages airway/ventilation and applies appropriate oxygen therapy in less than 3 minutes		*
Assesses circulation: radial/carotid pulse, skin color, temperature, condition, and turgor		*
Controls any major bleeding		*
Makes rapid transport decision		*
Obtains IV (2 if indicated), BGL, GCS, and complete vital signs		
RAPID TRAUMA ASSESSMENT (If patient is Trauma Alert or Load and Go)		
Assesses abdomen		
Rapidly palpates each extremity, assessing for obvious injuries and distal PMS		
Provides spinal motion restriction (SMR) on long backboard (LBB), checking posterior torso and legs		
Secures head LAST		
Identifies patient problem: musculoskeletal trauma (identify specific injuries)		*
Loads patient/initiates transport (to appropriate LZ or to appropriate facility) in less than 10 minutes		*
Reassesses ABCs and interventions		*
FOCUSED HISTORY AND PHYSICAL ASSESSMENT		
Reassesses interventions and further assesses injuries found		
Obtains vital signs and GCS (Glasgow Coma Score)		
Obtains SAMPLE history		
Inspects and palpates head, facial, and neck regions		
Inspects, palpates, and auscultates chest/thorax		
Inspects and palpates abdomen and pelvis		
Inspects and palpates upper and lower extremities checking distal PMS		
Inspects and palpates posterior torso		
Manages all injuries/wounds appropriately—splinting, bandaging, hemostasis, etc.		
Repeats initial assessment, vital signs, and evaluates trends		*
Evaluates response to interventions/treatments		*
Performs ongoing assessment (VS every 5 minutes for critical patient/every 15 minutes for stable patient)		
Gives radio report to receiving facility		
Turns over patient care with verbal report		*
Student exhibits competence with skill		

Any items in the Not Done column that are marked with an * are mandatory for the student to complete. A check mark in the Not Done column of an item with an * indicates that the student was unsuccessful and must attempt the skill again to assure competency. Examiners should use a different-color ink for the second attempt.

☐ Successful   ☐ Unsuccessful   Examiner Initials: _____

©2006 Prentice-Hall Inc.

Endotracheal Intubation with Suspected Cervical Spine— Musculoskeletal Trauma

Student: _____   **Examiner:** _____

Date: _____

	Done ✓	Not Done
Determines scene safety and utilizes appropriate PPE		*
Opens the airway manually with trauma jaw-thrust while assistant maintains C-spine SMR		*
Checks mouth for blood or potential airway obstruction		*
Suctions or removes loose teeth or foreign materials as needed		
Inserts simple airway adjunct (oropharyngeal airway)		
Directs assistant to ventilate patient with bag-valve-mask device (room air)		*
Observes chest rise/fall and auscultates bilaterally over lungs for baseline		*
Obtains effective ventilation in less than 30 seconds		*
Attaches oxygen reservoir to bag-valve-mask device and connects to high-flow oxygen		
Ventilates patient and evaluates chest wall/lung compliance		*
Directs assistant to preoxygenate patient with assistant maintaining C-spine SMR		*
Identifies/selects proper equipment for intubation		
Checks laryngoscope light and cuff of ET tube		
Removes all air from cuff and properly inserts stylet if used		
Directs assistant to face patient and establish cervical spine SMR from front		
Intubating paramedic sits behind patient on ground with legs straddling patient's shoulders		
Moves up until patient's head is secured		
Removes OPA and directs assistant to perform Sellick's maneuver		*
Opens mouth and gently inserts blade while sweeping tongue to side		*
Gently elevates mandible with laryngoscope and leans backward to visualize cords		*
Inserts ET tube and visualizes as tube is advanced through cords		*
"Threads" ET tube off stylet (if used), maintaining hold on ET tube as stylet removed		
Inflates cuff to proper pressure and disconnects syringe		*
Disconnects mask from bag-valve device and attaches to ET tube without releasing ET tube		
Directs ventilation of patient while maintaining Sellick's maneuver and holding ET tube in place		
Confirms proper placement by auscultation over epigastrium and bilaterally over each lung		*
Directs assistant to release cricoid pressure		*
Secures ET tube		*
Reassesses bilateral lung sounds and compliance		*
Uses secondary device to confirm tube placement		*
Assesses patient's response to intervention		*
Student exhibits competence with skill		

Any items in the Not Done column that are marked with an * are mandatory for the student to complete. A check mark in the Not Done column of an item with an * indicates that the student was unsuccessful and must attempt the skill again to assure competency. Examiners should use a different-color ink for the second attempt.

☐ Successful   ☐ Unsuccessful   Examiner Initials: _____

©2006 Prentice-Hall Inc.

Scenario IV Insertion—Musculoskeletal Trauma

Student: _____   Examiner: _____

Date: _____

	Done ✓	Not Done
Selects appropriate IV fluid, checking clarity, color, and expiration date		*
Selects appropriate catheter		
Selects appropriate administration set		
Properly inserts IV tubing into the IV bag		*
Prepares administration set (fills drip chamber and flushes tubing)		*
Cuts or tears tape (at any time before venipuncture)		*
Applies constricting band (checks distal pulse to assure NOT a tourniquet)		*
Palpates suitable vein		*
Cleanses site appropriately		*
Utilizes appropriate PPE		*
Inserts catheter with sterile technique		*
Verbalizes flash/blood return and advances catheter slightly farther		*
Occludes vein with finger at distal end of catheter and removes stylet		
Immediately disposes (or verbalizes disposal) of needle/sharp in proper container		
Obtains blood sample or connects IV tubing to catheter		
Obtains BGL (blood glucose level)		*
Releases constricting band		*
Runs IV for a brief period to ensure patency and adjusts flow rate as appropriate		*
Checks IV site for signs of infiltration		*
Secures catheter (tapes securely or verbalizes)		*
Attaches label with size of catheter, date, time, and "prehospital"		*
Assesses patient's response to intervention		*
Student exhibits competence with skill		

Any items in the Not Done column that are marked with an * are mandatory for the student to complete. A check mark in the Not Done column of an item with an * indicates that the student was unsuccessful and must attempt the skill again to assure competency. Examiners should use a different-color ink for the second attempt.

☐ Successful   ☐ Unsuccessful   Examiner Initials: _____

©2006 Prentice-Hall Inc.

Scenario Radio Report—Musculoskeletal Trauma

Student: _____   Examiner: _____

Date: _____

	Done ✓	Not Done
Requests and checks for open channel before speaking		
Presses transmit button 1 second before speaking		
Holds microphone 2–3 in. from mouth		
Speaks slowly and clearly		*
Speaks in a normal voice		
Briefly transmits: Agency, unit designation, identification/name		*
Briefly transmits: Patient's age, sex, weight		*
Briefly transmits: Scene description/mechanism of injury or medical problem		*
Briefly transmits: Chief complaint with brief history of *present* illness		*
Briefly transmits: Associated symptoms (unless able to be deferred to bedside report)		
Briefly transmits: Past medical history (usually deferred to bedside report)		
Briefly transmits: Vital signs		*
Briefly transmits: Level of consciousness/GCS on trauma		*
Briefly transmits: General appearance, distress, cardiac rhythm, blood glucose, and other pertinent findings unable to be deferred to bedside report		
Briefly transmits: Interventions by EMS AND response(s)		*
ETA (the more critical the patient, the earlier you need to notify the receiving facility)		
Does not waste airtime		
Protects privacy of patient		*
Echoes dispatch information and any physician orders		*
Writes down dispatch information or physician orders		
Confirms with facility that message is received		
Demonstrates/verbalizes ability to troubleshoot basic equipment malfunction		
Student exhibits competence with skill		

Any items in the Not Done column that are marked with an * are mandatory for the student to complete. A check mark in the Not Done column of an item with an * indicates that the student was unsuccessful and must attempt the skill again to assure competency. Examiners should use a different-color ink for the second attempt.

☐ Successful   ☐ Unsuccessful   Examiner Initials: _____

©2006 Prentice-Hall Inc.

Scenario Patient Care Report (PCR)—Musculoskeletal Trauma

Student: _____   **Examiner:** _____

Date: _____

	Done ✓	Not Done
Records all pertinent dispatch/scene data, using a consistent format		
Completely identifies all additional resources and personnel		
Documents chief complaint, signs/symptoms, position found, age, sex, and weight		
Identifies and records all pertinent, reportable clinical data for each patient		
Documents SAMPLE and OPQRST if applicable		
Records all pertinent negatives		
Records all pertinent denials		
Records accurate, consistent times and patient information		
Includes relevant oral statements of witnesses, bystanders, and patient in "quotes" when appropriate		
Documents initial assessment findings: airway, breathing, and circulation		
Documents any interventions in initial assessment with patient response		
Documents level of consciousness, GCS (if trauma), and VS		
Documents rapid trauma assessment if applicable		
Documents any interventions in rapid trauma assessment with patient response		
Documents focused history and physical assessment		
Documents any interventions in focused assessment with patient response		
Documents repeat VS (every 5 minutes for critical; every 15 minutes for stable)		
Repeats initial assessment and documents findings		
Records ALL treatments with times and patient response(s) in treatment section		
Documents field impression		
Documents transport to specific facility and transfer of care WITH VERBAL REPORT		
Uses correct grammar, abbreviations, spelling, and terminology		
Writes legibly		
Thoroughly documents refusals, denials of transport, and call cancellations		
Documents patient GCS of 15 PRIOR to signing refusal		
Documents advice given to refusal patient, including "call 9-1-1 for further problems"		
Properly corrects errors and omissions		
Writes cautiously, avoids jargon, opinions, inferences, or any derogatory/libelous remarks		
Signs run report		
Uses EMS supplement form if needed		
Student exhibits competence with skill		

Any items in the Not Done column should be evaluated with student. Check marks in this column do not necessarily mean student was unsuccessful as all lines are not completed on all patients. Evaluation of each PCR should be based on the scenario given.

Student must be able to write an EMS report with consistency and accuracy.

☐ Successful   ☐ Unsuccessful   Examiner Initials: _____

     ©2006 Prentice-Hall Inc.

Overall Scenario Management—Musculoskeletal Trauma

Student: _____   Examiner: _____

Date: _____   Scenario: _____

NOTE: This skill sheet is to be done after the student completes a scenario as the TEAM LEADER. It is to let the student know if he or she is beginning to "put it all together" and use critical thinking skills to manage an EMS call. PLEASE notice that it is graded on a different basis than the basic lab skill sheet.

	Done ✓	Needs to Improve
SCENE MANAGEMENT		
Recognized hazards and controlled scene—safety, crowd, and patient issues		
Recognized hazards, but did not control the scene		
Unsuccessfully attempted to manage the scene	*	
Did not evaluate the scene and took no control of the scene	*	
PATIENT ASSESSMENT		
Performed a timely, organized complete patient assessment		
Performed complete initial, focused, and ongoing assessments, but in a disorganized manner		
Performed an incomplete assessment	*	
Did not perform an initial assessment	*	
PATIENT MANAGEMENT		
Evaluated assessment findings to manage all aspects of patient condition		
Managed the patient's presenting signs and symptoms without considering all of assessment		
Inadequately managed the patient	*	
Did not manage life-threatening conditions	*	
COMMUNICATION		
Communicated well with crew, patient, family, bystanders, and assisting agencies		
Communicated well with patient and crew		
Communicated with patient and crew, but poor communication skills	*	
Unable to communicate effectively	*	
REPORT AND TRANSFER OF CARE		
Identified correct destination for patient transport, gave accurate, brief report over radio, and provided full report at bedside demonstrating thorough understanding of patient condition and pathophysiological processes		
Identified correct destination and gave accurate radio and bedside report, but did not demonstrate understanding of patient condition and pathophysiological processes		
Identified correct destination, but provided inadequate radio and bedside report	*	
Identified inappropriate destination or provided no radio or bedside report	*	
Student exhibits competence with skill		

Any items that are marked with an * indicate the student needs to improve and a check mark should be placed in the right-hand column. A check mark in the right-hand column indicates that the student was unsuccessful and must attempt the skill again to assure competency. Examiners should use a different-color ink for the second attempt.

☐ Successful   ☐ Unsuccessful   Examiner Initials: _____

©2006 Prentice-Hall Inc.

Patient Assessment: Trauma—Shock/Hemorrhage

Student: _____   Examiner: _____

Date: _____   Scenario: _____

	Done ✓	Not Done
Assesses scene safety and utilizes appropriate PPE		*
OVERALL SCENE EVALUATION		
Trauma—assesses mechanism of injury/if medical component determines nature of illness		*
Determines the number of patients, location, obstacles, and requests any additional resources as needed		
Verbalizes general impression of the patient as approaches		*
Stabilizes C-spine/spinal motion restriction (SMR) of spine		*
INITIAL ASSESSMENT/RESUSCITATION		
Determines responsiveness/level of consciousness/AVPU		*
Opens airway with appropriate technique and assesses airway/ventilation		*
Manages airway/ventilation and applies appropriate oxygen therapy in less than 3 minutes		*
Assesses circulation: radial/carotid pulse, skin color, temperature, condition, and turgor		*
Controls any major bleeding		*
Makes rapid transport decision		*
Obtains IV (2 if indicated), BGL, GCS, and complete vital signs		
RAPID TRAUMA ASSESSMENT (If patient is Trauma Alert or Load and Go)		
Assesses abdomen		
Rapidly palpates each extremity, assessing for obvious injuries and distal PMS		
Provides spinal motion restriction (SMR) on long backboard (LBB), checking posterior torso and legs		
Secures head LAST		
Identifies patient problem: shock/hemorrhage (specify type and stage of shock)		*
Loads patient/initiates transport (to appropriate LZ or to appropriate facility) in less than 10 minutes		*
Reassesses ABCs and interventions		*
FOCUSED HISTORY AND PHYSICAL ASSESSMENT		
Reassesses interventions and further assesses injuries found		
Obtains vital signs and GCS (Glasgow Coma Score)		
Obtains SAMPLE history		
Inspects and palpates head, facial, and neck regions		
Inspects, palpates, and auscultates chest/thorax		
Inspects and palpates abdomen and pelvis		
Inspects and palpates upper and lower extremities, checking distal PMS		
Inspects and palpates posterior torso		
Manages all injuries/wounds appropriately—identifies type of hemorrhage		
Repeats initial assessment, vital signs, and evaluates trends		*
Evaluates response to interventions/treatments		*
Performs ongoing assessment (VS every 5 minutes for critical patient/every 15 minutes for stable patient)		
Gives radio report to receiving facility		
Turns over patient care with verbal report		*
Student exhibits competence with skill		

Any items in the Not Done column that are marked with an * are mandatory for the student to complete. A check mark in the Not Done column of an item with an * indicates that the student was unsuccessful and must attempt the skill again to assure competency. Examiners should use a different-color ink for the second attempt.

☐ Successful   ☐ Unsuccessful   Examiner Initials: _____

    ©2006 Prentice-Hall Inc.

Endotracheal Intubation with Suspected Cervical Spine—Shock/Hemorrhage

Student: _____   **Examiner:** _____

Date: _____

	Done ✓	Not Done
Determines scene safety and utilizes appropriate PPE		*
Opens the airway manually with trauma jaw-thrust while assistant maintains C-spine SMR		*
Checks mouth for blood or potential airway obstruction		*
Suctions or removes loose teeth or foreign materials as needed		
Inserts simple airway adjunct (oropharyngeal airway)		
Directs assistant to ventilate patient with bag-valve-mask device (room air)		*
Observes chest rise/fall and auscultates bilaterally over lungs for baseline		*
Obtains effective ventilation in less than 30 seconds		*
Attaches oxygen reservoir to bag-valve-mask device and connects to high-flow oxygen		
Ventilates patient and evaluates chest wall/lung compliance		*
Directs assistant to preoxygenate patient with assistant maintaining C-spine SMR		*
Identifies/selects proper equipment for intubation		
Checks laryngoscope light and cuff of ET tube		
Removes all air from cuff and properly inserts stylet if used		
Directs assistant to face patient and establish cervical spine SMR from front		
Intubating paramedic sits behind patient on ground with legs straddling patient's shoulders		
Moves up until patient's head is secured		
Removes OPA and directs assistant to perform Sellick's maneuver		*
Opens mouth and gently inserts blade while sweeping tongue to side		*
Gently elevates mandible with laryngoscope and leans backward to visualize cords		*
Inserts ET tube and visualizes as tube is advanced through cords		*
"Threads" ET tube off stylet (if used), maintaining hold on ET tube as stylet removed		
Inflates cuff to proper pressure and disconnects syringe		*
Disconnects mask from bag-valve device and attaches to ET tube without releasing ET tube		
Directs ventilation of patient while maintaining Sellick's maneuver and holding ET tube in place		
Confirms proper placement by auscultation over epigastrium and bilaterally over each lung		*
Directs assistant to release cricoid pressure		*
Secures ET tube		*
Reassesses bilateral lung sounds and compliance		*
Uses secondary device to confirm tube placement		*
Assesses patient's response to intervention		*
Student exhibits competence with skill		

Any items in the Not Done column that are marked with an * are mandatory for the student to complete. A check mark in the Not Done column of an item with an * indicates that the student was unsuccessful and must attempt the skill again to assure competency. Examiners should use a different-color ink for the second attempt.

☐ Successful   ☐ Unsuccessful   Examiner Initials: _____

Scenario IV Insertion—Shock/Hemorrhage

Student: _____   Examiner: _____

Date: _____

	Done ✓	Not Done
Selects appropriate IV fluid, checking clarity, color, and expiration date		*
Selects appropriate catheter		
Selects appropriate administration set		
Properly inserts IV tubing into the IV bag		*
Prepares administration set (fills drip chamber and flushes tubing)		*
Cuts or tears tape (at any time before venipuncture)		*
Applies constricting band (checks distal pulse to assure NOT a tourniquet)		*
Palpates suitable vein		*
Cleanses site appropriately		*
Utilizes appropriate PPE		*
Inserts catheter with sterile technique		*
Verbalizes flash/blood return and advances catheter slightly farther		*
Occludes vein with finger at distal end of catheter and removes stylet		
Immediately disposes (or verbalizes disposal) of needle/sharp in proper container		
Obtains blood sample or connects IV tubing to catheter		
Obtains BGL (blood glucose level)		*
Releases constricting band		*
Runs IV for a brief period to ensure patency and adjusts flow rate as appropriate		*
Checks IV site for signs of infiltration		*
Secures catheter (tapes securely or verbalizes)		*
Attaches label with size of catheter, date, time, and "prehospital"		*
Assesses patient's response to intervention		*
Student exhibits competence with skill		

Any items in the Not Done column that are marked with an * are mandatory for the student to complete. A check mark in the Not Done column of an item with an * indicates that the student was unsuccessful and must attempt the skill again to assure competency. Examiners should use a different-color ink for the second attempt.

☐ Successful   ☐ Unsuccessful   Examiner Initials: _____

©2006 Prentice-Hall Inc.

Scenario Radio Report—Shock/Hemorrhage

Student: _____   **Examiner:** _____

Date: _____

	Done ✓	Not Done
Requests and checks for open channel before speaking		
Presses transmit button 1 second before speaking		
Holds microphone 2–3 in. from mouth		
Speaks slowly and clearly		*
Speaks in a normal voice		
Briefly transmits: Agency, unit designation, identification/name		*
Briefly transmits: Patient's age, sex, weight		*
Briefly transmits: Scene description/mechanism of injury or medical problem		*
Briefly transmits: Chief complaint with brief history of *present* illness		*
Briefly transmits: Associated symptoms (unless able to be deferred to bedside report)		
Briefly transmits: Past medical history (usually deferred to bedside report)		
Briefly transmits: Vital signs		*
Briefly transmits: Level of consciousness/GCS on trauma		*
Briefly transmits: General appearance, distress, cardiac rhythm, blood glucose, and other pertinent findings unable to be deferred to bedside report		
Briefly transmits: Interventions by EMS AND response(s)		*
ETA (the more critical the patient, the earlier you need to notify the receiving facility)		
Does not waste airtime		
Protects privacy of patient		*
Echoes dispatch information and any physician orders		*
Writes down dispatch information or physician orders		
Confirms with facility that message is received		
Demonstrates/verbalizes ability to troubleshoot basic equipment malfunction		
Student exhibits competence with skill		

Any items in the Not Done column that are marked with an * are mandatory for the student to complete. A check mark in the Not Done column of an item with an * indicates that the student was unsuccessful and must attempt the skill again to assure competency. Examiners should use a different-color ink for the second attempt.

☐ Successful   ☐ Unsuccessful   Examiner Initials: _____

©2006 Prentice-Hall Inc.

Scenario Patient Care Report (PCR)—Shock/Hemorrhage

Student: _____   Examiner: _____

Date: _____

	Done ✓	Not Done
Records all pertinent dispatch/scene data, using a consistent format		
Completely identifies all additional resources and personnel		
Documents chief complaint, signs/symptoms, position found, age, sex, and weight		
Identifies and records all pertinent, reportable clinical data for each patient		
Documents SAMPLE and OPQRST if applicable		
Records all pertinent negatives		
Records all pertinent denials		
Records accurate, consistent times and patient information		
Includes relevant oral statements of witnesses, bystanders, and patient in "quotes" when appropriate		
Documents initial assessment findings: airway, breathing, and circulation		
Documents any interventions in initial assessment with patient response		
Documents level of consciousness, GCS (if trauma), and VS		
Documents rapid trauma assessment if applicable		
Documents any interventions in rapid trauma assessment with patient response		
Documents focused history and physical assessment		
Documents any interventions in focused assessment with patient response		
Documents repeat VS (every 5 minutes for critical; every 15 minutes for stable)		
Repeats initial assessment and documents findings		
Records ALL treatments with times and patient response(s) in treatment section		
Documents field impression		
Documents transport to specific facility and transfer of care WITH VERBAL REPORT		
Uses correct grammar, abbreviations, spelling, and terminology		
Writes legibly		
Thoroughly documents refusals, denials of transport, and call cancellations		
Documents patient GCS of 15 PRIOR to signing refusal		
Documents advice given to refusal patient, including "call 9-1-1 for further problems"		
Properly corrects errors and omissions		
Writes cautiously, avoids jargon, opinions, inferences, or any derogatory/libelous remarks		
Signs run report		
Uses EMS supplement form if needed		
Student exhibits competence with skill		

Any items in the Not Done column should be evaluated with student. Check marks in this column do not necessarily mean student was unsuccessful as all lines are not completed on all patients. Evaluation of each PCR should be based on the scenario given.

Student must be able to write an EMS report with consistency and accuracy.

☐ Successful   ☐ Unsuccessful   Examiner Initials: _____

©2006 Prentice-Hall Inc.

Overall Scenario Management—Shock/Hemorrhage

Student: _____   Examiner: _____

Date: _____   Scenario: _____

NOTE: This skill sheet is to be done after the student completes a scenario as the TEAM LEADER. It is to let the student know if he or she is beginning to "put it all together" and use critical thinking skills to manage an EMS call. PLEASE notice that it is graded on a different basis than the basic lab skill sheet.

	Done ✓	Needs to Improve
SCENE MANAGEMENT		
Recognized hazards and controlled scene—safety, crowd, and patient issues		
Recognized hazards, but did not control the scene		
Unsuccessfully attempted to manage the scene	*	
Did not evaluate the scene and took no control of the scene	*	
PATIENT ASSESSMENT		
Performed a timely, organized complete patient assessment		
Performed complete initial, focused, and ongoing assessments, but in a disorganized manner		
Performed an incomplete assessment	*	
Did not perform an initial assessment	*	
PATIENT MANAGEMENT		
Evaluated assessment findings to manage all aspects of patient condition		
Managed the patient's presenting signs and symptoms without considering all of assessment		
Inadequately managed the patient	*	
Did not manage life-threatening conditions	*	
COMMUNICATION		
Communicated well with crew, patient, family, bystanders, and assisting agencies		
Communicated well with patient and crew		
Communicated with patient and crew, but poor communication skills	*	
Unable to communicate effectively	*	
REPORT AND TRANSFER OF CARE		
Identified correct destination for patient transport, gave accurate, brief report over radio, and provided full report at bedside demonstrating thorough understanding of patient condition and pathophysiological processes		
Identified correct destination and gave accurate radio and bedside report, but did not demonstrate understanding of patient condition and pathophysiological processes		
Identified correct destination, but provided inadequate radio and bedside report	*	
Identified inappropriate destination or provided no radio or bedside report	*	
Student exhibits competence with skill		

Any items that are marked with an * indicate the student needs to improve and a check mark should be placed in the right-hand column. A check mark in the right-hand column indicates that the student was unsuccessful and must attempt the skill again to assure competency. Examiners should use a different-color ink for the second attempt.

☐ Successful   ☐ Unsuccessful   Examiner Initials: _____

Patient Assessment: Trauma—Soft Tissue Trauma

Student: _____   Examiner: _____

Date: _____   Scenario: _____

	Done ✓	Not Done
Assesses scene safety and utilizes appropriate PPE		*
OVERALL SCENE EVALUATION		
Trauma—assesses mechanism of injury/if medical component determines nature of illness		*
Determines the number of patients, location, obstacles, and requests any additional resources as needed		
Verbalizes general impression of the patient as approaches		*
Stabilizes C-spine/spinal motion restriction (SMR) of spine		*
INITIAL ASSESSMENT/RESUSCITATION		
Determines responsiveness/level of consciousness/AVPU		*
Opens airway with appropriate technique and assesses airway/ventilation		*
Manages airway/ventilation and applies appropriate oxygen therapy in less than 3 minutes		*
Assesses circulation: radial/carotid pulse, skin color, temperature, condition, and turgor		*
Controls any major bleeding		*
Makes rapid transport decision		*
Obtains IV (2 if indicated), BGL, GCS, and complete vital signs		
RAPID TRAUMA ASSESSMENT (If patient is Trauma Alert or Load and Go)		
Assesses abdomen		
Rapidly palpates each extremity, assessing for obvious injuries and distal PMS		
Provides spinal motion restriction (SMR) on long backboard (LBB), checking posterior torso and legs		
Secures head LAST		
Identifies patient problem: soft tissue trauma (specify type)		*
Loads patient/initiates transport (to appropriate LZ or to appropriate facility) in less than 10 minutes		*
Reassesses ABCs and interventions		*
FOCUSED HISTORY AND PHYSICAL ASSESSMENT		
Reassesses interventions and further assesses injuries found		
Obtains vital signs and GCS (Glasgow Coma Score)		
Obtains SAMPLE history		
Inspects and palpates head, facial, and neck regions		
Inspects, palpates, and auscultates chest/thorax		
Inspects and palpates abdomen and pelvis		
Inspects and palpates upper and lower extremities, checking distal PMS		
Inspects and palpates posterior torso		
Manages all injuries/wounds appropriately—specific to type of soft tissue trauma		
Repeats initial assessment, vital signs, and evaluates trends		*
Evaluates response to interventions/treatments		*
Performs ongoing assessment (VS every 5 minutes for critical patient/every 15 minutes for stable patient)		
Gives radio report to receiving facility		
Turns over patient care with verbal report		*
Student exhibits competence with skill		

Any items in the Not Done column that are marked with an * are mandatory for the student to complete. A check mark in the Not Done column of an item with an * indicates that the student was unsuccessful and must attempt the skill again to assure competency. Examiners should use a different-color ink for the second attempt.

☐ Successful   ☐ Unsuccessful   Examiner Initials: _____

©2006 Prentice-Hall Inc.

Scenario IV Insertion—Soft Tissue Trauma

Student: _____   Examiner: _____

Date: _____

	Done ✓	Not Done
Selects appropriate IV fluid, checking clarity, color, and expiration date		*
Selects appropriate catheter		
Selects appropriate administration set		
Properly inserts IV tubing into the IV bag		*
Prepares administration set (fills drip chamber and flushes tubing)		*
Cuts or tears tape (at any time before venipuncture)		*
Applies constricting band (checks distal pulse to assure NOT a tourniquet)		*
Palpates suitable vein		*
Cleanses site appropriately		*
Utilizes appropriate PPE		*
Inserts catheter with sterile technique		*
Verbalizes flash/blood return and advances catheter slightly farther		*
Occludes vein with finger at distal end of catheter and removes stylet		
Immediately disposes (or verbalizes disposal) of needle/sharp in proper container		
Obtains blood sample or connects IV tubing to catheter		
Obtains BGL (blood glucose level)		*
Releases constricting band		*
Runs IV for a brief period to ensure patency and adjusts flow rate as appropriate		*
Checks IV site for signs of infiltration		*
Secures catheter (tapes securely or verbalizes)		*
Attaches label with size of catheter, date, time, and "prehospital"		*
Assesses patient's response to intervention		*
Student exhibits competence with skill		

Any items in the Not Done column that are marked with an * are mandatory for the student to complete. A check mark in the Not Done column of an item with an * indicates that the student was unsuccessful and must attempt the skill again to assure competency. Examiners should use a different-color ink for the second attempt.

☐ Successful   ☐ Unsuccessful   Examiner Initials: _____

©2006 Prentice-Hall Inc.

Scenario Radio Report—Soft Tissue Trauma

Student: _____   **Examiner:** _____

Date: _____

	Done ✓	Not Done
Requests and checks for open channel before speaking		
Presses transmit button 1 second before speaking		
Holds microphone 2–3 in. from mouth		
Speaks slowly and clearly		*
Speaks in a normal voice		
Briefly transmits: Agency, unit designation, identification/name		*
Briefly transmits: Patient's age, sex, weight		*
Briefly transmits: Scene description/mechanism of injury or medical problem		*
Briefly transmits: Chief complaint with brief history of *present* illness		*
Briefly transmits: Associated symptoms (unless able to be deferred to bedside report)		
Briefly transmits: Past medical history (usually deferred to bedside report)		
Briefly transmits: Vital signs		*
Briefly transmits: Level of consciousness/GCS on trauma		*
Briefly transmits: General appearance, distress, cardiac rhythm, blood glucose, and other pertinent findings unable to be deferred to bedside report		
Briefly transmits: Interventions by EMS AND response(s)		*
ETA (the more critical the patient, the earlier you need to notify the receiving facility)		
Does not waste airtime		
Protects privacy of patient		*
Echoes dispatch information and any physician orders		*
Writes down dispatch information or physician orders		
Confirms with facility that message is received		
Demonstrates/verbalizes ability to troubleshoot basic equipment malfunction		
Student exhibits competence with skill		

Any items in the Not Done column that are marked with an * are mandatory for the student to complete. A check mark in the Not Done column of an item with an * indicates that the student was unsuccessful and must attempt the skill again to assure competency. Examiners should use a different-color ink for the second attempt.

☐ Successful   ☐ Unsuccessful   Examiner Initials: _____

©2006 Prentice-Hall Inc.

Scenario Patient Care Report (PCR)—Soft Tissue Trauma

Student: _____   **Examiner:** _____

Date: _____

	Done ✓	Not Done
Records all pertinent dispatch/scene data, using a consistent format		
Completely identifies all additional resources and personnel		
Documents chief complaint, signs/symptoms, position found, age, sex, and weight		
Identifies and records all pertinent, reportable clinical data for each patient		
Documents SAMPLE and OPQRST if applicable		
Records all pertinent negatives		
Records all pertinent denials		
Records accurate, consistent times and patient information		
Includes relevant oral statements of witnesses, bystanders, and patient in "quotes" when appropriate		
Documents initial assessment findings: airway, breathing, and circulation		
Documents any interventions in initial assessment with patient response		
Documents level of consciousness, GCS (if trauma), and VS		
Documents rapid trauma assessment if applicable		
Documents any interventions in rapid trauma assessment with patient response		
Documents focused history and physical assessment		
Documents any interventions in focused assessment with patient response		
Documents repeat VS (every 5 minutes for critical; every 15 minutes for stable)		
Repeats initial assessment and documents findings		
Records ALL treatments with times and patient response(s) in treatment section		
Documents field impression		
Documents transport to specific facility and transfer of care WITH VERBAL REPORT		
Uses correct grammar, abbreviations, spelling, and terminology		
Writes legibly		
Thoroughly documents refusals, denials of transport, and call cancellations		
Documents patient GCS of 15 PRIOR to signing refusal		
Documents advice given to refusal patient, including "call 9-1-1 for further problems"		
Properly corrects errors and omissions		
Writes cautiously, avoids jargon, opinions, inferences, or any derogatory/libelous remarks		
Signs run report		
Uses EMS supplement form if needed		
Student exhibits competence with skill		

Any items in the Not Done column should be evaluated with student. Check marks in this column do not necessarily mean student was unsuccessful as all lines are not completed on all patients. Evaluation of each PCR should be based on the scenario given.

Student must be able to write an EMS report with consistency and accuracy.

☐ Successful   ☐ Unsuccessful   Examiner Initials: _____

Overall Scenario Management—Soft Tissue Trauma

Student: _____   Examiner: _____

Date: _____   Scenario: _____

NOTE: This skill sheet is to be done after the student completes a scenario as the TEAM LEADER. It is to let the student know if he or she is beginning to "put it all together" and use critical thinking skills to manage an EMS call. PLEASE notice that it is graded on a different basis than the basic lab skill sheet.

	Done ✓	Needs to Improve
SCENE MANAGEMENT		
Recognized hazards and controlled scene—safety, crowd, and patient issues		
Recognized hazards, but did not control the scene		
Unsuccessfully attempted to manage the scene	*	
Did not evaluate the scene and took no control of the scene	*	
PATIENT ASSESSMENT		
Performed a timely, organized complete patient assessment		
Performed complete initial, focused, and ongoing assessments, but in a disorganized manner		
Performed an incomplete assessment	*	
Did not perform an initial assessment	*	
PATIENT MANAGEMENT		
Evaluated assessment findings to manage all aspects of patient condition		
Managed the patient's presenting signs and symptoms without considering all of assessment		
Inadequately managed the patient	*	
Did not manage life-threatening conditions	*	
COMMUNICATION		
Communicated well with crew, patient, family, bystanders, and assisting agencies		
Communicated well with patient and crew		
Communicated with patient and crew, but poor communication skills	*	
Unable to communicate effectively	*	
REPORT AND TRANSFER OF CARE		
Identified correct destination for patient transport, gave accurate, brief report over radio, and provided full report at bedside demonstrating thorough understanding of patient condition and pathophysiological processes		
Identified correct destination and gave accurate radio and bedside report, but did not demonstrate understanding of patient condition and pathophysiological processes		
Identified correct destination, but provided inadequate radio and bedside report	*	
Identified inappropriate destination or provided no radio or bedside report	*	
Student exhibits competence with skill		

Any items that are marked with an * indicate the student needs to improve and a check mark should be placed in the right-hand column. A check mark in the right-hand column indicates that the student was unsuccessful and must attempt the skill again to assure competency. Examiners should use a different-color ink for the second attempt.

☐ Successful   ☐ Unsuccessful   Examiner Initials: _____

©2006 Prentice-Hall Inc.

Patient Assessment: Trauma—Spinal Trauma

Student: _____   **Examiner:** _____

Date: _____   **Scenario:** _____

	Done ✓	Not Done
Assesses scene safety and utilizes appropriate PPE		*
OVERALL SCENE EVALUATION		
Trauma—assesses mechanism of injury/if medical component determines nature of illness		*
Determines the number of patients, location, obstacles, and requests any additional resources as needed		
Verbalizes general impression of the patient as approaches		*
Stabilizes C-spine/spinal motion restriction (SMR) of spine		*
INITIAL ASSESSMENT/RESUSCITATION		
Determines responsiveness/level of consciousness/AVPU		*
Opens airway with appropriate technique and assesses airway/ventilation		*
Manages airway/ventilation and applies appropriate oxygen therapy in less than 3 minutes		*
Assesses circulation: radial/carotid pulse, skin color, temperature, condition, and turgor		*
Controls any major bleeding		*
Makes rapid transport decision		*
Obtains IV (2 if indicated), BGL, GCS, and complete vital signs		
RAPID TRAUMA ASSESSMENT (If patient is Trauma Alert or Load and Go)		
Assesses abdomen		
Rapidly palpates each extremity, assessing for obvious injuries and distal PMS		
Provides spinal motion restriction (SMR) on long backboard (LBB), checking posterior torso and legs		
Secures head LAST		
Identifies patient problem: spinal trauma—verbalizes monitoring for Cushing's Triad in case head involved		*
Loads patient/initiates transport (to appropriate LZ or to appropriate facility) in less than 10 minutes		*
Reassesses ABCs and interventions		*
FOCUSED HISTORY AND PHYSICAL ASSESSMENT		
Reassesses interventions and further assesses injuries found		
Obtains vital signs and GCS (Glasgow Coma Score)		
Obtains SAMPLE history		
Inspects and palpates head, facial, and neck regions		
Inspects, palpates, and auscultates chest/thorax		
Inspects and palpates abdomen and pelvis		
Inspects and palpates upper and lower extremities, checking distal PMS		
Inspects and palpates posterior torso		
Manages all injuries/wounds appropriately		
Repeats initial assessment, vital signs, and evaluates trends		*
Evaluates response to interventions/treatments		*
Performs ongoing assessment (VS every 5 minutes for critical patient/every 15 minutes for stable patient)		
Gives radio report to receiving facility		
Turns over patient care with verbal report		*
Student exhibits competence with skill		

Any items in the Not Done column that are marked with an * are mandatory for the student to complete. A check mark in the Not Done column of an item with an * indicates that the student was unsuccessful and must attempt the skill again to assure competency. Examiners should use a different-color ink for the second attempt.

☐ Successful   ☐ Unsuccessful   Examiner Initials: _____

©2006 Prentice-Hall Inc.

Endotracheal Intubation with Suspected Cervical Spine—Spinal Trauma

Student: _____   Examiner:_____

Date: _____

	Done ✓	Not Done
Determines scene safety and utilizes appropriate PPE		*
Opens the airway manually with trauma jaw-thrust while assistant maintains C-spine SMR		*
Checks mouth for blood or potential airway obstruction		*
Suctions or removes loose teeth or foreign materials as needed		
Inserts simple airway adjunct (oropharyngeal airway)		
Directs assistant to ventilate patient with bag-valve-mask device (room air)		*
Observes chest rise/fall and auscultates bilaterally over lungs for baseline		*
Obtains effective ventilation in less than 30 seconds		*
Attaches oxygen reservoir to bag-valve-mask device and connects to high-flow oxygen		
Ventilates patient and evaluates chest wall/lung compliance		*
Directs assistant to preoxygenate patient with assistant maintaining C-spine SMR		*
Identifies/selects proper equipment for intubation		
Checks laryngoscope light and cuff of ET tube		
Removes all air from cuff and properly inserts stylet if used		
Directs assistant to face patient and establish cervical spine SMR from front		
Intubating paramedic sits behind patient on ground with legs straddling patient's shoulders		
Moves up until patient's head is secured		
Removes OPA and directs assistant to perform Sellick's maneuver		*
Opens mouth and gently inserts blade while sweeping tongue to side		*
Gently elevates mandible with laryngoscope and leans backward to visualize cords		*
Inserts ET tube and visualizes as tube is advanced through cords		*
"Threads" ET tube off stylet (if used), maintaining hold on ET tube as stylet removed		
Inflates cuff to proper pressure and disconnects syringe		*
Disconnects mask from bag-valve device and attaches to ET tube without releasing ET tube		
Directs ventilation of patient while maintaining Sellick's maneuver and holding ET tube in place		
Confirms proper placement by auscultation over epigastrium and bilaterally over each lung		*
Directs assistant to release cricoid pressure		*
Secures ET tube		*
Reassesses bilateral lung sounds and compliance		*
Uses secondary device to confirm tube placement		*
Assesses patient's response to intervention		*
Student exhibits competence with skill		

Any items in the Not Done column that are marked with an * are mandatory for the student to complete. A check mark in the Not Done column of an item with an * indicates that the student was unsuccessful and must attempt the skill again to assure competency. Examiners should use a different-color ink for the second attempt.

☐ Successful   ☐ Unsuccessful   Examiner Initials: _____

©2006 Prentice-Hall Inc.

Scenario IV Insertion—Spinal Trauma

Student: _____   **Examiner:** _____

Date: _____

	Done ✓	Not Done
Selects appropriate IV fluid, checking clarity, color, and expiration date		*
Selects appropriate catheter		
Selects appropriate administration set		
Properly inserts IV tubing into the IV bag		*
Prepares administration set (fills drip chamber and flushes tubing)		*
Cuts or tears tape (at any time before venipuncture)		*
Applies constricting band (checks distal pulse to assure NOT a tourniquet)		*
Palpates suitable vein		*
Cleanses site appropriately		*
Utilizes appropriate PPE		*
Inserts catheter with sterile technique		*
Verbalizes flash/blood return and advances catheter slightly farther		*
Occludes vein with finger at distal end of catheter and removes stylet		
Immediately disposes (or verbalizes disposal) of needle/sharp in proper container		
Obtains blood sample or connects IV tubing to catheter		
Obtains BGL (blood glucose level)		*
Releases constricting band		*
Runs IV for a brief period to ensure patency and adjusts flow rate as appropriate		*
Checks IV site for signs of infiltration		*
Secures catheter (tapes securely or verbalizes)		*
Attaches label with size of catheter, date, time, and "prehospital"		*
Assesses patient's response to intervention		*
Student exhibits competence with skill		

Any items in the Not Done column that are marked with an * are mandatory for the student to complete. A check mark in the Not Done column of an item with an * indicates that the student was unsuccessful and must attempt the skill again to assure competency. Examiners should use a different-color ink for the second attempt.

☐ Successful   ☐ Unsuccessful   Examiner Initials: _____

Scenario Radio Report—Spinal Trauma

Student: _____   **Examiner:** _____

Date: _____

	Done ✓	Not Done
Requests and checks for open channel before speaking		
Presses transmit button 1 second before speaking		
Holds microphone 2–3 in. from mouth		
Speaks slowly and clearly		*
Speaks in a normal voice		
Briefly transmits: Agency, unit designation, identification/name		*
Briefly transmits: Patient's age, sex, weight		*
Briefly transmits: Scene description/mechanism of injury or medical problem		*
Briefly transmits: Chief complaint with brief history of *present* illness		*
Briefly transmits: Associated symptoms (unless able to be deferred to bedside report)		
Briefly transmits: Past medical history (usually deferred to bedside report)		
Briefly transmits: Vital signs		*
Briefly transmits: Level of consciousness/GCS on trauma		*
Briefly transmits: General appearance, distress, cardiac rhythm, blood glucose, and other pertinent findings unable to be deferred to bedside report		
Briefly transmits: Interventions by EMS AND response(s)		*
ETA (the more critical the patient, the earlier you need to notify the receiving facility)		
Does not waste airtime		
Protects privacy of patient		*
Echoes dispatch information and any physician orders		*
Writes down dispatch information or physician orders		
Confirms with facility that message is received		
Demonstrates/verbalizes ability to troubleshoot basic equipment malfunction		
Student exhibits competence with skill		

Any items in the Not Done column that are marked with an * are mandatory for the student to complete. A check mark in the Not Done column of an item with an * indicates that the student was unsuccessful and must attempt the skill again to assure competency. Examiners should use a different-color ink for the second attempt.

☐ Successful   ☐ Unsuccessful   Examiner Initials: _____

©2006 Prentice-Hall Inc.

Scenario Patient Care Report (PCR)—Spinal Trauma

Student: _____   **Examiner:** _____

Date: _____

	Done ✓	Not Done
Records all pertinent dispatch/scene data, using a consistent format		
Completely identifies all additional resources and personnel		
Documents chief complaint, signs/symptoms, position found, age, sex, and weight		
Identifies and records all pertinent, reportable clinical data for each patient		
Documents SAMPLE and OPQRST if applicable		
Records all pertinent negatives		
Records all pertinent denials		
Records accurate, consistent times and patient information		
Includes relevant oral statements of witnesses, bystanders, and patient in "quotes" when appropriate		
Documents initial assessment findings: airway, breathing, and circulation		
Documents any interventions in initial assessment with patient response		
Documents level of consciousness, GCS (if trauma), and VS		
Documents rapid trauma assessment if applicable		
Documents any interventions in rapid trauma assessment with patient response		
Documents focused history and physical assessment		
Documents any interventions in focused assessment with patient response		
Documents repeat VS (every 5 minutes for critical; every 15 minutes for stable)		
Repeats initial assessment and documents findings		
Records ALL treatments with times and patient response(s) in treatment section		
Documents field impression		
Documents transport to specific facility and transfer of care WITH VERBAL REPORT		
Uses correct grammar, abbreviations, spelling, and terminology		
Writes legibly		
Thoroughly documents refusals, denials of transport, and call cancellations		
Documents patient GCS of 15 PRIOR to signing refusal		
Documents advice given to refusal patient, including "call 9-1-1 for further problems"		
Properly corrects errors and omissions		
Writes cautiously, avoids jargon, opinions, inferences, or any derogatory/libelous remarks		
Signs run report		
Uses EMS supplement form if needed		
Student exhibits competence with skill		

Any items in the Not Done column should be evaluated with student. Check marks in this column do not necessarily mean student was unsuccessful as all lines are not completed on all patients. Evaluation of each PCR should be based on the scenario given.

Student must be able to write an EMS report with consistency and accuracy.

☐ Successful   ☐ Unsuccessful   Examiner Initials: _____

©2006 Prentice-Hall Inc.

Overall Scenario Management—Spinal Trauma

Student: _____   Examiner:_____

Date: _____   Scenario: _____

NOTE: This skill sheet is to be done after the student completes a scenario as the TEAM LEADER. It is to let the student know if he or she is beginning to "put it all together" and use critical thinking skills to manage an EMS call. PLEASE notice that it is graded on a different basis than the basic lab skill sheet.

	Done ✓	Needs to Improve
SCENE MANAGEMENT		
Recognized hazards and controlled scene—safety, crowd, and patient issues		
Recognized hazards, but did not control the scene		
Unsuccessfully attempted to manage the scene	*	
Did not evaluate the scene and took no control of the scene	*	
PATIENT ASSESSMENT		
Performed a timely, organized complete patient assessment		
Performed complete initial, focused, and ongoing assessments, but in a disorganized manner		
Performed an incomplete assessment	*	
Did not perform an initial assessment	*	
PATIENT MANAGEMENT		
Evaluated assessment findings to manage all aspects of patient condition		
Managed the patient's presenting signs and symptoms without considering all of assessment		
Inadequately managed the patient	*	
Did not manage life-threatening conditions	*	
COMMUNICATION		
Communicated well with crew, patient, family, bystanders, and assisting agencies		
Communicated well with patient and crew		
Communicated with patient and crew, but poor communication skills	*	
Unable to communicate effectively	*	
REPORT AND TRANSFER OF CARE		
Identified correct destination for patient transport, gave accurate, brief report over radio, and provided full report at bedside demonstrating thorough understanding of patient condition and pathophysiological processes		
Identified correct destination and gave accurate radio and bedside report, but did not demonstrate understanding of patient condition and pathophysiological processes		
Identified correct destination, but provided inadequate radio and bedside report	*	
Identified inappropriate destination or provided no radio or bedside report	*	
Student exhibits competence with skill		

Any items that are marked with an * indicate the student needs to improve and a check mark should be placed in the right-hand column. A check mark in the right-hand column indicates that the student was unsuccessful and must attempt the skill again to assure competency. Examiners should use a different-color ink for the second attempt.

☐ Successful   ☐ Unsuccessful   Examiner Initials: _____

          ©2006 Prentice-Hall Inc.

Patient Assessment: Trauma—Thoracic Trauma

Student: _____   **Examiner:** _____

Date: _____   **Scenario:** _____

	Done ✓	Not Done
Assesses scene safety and utilizes appropriate PPE		*
OVERALL SCENE EVALUATION		
Trauma—assesses mechanism of injury/if medical component determines nature of illness		*
Determines the number of patients, location, obstacles, and requests any additional resources as needed		
Verbalizes general impression of the patient as approaches		*
Stabilizes C-spine/spinal motion restriction (SMR) of spine		*
INITIAL ASSESSMENT/RESUSCITATION		
Determines responsiveness/level of consciousness/AVPU		*
Opens airway with appropriate technique and assesses airway/ventilation		*
Manages airway/ventilation and applies oxygen therapy in less than 3 minutes (***occlusive dsg for open chest***)		*
Assesses circulation: radial/carotid pulse, skin color, temperature, condition, and turgor		*
Controls any major bleeding		*
Makes rapid transport decision		*
Obtains IV (2 if indicated), BGL, GCS, and complete vital signs		
RAPID TRAUMA ASSESSMENT (If patient is Trauma Alert or Load And Go)		
Assesses abdomen		
Rapidly palpates each extremity, assessing for obvious injuries and distal PMS		
Provides spinal motion restriction (SMR) on long backboard (LBB), checking posterior torso and legs		
Secures head LAST		
Identifies patient problem: thoracic trauma		*
Loads patient/initiates transport (to appropriate LZ or to appropriate facility) in less than 10 minutes		*
Reassesses ABCs and interventions		*
FOCUSED HISTORY AND PHYSICAL ASSESSMENT		
Reassesses interventions and further assesses injuries found		
Obtains vital signs and GCS (Glasgow Coma Score)		
Obtains SAMPLE history		
Inspects and palpates head, facial, and neck regions		
Inspects, palpates, and auscultates chest/thorax		
Inspects and palpates abdomen and pelvis		
Inspects and palpates upper and lower extremities, checking distal PMS		
Inspects and palpates posterior torso		
Manages all injuries/wounds appropriately—monitors closely for potential ventilation compromise		
Repeats initial assessment, vital signs, and evaluates trends		*
Evaluates response to interventions/treatments		*
Performs ongoing assessment (VS every 5 minutes for critical patient/every 15 minutes for stable patient)		
Gives radio report to receiving facility		
Turns over patient care with verbal report		*
Student exhibits competence with skill		

Any items in the Not Done column that are marked with an * are mandatory for the student to complete. A check mark in the Not Done column of an item with an * indicates that the student was unsuccessful and must attempt the skill again to assure competency. Examiners should use a different-color ink for the second attempt.

☐ Successful   ☐ Unsuccessful   Examiner Initials: _____

Endotracheal Intubation with Suspected Cervical Spine—Thoracic Trauma

Student: _____   Examiner: _____

Date: _____

	Done ✓	Not Done
Determines scene safety and utilizes appropriate PPE		*
Opens the airway manually with trauma jaw-thrust while assistant maintains C-spine SMR		*
Checks mouth for blood or potential airway obstruction		*
Suctions or removes loose teeth or foreign materials as needed		
Inserts simple airway adjunct (oropharyngeal airway)		
Directs assistant to ventilate patient with bag-valve-mask device (room air)		*
Observes chest rise/fall and auscultates bilaterally over lungs for baseline		*
Obtains effective ventilation in less than 30 seconds		*
Attaches oxygen reservoir to bag-valve-mask device and connects to high-flow oxygen		
Ventilates patient and evaluates chest wall/lung compliance		*
Directs assistant to preoxygenate patient with assistant maintaining C-spine SMR		*
Identifies/selects proper equipment for intubation		
Checks laryngoscope light and cuff of ET tube		
Removes all air from cuff and properly inserts stylet if used		
Directs assistant to face patient and establish cervical spine SMR from front		
Intubating paramedic sits behind patient on ground with legs straddling patient's shoulders		
Moves up until patient's head is secured		
Removes OPA and directs assistant to perform Sellick's maneuver		*
Opens mouth and gently inserts blade while sweeping tongue to side		*
Gently elevates mandible with laryngoscope and leans backward to visualize cords		*
Inserts ET tube and visualizes as tube is advanced through cords		*
"Threads" ET tube off stylet (if used), maintaining hold on ET tube as stylet removed		
Inflates cuff to proper pressure and disconnects syringe		*
Disconnects mask from bag-valve device and attaches to ET tube without releasing ET tube		
Directs ventilation of patient while maintaining Sellick's maneuver and holding ET tube in place		
Confirms proper placement by auscultation over epigastrium and bilaterally over each lung		*
Directs assistant to release cricoid pressure		*
Secures ET tube		*
Reassesses bilateral lung sounds and compliance		*
Uses secondary device to confirm tube placement		*
Assesses patient's response to intervention		*
Student exhibits competence with skill		

Any items in the Not Done column that are marked with an * are mandatory for the student to complete. A check mark in the Not Done column of an item with an * indicates that the student was unsuccessful and must attempt the skill again to assure competency. Examiners should use a different-color ink for the second attempt.

☐ Successful   ☐ Unsuccessful   Examiner Initials: _____

    ©2006 Prentice-Hall Inc.

Scenario IV Insertion—Thoracic Trauma

Student: _____

Examiner: _____

Date: _____

	Done ✓	Not Done
Selects appropriate IV fluid, checking clarity, color, and expiration date		*
Selects appropriate catheter		
Selects appropriate administration set		
Properly inserts IV tubing into the IV bag		*
Prepares administration set (fills drip chamber and flushes tubing)		*
Cuts or tears tape (at any time before venipuncture)		*
Applies constricting band (checks distal pulse to assure NOT a tourniquet)		*
Palpates suitable vein		*
Cleanses site appropriately		*
Utilizes appropriate PPE		*
Inserts catheter with sterile technique		*
Verbalizes flash/blood return and advances catheter slightly farther		*
Occludes vein with finger at distal end of catheter and removes stylet		
Immediately disposes (or verbalizes disposal) of needle/sharp in proper container		
Obtains blood sample or connects IV tubing to catheter		
Obtains BGL (blood glucose level)		*
Releases constricting band		*
Runs IV for a brief period to ensure patency and adjusts flow rate as appropriate		*
Checks IV site for signs of infiltration		*
Secures catheter (tapes securely or verbalizes)		*
Attaches label with size of catheter, date, time, and "prehospital"		*
Assesses patient's response to intervention		*
Student exhibits competence with skill		

Any items in the Not Done column that are marked with an * are mandatory for the student to complete. A check mark in the Not Done column of an item with an * indicates that the student was unsuccessful and must attempt the skill again to assure competency. Examiners should use a different-color ink for the second attempt.

☐ Successful   ☐ Unsuccessful   Examiner Initials: _____

©2006 Prentice-Hall Inc.

Scenario Radio Report—Thoracic Trauma

Student: _____   **Examiner:** _____

Date: _____

	Done ✓	Not Done
Requests and checks for open channel before speaking		
Presses transmit button 1 second before speaking		
Holds microphone 2–3 in. from mouth		
Speaks slowly and clearly		*
Speaks in a normal voice		
Briefly transmits: Agency, unit designation, identification/name		*
Briefly transmits: Patient's age, sex, weight		*
Briefly transmits: Scene description/mechanism of injury or medical problem		*
Briefly transmits: Chief complaint with brief history of *present* illness		*
Briefly transmits: Associated symptoms (unless able to be deferred to bedside report)		
Briefly transmits: Past medical history (usually deferred to bedside report)		
Briefly transmits: Vital signs		*
Briefly transmits: Level of consciousness/GCS on trauma		*
Briefly transmits: General appearance, distress, cardiac rhythm, blood glucose, and other pertinent findings unable to be deferred to bedside report		
Briefly transmits: Interventions by EMS AND response(s)		*
ETA (the more critical the patient, the earlier you need to notify the receiving facility)		
Does not waste airtime		
Protects privacy of patient		*
Echoes dispatch information and any physician orders		*
Writes down dispatch information or physician orders		
Confirms with facility that message is received		
Demonstrates/verbalizes ability to troubleshoot basic equipment malfunction		
Student exhibits competence with skill		

Any items in the Not Done column that are marked with an * are mandatory for the student to complete. A check mark in the Not Done column of an item with an * indicates that the student was unsuccessful and must attempt the skill again to assure competency. Examiners should use a different-color ink for the second attempt.

☐ Successful   ☐ Unsuccessful   Examiner Initials: _____

©2006 Prentice-Hall Inc.

Scenario Patient Care Report (PCR)—Thoracic Trauma

Student: _____   **Examiner:** _____

Date: _____

	Done ✓	Not Done
Records all pertinent dispatch/scene data, using a consistent format		
Completely identifies all additional resources and personnel		
Documents chief complaint, signs/symptoms, position found, age, sex, and weight		
Identifies and records all pertinent, reportable clinical data for each patient		
Documents SAMPLE and OPQRST if applicable		
Records all pertinent negatives		
Records all pertinent denials		
Records accurate, consistent times and patient information		
Includes relevant oral statements of witnesses, bystanders, and patient in "quotes" when appropriate		
Documents initial assessment findings: airway, breathing, and circulation		
Documents any interventions in initial assessment with patient response		
Documents level of consciousness, GCS (if trauma), and VS		
Documents rapid trauma assessment if applicable		
Documents any interventions in rapid trauma assessment with patient response		
Documents focused history and physical assessment		
Documents any interventions in focused assessment with patient response		
Documents repeat VS (every 5 minutes for critical; every 15 minutes for stable)		
Repeats initial assessment and documents findings		
Records ALL treatments with times and patient response(s) in treatment section		
Documents field impression		
Documents transport to specific facility and transfer of care WITH VERBAL REPORT		
Uses correct grammar, abbreviations, spelling, and terminology		
Writes legibly		
Thoroughly documents refusals, denials of transport, and call cancellations		
Documents patient GCS of 15 PRIOR to signing refusal		
Documents advice given to refusal patient, including "call 9-1-1 for further problems"		
Properly corrects errors and omissions		
Writes cautiously, avoids jargon, opinions, inferences, or any derogatory/libelous remarks		
Signs run report		
Uses EMS supplement form if needed		
Student exhibits competence with skill		

Any items in the Not Done column should be evaluated with student. Check marks in this column do not necessarily mean student was unsuccessful as all lines are not completed on all patients. Evaluation of each PCR should be based on the scenario given.

Student must be able to write an EMS report with consistency and accuracy.

☐ Successful   ☐ Unsuccessful   Examiner Initials: _____

Overall Scenario Management—Thoracic Trauma

Student: _____   Examiner:_____

Date: _____   Scenario: _____

NOTE: This skill sheet is to be done after the student completes a scenario as the TEAM LEADER. It is to let the student know if he or she is beginning to "put it all together" and use critical thinking skills to manage an EMS call. PLEASE notice that it is graded on a different basis than the basic lab skill sheet.

	Done ✓	Needs to Improve
SCENE MANAGEMENT		
Recognized hazards and controlled scene—safety, crowd, and patient issues		
Recognized hazards, but did not control the scene		
Unsuccessfully attempted to manage the scene	*	
Did not evaluate the scene and took no control of the scene	*	
PATIENT ASSESSMENT		
Performed a timely, organized complete patient assessment		
Performed complete initial, focused, and ongoing assessments, but in a disorganized manner		
Performed an incomplete assessment	*	
Did not perform an initial assessment	*	
PATIENT MANAGEMENT		
Evaluated assessment findings to manage all aspects of patient condition		
Managed the patient's presenting signs and symptoms without considering all of assessment		
Inadequately managed the patient	*	
Did not manage life-threatening conditions	*	
COMMUNICATION		
Communicated well with crew, patient, family, bystanders, and assisting agencies		
Communicated well with patient and crew		
Communicated with patient and crew, but poor communication skills	*	
Unable to communicate effectively	*	
REPORT AND TRANSFER OF CARE		
Identified correct destination for patient transport, gave accurate, brief report over radio, and provided full report at bedside demonstrating thorough understanding of patient condition and pathophysiological processes		
Identified correct destination and gave accurate radio and bedside report, but did not demonstrate understanding of patient condition and pathophysiological processes		
Identified correct destination, but provided inadequate radio and bedside report	*	
Identified inappropriate destination or provided no radio or bedside report	*	
Student exhibits competence with skill		

Any items that are marked with an * indicate the student needs to improve and a check mark should be placed in the right-hand column. A check mark in the right-hand column indicates that the student was unsuccessful and must attempt the skill again to assure competency. Examiners should use a different-color ink for the second attempt.

☐ Successful   ☐ Unsuccessful   Examiner Initials: _____

©2006 Prentice-Hall Inc.

Patient Assessment: Trauma—Trauma Mix

Student: _____   Examiner: _____

Date: _____   Scenario: _____

	Done ✓	Not Done
Assesses scene safety and utilizes appropriate PPE		*
OVERALL SCENE EVALUATION		
Trauma—assesses mechanism of injury/if medical component determines nature of illness		*
Determines the number of patients, location, obstacles, and requests any additional resources as needed		
Verbalizes general impression of the patient as approaches		*
Stabilizes C-spine/spinal motion restriction (SMR) of spine		*
INITIAL ASSESSMENT/RESUSCITATION		
Determines responsiveness/level of consciousness/AVPU		*
Opens airway with appropriate technique and assesses airway/ventilation		*
Manages airway/ventilation and applies appropriate oxygen therapy in less than 3 minutes		*
Assesses circulation: radial/carotid pulse, skin color, temperature, condition, and turgor		*
Controls any major bleeding		*
Makes rapid transport decision		*
Obtains IV (2 if indicated), BGL, GCS, and complete vital signs		
RAPID TRAUMA ASSESSMENT (If patient is Trauma Alert or Load and Go)		
Assesses abdomen		
Rapidly palpates each extremity, assessing for obvious injuries and distal PMS		
Provides spinal motion restriction (SMR) on long backboard (LBB), checking posterior torso and legs		
Secures head LAST		
Identifies patient problem: specify trauma		*
Loads patient/initiates transport (to appropriate LZ or to appropriate facility) in less than 10 minutes		*
Reassesses ABCs and interventions		*
FOCUSED HISTORY AND PHYSICAL ASSESSMENT		
Reassesses interventions and further assesses injuries found		
Obtains vital signs and GCS (Glasgow Coma Score)		
Obtains SAMPLE history		
Inspects and palpates head, facial, and neck regions		
Inspects, palpates, and auscultates chest/thorax		
Inspects and palpates abdomen and pelvis		
Inspects and palpates upper and lower extremities, checking distal PMS		
Inspects and palpates posterior torso		
Manages all injuries/wounds appropriately		
Repeats initial assessment, vital signs, and evaluates trends		*
Evaluates response to interventions/treatments		*
Performs ongoing assessment (VS every 5 minutes for critical patient/every 15 minutes for stable patient)		
Gives radio report to receiving facility		
Turns over patient care with verbal report		*
Student exhibits competence with skill		

Any items in the Not Done column that are marked with an * are mandatory for the student to complete. A check mark in the Not Done column of an item with an * indicates that the student was unsuccessful and must attempt the skill again to assure competency. Examiners should use a different-color ink for the second attempt.

☐ Successful   ☐ Unsuccessful   Examiner Initials: _____

©2006 Prentice-Hall Inc.

Endotracheal Intubation with Suspected Cervical Spine—Trauma Mix

Student: _____   Examiner: _____

Date: _____

	Done ✓	Not Done
Determines scene safety and utilizes appropriate PPE		*
Opens the airway manually with trauma jaw-thrust while assistant maintains C-spine SMR		*
Checks mouth for blood or potential airway obstruction		*
Suctions or removes loose teeth or foreign materials as needed		
Inserts simple airway adjunct (oropharyngeal airway)		
Directs assistant to ventilate patient with bag-valve-mask device (room air)		*
Observes chest rise/fall and auscultates bilaterally over lungs for baseline		*
Obtains effective ventilation in less than 30 seconds		*
Attaches oxygen reservoir to bag-valve-mask device and connects to high-flow oxygen		
Ventilates patient and evaluates chest wall/lung compliance		*
Directs assistant to preoxygenate patient with assistant maintaining C-spine SMR		*
Identifies/selects proper equipment for intubation		
Checks laryngoscope light and cuff of ET tube		
Removes all air from cuff and properly inserts stylet if used		
Directs assistant to face patient and establish cervical spine SMR from front		
Intubating paramedic sits behind patient on ground with legs straddling patient's shoulders		
Moves up until patient's head is secured		
Removes OPA and directs assistant to perform Sellick's maneuver		*
Opens mouth and gently inserts blade while sweeping tongue to side		*
Gently elevates mandible with laryngoscope and leans backward to visualize cords		*
Inserts ET tube and visualizes as tube is advanced through cords		*
"Threads" ET tube off stylet (if used), maintaining hold on ET tube as stylet removed		
Inflates cuff to proper pressure and disconnects syringe		*
Disconnects mask from bag-valve device and attaches to ET tube without releasing ET tube		
Directs ventilation of patient while maintaining Sellick's maneuver and holding ET tube in place		
Confirms proper placement by auscultation over epigastrium and bilaterally over each lung		*
Directs assistant to release cricoid pressure		*
Secures ET tube		*
Reassesses bilateral lung sounds and compliance		*
Uses secondary device to confirm tube placement		*
Assesses patient's response to intervention		*
Student exhibits competence with skill		

Any items in the Not Done column that are marked with an * are mandatory for the student to complete. A check mark in the Not Done column of an item with an * indicates that the student was unsuccessful and must attempt the skill again to assure competency. Examiners should use a different-color ink for the second attempt.

☐ Successful   ☐ Unsuccessful   Examiner Initials: _____

©2006 Prentice-Hall Inc.

Scenario IV Insertion—Trauma Mix

Student: _____   **Examiner:** _____

Date: _____

	Done ✓	Not Done
Selects appropriate IV fluid, checking clarity, color, and expiration date		*
Selects appropriate catheter		
Selects appropriate administration set		
Properly inserts IV tubing into the IV bag		*
Prepares administration set (fills drip chamber and flushes tubing)		*
Cuts or tears tape (at any time before venipuncture)		*
Applies constricting band (checks distal pulse to assure NOT a tourniquet)		*
Palpates suitable vein		*
Cleanses site appropriately		*
Utilizes appropriate PPE		*
Inserts catheter with sterile technique		*
Verbalizes flash/blood return and advances catheter slightly farther		*
Occludes vein with finger at distal end of catheter and removes stylet		
Immediately disposes (or verbalizes disposal) of needle/sharp in proper container		
Obtains blood sample or connects IV tubing to catheter		
Obtains BGL (blood glucose level)		*
Releases constricting band		*
Runs IV for a brief period to ensure patency and adjusts flow rate as appropriate		*
Checks IV site for signs of infiltration		*
Secures catheter (tapes securely or verbalizes)		*
Attaches label with size of catheter, date, time, and "prehospital"		*
Assesses patient's response to intervention		*
Student exhibits competence with skill		

Any items in the Not Done column that are marked with an * are mandatory for the student to complete. A check mark in the Not Done column of an item with an * indicates that the student was unsuccessful and must attempt the skill again to assure competency. Examiners should use a different-color ink for the second attempt.

☐ Successful   ☐ Unsuccessful   Examiner Initials: _____

Scenario Radio Report—Trauma Mix

Student: _____   **Examiner:** _____

Date: _____

	Done ✓	Not Done
Requests and checks for open channel before speaking		
Presses transmit button 1 second before speaking		
Holds microphone 2–3 in. from mouth		
Speaks slowly and clearly		*
Speaks in a normal voice		
Briefly transmits: Agency, unit designation, identification/name		*
Briefly transmits: Patient's age, sex, weight		*
Briefly transmits: Scene description/mechanism of injury or medical problem		*
Briefly transmits: Chief complaint with brief history of *present* illness		*
Briefly transmits: Associated symptoms (unless able to be deferred to bedside report)		
Briefly transmits: Past medical history (usually deferred to bedside report)		
Briefly transmits: Vital signs		*
Briefly transmits: Level of consciousness/GCS on trauma		*
Briefly transmits: General appearance, distress, cardiac rhythm, blood glucose, and other pertinent findings unable to be deferred to bedside report		
Briefly transmits: Interventions by EMS AND response(s)		*
ETA (the more critical the patient, the earlier you need to notify the receiving facility)		
Does not waste airtime		
Protects privacy of patient		*
Echoes dispatch information and any physician orders		*
Writes down dispatch information or physician orders		
Confirms with facility that message is received		
Demonstrates/verbalizes ability to troubleshoot basic equipment malfunction		
Student exhibits competence with skill		

Any items in the Not Done column that are marked with an * are mandatory for the student to complete. A check mark in the Not Done column of an item with an * indicates that the student was unsuccessful and must attempt the skill again to assure competency. Examiners should use a different-color ink for the second attempt.

☐ Successful   ☐ Unsuccessful   Examiner Initials: _____

©2006 Prentice-Hall Inc.

Scenario Patient Care Report (PCR)—Trauma Mix

Student: _____   **Examiner:** _____

Date: _____

	Done ✓	Not Done
Records all pertinent dispatch/scene data, using a consistent format		
Completely identifies all additional resources and personnel		
Documents chief complaint, signs/symptoms, position found, age, sex, and weight		
Identifies and records all pertinent, reportable clinical data for each patient		
Documents SAMPLE and OPQRST if applicable		
Records all pertinent negatives		
Records all pertinent denials		
Records accurate, consistent times and patient information		
Includes relevant oral statements of witnesses, bystanders, and patient in "quotes" when appropriate		
Documents initial assessment findings: airway, breathing, and circulation		
Documents any interventions in initial assessment with patient response		
Documents level of consciousness, GCS (if trauma), and VS		
Documents rapid trauma assessment if applicable		
Documents any interventions in rapid trauma assessment with patient response		
Documents focused history and physical assessment		
Documents any interventions in focused assessment with patient response		
Documents repeat VS (every 5 minutes for critical; every 15 minutes for stable)		
Repeats initial assessment and documents findings		
Records ALL treatments with times and patient response(s) in treatment section		
Documents field impression		
Documents transport to specific facility and transfer of care WITH VERBAL REPORT		
Uses correct grammar, abbreviations, spelling, and terminology		
Writes legibly		
Thoroughly documents refusals, denials of transport, and call cancellations		
Documents patient GCS of 15 PRIOR to signing refusal		
Documents advice given to refusal patient, including "call 9-1-1 for further problems"		
Properly corrects errors and omissions		
Writes cautiously, avoids jargon, opinions, inferences, or any derogatory/libelous remarks		
Signs run report		
Uses EMS supplement form if needed		
Student exhibits competence with skill		

Any items in the Not Done column should be evaluated with student. Check marks in this column do not necessarily mean student was unsuccessful as all lines are not completed on all patients. Evaluation of each PCR should be based on the scenario given.

Student must be able to write an EMS report with consistency and accuracy.

☐ Successful   ☐ Unsuccessful   Examiner Initials: _____

©2006 Prentice-Hall Inc.

Overall Scenario Management—Trauma Mix

Student: _____   Examiner: _____

Date: _____   Scenario: _____

NOTE: This skill sheet is to be done after the student completes a scenario as the TEAM LEADER. It is to let the student know if he or she is beginning to "put it all together" and use critical thinking skills to manage an EMS call. PLEASE notice that it is graded on a different basis than the basic lab skill sheet.

	Done ✓	Needs to Improve
SCENE MANAGEMENT		
Recognized hazards and controlled scene—safety, crowd, and patient issues		
Recognized hazards, but did not control the scene		
Unsuccessfully attempted to manage the scene	*	
Did not evaluate the scene and took no control of the scene	*	
PATIENT ASSESSMENT		
Performed a timely, organized complete patient assessment		
Performed complete initial, focused, and ongoing assessments, but in a disorganized manner		
Performed an incomplete assessment	*	
Did not perform an initial assessment	*	
PATIENT MANAGEMENT		
Evaluated assessment findings to manage all aspects of patient condition		
Managed the patient's presenting signs and symptoms without considering all of assessment		
Inadequately managed the patient	*	
Did not manage life-threatening conditions	*	
COMMUNICATION		
Communicated well with crew, patient, family, bystanders, and assisting agencies		
Communicated well with patient and crew		
Communicated with patient and crew, but poor communication skills	*	
Unable to communicate effectively	*	
REPORT AND TRANSFER OF CARE		
Identified correct destination for patient transport, gave accurate, brief report over radio, and provided full report at bedside demonstrating thorough understanding of patient condition and pathophysiological processes		
Identified correct destination and gave accurate radio and bedside report, but did not demonstrate understanding of patient condition and pathophysiological processes		
Identified correct destination, but provided inadequate radio and bedside report	*	
Identified inappropriate destination or provided no radio or bedside report	*	
Student exhibits competence with skill		

Any items that are marked with an * indicate the student needs to improve and a check mark should be placed in the right-hand column. A check mark in the right-hand column indicates that the student was unsuccessful and must attempt the skill again to assure competency. Examiners should use a different-color ink for the second attempt.

☐ Successful   ☐ Unsuccessful   Examiner Initials: _____

©2006 Prentice-Hall Inc.

Patient Assessment: Trauma—Trauma Mix

Student: _____   Examiner: _____

Date: _____   Scenario: _____

	Done ✓	Not Done
Assesses scene safety and utilizes appropriate PPE		*
OVERALL SCENE EVALUATION		
Trauma—assesses mechanism of injury/if medical component determines nature of illness		*
Determines the number of patients, location, obstacles, and requests any additional resources as needed		
Verbalizes general impression of the patient as approaches		*
Stabilizes C-spine/spinal motion restriction (SMR) of spine		*
INITIAL ASSESSMENT/RESUSCITATION		
Determines responsiveness/level of consciousness/AVPU		*
Opens airway with appropriate technique and assesses airway/ventilation		*
Manages airway/ventilation and applies appropriate oxygen therapy in less than 3 minutes		*
Assesses circulation: radial/carotid pulse, skin color, temperature, condition, and turgor		*
Controls any major bleeding		*
Makes rapid transport decision		*
Obtains IV (2 if indicated), BGL, GCS, and complete vital signs		
RAPID TRAUMA ASSESSMENT (If patient is Trauma Alert or Load and Go)		
Assesses abdomen		
Rapidly palpates each extremity, assessing for obvious injuries and distal PMS		
Provides spinal motion restriction (SMR) on long backboard (LBB), checking posterior torso and legs		
Secures head LAST		
Identifies patient problem: identify specific trauma		*
Loads patient/initiates transport (to appropriate LZ or to appropriate facility) in less than 10 minutes		*
Reassesses ABCs and interventions		*
FOCUSED HISTORY AND PHYSICAL ASSESSMENT		
Reassesses interventions and further assesses injuries found		
Obtains vital signs and GCS (Glasgow Coma Score)		
Obtains SAMPLE history		
Inspects and palpates head, facial, and neck regions		
Inspects, palpates, and auscultates chest/thorax		
Inspects and palpates abdomen and pelvis		
Inspects and palpates upper and lower extremities, checking distal PMS		
Inspects and palpates posterior torso		
Manages all injuries/wounds appropriately		
Repeats initial assessment, vital signs, and evaluates trends		*
Evaluates response to interventions/treatments		*
Performs ongoing assessment (VS every 5 minutes for critical patient/every 15 minutes for stable patient)		
Gives radio report to receiving facility		
Turns over patient care with verbal report		*
Student exhibits competence with skill		

Any items in the Not Done column that are marked with an * are mandatory for the student to complete. A check mark in the Not Done column of an item with an * indicates that the student was unsuccessful and must attempt the skill again to assure competency. Examiners should use a different-color ink for the second attempt.

☐ Successful   ☐ Unsuccessful   Examiner Initials: _____

Endotracheal Intubation with Suspected Cervical Spine—Trauma Mix

Student: _____   Examiner: _____

Date: _____

	Done ✓	Not Done
Determines scene safety and utilizes appropriate PPE		*
Opens the airway manually with trauma jaw-thrust while assistant maintains C-spine SMR		*
Checks mouth for blood or potential airway obstruction		*
Suctions or removes loose teeth or foreign materials as needed		
Inserts simple airway adjunct (oropharyngeal airway)		
Directs assistant to ventilate patient with bag-valve-mask device (room air)		*
Observes chest rise/fall and auscultates bilaterally over lungs for baseline		*
Obtains effective ventilation in less than 30 seconds		*
Attaches oxygen reservoir to bag-valve-mask device and connects to high-flow oxygen		
Ventilates patient and evaluates chest wall/lung compliance		*
Directs assistant to preoxygenate patient with assistant maintaining C-spine SMR		*
Identifies/selects proper equipment for intubation		
Checks laryngoscope light and cuff of ET tube		
Removes all air from cuff and properly inserts stylet if used		
Directs assistant to face patient and establish cervical spine SMR from front		
Intubating paramedic sits behind patient on ground with legs straddling patient's shoulders		
Moves up until patient's head is secured		
Removes OPA and directs assistant to perform Sellick's maneuver		*
Opens mouth and gently inserts blade while sweeping tongue to side		*
Gently elevates mandible with laryngoscope and leans backward to visualize cords		*
Inserts ET tube and visualizes as tube is advanced through cords		*
"Threads" ET tube off stylet (if used), maintaining hold on ET tube as stylet removed		
Inflates cuff to proper pressure and disconnects syringe		*
Disconnects mask from bag-valve device and attaches to ET tube without releasing ET tube		
Directs ventilation of patient while maintaining Sellick's maneuver and holding ET tube in place		
Confirms proper placement by auscultation over epigastrium and bilaterally over each lung		*
Directs assistant to release cricoid pressure		*
Secures ET tube		*
Reassesses bilateral lung sounds and compliance		*
Uses secondary device to confirm tube placement		*
Assesses patient's response to intervention		*
Student exhibits competence with skill		

Any items in the Not Done column that are marked with an * are mandatory for the student to complete. A check mark in the Not Done column of an item with an * indicates that the student was unsuccessful and must attempt the skill again to assure competency. Examiners should use a different-color ink for the second attempt.

☐ Successful   ☐ Unsuccessful   Examiner Initials: _____

©2006 Prentice-Hall Inc.

Scenario IV Insertion—Trauma Mix

Student: _____   **Examiner:** _____

Date: _____

	Done ✓	Not Done
Selects appropriate IV fluid, checking clarity, color, and expiration date		*
Selects appropriate catheter		
Selects appropriate administration set		
Properly inserts IV tubing into the IV bag		*
Prepares administration set (fills drip chamber and flushes tubing)		*
Cuts or tears tape (at any time before venipuncture)		*
Applies constricting band (checks distal pulse to assure NOT a tourniquet)		*
Palpates suitable vein		*
Cleanses site appropriately		*
Utilizes appropriate PPE		*
Inserts catheter with sterile technique		*
Verbalizes flash/blood return and advances catheter slightly farther		*
Occludes vein with finger at distal end of catheter and removes stylet		
Immediately disposes (or verbalizes disposal) of needle/sharp in proper container		
Obtains blood sample or connects IV tubing to catheter		
Obtains BGL (blood glucose level)		*
Releases constricting band		*
Runs IV for a brief period to ensure patency and adjusts flow rate as appropriate		*
Checks IV site for signs of infiltration		*
Secures catheter (tapes securely or verbalizes)		*
Attaches label with size of catheter, date, time, and "prehospital"		*
Assesses patient's response to intervention		*
Student exhibits competence with skill		

Any items in the Not Done column that are marked with an * are mandatory for the student to complete. A check mark in the Not Done column of an item with an * indicates that the student was unsuccessful and must attempt the skill again to assure competency. Examiners should use a different-color ink for the second attempt.

☐ Successful   ☐ Unsuccessful   Examiner Initials: _____

©2006 Prentice-Hall Inc.

Scenario Radio Report—Trauma Mix

Student: _____   **Examiner:**_____

Date: _____

	Done ✓	Not Done
Requests and checks for open channel before speaking		
Presses transmit button 1 second before speaking		
Holds microphone 2–3 in. from mouth		
Speaks slowly and clearly		*
Speaks in a normal voice		
Briefly transmits: Agency, unit designation, identification/name		*
Briefly transmits: Patient's age, sex, weight		*
Briefly transmits: Scene description/mechanism of injury or medical problem		*
Briefly transmits: Chief complaint with brief history of *present* illness		*
Briefly transmits: Associated symptoms (unless able to be deferred to bedside report)		
Briefly transmits: Past medical history (usually deferred to bedside report)		
Briefly transmits: Vital signs		*
Briefly transmits: Level of consciousness/GCS on trauma		*
Briefly transmits: General appearance, distress, cardiac rhythm, blood glucose, and other pertinent findings unable to be deferred to bedside report		
Briefly transmits: Interventions by EMS AND response(s)		*
ETA (the more critical the patient, the earlier you need to notify the receiving facility)		
Does not waste airtime		
Protects privacy of patient		*
Echoes dispatch information and any physician orders		*
Writes down dispatch information or physician orders		
Confirms with facility that message is received		
Demonstrates/verbalizes ability to troubleshoot basic equipment malfunction		
Student exhibits competence with skill		

Any items in the Not Done column that are marked with an * are mandatory for the student to complete. A check mark in the Not Done column of an item with an * indicates that the student was unsuccessful and must attempt the skill again to assure competency. Examiners should use a different-color ink for the second attempt.

☐ Successful   ☐ Unsuccessful   Examiner Initials: _____

©2006 Prentice-Hall Inc.

Scenario Patient Care Report (PCR)—Trauma Mix

Student: _____   **Examiner:**_____

Date: _____

	Done ✓	Not Done
Records all pertinent dispatch/scene data, using a consistent format		
Completely identifies all additional resources and personnel		
Documents chief complaint, signs/symptoms, position found, age, sex, and weight		
Identifies and records all pertinent, reportable clinical data for each patient		
Documents SAMPLE and OPQRST if applicable		
Records all pertinent negatives		
Records all pertinent denials		
Records accurate, consistent times and patient information		
Includes relevant oral statements of witnesses, bystanders, and patient in "quotes" when appropriate		
Documents initial assessment findings: airway, breathing, and circulation		
Documents any interventions in initial assessment with patient response		
Documents level of consciousness, GCS (if trauma), and VS		
Documents rapid trauma assessment if applicable		
Documents any interventions in rapid trauma assessment with patient response		
Documents focused history and physical assessment		
Documents any interventions in focused assessment with patient response		
Documents repeat VS (every 5 minutes for critical; every 15 minutes for stable)		
Repeats initial assessment and documents findings		
Records ALL treatments with times and patient response(s) in treatment section		
Documents field impression		
Documents transport to specific facility and transfer of care WITH VERBAL REPORT		
Uses correct grammar, abbreviations, spelling, and terminology		
Writes legibly		
Thoroughly documents refusals, denials of transport, and call cancellations		
Documents patient GCS of 15 PRIOR to signing refusal		
Documents advice given to refusal patient, including "call 9-1-1 for further problems"		
Properly corrects errors and omissions		
Writes cautiously, avoids jargon, opinions, inferences, or any derogatory/libelous remarks		
Signs run report		
Uses EMS supplement form if needed		
Student exhibits competence with skill		

Any items in the Not Done column should be evaluated with student. Check marks in this column do not necessarily mean student was unsuccessful as all lines are not completed on all patients. Evaluation of each PCR should be based on the scenario given.

Student must be able to write an EMS report with consistency and accuracy.

☐ Successful   ☐ Unsuccessful   Examiner Initials: _____

©2006 Prentice-Hall Inc.

Overall Scenario Management—Trauma Mix

Student: _____   Examiner:_____

Date: _____   Scenario: _____

NOTE: This skill sheet is to be done after the student completes a scenario as the TEAM LEADER. It is to let the student know if he or she is beginning to "put it all together" and use critical thinking skills to manage an EMS call. PLEASE notice that it is graded on a different basis than the basic lab skill sheet.

	Done ✓	Needs to Improve
SCENE MANAGEMENT		
Recognized hazards and controlled scene—safety, crowd, and patient issues		
Recognized hazards, but did not control the scene		
Unsuccessfully attempted to manage the scene	*	
Did not evaluate the scene and took no control of the scene	*	
PATIENT ASSESSMENT		
Performed a timely, organized complete patient assessment		
Performed complete initial, focused, and ongoing assessments, but in a disorganized manner		
Performed an incomplete assessment	*	
Did not perform an initial assessment	*	
PATIENT MANAGEMENT		
Evaluated assessment findings to manage all aspects of patient condition		
Managed the patient's presenting signs and symptoms without considering all of assessment		
Inadequately managed the patient	*	
Did not manage life-threatening conditions	*	
COMMUNICATION		
Communicated well with crew, patient, family, bystanders, and assisting agencies		
Communicated well with patient and crew		
Communicated with patient and crew, but poor communication skills	*	
Unable to communicate effectively	*	
REPORT AND TRANSFER OF CARE		
Identified correct destination for patient transport, gave accurate, brief report over radio, and provided full report at bedside demonstrating thorough understanding of patient condition and pathophysiological processes		
Identified correct destination and gave accurate radio and bedside report, but did not demonstrate understanding of patient condition and pathophysiological processes		
Identified correct destination, but provided inadequate radio and bedside report	*	
Identified inappropriate destination or provided no radio or bedside report	*	
Student exhibits competence with skill		

Any items that are marked with an * indicate the student needs to improve and a check mark should be placed in the right-hand column. A check mark in the right-hand column indicates that the student was unsuccessful and must attempt the skill again to assure competency. Examiners should use a different-color ink for the second attempt.

☐ Successful   ☐ Unsuccessful   Examiner Initials: _____

©2006 Prentice-Hall Inc.

Patient Assessment: Trauma—Trauma Arrest

Student: _____   **Examiner:** _____

Date: _____   **Scenario:** _____

	Done ✓	Not Done
Assesses scene safety and utilizes appropriate PPE		*
OVERALL SCENE EVALUATION		
Trauma—assesses mechanism of injury/if medical component determines nature of illness		*
Determines the number of patients, location, obstacles, and requests any additional resources as needed		
Verbalizes general impression of the patient as approaches		*
Stabilizes C-spine/spinal motion restriction (SMR) of spine		*
INITIAL ASSESSMENT/RESUSCITATION		
Determines responsiveness/level of consciousness/AVPU		*
Opens airway with appropriate technique and assesses airway/ventilation		*
Manages airway/ventilation and applies appropriate oxygen therapy in less than 3 minutes		*
Assesses circulation: radial/carotid pulse, skin color, temperature, condition, and turgor		*
Controls any major bleeding		*
Initiates ACLS protocols, makes rapid transport decision		*
Obtains 2 large-bore IV lines, BGL, GCS, and complete vital signs		
RAPID TRAUMA ASSESSMENT (If patient is Trauma Alert or Load and Go)		
Assesses abdomen		
Rapidly palpates each extremity, assessing for obvious injuries and distal PMS		
Provides spinal motion restriction (SMR) on long backboard (LBB), checking posterior torso and legs		
Secures head LAST		
Identifies patient problem: trauma arrest		*
Loads patient/initiates transport (to appropriate LZ or to appropriate facility) in less than 10 minutes		*
Reassesses ABCs and interventions		*
FOCUSED HISTORY AND PHYSICAL ASSESSMENT		
Reassesses interventions and further assesses injuries found if patient responds to ALS interventions		
Obtains vital signs and GCS (Glasgow Coma Score)		
Obtains SAMPLE history		
Inspects and palpates head, facial, and neck regions		
Inspects, palpates, and auscultates chest/thorax		
Inspects and palpates abdomen and pelvis		
Inspects and palpates upper and lower extremities, checking distal PMS		
Inspects and palpates posterior torso		
Manages all injuries/wounds appropriately—follow ACLS for cardiac portion		
Repeats initial assessment, vital signs, and evaluates trends		*
Evaluates response to interventions/treatments		*
Performs ongoing assessment (VS every 5 minutes for critical patient)		
Gives radio report to receiving facility		
Turns over patient care with verbal report		*
Student exhibits competence with skill		

Any items in the Not Done column that are marked with an * are mandatory for the student to complete. A check mark in the Not Done column of an item with an * indicates that the student was unsuccessful and must attempt the skill again to assure competency. Examiners should use a different-color ink for the second attempt.

☐ Successful   ☐ Unsuccessful   Examiner Initials: _____

Endotracheal Intubation with Suspected Cervical Spine—Trauma Arrest

Student: _____   Examiner: _____

Date: _____

	Done ✓	Not Done
Determines scene safety and utilizes appropriate PPE		*
Opens the airway manually with trauma jaw-thrust while assistant maintains C-spine SMR		*
Checks mouth for blood or potential airway obstruction		*
Suctions or removes loose teeth or foreign materials as needed		
Inserts simple airway adjunct (oropharyngeal airway)		
Directs assistant to ventilate patient with bag-valve-mask device (room air)		*
Observes chest rise/fall and auscultates bilaterally over lungs for baseline		*
Obtains effective ventilation in less than 30 seconds		*
Attaches oxygen reservoir to bag-valve-mask device and connects to high-flow oxygen		
Ventilates patient and evaluates chest wall/lung compliance		*
Directs assistant to preoxygenate patient with assistant maintaining C-spine SMR		*
Identifies/selects proper equipment for intubation		
Checks laryngoscope light and cuff of ET tube		
Removes all air from cuff and properly inserts stylet if used		
Directs assistant to face patient and establish cervical spine SMR from front		
Intubating paramedic sits behind patient on ground with legs straddling patient's shoulders		
Moves up until patient's head is secured		
Removes OPA and directs assistant to perform Sellick's maneuver		*
Opens mouth and gently inserts blade while sweeping tongue to side		*
Gently elevates mandible with laryngoscope and leans backward to visualize cords		*
Inserts ET tube and visualizes as tube is advanced through cords		*
"Threads" ET tube off stylet (if used), maintaining hold on ET tube as stylet removed		
Inflates cuff to proper pressure and disconnects syringe		*
Disconnects mask from bag-valve device and attaches to ET tube without releasing ET tube		
Directs ventilation of patient while maintaining Sellick's maneuver and holding ET tube in place		
Confirms proper placement by auscultation over epigastrium and bilaterally over each lung		*
Directs assistant to release cricoid pressure		*
Secures ET tube		*
Reassesses bilateral lung sounds and compliance		*
Uses secondary device to confirm tube placement		*
Assesses patient's response to intervention		*
Student exhibits competence with skill		

Any items in the Not Done column that are marked with an * are mandatory for the student to complete. A check mark in the Not Done column of an item with an * indicates that the student was unsuccessful and must attempt the skill again to assure competency. Examiners should use a different-color ink for the second attempt.

☐ Successful   ☐ Unsuccessful   Examiner Initials: _____

©2006 Prentice-Hall Inc.

Scenario IV Insertion—Trauma Arrest

Student: _____   Examiner: _____

Date: _____

	Done ✓	Not Done
Selects appropriate IV fluid, checking clarity, color, and expiration date		*
Selects appropriate catheter		
Selects appropriate administration set		
Properly inserts IV tubing into the IV bag		*
Prepares administration set (fills drip chamber and flushes tubing)		*
Cuts or tears tape (at any time before venipuncture)		*
Applies constricting band (checks distal pulse to assure NOT a tourniquet)		*
Palpates suitable vein		*
Cleanses site appropriately		*
Utilizes appropriate PPE		*
Inserts catheter with sterile technique		*
Verbalizes flash/blood return and advances catheter slightly farther		*
Occludes vein with finger at distal end of catheter and removes stylet		
Immediately disposes (or verbalizes disposal) of needle/sharp in proper container		
Obtains blood sample or connects IV tubing to catheter		
Obtains BGL (blood glucose level)		*
Releases constricting band		*
Runs IV for a brief period to ensure patency and adjusts flow rate as appropriate		*
Checks IV site for signs of infiltration		*
Secures catheter (tapes securely or verbalizes)		*
Attaches label with size of catheter, date, time, and "prehospital"		*
Assesses patient's response to intervention		*
Student exhibits competence with skill		

Any items in the Not Done column that are marked with an * are mandatory for the student to complete. A check mark in the Not Done column of an item with an * indicates that the student was unsuccessful and must attempt the skill again to assure competency. Examiners should use a different-color ink for the second attempt.

☐ Successful   ☐ Unsuccessful   Examiner Initials: _____

©2006 Prentice-Hall Inc.

Scenario Radio Report—Trauma Arrest

Student: _____   **Examiner:** _____

Date: _____

	Done ✓	Not Done
Requests and checks for open channel before speaking		
Presses transmit button 1 second before speaking		
Holds microphone 2–3 in. from mouth		
Speaks slowly and clearly		*
Speaks in a normal voice		
Briefly transmits: Agency, unit designation, identification/name		*
Briefly transmits: Patient's age, sex, weight		*
Briefly transmits: Scene description/mechanism of injury or medical problem		*
Briefly transmits: Chief complaint with brief history of *present* illness		*
Briefly transmits: Associated symptoms (unless able to be deferred to bedside report)		
Briefly transmits: Past medical history (usually deferred to bedside report)		
Briefly transmits: Vital signs		*
Briefly transmits: Level of consciousness/GCS on trauma		*
Briefly transmits: General appearance, distress, cardiac rhythm, blood glucose, and other pertinent findings unable to be deferred to bedside report		
Briefly transmits: Interventions by EMS AND response(s)		*
ETA (the more critical the patient, the earlier you need to notify the receiving facility)		
Does not waste airtime		
Protects privacy of patient		*
Echoes dispatch information and any physician orders		*
Writes down dispatch information or physician orders		
Confirms with facility that message is received		
Demonstrates/verbalizes ability to troubleshoot basic equipment malfunction		
Student exhibits competence with skill		

Any items in the Not Done column that are marked with an * are mandatory for the student to complete. A check mark in the Not Done column of an item with an * indicates that the student was unsuccessful and must attempt the skill again to assure competency. Examiners should use a different-color ink for the second attempt.

☐ Successful   ☐ Unsuccessful   Examiner Initials: _____

©2006 Prentice-Hall Inc.

Scenario Patient Care Report (PCR)—Trauma Arrest

Student: _____   **Examiner:** _____

Date: _____

	Done ✓	Not Done
Records all pertinent dispatch/scene data, using a consistent format		
Completely identifies all additional resources and personnel		
Documents chief complaint, signs/symptoms, position found, age, sex, and weight		
Identifies and records all pertinent, reportable clinical data for each patient		
Documents SAMPLE and OPQRST if applicable		
Records all pertinent negatives		
Records all pertinent denials		
Records accurate, consistent times and patient information		
Includes relevant oral statements of witnesses, bystanders, and patient in "quotes" when appropriate		
Documents initial assessment findings: airway, breathing, and circulation		
Documents any interventions in initial assessment with patient response		
Documents level of consciousness, GCS (if trauma), and VS		
Documents rapid trauma assessment if applicable		
Documents any interventions in rapid trauma assessment with patient response		
Documents focused history and physical assessment		
Documents any interventions in focused assessment with patient response		
Documents repeat VS (every 5 minutes for critical; every 15 minutes for stable)		
Repeats initial assessment and documents findings		
Records ALL treatments with times and patient response(s) in treatment section		
Documents field impression		
Documents transport to specific facility and transfer of care WITH VERBAL REPORT		
Uses correct grammar, abbreviations, spelling, and terminology		
Writes legibly		
Thoroughly documents refusals, denials of transport, and call cancellations		
Documents patient GCS of 15 PRIOR to signing refusal		
Documents advice given to refusal patient, including "call 9-1-1 for further problems"		
Properly corrects errors and omissions		
Writes cautiously, avoids jargon, opinions, inferences, or any derogatory/libelous remarks		
Signs run report		
Uses EMS supplement form if needed		
Student exhibits competence with skill		

Any items in the Not Done column should be evaluated with student. Check marks in this column do not necessarily mean student was unsuccessful as all lines are not completed on all patients. Evaluation of each PCR should be based on the scenario given.

Student must be able to write an EMS report with consistency and accuracy.

☐ Successful   ☐ Unsuccessful   Examiner Initials: _____

Overall Scenario Management—Trauma Arrest

Student: _____   Examiner: _____

Date: _____   Scenario: _____

NOTE: This skill sheet is to be done after the student completes a scenario as the TEAM LEADER. It is to let the student know if he or she is beginning to "put it all together" and use critical thinking skills to manage an EMS call. PLEASE notice that it is graded on a different basis than the basic lab skill sheet.

	Done ✓	Needs to Improve
SCENE MANAGEMENT		
Recognized hazards and controlled scene—safety, crowd, and patient issues		
Recognized hazards, but did not control the scene		
Unsuccessfully attempted to manage the scene	*	
Did not evaluate the scene and took no control of the scene	*	
PATIENT ASSESSMENT		
Performed a timely, organized complete patient assessment		
Performed complete initial, focused, and ongoing assessments, but in a disorganized manner		
Performed an incomplete assessment	*	
Did not perform an initial assessment	*	
PATIENT MANAGEMENT		
Evaluated assessment findings to manage all aspects of patient condition		
Managed the patient's presenting signs and symptoms without considering all of assessment		
Inadequately managed the patient	*	
Did not manage life-threatening conditions	*	
COMMUNICATION		
Communicated well with crew, patient, family, bystanders, and assisting agencies		
Communicated well with patient and crew		
Communicated with patient and crew, but poor communication skills	*	
Unable to communicate effectively	*	
REPORT AND TRANSFER OF CARE		
Identified correct destination for patient transport, gave accurate, brief report over radio, and provided full report at bedside demonstrating thorough understanding of patient condition and pathophysiological processes		
Identified correct destination and gave accurate radio and bedside report, but did not demonstrate understanding of patient condition and pathophysiological processes		
Identified correct destination, but provided inadequate radio and bedside report	*	
Identified inappropriate destination or provided no radio or bedside report	*	
Student exhibits competence with skill		

Any items that are marked with an * indicate the student needs to improve and a check mark should be placed in the right-hand column. A check mark in the right-hand column indicates that the student was unsuccessful and must attempt the skill again to assure competency. Examiners should use a different-color ink for the second attempt.

☐ Successful   ☐ Unsuccessful   Examiner Initials: _____

©2006 Prentice-Hall Inc.

DAILY DISCUSSIONS AND PERTINENT POINTS—TRAUMA

Student: _____   Date: _____

Instructor: _____

	Instructor Initials
Identify local municipal and community resources available for physical or socioeconomic crises.	
List the general and specific environmental parameters that should be inspected to assess a patient's need for preventative information and direction.	
Identify the role of EMS in local municipal and community prevention programs.	
Identify the local prevention programs that promote safety for all age populations.	
Identify patient situations in which the paramedic can intervene in a preventative manner.	
Relate pulse pressure changes to perfusion status.	
Discuss the management of external hemorrhage.	
Differentiate between controlled and uncontrolled hemorrhage.	
Differentiate between the administration rate and amount of IV fluid in a patient with controlled versus uncontrolled hemorrhage.	
Apply epidemiology to develop prevention strategies for hemorrhage and shock.	
Defend the rationale explaining why immediate life threats must take priority over wound closure.	
Defend the management regimens for various soft tissue injuries.	
Defend why immediate life-threatening conditions take priority over soft tissue management.	
Value the importance of a thorough assessment for patients with soft tissue injuries.	
Attend to the feelings that the patient with a soft tissue injury may experience.	
Appreciate the importance of good follow-up care for patients receiving sutures.	
Understand the value of the written report for soft tissue injuries, in the continuum of patient care.	
Value the changes of a patient's self-image associated with a burn injury.	
Value the impact of managing a burn patient.	
Advocate empathy for a burn-injured patient.	
Assess safety at a burn injury incident.	
Characterize mortality and morbidity based on the pathophysiology and assessment findings of a patient with a burn injury.	
Value and defend the sense of urgency in burn injuries.	
Serve as a role model for universal precautions and BSI (appropriate PPE) in lab and clinical areas.	
Describe the special considerations involved in femur fracture management.	
Advocate the use of a thorough assessment to determine the proper treatment plan for a patient with a suspected musculoskeletal injury.	
Advocate the use of pain management in the treatment of musculoskeletal injuries.	
Advocate the use of a thorough assessment when determining the proper management modality for spine injuries.	
Value the implications of failing to properly restrict motion in a spine-injured patient.	
Advocate the use of a thorough assessment to determine a differential diagnosis and treatment plan for thoracic trauma.	
Advocate the use of a thorough scene survey to determine the forces involved in thoracic trauma.	
Value the implications of failing to properly diagnose thoracic trauma.	
Value the implications of failing to initiate timely interventions for patients with thoracic trauma.	
Apply the epidemiologic principles to develop prevention strategies for abdominal injuries.	
Integrate the pathophysiological principles to the assessment of a patient with abdominal injuries.	
Advocate the use of a thorough assessment to determine a differential diagnosis and treatment plan for abdominal trauma.	
Advocate the use of a thorough scene survey to determine the forces involved in abdominal trauma.	
Value the implications of failing to properly diagnose abdominal trauma and initiate timely interventions for patients with abdominal trauma.	
Discuss the physiologic changes associated with the pneumatic anti-shock garment (PASG).	
Discuss the indications and contraindications for the application and inflation of the PASG.	
Discuss the usefulness of the PASG in the management of fractures.	
Characterize the feelings of a patient who regains consciousness among strangers.	
Formulate means of conveying empathy to patients whose ability to communicate is limited by their condition.	

SECTION 6

Medical

Fabulous Factoids

Skill Sheets

Daily Discussions and Pertinent Points

FABULOUS FACTOIDS—MEDICAL

Neurotics build castles in the clouds. Psychotics live in them.

Sigmund Freud had a morbid fear of ferns.

Sleepwalking is hereditary.

In 19th-century England, attempting suicide was a crime punishable by death.

The acute abdomen cannot be properly assessed without visualizing the abdomen or placing the patient supine for palpation.

The most common cause of UGI bleeding is PUD (peptic ulcer disease). Some 80% of UGI bleeds stop by themselves.

Stomach acid can dissolve razor blades.

The average adult eats 1,400 to 2,000 pounds of food per year.

Every day, Americans eat an estimated 18 acres of pizza, which was, incidentally, invented by the Greeks, not the Italians.

The most common cause of an acute abdomen is appendicitis.

The two most commonly missed diagnoses, who are wrongfully discharged from EDs, are acute appendicitis and acute intestinal obstruction.

Decrease in LOC in a patient with previously good mental function suggests ARF (acute renal failure) and a potential threat to life.

Causes of prerenal ARF (inadequate renal perfusion) include heatstroke and burns.

In some unusual circumstances dialysis has been used to treat specific poisonings.

Use care and caution when caring for hemodialysis patients. Two of the most common complications are bleeding from the needle puncture site and local infection.

Personal and family history play an important role in the diagnosis of kidney stones.

Viruses were discovered by Dmitry Ivanovsky, a Russian scientist, in 1892.

Any child under age 2 with a high-grade fever has meningitis until proven otherwise.

Influenza was first recorded in Paris in 1414, but first described by Hippocrates in 412 B.C.

People born before 1957 are probably immune to measles.

About 12 million people in the United States contract a sexually transmitted disease each year.

Strokes caused by thrombus formation frequently occur when sleeping. Why? (legs elevated—circulation improved—thrombus becomes embolus)

Always do GCS on suspected stroke along with MEND/neuro/regionally accepted stroke scale/exam.

Crocodile-tear syndrome is a nerve disorder that makes people cry when they eat.

Many endocrine emergencies in the field present as altered mental status, especially with insulin-related disorders.

DUMBELS for signs and symptoms of acute cholinergic poisoning:

Diarrhea

Urination

Miosis

Bronchospasm

Emesis

Lacrimation

Salivation

Another mnemonic for signs and symptoms of acute cholinergic poisoning is SLUDGEM:

Salivation

Lacrimation

Urination

Diarrhea

GI upset

Emesis

Miosis

There are 2,600 black widow spider bites each year, over half with serious reactions. Black widow is leading cause of spider deaths in the United States. What is the antidote? (calcium gluconate)

To distinguish a coral snake refer to color rings: Red touch Yellow = Kill a Fellow; Red touch Black = Venom Lack.

No one is dead until he or she is warm and dead. Lowest documented resuscitation temperature = 18°C.

Remember, the abdomen is the last place to get cold. A cold abdomen upon deep palpation means profound hypothermia.

Most common cause of missed hypothermia is a thermometer that doesn't measure hypothermia.

Cerebral blood flow decreases 6–7% for each 1°C drop in temperature.

It takes approximately 25 seconds for the mammalian dive reflex to work in adults and 45 seconds in children less than 5 years old.

©2006 Prentice-Hall Inc.

Endocrine system problems result from either too much or too little secretion of a specific hormone or other chemical substance.

Hormones released from the *anterior pituitary*:

At the movies,

> Alan—ACTH
> Fondled—FSH
> Lisa—LH ⟩ Target Organs/Glands
> Many—MSH
> Times—TSH

(Rated)☺

> P—Prolactin
> G—Growth Hormone ⟩ Target Tissues

This mnemonic might be offensive to some students. It is NOT meant to infer or insult, but it has proven to be very memorable to students because of its "risque" nature.

(Because if Alan did anything else—it would be rated X!)

Hormones released from the *posterior pituitary*:

> A—ADH
> O—Oxytocin

The 3 Ps of diabetes mellitus are

> Polydipsia
> Polyphagia
> Polyuria

Thyroid disease is common. However, life-threatening extremes (myxedema and thyroid storm) are rare (1–2%).

Drugs of the Section (see Emergency Drug Quiz Key, p. xxxiv):

Haldol
Valium
Calcium Chloride
Sodium Bicarbonate

Pathophysiologies of the Section: 6.01–6.50 (see Checklist, pp. 596–597)

SKILL SHEETS

Patient Restraints

Student: _____   Examiner: _____

Date: _____

	Done ✓	Not Done
Utilizes appropriate PPE		*
Verbalizes proper indications for use of restraints		
Calmly explains procedure to patient		

Prepares equipment
    Soft wrist restraints for unresponsive patient
    Leather four-point restraints for combative patient		

Assures adequate personnel available for restraint application		*
Places patient supine		*
Applies soft wrist restraints, checking distal PMS before and after application, OR pads beneath leather restraint one extremity at a time, checking distal PMS before and after		*
Places sheet restraint or padded strap across chest, securing combative patient to stretcher		*
Reassesses patient after restraints in place		*
Monitors restrained patient continuously		*
Documents indications, assessment findings, and continuous monitoring		*
Student exhibits competence with skill		

Any items in the Not Done column that are marked with an * are mandatory for the student to complete. A check mark in the Not Done column of an item with an * indicates that the student was unsuccessful and must attempt the skill again to assure competency. Examiners should use a different-color ink for the second attempt.

☐ Successful   ☐ Unsuccessful   Examiner Initials: _____

©2006 Prentice-Hall Inc.

ALS Emergency Care for Heat Disorders

Student: _____   Examiner: _____

Date: _____

Heat Cramps	Done ✓	Not Done
Utilizes appropriate PPE		*
Removes patient from hot environment		*
Places patient in a cool, shaded, or air-conditioned environment		
Administers oral fluids if patient is alert and able to swallow, or an IV of NS		*
Assesses patient's response to intervention		*
Student exhibits competence with skill		

Heat Exhaustion		
Utilizes appropriate PPE		*
Removes patient from hot environment		*
Places patient in a cool, shaded, or air-conditioned environment		
Administers oral fluids if patient is alert and able to swallow, or an IV of NS		*
Places patient in supine position		*
Removes some clothing and fans the patient, but does not chill the patient		*
Treats for shock if shock is suspected		
Assesses patient's response to intervention		*
Student exhibits competence with skill		

Heatstroke		
Utilizes appropriate PPE		*
Removes patient from hot environment		*
Places patient in a cool, shaded, or air-conditioned environment		
Recognizes true emergency and initiates rapid transport		*
Initiates rapid active cooling en route to hospital by removing patient's clothing		*
Covers patient with sheets soaked in tepid water		*
Cools body temperature to no lower than 102°F/30°C		*
Administers high-flow oxygen by nonrebreather mask		
Administers oral fluids if patient is alert and able to swallow		
Begins one or two IVs of NS wide open		*
Monitors EKG		*
Monitors body temperature		*
Assesses patient's response to intervention		*
Student exhibits competence with skill		

Any items in the Not Done column that are marked with an * are mandatory for the student to complete. A check mark in the Not Done column of an item with an * indicates that the student was unsuccessful and must attempt the skill again to assure competency. Examiners should use a different-color ink for the second attempt.

☐ Successful   ☐ Unsuccessful   Examiner Initials: _____

©2006 Prentice-Hall Inc.

ALS Recognition and Treatment of Hypothermia

Student: _____   Examiner: _____

Date: _____

Mild Hypothermia	Done ✓	Not Done
Utilizes appropriate PPE		*
Recognizes mild hypothermia/verbalizes core temperature above 90°F or 32°C		*
Observes for shivering		*
Verbalizes checking level of consciousness as may be lethargic and somewhat dulled or AAO × 4		*
Observes for uncoordinated or stiff and stumbling gait		*
Removes from environment (heat on) and removes any wet clothing/wraps in DRY blankets		*
Gives warm liquids, avoiding caffeine, stimulants, or alcohol		
Assesses patient's response to intervention		*
Student exhibits competence with skill		

Severe Hypothermia	Done ✓	Not Done
Utilizes appropriate PPE		*
Recognizes severe hypothermia/verbalizes core temperature less than 90°F or 32°C		*
Verbalizes shivering will usually stop by this stage and physical activity will be uncoordinated		
Checks level of consciousness as patient will be stuporous and complete coma will follow		
Removes from environment (heat on) and removes any wet clothing/wraps in dry blankets		*
Places patient in supine position on cardiac monitor and looks for "J" waves (Osborne waves)		*
Initiates rapid transport for active rewarming in the hospital environment		*
Observes for atrial fibrillation, bradycardia, and/or ventricular fibrillation		*
Initiates 2 large-bore IVs of WARMED crystalloid		*
Does NOT allow rough handling as may initiate ventricular fibrillation		*
Monitors core temperature with hypothermia thermometer		
Monitors cardiac rhythm during transport		*
Assesses patient's response to interventions		*
Verbalizes **active** rewarming should not be attempted unless transport time exceeds 15 minutes		*
Student exhibits competence with skill		

Any items in the Not Done column that are marked with an * are mandatory for the student to complete. A check mark in the Not Done column of an item with an * indicates that the student was unsuccessful and must attempt the skill again to assure competency. Examiners should use a different-color ink for the second attempt.

☐ Successful   ☐ Unsuccessful   Examiner Initials: _____

©2006 Prentice-Hall Inc.

Patient Assessment: Medical—Abdominal

Student: _____   Examiner: _____

Date: _____   Scenario: _____

	Done ✓	Not Done
Assesses scene safety and utilizes appropriate PPE		*
OVERALL SCENE EVALUATION		
Medical—determines nature of illness/if trauma involved determines MOI		*
Determines the number of patients, location, obstacles, and requests any additional resources as needed		
Verbalizes general impression of the patient as approaches		*
Considers stabilization/spinal motion restriction of spine if trauma involved		*
INITIAL ASSESSMENT		
Determines responsiveness/level of consciousness/AVPU		*
Opens airway with appropriate technique and assesses airway/ventilation		*
Manages airway/ventilation and applies appropriate oxygen therapy in less than 3 minutes		*
Assesses circulation: radial/carotid pulse, skin color, temperature, condition, and turgor		*
Controls any major bleeding		*
Makes rapid transport decision if indicated		
Initiates IV, obtains BGL, GCS, and complete vital signs		
FOCUSED HISTORY AND PHYSICAL EXAMINATION/RAPID ASSESSMENT		
Obtains SAMPLE history		
Obtains OPQRST for differential diagnosis		
Obtains associated symptoms, pertinent negatives/denials		
Evaluates decision to perform focused exam or completes rapid assessment		*
Vital signs including AVPU (and GCS if trauma)		*
Assesses cardiovascular system including heart sounds, peripheral edema, and peripheral perfusion		*
Assesses pulmonary system including reassessing airway, ventilation, breath sounds, pulse oximetry, chest wall excursion, accessory muscle use, or other signs of distress		*
Assesses neurological system including speech, droop, drift, if applicable, and distal movement and sensation		*
Assesses musculoskeletal and integumentary systems		
Assesses behavioral, psychological, and social aspects of patient and situation		
States field impression of patient—abdominal problem (states suspected differential diagnosis)		*
Verbalizes treatment plan for patient and calls for appropriate intervention(s)—IVs, no pain meds recommended for undiagnosed abdominal pain, nothing by mouth		*
Reevaluates transport decision		
ONGOING ASSESSMENT		
Repeats initial assessment		*
Repeats vital signs and evaluates trends		*
Evaluates response to treatments		*
Repeats focused assessment regarding patient complaint or injuries		
Gives radio report to receiving facility		
Turns over patient care with verbal report		*
Student exhibits competence with skill		

Any items in the Not Done column that are marked with an * are mandatory for the student to complete. A check mark in the Not Done column of an item with an * indicates that the student was unsuccessful and must attempt the skill again to assure competency. Examiners should use a different-color ink for the second attempt.

☐ Successful   ☐ Unsuccessful   Examiner Initials: _____

©2006 Prentice-Hall Inc.

Scenario Intubation—Abdominal

Student: _____   Examiner:_____

Date: _____

	Done ✓	Not Done
Assesses scene safety and utilizes appropriate PPE		*
Manually opens the airway with technique appropriate for patient condition		*
Checks mouth for blood or potential airway obstruction		*
Suctions or removes loose teeth or foreign materials as needed		
Inserts simple adjunct (oropharyngeal or nasopharyngeal airway)		
Directs assistant to ventilate patient with bag-valve-mask device (room air)		*
Observes chest rise/fall and auscultates bilaterally over lungs for baseline		*
Obtains effective ventilation in less than 30 seconds		*
Attaches oxygen reservoir to bag-valve-mask device and connects to high-flow oxygen		
Ventilates patient and evaluates chest wall/lung compliance		*
Directs assistant to preoxygenate patient		*
Identifies/selects proper equipment for intubation		
Checks laryngoscope light and cuff of ET tube		
Removes all air from cuff and properly inserts stylet if used		
Removes airway adjunct		
Positions patient's head properly and has assistant perform Sellick's maneuver		*
Opens mouth and gently inserts blade while sweeping tongue to side		*
Has assistant maintain Sellick's pressure		
Gently elevates mandible with laryngoscope and visualizes cords		*
Introduces ET tube to side of blade and visualizes tube passing through cords		*
"Threads" ET tube off stylet (if used), maintaining hold on ET tube as stylet removed		
Inflates cuff to proper pressure and disconnects syringe		*
Disconnects mask from bag-valve device and attaches to ET tube without releasing ET tube		
Directs ventilation of patient while maintaining Sellick's maneuver and holding ET tube in place		
Confirms proper placement by auscultation over epigastrium and bilaterally over each lung		*
Directs assistant to release cricoid pressure		*
Secures ET tube		*
Reassesses bilateral lung sounds and compliance		*
Uses secondary device to confirm tube placement		*
Assesses patient's response to intervention		*
Student exhibits competence with skill		

Any items in the Not Done column that are marked with an * are mandatory for the student to complete. A check mark in the Not Done column of an item with an * indicates that the student was unsuccessful and must attempt the skill again to assure competency. Examiners should use a different-color ink for the second attempt.

☐ Successful   ☐ Unsuccessful   Examiner Initials: _____

©2006 Prentice-Hall Inc.

Scenario IV Insertion—Abdominal

Student: _____   Examiner:_____

Date: _____

	Done ✓	Not Done
Selects appropriate IV fluid, checking clarity, color, and expiration date		*
Selects appropriate catheter		
Selects appropriate administration set		
Properly inserts IV tubing into the IV bag		*
Prepares administration set (fills drip chamber and flushes tubing)		*
Cuts or tears tape (at any time before venipuncture)		*
Applies constricting band (checks distal pulse to assure NOT a tourniquet)		*
Palpates suitable vein		*
Cleanses site appropriately		*
Utilizes appropriate PPE		*
Inserts catheter with sterile technique		*
Verbalizes flash/blood return and advances catheter slightly farther		*
Occludes vein with finger at distal end of catheter and removes stylet		
Immediately disposes (or verbalizes disposal) of needle/sharp in proper container		
Obtains blood sample or connects IV tubing to catheter		
Obtains BGL (blood glucose level)		*
Releases constricting band		*
Runs IV for a brief period to ensure patency and adjusts flow rate as appropriate		*
Checks IV site for signs of infiltration		*
Secures catheter (tapes securely or verbalizes)		*
Attaches label with size of catheter, date, time, and "prehospital"		*
Assesses patient's response to intervention		*
Student exhibits competence with skill		

Any items in the Not Done column that are marked with an * are mandatory for the student to complete. A check mark in the Not Done column of an item with an * indicates that the student was unsuccessful and must attempt the skill again to assure competency. Examiners should use a different-color ink for the second attempt.

☐ Successful   ☐ Unsuccessful   Examiner Initials: _____

©2006 Prentice-Hall Inc.

Scenario Radio Report—Abdominal

Student: _____   **Examiner:** _____

Date: _____

	Done ✓	Not Done
Requests and checks for open channel before speaking		
Presses transmit button 1 second before speaking		
Holds microphone 2–3 in. from mouth		
Speaks slowly and clearly		*
Speaks in a normal voice		
Briefly transmits: Agency, unit designation, identification/name		*
Briefly transmits: Patient's age, sex, weight		*
Briefly transmits: Scene description/mechanism of injury or medical problem		*
Briefly transmits: Chief complaint with brief history of *present* illness		*
Briefly transmits: Associated symptoms (unless able to be deferred to bedside report)		
Briefly transmits: Past medical history (usually deferred to bedside report)		
Briefly transmits: Vital signs		*
Briefly transmits: Level of consciousness/GCS on trauma		*
Briefly transmits: General appearance, distress, cardiac rhythm, blood glucose, and other pertinent findings unable to be deferred to bedside report		
Briefly transmits: Interventions by EMS AND response(s)		*
ETA (the more critical the patient, the earlier you need to notify the receiving facility)		
Does not waste airtime		
Protects privacy of patient		*
Echoes dispatch information and any physician orders		*
Writes down dispatch information or physician orders		
Confirms with facility that message is received		
Demonstrates/verbalizes ability to troubleshoot basic equipment malfunction		
Student exhibits competence with skill		

Any items in the Not Done column that are marked with an * are mandatory for the student to complete. A check mark in the Not Done column of an item with an * indicates that the student was unsuccessful and must attempt the skill again to assure competency. Examiners should use a different-color ink for the second attempt.

☐ Successful   ☐ Unsuccessful   Examiner Initials: _____

©2006 Prentice-Hall Inc.

Scenario Patient Care Report (PCR)—Abdominal

Student: _____   Examiner: _____

Date: _____

	Done ✓	Not Done
Records all pertinent dispatch/scene data, using a consistent format		
Completely identifies all additional resources and personnel		
Documents chief complaint, signs/symptoms, position found, age, sex, and weight		
Identifies and records all pertinent, reportable clinical data for each patient		
Documents SAMPLE and OPQRST if applicable		
Records all pertinent negatives		
Records all pertinent denials		
Records accurate, consistent times and patient information		
Includes relevant oral statements of witnesses, bystanders, and patient in "quotes" when appropriate		
Documents initial assessment findings: airway, breathing, and circulation		
Documents any interventions in initial assessment with patient response		
Documents level of consciousness, GCS (if trauma), and VS		
Documents rapid trauma assessment if applicable		
Documents any interventions in rapid trauma assessment with patient response		
Documents focused history and physical assessment		
Documents any interventions in focused assessment with patient response		
Documents repeat VS (every 5 minutes for critical; every 15 minutes for stable)		
Repeats initial assessment and documents findings		
Records ALL treatments with times and patient response(s) in treatment section		
Documents field impression		
Documents transport to specific facility and transfer of care WITH VERBAL REPORT		
Uses correct grammar, abbreviations, spelling, and terminology		
Writes legibly		
Thoroughly documents refusals, denials of transport, and call cancellations		
Documents patient GCS of 15 PRIOR to signing refusal		
Documents advice given to refusal patient, including "call 9-1-1 for further problems"		
Properly corrects errors and omissions		
Writes cautiously, avoids jargon, opinions, inferences, or any derogatory/libelous remarks		
Signs run report		
Uses EMS supplement form if needed		
Student exhibits competence with skill		

Any items in the Not Done column should be evaluated with student. Check marks in this column do not necessarily mean student was unsuccessful as all lines are not completed on all patients. Evaluation of each PCR should be based on the scenario given.

Student must be able to write an EMS report with consistency and accuracy.

☐ Successful   ☐ Unsuccessful   Examiner Initials: _____

Overall Scenario Management—Abdominal

Student: _____   Examiner: _____

Date: _____   Scenario: _____

NOTE: This skill sheet is to be done after the student completes a scenario as the **TEAM LEADER**. It is to let the student know if he or she is beginning to "put it all together" and use critical thinking skills to manage an EMS call. PLEASE notice that it is graded on a different basis than the basic lab skill sheet.

	Done ✓	Needs to Improve
SCENE MANAGEMENT		
Recognized hazards and controlled scene—safety, crowd, and patient issues		
Recognized hazards, but did not control the scene		
Unsuccessfully attempted to manage the scene	*	
Did not evaluate the scene and took no control of the scene	*	
PATIENT ASSESSMENT		
Performed a timely, organized complete patient assessment		
Performed complete initial, focused, and ongoing assessments, but in a disorganized manner		
Performed an incomplete assessment	*	
Did not perform an initial assessment	*	
PATIENT MANAGEMENT		
Evaluated assessment findings to manage all aspects of patient condition		
Managed the patient's presenting signs and symptoms without considering all of assessment		
Inadequately managed the patient	*	
Did not manage life-threatening conditions	*	
COMMUNICATION		
Communicated well with crew, patient, family, bystanders, and assisting agencies		
Communicated well with patient and crew		
Communicated with patient and crew, but poor communication skills	*	
Unable to communicate effectively	*	
REPORT AND TRANSFER OF CARE		
Identified correct destination for patient transport, gave accurate, brief report over radio, and provided full report at bedside demonstrating thorough understanding of patient condition and pathophysiological processes		
Identified correct destination and gave accurate radio and bedside report, but did not demonstrate understanding of patient condition and pathophysiological processes		
Identified correct destination, but provided inadequate radio and bedside report	*	
Identified inappropriate destination or provided no radio or bedside report	*	
Student exhibits competence with skill		

Any items that are marked with an * indicate the student needs to improve and a check mark should be placed in the right-hand column. A check mark in the right-hand column indicates that the student was unsuccessful and must attempt the skill again to assure competency. Examiners should use a different-color ink for the second attempt.

☐ Successful   ☐ Unsuccessful   Examiner Initials: _____

©2006 Prentice-Hall Inc.

Patient Assessment: Medical—Abdominal

Student: _____   Examiner: _____

Date: _____   Scenario: _____

	Done ✓	Not Done
Assesses scene safety and utilizes appropriate PPE		*
OVERALL SCENE EVALUATION		
Medical—determines nature of illness/if trauma involved determines MOI		*
Determines the number of patients, location, obstacles, and requests any additional resources as needed		
Verbalizes general impression of the patient as approaches		*
Considers stabilization/spinal motion restriction of spine if trauma involved		*
INITIAL ASSESSMENT		
Determines responsiveness/level of consciousness/AVPU		*
Opens airway with appropriate technique and assesses airway/ventilation		*
Manages airway/ventilation and applies appropriate oxygen therapy in less than 3 minutes		*
Assesses circulation: radial/carotid pulse, skin color, temperature, condition, and turgor		*
Controls any major bleeding		*
Makes rapid transport decision if indicated		
Initiates IV, obtains BGL, GCS, and complete vital signs		
FOCUSED HISTORY AND PHYSICAL EXAMINATION / RAPID ASSESSMENT		
Obtains SAMPLE history		
Obtains OPQRST for differential diagnosis		
Obtains associated symptoms, pertinent negatives/denials		
Evaluates decision to perform focused exam or completes rapid assessment		*
Vital signs including AVPU (and GCS if trauma)		*
Assesses cardiovascular system including heart sounds, peripheral edema, and peripheral perfusion		*
Assesses pulmonary system including reassessing airway, ventilation, breath sounds, pulse oximetry, chest wall excursion, accessory muscle use, or other signs of distress		*
Assesses neurological system including speech, droop, drift, if applicable, and distal movement and sensation		*
Assesses musculoskeletal and integumentary systems		
Assesses behavioral, psychological, and social aspects of patient and situation		
States field impression of patient—abdominal problem (states suspected differential diagnosis)		*
Verbalizes treatment plan for patient and calls for appropriate intervention(s)—IVs		*
Reevaluates transport decision		
ONGOING ASSESSMENT		
Repeats initial assessment		*
Repeats vital signs and evaluates trends		*
Evaluates response to treatments		*
Repeats focused assessment regarding patient complaint or injuries		
Gives radio report to receiving facility		
Turns over patient care with verbal report		*
Student exhibits competence with skill		

Any items in the Not Done column that are marked with an * are mandatory for the student to complete. A check mark in the Not Done column of an item with an * indicates that the student was unsuccessful and must attempt the skill again to assure competency. Examiners should use a different-color ink for the second attempt.

☐ Successful   ☐ Unsuccessful   Examiner Initials: _____

Scenario IV Insertion—Abdominal

Student: _____   **Examiner:** _____

Date: _____

	Done ✓	Not Done
Selects appropriate IV fluid, checking clarity, color, and expiration date		*
Selects appropriate catheter		
Selects appropriate administration set		
Properly inserts IV tubing into the IV bag		*
Prepares administration set (fills drip chamber and flushes tubing)		*
Cuts or tears tape (at any time before venipuncture)		*
Applies constricting band (checks distal pulse to assure NOT a tourniquet)		*
Palpates suitable vein		*
Cleanses site appropriately		*
Utilizes appropriate PPE		*
Inserts catheter with sterile technique		*
Verbalizes flash/blood return and advances catheter slightly farther		*
Occludes vein with finger at distal end of catheter and removes stylet		
Immediately disposes (or verbalizes disposal) of needle/sharp in proper container		
Obtains blood sample or connects IV tubing to catheter		
Obtains BGL (blood glucose level)		*
Releases constricting band		*
Runs IV for a brief period to ensure patency and adjusts flow rate as appropriate		*
Checks IV site for signs of infiltration		*
Secures catheter (tapes securely or verbalizes)		*
Attaches label with size of catheter, date, time, and "prehospital"		*
Assesses patient's response to intervention		*
Student exhibits competence with skill		

Any items in the Not Done column that are marked with an * are mandatory for the student to complete. A check mark in the Not Done column of an item with an * indicates that the student was unsuccessful and must attempt the skill again to assure competency. Examiners should use a different-color ink for the second attempt.

☐ Successful   ☐ Unsuccessful   Examiner Initials: _____

Scenario Radio Report—Abdominal

Student: _____   **Examiner:** _____

Date: _____

	Done ✓	Not Done
Requests and checks for open channel before speaking		
Presses transmit button 1 second before speaking		
Holds microphone 2–3 in. from mouth		
Speaks slowly and clearly		*
Speaks in a normal voice		
Briefly transmits: Agency, unit designation, identification/name		*
Briefly transmits: Patient's age, sex, weight		*
Briefly transmits: Scene description/mechanism of injury or medical problem		*
Briefly transmits: Chief complaint with brief history of *present* illness		*
Briefly transmits: Associated symptoms (unless able to be deferred to bedside report)		
Briefly transmits: Past medical history (usually deferred to bedside report)		
Briefly transmits: Vital signs		*
Briefly transmits: Level of consciousness/GCS on trauma		*
Briefly transmits: General appearance, distress, cardiac rhythm, blood glucose, and other pertinent findings unable to be deferred to bedside report		
Briefly transmits: Interventions by EMS AND response(s)		*
ETA (the more critical the patient, the earlier you need to notify the receiving facility)		
Does not waste airtime		
Protects privacy of patient		*
Echoes dispatch information and any physician orders		*
Writes down dispatch information or physician orders		
Confirms with facility that message is received		
Demonstrates/verbalizes ability to troubleshoot basic equipment malfunction		
Student exhibits competence with skill		

Any items in the Not Done column that are marked with an * are mandatory for the student to complete. A check mark in the Not Done column of an item with an * indicates that the student was unsuccessful and must attempt the skill again to assure competency. Examiners should use a different-color ink for the second attempt.

☐ Successful   ☐ Unsuccessful   Examiner Initials: _____

©2006 Prentice-Hall Inc.

Scenario Patient Care Report (PCR)—Abdominal

Student: _____   Examiner: _____

Date: _____

	Done ✓	Not Done
Records all pertinent dispatch/scene data, using a consistent format		
Completely identifies all additional resources and personnel		
Documents chief complaint, signs/symptoms, position found, age, sex, and weight		
Identifies and records all pertinent, reportable clinical data for each patient		
Documents SAMPLE and OPQRST if applicable		
Records all pertinent negatives		
Records all pertinent denials		
Records accurate, consistent times and patient information		
Includes relevant oral statements of witnesses, bystanders, and patient in "quotes" when appropriate		
Documents initial assessment findings: airway, breathing, and circulation		
Documents any interventions in initial assessment with patient response		
Documents level of consciousness, GCS (if trauma), and VS		
Documents rapid trauma assessment if applicable		
Documents any interventions in rapid trauma assessment with patient response		
Documents focused history and physical assessment		
Documents any interventions in focused assessment with patient response		
Documents repeat VS (every 5 minutes for critical; every 15 minutes for stable)		
Repeats initial assessment and documents findings		
Records ALL treatments with times and patient response(s) in treatment section		
Documents field impression		
Documents transport to specific facility and transfer of care WITH VERBAL REPORT		
Uses correct grammar, abbreviations, spelling, and terminology		
Writes legibly		
Thoroughly documents refusals, denials of transport, and call cancellations		
Documents patient GCS of 15 PRIOR to signing refusal		
Documents advice given to refusal patient, including "call 9-1-1 for further problems"		
Properly corrects errors and omissions		
Writes cautiously, avoids jargon, opinions, inferences, or any derogatory/libelous remarks		
Signs run report		
Uses EMS supplement form if needed		
Student exhibits competence with skill		

Any items in the Not Done column should be evaluated with student. Check marks in this column do not necessarily mean student was unsuccessful as all lines are not completed on all patients. Evaluation of each PCR should be based on the scenario given.

Student must be able to write an EMS report with consistency and accuracy.

☐ Successful   ☐ Unsuccessful   Examiner Initials: _____

©2006 Prentice-Hall Inc.

Overall Scenario Management—Abdominal

Student: _____   Examiner: _____

Date: _____   Scenario: _____

NOTE: This skill sheet is to be done after the student completes a scenario as the TEAM LEADER. It is to let the student know if he or she is beginning to "put it all together" and use critical thinking skills to manage an EMS call. PLEASE notice that it is graded on a different basis than the basic lab skill sheet.

	Done ✓	Needs to Improve
SCENE MANAGEMENT		
Recognized hazards and controlled scene—safety, crowd, and patient issues		
Recognized hazards, but did not control the scene		
Unsuccessfully attempted to manage the scene	*	
Did not evaluate the scene and took no control of the scene	*	
PATIENT ASSESSMENT		
Performed a timely, organized complete patient assessment		
Performed complete initial, focused, and ongoing assessments, but in a disorganized manner		
Performed an incomplete assessment	*	
Did not perform an initial assessment	*	
PATIENT MANAGEMENT		
Evaluated assessment findings to manage all aspects of patient condition		
Managed the patient's presenting signs and symptoms without considering all of assessment		
Inadequately managed the patient	*	
Did not manage life-threatening conditions	*	
COMMUNICATION		
Communicated well with crew, patient, family, bystanders, and assisting agencies		
Communicated well with patient and crew		
Communicated with patient and crew, but poor communication skills	*	
Unable to communicate effectively	*	
REPORT AND TRANSFER OF CARE		
Identified correct destination for patient transport, gave accurate, brief report over radio, and provided full report at bedside demonstrating thorough understanding of patient condition and pathophysiological processes		
Identified correct destination and gave accurate radio and bedside report, but did not demonstrate understanding of patient condition and pathophysiological processes		
Identified correct destination, but provided inadequate radio and bedside report	*	
Identified inappropriate destination or provided no radio or bedside report	*	
Student exhibits competence with skill		

Any items that are marked with an * indicate the student needs to improve and a check mark should be placed in the right-hand column. A check mark in the right-hand column indicates that the student was unsuccessful and must attempt the skill again to assure competency. Examiners should use a different-color ink for the second attempt.

☐ Successful   ☐ Unsuccessful   Examiner Initials: _____

©2006 Prentice-Hall Inc.

Patient Assessment: Medical—Altered Level of Consciousness (LOC)

Student: _____   Examiner: _____

Date: _____   Scenario: _____

	Done ✓	Not Done
Assesses scene safety and utilizes appropriate PPE		*
OVERALL SCENE EVALUATION		
Medical—determines nature of illness/if trauma involved determines MOI		*
Determines the number of patients, location, obstacles, and requests any additional resources as needed		
Verbalizes general impression of the patient as approaches		*
Considers stabilization/spinal motion restriction of spine if trauma involved		*
INITIAL ASSESSMENT		
Determines responsiveness/level of consciousness/AVPU		*
Opens airway with appropriate technique and assesses airway/ventilation		*
Manages airway/ventilation and applies appropriate oxygen therapy in less than 3 minutes		*
Assesses circulation: radial/carotid pulse, skin color, temperature, condition, and turgor		*
Controls any major bleeding		*
Makes rapid transport decision if indicated		
Initiates IV, **obtains BGL,** GCS, and complete vital signs		*
FOCUSED HISTORY AND PHYSICAL EXAMINATION/RAPID ASSESSMENT		
Obtains SAMPLE history		
Obtains OPQRST for differential diagnosis		
Obtains associated symptoms, pertinent negatives/denials		
Evaluates decision to perform focused exam or completes rapid assessment		*
Vital signs including AVPU (and GCS if trauma)		*
Assesses cardiovascular system including heart sounds, peripheral edema, and peripheral perfusion		*
Assesses pulmonary system including reassessing airway, ventilation, breath sounds, pulse oximetry, chest wall excursion, accessory muscle use, or other signs of distress		*
Assesses neurological system including **speech, droop, drift,** if applicable, and distal movement and sensation		*
Assesses musculoskeletal and integumentary systems		
Assesses behavioral, psychological, and social aspects of patient and situation		
States field impression of patient—altered LOC (states suspected differential diagnosis AEIOU-TIPS)		*
Verbalizes treatment plan for patient and calls for appropriate intervention(s)—IVs, treat cause		*
Reevaluates transport decision		
ONGOING ASSESSMENT		
Repeats initial assessment		*
Repeats vital signs and evaluates trends		*
Evaluates response to treatments		*
Repeats focused assessment regarding patient complaint or injuries		
Gives radio report to receiving facility		
Turns over patient care with verbal report		*
Student exhibits competence with skill		

Any items in the Not Done column that are marked with an * are mandatory for the student to complete. A check mark in the Not Done column of an item with an * indicates that the student was unsuccessful and must attempt the skill again to assure competency. Examiners should use a different-color ink for the second attempt.

☐ Successful   ☐ Unsuccessful   Examiner Initials: _____

   ©2006 Prentice-Hall Inc.

Scenario Intubation—Altered LOC

Student: _____   Examiner: _____

Date: _____

	Done ✓	Not Done
Assesses scene safety and utilizes appropriate PPE		*
Manually opens the airway with technique appropriate for patient condition		*
Checks mouth for blood or potential airway obstruction		*
Suctions or removes loose teeth or foreign materials as needed		
Inserts simple adjunct (oropharyngeal or nasopharyngeal airway)		
Directs assistant to ventilate patient with bag-valve-mask device (room air)		*
Observes chest rise/fall and auscultates bilaterally over lungs for baseline		*
Obtains effective ventilation in less than 30 seconds		*
Attaches oxygen reservoir to bag-valve-mask device and connects to high-flow oxygen		
Ventilates patient and evaluates chest wall/lung compliance		*
Directs assistant to preoxygenate patient		*
Identifies/selects proper equipment for intubation		
Checks laryngoscope light and cuff of ET tube		
Removes all air from cuff and properly inserts stylet if used		
Removes airway adjunct		
Positions patient's head properly and has assistant perform Sellick's maneuver		*
Opens mouth and gently inserts blade while sweeping tongue to side		*
Has assistant maintain Sellick's pressure		
Gently elevates mandible with laryngoscope and visualizes cords		*
Introduces ET tube to side of blade and visualizes tube passing through cords		*
"Threads" ET tube off stylet (if used), maintaining hold on ET tube as stylet removed		
Inflates cuff to proper pressure and disconnects syringe		*
Disconnects mask from bag-valve device and attaches to ET tube without releasing ET tube		
Directs ventilation of patient while maintaining Sellick's maneuver and holding ET tube in place		
Confirms proper placement by auscultation over epigastrium and bilaterally over each lung		*
Directs assistant to release cricoid pressure		*
Secures ET tube		*
Reassesses bilateral lung sounds and compliance		*
Uses secondary device to confirm tube placement		*
Assesses patient's response to intervention		*
Student exhibits competence with skill		

Any items in the Not Done column that are marked with an * are mandatory for the student to complete. A check mark in the Not Done column of an item with an * indicates that the student was unsuccessful and must attempt the skill again to assure competency. Examiners should use a different-color ink for the second attempt.

☐ Successful   ☐ Unsuccessful   Examiner Initials: _____

©2006 Prentice-Hall Inc.

Scenario IV Insertion—Altered LOC

Student: _____   Examiner: _____

Date: _____

	Done ✓	Not Done
Selects appropriate IV fluid, checking clarity, color, and expiration date		*
Selects appropriate catheter		
Selects appropriate administration set		
Properly inserts IV tubing into the IV bag		*
Prepares administration set (fills drip chamber and flushes tubing)		*
Cuts or tears tape (at any time before venipuncture)		*
Applies constricting band (checks distal pulse to assure NOT a tourniquet)		*
Palpates suitable vein		*
Cleanses site appropriately		*
Utilizes appropriate PPE		*
Inserts catheter with sterile technique		*
Verbalizes flash/blood return and advances catheter slightly farther		*
Occludes vein with finger at distal end of catheter and removes stylet		
Immediately disposes (or verbalizes disposal) of needle/sharp in proper container		
Obtains blood sample or connects IV tubing to catheter		
Obtains BGL (blood glucose level)		*
Releases constricting band		*
Runs IV for a brief period to ensure patency and adjusts flow rate as appropriate		*
Checks IV site for signs of infiltration		*
Secures catheter (tapes securely or verbalizes)		*
Attaches label with size of catheter, date, time, and "prehospital"		*
Assesses patient's response to intervention		*
Student exhibits competence with skill		

Any items in the Not Done column that are marked with an * are mandatory for the student to complete. A check mark in the Not Done column of an item with an * indicates that the student was unsuccessful and must attempt the skill again to assure competency. Examiners should use a different-color ink for the second attempt.

☐ Successful   ☐ Unsuccessful   Examiner Initials: _____

©2006 Prentice-Hall Inc.

Scenario Radio Report—Altered LOC

Student: _____   **Examiner:** _____

Date: _____

	Done ✓	Not Done
Requests and checks for open channel before speaking		
Presses transmit button 1 second before speaking		
Holds microphone 2–3 in. from mouth		
Speaks slowly and clearly		*
Speaks in a normal voice		
Briefly transmits: Agency, unit designation, identification/name		*
Briefly transmits: Patient's age, sex, weight		*
Briefly transmits: Scene description/mechanism of injury or medical problem		*
Briefly transmits: Chief complaint with brief history of *present* illness		*
Briefly transmits: Associated symptoms (unless able to be deferred to bedside report)		
Briefly transmits: Past medical history (usually deferred to bedside report)		
Briefly transmits: Vital signs		*
Briefly transmits: Level of consciousness/GCS on trauma		*
Briefly transmits: General appearance, distress, cardiac rhythm, blood glucose, and other pertinent findings unable to be deferred to bedside report		
Briefly transmits: Interventions by EMS AND response(s)		*
ETA (the more critical the patient, the earlier you need to notify the receiving facility)		
Does not waste airtime		
Protects privacy of patient		*
Echoes dispatch information and any physician orders		*
Writes down dispatch information or physician orders		
Confirms with facility that message is received		
Demonstrates/verbalizes ability to troubleshoot basic equipment malfunction		
Student exhibits competence with skill		

Any items in the Not Done column that are marked with an * are mandatory for the student to complete. A check mark in the Not Done column of an item with an * indicates that the student was unsuccessful and must attempt the skill again to assure competency. Examiners should use a different-color ink for the second attempt.

☐ Successful   ☐ Unsuccessful   Examiner Initials: _____

©2006 Prentice-Hall Inc.

Scenario Patient Care Report (PCR)—Altered LOC

Student: _____   Examiner: _____

Date: _____

	Done ✓	Not Done
Records all pertinent dispatch/scene data, using a consistent format		
Completely identifies all additional resources and personnel		
Documents chief complaint, signs/symptoms, position found, age, sex, and weight		
Identifies and records all pertinent, reportable clinical data for each patient		
Documents SAMPLE and OPQRST if applicable		
Records all pertinent negatives		
Records all pertinent denials		
Records accurate, consistent times and patient information		
Includes relevant oral statements of witnesses, bystanders, and patient in "quotes" when appropriate		
Documents initial assessment findings: airway, breathing, and circulation		
Documents any interventions in initial assessment with patient response		
Documents level of consciousness, GCS (if trauma), and VS		
Documents rapid trauma assessment if applicable		
Documents any interventions in rapid trauma assessment with patient response		
Documents focused history and physical assessment		
Documents any interventions in focused assessment with patient response		
Documents repeat VS (every 5 minutes for critical; every 15 minutes for stable)		
Repeats initial assessment and documents findings		
Records ALL treatments with times and patient response(s) in treatment section		
Documents field impression		
Documents transport to specific facility and transfer of care WITH VERBAL REPORT		
Uses correct grammar, abbreviations, spelling, and terminology		
Writes legibly		
Thoroughly documents refusals, denials of transport, and call cancellations		
Documents patient GCS of 15 PRIOR to signing refusal		
Documents advice given to refusal patient, including "call 9-1-1 for further problems"		
Properly corrects errors and omissions		
Writes cautiously, avoids jargon, opinions, inferences, or any derogatory/libelous remarks		
Signs run report		
Uses EMS supplement form if needed		
Student exhibits competence with skill		

Any items in the Not Done column should be evaluated with student. Check marks in this column do not necessarily mean student was unsuccessful as all lines are not completed on all patients. Evaluation of each PCR should be based on the scenario given.

Student must be able to write an EMS report with consistency and accuracy.

☐ Successful   ☐ Unsuccessful   Examiner Initials: _____

©2006 Prentice-Hall Inc.

Overall Scenario Management—Altered LOC

Student: _____   Examiner: _____

Date: _____   Scenario: _____

NOTE: This skill sheet is to be done after the student completes a scenario as the TEAM LEADER. It is to let the student know if he or she is beginning to "put it all together" and use critical thinking skills to manage an EMS call. PLEASE notice that it is graded on a different basis than the basic lab skill sheet.

	Done ✓	Needs to Improve
SCENE MANAGEMENT		
Recognized hazards and controlled scene—safety, crowd, and patient issues		
Recognized hazards, but did not control the scene		
Unsuccessfully attempted to manage the scene	*	
Did not evaluate the scene and took no control of the scene	*	
PATIENT ASSESSMENT		
Performed a timely, organized complete patient assessment		
Performed complete initial, focused, and ongoing assessments, but in a disorganized manner		
Performed an incomplete assessment	*	
Did not perform an initial assessment	*	
PATIENT MANAGEMENT		
Evaluated assessment findings to manage all aspects of patient condition		
Managed the patient's presenting signs and symptoms without considering all of assessment		
Inadequately managed the patient	*	
Did not manage life-threatening conditions	*	
COMMUNICATION		
Communicated well with crew, patient, family, bystanders, and assisting agencies		
Communicated well with patient and crew		
Communicated with patient and crew, but poor communication skills	*	
Unable to communicate effectively	*	
REPORT AND TRANSFER OF CARE		
Identified correct destination for patient transport, gave accurate, brief report over radio, and provided full report at bedside demonstrating thorough understanding of patient condition and pathophysiological processes		
Identified correct destination and gave accurate radio and bedside report, but did not demonstrate understanding of patient condition and pathophysiological processes		
Identified correct destination, but provided inadequate radio and bedside report	*	
Identified inappropriate destination or provided no radio or bedside report	*	
Student exhibits competence with skill		

Any items that are marked with an * indicate the student needs to improve and a check mark should be placed in the right-hand column. A check mark in the right-hand column indicates that the student was unsuccessful and must attempt the skill again to assure competency. Examiners should use a different-color ink for the second attempt.

☐ Successful   ☐ Unsuccessful   Examiner Initials: _____

©2006 Prentice-Hall Inc.

Patient Assessment: Medical—Behavioral

Student: _____   Examiner: _____

Date: _____   Scenario: _____

	Done ✓	Not Done
Assesses scene safety and utilizes appropriate PPE		*
OVERALL SCENE EVALUATION		
Medical—determines nature of illness/if trauma involved determines MOI		*
Determines the number of patients, location, obstacles, and requests any additional resources as needed		
Verbalizes general impression of the patient as approaches		*
Considers stabilization/spinal motion restriction of spine if trauma involved		*
INITIAL ASSESSMENT		
Determines responsiveness/level of consciousness/AVPU		*
Opens airway with appropriate technique and assesses airway/ventilation		*
Manages airway/ventilation and applies appropriate oxygen therapy in less than 3 minutes		*
Assesses circulation: radial/carotid pulse, skin color, temperature, condition, and turgor		*
Controls any major bleeding		*
Makes rapid transport decision if indicated		
Initiates IV, **obtains BGL**, GCS, and complete vital signs		*
FOCUSED HISTORY AND PHYSICAL EXAMINATION/RAPID ASSESSMENT		
Obtains SAMPLE history		
Obtains OPQRST for differential diagnosis		
Obtains associated symptoms, pertinent negatives/denials		
Evaluates decision to perform focused exam or completes rapid assessment		*
Vital signs including AVPU (and GCS if trauma)		*
Assesses cardiovascular system including heart sounds, peripheral edema, and peripheral perfusion		*
Assesses pulmonary system including reassessing airway, ventilation, breath sounds, pulse oximetry, chest wall excursion, accessory muscle use, or other signs of distress		*
Assesses neurological system including speech, droop, drift, if applicable, and distal movement and sensation		*
Assesses musculoskeletal and integumentary systems		
Assesses behavioral, psychological, and social aspects of patient and situation		
States field impression of patient—behavioral problem (rules out medical diagnosis)		*
Verbalizes treatment plan for patient and calls for appropriate intervention(s)—IVs, potential safety issues		*
Reevaluates transport decision		
ONGOING ASSESSMENT		
Repeats initial assessment		*
Repeats vital signs and evaluates trends		*
Evaluates response to treatments		*
Repeats focused assessment regarding patient complaint or injuries		
Gives radio report to receiving facility		
Turns over patient care with verbal report		*
Student exhibits competence with skill		

Any items in the Not Done column that are marked with an * are mandatory for the student to complete. A check mark in the Not Done column of an item with an * indicates that the student was unsuccessful and must attempt the skill again to assure competency. Examiners should use a different-color ink for the second attempt.

☐ Successful   ☐ Unsuccessful   Examiner Initials: _____

©2006 Prentice-Hall Inc.

Scenario Intubation—Behavioral

Student: _____   **Examiner:** _____

Date: _____

	Done ✓	Not Done
Assesses scene safety and utilizes appropriate PPE		*
Manually opens the airway with technique appropriate for patient condition		*
Checks mouth for blood or potential airway obstruction		*
Suctions or removes loose teeth or foreign materials as needed		
Inserts simple adjunct (oropharyngeal or nasopharyngeal airway)		
Directs assistant to ventilate patient with bag-valve-mask device (room air)		*
Observes chest rise/fall and auscultates bilaterally over lungs for baseline		*
Obtains effective ventilation in less than 30 seconds		*
Attaches oxygen reservoir to bag-valve-mask device and connects to high-flow oxygen		
Ventilates patient and evaluates chest wall/lung compliance		*
Directs assistant to preoxygenate patient		*
Identifies/selects proper equipment for intubation		
Checks laryngoscope light and cuff of ET tube		
Removes all air from cuff and properly inserts stylet if used		
Removes airway adjunct		
Positions patient's head properly and has assistant perform Sellick's maneuver		*
Opens mouth and gently inserts blade while sweeping tongue to side		*
Has assistant maintain Sellick's pressure		
Gently elevates mandible with laryngoscope and visualizes cords		*
Introduces ET tube to side of blade and visualizes tube passing through cords		*
"Threads" ET tube off stylet (if used), maintaining hold on ET tube as stylet removed		
Inflates cuff to proper pressure and disconnects syringe		*
Disconnects mask from bag-valve device and attaches to ET tube without releasing ET tube		
Directs ventilation of patient while maintaining Sellick's maneuver and holding ET tube in place		
Confirms proper placement by auscultation over epigastrium and bilaterally over each lung		*
Directs assistant to release cricoid pressure		*
Secures ET tube		*
Reassesses bilateral lung sounds and compliance		*
Uses secondary device to confirm tube placement		*
Assesses patient's response to intervention		*
Student exhibits competence with skill		

Any items in the Not Done column that are marked with an * are mandatory for the student to complete. A check mark in the Not Done column of an item with an * indicates that the student was unsuccessful and must attempt the skill again to assure competency. Examiners should use a different-color ink for the second attempt.

☐ Successful   ☐ Unsuccessful   Examiner Initials: _____

Scenario IV Insertion—Behavioral

Student: _____   Examiner: _____

Date: _____

	Done ✓	Not Done
Selects appropriate IV fluid, checking clarity, color, and expiration date		*
Selects appropriate catheter		
Selects appropriate administration set		
Properly inserts IV tubing into the IV bag		*
Prepares administration set (fills drip chamber and flushes tubing)		*
Cuts or tears tape (at any time before venipuncture)		*
Applies constricting band (checks distal pulse to assure NOT a tourniquet)		*
Palpates suitable vein		*
Cleanses site appropriately		*
Utilizes appropriate PPE		*
Inserts catheter with sterile technique		*
Verbalizes flash/blood return and advances catheter slightly farther		*
Occludes vein with finger at distal end of catheter and removes stylet		
Immediately disposes (or verbalizes disposal) of needle/sharp in proper container		
Obtains blood sample or connects IV tubing to catheter		
Obtains BGL (blood glucose level)		*
Releases constricting band		*
Runs IV for a brief period to ensure patency and adjusts flow rate as appropriate		*
Checks IV site for signs of infiltration		*
Secures catheter (tapes securely or verbalizes)		*
Attaches label with size of catheter, date, time, and "prehospital"		*
Assesses patient's response to intervention		*
Student exhibits competence with skill		

Any items in the Not Done column that are marked with an * are mandatory for the student to complete. A check mark in the Not Done column of an item with an * indicates that the student was unsuccessful and must attempt the skill again to assure competency. Examiners should use a different-color ink for the second attempt.

☐ Successful   ☐ Unsuccessful   Examiner Initials: _____

©2006 Prentice-Hall Inc.

Scenario Radio Report—Behavioral

Student: _____   **Examiner:** _____

Date: _____

	Done ✓	Not Done
Requests and checks for open channel before speaking		
Presses transmit button 1 second before speaking		
Holds microphone 2–3 in. from mouth		
Speaks slowly and clearly		*
Speaks in a normal voice		
Briefly transmits: Agency, unit designation, identification/name		*
Briefly transmits: Patient's age, sex, weight		*
Briefly transmits: Scene description/mechanism of injury or medical problem		*
Briefly transmits: Chief complaint with brief history of *present* illness		*
Briefly transmits: Associated symptoms (unless able to be deferred to bedside report)		
Briefly transmits: Past medical history (usually deferred to bedside report)		
Briefly transmits: Vital signs		*
Briefly transmits: Level of consciousness/GCS on trauma		*
Briefly transmits: General appearance, distress, cardiac rhythm, blood glucose, and other pertinent findings unable to be deferred to bedside report		
Briefly transmits: Interventions by EMS AND response(s)		*
ETA (the more critical the patient, the earlier you need to notify the receiving facility)		
Does not waste airtime		
Protects privacy of patient		*
Echoes dispatch information and any physician orders		*
Writes down dispatch information or physician orders		
Confirms with facility that message is received and advises of potential safety issues		
Demonstrates/verbalizes ability to troubleshoot basic equipment malfunction		
Student exhibits competence with skill		

Any items in the Not Done column that are marked with an * are mandatory for the student to complete. A check mark in the Not Done column of an item with an * indicates that the student was unsuccessful and must attempt the skill again to assure competency. Examiners should use a different-color ink for the second attempt.

☐ Successful   ☐ Unsuccessful   Examiner Initials: _____

Scenario Patient Care Report (PCR)—Behavioral

Student: _____   **Examiner:** _____

Date: _____

	Done ✓	Not Done
Records all pertinent dispatch/scene data, using a consistent format		
Completely identifies all additional resources and personnel		
Documents chief complaint, signs/symptoms, position found, age, sex, and weight		
Identifies and records all pertinent, reportable clinical data for each patient		
Documents SAMPLE and OPQRST if applicable		
Records all pertinent negatives		
Records all pertinent denials		
Records accurate, consistent times and patient information		
Includes relevant oral statements of witnesses, bystanders, and patient in "quotes" when appropriate		
Documents initial assessment findings: airway, breathing, and circulation		
Documents any interventions in initial assessment with patient response		
Documents level of consciousness, GCS (if trauma), and VS		
Documents rapid trauma assessment if applicable		
Documents any interventions in rapid trauma assessment with patient response		
Documents focused history and physical assessment		
Documents any interventions in focused assessment with patient response		
Documents repeat VS (every 5 minutes for critical; every 15 minutes for stable)		
Repeats initial assessment and documents findings		
Records ALL treatments with times and patient response(s) in treatment section		
Documents field impression		
Documents transport to specific facility and transfer of care WITH VERBAL REPORT		
Uses correct grammar, abbreviations, spelling, and terminology		
Writes legibly		
Thoroughly documents refusals, denials of transport, and call cancellations		
Documents patient GCS of 15 PRIOR to signing refusal		
Documents advice given to refusal patient, including "call 9-1-1 for further problems"		
Properly corrects errors and omissions		
Writes cautiously, avoids jargon, opinions, inferences, or any derogatory/libelous remarks		
Signs run report		
Uses EMS supplement form if needed		
Student exhibits competence with skill		

Any items in the Not Done column should be evaluated with student. Check marks in this column do not necessarily mean student was unsuccessful as all lines are not completed on all patients. Evaluation of each PCR should be based on the scenario given.

Student must be able to write an EMS report with consistency and accuracy.

☐ Successful   ☐ Unsuccessful   Examiner Initials: _____

©2006 Prentice-Hall Inc.

Overall Scenario Management—Behavioral

Student: _____   Examiner: _____

Date: _____   Scenario: _____

NOTE: This skill sheet is to be done after the student completes a scenario as the TEAM LEADER. It is to let the student know if he or she is beginning to "put it all together" and use critical thinking skills to manage an EMS call. PLEASE notice that it is graded on a different basis than the basic lab skill sheet.

	Done ✓	Needs to Improve
SCENE MANAGEMENT		
Recognized hazards and controlled scene—safety, crowd, and patient issues		
Recognized hazards, but did not control the scene		
Unsuccessfully attempted to manage the scene	*	
Did not evaluate the scene and took no control of the scene	*	
PATIENT ASSESSMENT		
Performed a timely, organized complete patient assessment		
Performed complete initial, focused, and ongoing assessments, but in a disorganized manner		
Performed an incomplete assessment	*	
Did not perform an initial assessment	*	
PATIENT MANAGEMENT		
Evaluated assessment findings to manage all aspects of patient condition		
Managed the patient's presenting signs and symptoms without considering all of assessment		
Inadequately managed the patient	*	
Did not manage life-threatening conditions	*	
COMMUNICATION		
Communicated well with crew, patient, family, bystanders, and assisting agencies		
Communicated well with patient and crew		
Communicated with patient and crew, but poor communication skills	*	
Unable to communicate effectively	*	
REPORT AND TRANSFER OF CARE		
Identified correct destination for patient transport, gave accurate, brief report over radio, and provided full report at bedside demonstrating thorough understanding of patient condition and pathophysiological processes		
Identified correct destination and gave accurate radio and bedside report, but did not demonstrate understanding of patient condition and pathophysiological processes		
Identified correct destination, but provided inadequate radio and bedside report	*	
Identified inappropriate destination or provided no radio or bedside report	*	
Student exhibits competence with skill		

Any items that are marked with an * indicate the student needs to improve and a check mark should be placed in the right-hand column. A check mark in the right-hand column indicates that the student was unsuccessful and must attempt the skill again to assure competency. Examiners should use a different-color ink for the second attempt.

☐ Successful   ☐ Unsuccessful   Examiner Initials: _____

©2006 Prentice-Hall Inc.

Patient Assessment: Medical—Behavioral

Student: _____   Examiner: _____

Date: _____   Scenario: _____

	Done ✓	Not Done
Assesses scene safety and utilizes appropriate PPE		*
OVERALL SCENE EVALUATION		
Medical—determines nature of illness/if trauma involved determines MOI		*
Determines the number of patients, location, obstacles, and requests any additional resources as needed		
Verbalizes general impression of the patient as approaches		*
Considers stabilization/spinal motion restriction of spine if trauma involved		*
INITIAL ASSESSMENT		
Determines responsiveness/level of consciousness/AVPU		*
Opens airway with appropriate technique and assesses airway/ventilation		*
Manages airway/ventilation and applies appropriate oxygen therapy in less than 3 minutes		*
Assesses circulation: radial/carotid pulse, skin color, temperature, condition, and turgor		*
Controls any major bleeding		*
Makes rapid transport decision if indicated		
Initiates IV, **obtains BGL,** GCS, and complete vital signs		*
FOCUSED HISTORY AND PHYSICAL EXAMINATION/RAPID ASSESSMENT		
Obtains SAMPLE history		
Obtains OPQRST for differential diagnosis		
Obtains associated symptoms, pertinent negatives/denials		
Evaluates decision to perform focused exam or completes rapid assessment		*
Vital signs including AVPU (and GCS if trauma)		*
Assesses cardiovascular system including heart sounds, peripheral edema, and peripheral perfusion		*
Assesses pulmonary system including reassessing airway, ventilation, breath sounds, pulse oximetry, chest wall excursion, accessory muscle use, or other signs of distress		*
Assesses neurological system including speech, droop, drift, if applicable, and distal movement and sensation		*
Assesses musculoskeletal and integumentary systems		
Assesses behavioral, psychological, and social aspects of patient and situation		
States field impression of patient—behavioral problem (rules out medical diagnosis)		*
Verbalizes treatment plan for patient and calls for appropriate intervention(s)—IVs, potential safety issues		*
Reevaluates transport decision		
ONGOING ASSESSMENT		
Repeats initial assessment		*
Repeats vital signs and evaluates trends		*
Evaluates response to treatments		*
Repeats focused assessment regarding patient complaint or injuries		
Gives radio report to receiving facility		
Turns over patient care with verbal report		*
Student exhibits competence with skill		

Any items in the Not Done column that are marked with an * are mandatory for the student to complete. A check mark in the Not Done column of an item with an * indicates that the student was unsuccessful and must attempt the skill again to assure competency. Examiners should use a different-color ink for the second attempt.

☐ Successful   ☐ Unsuccessful   Examiner Initials: _____

©2006 Prentice-Hall Inc.

Scenario Intubation—Behavioral

Student: _____   Examiner: _____

Date: _____

	Done ✓	Not Done
Assesses scene safety and utilizes appropriate PPE		*
Manually opens the airway with technique appropriate for patient condition		*
Checks mouth for blood or potential airway obstruction		*
Suctions or removes loose teeth or foreign materials as needed		
Inserts simple adjunct (oropharyngeal or nasopharyngeal airway)		
Directs assistant to ventilate patient with bag-valve-mask device (room air)		*
Observes chest rise/fall and auscultates bilaterally over lungs for baseline		*
Obtains effective ventilation in less than 30 seconds		*
Attaches oxygen reservoir to bag-valve-mask device and connects to high-flow oxygen		
Ventilates patient and evaluates chest wall/lung compliance		*
Directs assistant to preoxygenate patient		*
Identifies/selects proper equipment for intubation		
Checks laryngoscope light and cuff of ET tube		
Removes all air from cuff and properly inserts stylet if used		
Removes airway adjunct		
Positions patient's head properly and has assistant perform Sellick's maneuver		*
Opens mouth and gently inserts blade while sweeping tongue to side		*
Has assistant maintain Sellick's pressure		
Gently elevates mandible with laryngoscope and visualizes cords		*
Introduces ET tube to side of blade and visualizes tube passing through cords		*
"Threads" ET tube off stylet (if used), maintaining hold on ET tube as stylet removed		
Inflates cuff to proper pressure and disconnects syringe		*
Disconnects mask from bag-valve device and attaches to ET tube without releasing ET tube		
Directs ventilation of patient while maintaining Sellick's maneuver and holding ET tube in place		
Confirms proper placement by auscultation over epigastrium and bilaterally over each lung		*
Directs assistant to release cricoid pressure		*
Secures ET tube		*
Reassesses bilateral lung sounds and compliance		*
Uses secondary device to confirm tube placement		*
Assesses patient's response to intervention		*
Student exhibits competence with skill		

Any items in the Not Done column that are marked with an * are mandatory for the student to complete. A check mark in the Not Done column of an item with an * indicates that the student was unsuccessful and must attempt the skill again to assure competency. Examiners should use a different-color ink for the second attempt.

☐ Successful   ☐ Unsuccessful   Examiner Initials: _____

©2006 Prentice-Hall Inc.

Scenario IV Insertion—Behavioral

Student: _____ Examiner: _____

Date: _____

	Done ✓	Not Done
Selects appropriate IV fluid, checking clarity, color, and expiration date		*
Selects appropriate catheter		
Selects appropriate administration set		
Properly inserts IV tubing into the IV bag		*
Prepares administration set (fills drip chamber and flushes tubing)		*
Cuts or tears tape (at any time before venipuncture)		*
Applies constricting band (checks distal pulse to assure NOT a tourniquet)		*
Palpates suitable vein		*
Cleanses site appropriately		*
Utilizes appropriate PPE		*
Inserts catheter with sterile technique		*
Verbalizes flash/blood return and advances catheter slightly farther		*
Occludes vein with finger at distal end of catheter and removes stylet		
Immediately disposes (or verbalizes disposal) of needle/sharp in proper container		
Obtains blood sample or connects IV tubing to catheter		
Obtains BGL (blood glucose level)		*
Releases constricting band		*
Runs IV for a brief period to ensure patency and adjusts flow rate as appropriate		*
Checks IV site for signs of infiltration		*
Secures catheter (tapes securely or verbalizes)		*
Attaches label with size of catheter, date, time, and "prehospital"		*
Assesses patient's response to intervention		*
Student exhibits competence with skill		

Any items in the Not Done column that are marked with an * are mandatory for the student to complete. A check mark in the Not Done column of an item with an * indicates that the student was unsuccessful and must attempt the skill again to assure competency. Examiners should use a different-color ink for the second attempt.

☐ Successful   ☐ Unsuccessful   Examiner Initials: _____

©2006 Prentice-Hall Inc.

Scenario Radio Report—Behavioral

Student: _____   **Examiner:** _____

Date: _____

	Done ✓	Not Done
Requests and checks for open channel before speaking		
Presses transmit button 1 second before speaking		
Holds microphone 2–3 in. from mouth		
Speaks slowly and clearly		*
Speaks in a normal voice		
Briefly transmits: Agency, unit designation, identification/name		*
Briefly transmits: Patient's age, sex, weight		*
Briefly transmits: Scene description/mechanism of injury or medical problem		*
Briefly transmits: Chief complaint with brief history of *present* illness		*
Briefly transmits: Associated symptoms (unless able to be deferred to bedside report)		
Briefly transmits: Past medical history (usually deferred to bedside report)		
Briefly transmits: Vital signs		*
Briefly transmits: Level of consciousness/GCS on trauma		*
Briefly transmits: General appearance, distress, cardiac rhythm, blood glucose, and other pertinent findings unable to be deferred to bedside report		
Briefly transmits: Interventions by EMS AND response(s)		*
ETA (the more critical the patient, the earlier you need to notify the receiving facility)		
Does not waste airtime		
Protects privacy of patient		*
Echoes dispatch information and any physician orders		*
Writes down dispatch information or physician orders		
Confirms with facility that message is received and advises of potential safety issues		
Demonstrates/verbalizes ability to troubleshoot basic equipment malfunction		
Student exhibits competence with skill		

Any items in the Not Done column that are marked with an * are mandatory for the student to complete. A check mark in the Not Done column of an item with an * indicates that the student was unsuccessful and must attempt the skill again to assure competency. Examiners should use a different-color ink for the second attempt.

☐ Successful   ☐ Unsuccessful   Examiner Initials: _____

©2006 Prentice-Hall Inc.

Scenario Patient Care Report (PCR)—Behavioral

Student: _____ **Examiner:** _____

Date: _____

	Done ✓	Not Done
Records all pertinent dispatch/scene data, using a consistent format		
Completely identifies all additional resources and personnel		
Documents chief complaint, signs/symptoms, position found, age, sex, and weight		
Identifies and records all pertinent, reportable clinical data for each patient		
Documents SAMPLE and OPQRST if applicable		
Records all pertinent negatives		
Records all pertinent denials		
Records accurate, consistent times and patient information		
Includes relevant oral statements of witnesses, bystanders, and patient in "quotes" when appropriate		
Documents initial assessment findings: airway, breathing, and circulation		
Documents any interventions in initial assessment with patient response		
Documents level of consciousness, GCS (if trauma), and VS		
Documents rapid trauma assessment if applicable		
Documents any interventions in rapid trauma assessment with patient response		
Documents focused history and physical assessment		
Documents any interventions in focused assessment with patient response		
Documents repeat VS (every 5 minutes for critical; every 15 minutes for stable)		
Repeats initial assessment and documents findings		
Records ALL treatments with times and patient response(s) in treatment section		
Documents field impression		
Documents transport to specific facility and transfer of care WITH VERBAL REPORT		
Uses correct grammar, abbreviations, spelling, and terminology		
Writes legibly		
Thoroughly documents refusals, denials of transport, and call cancellations		
Documents patient GCS of 15 PRIOR to signing refusal		
Documents advice given to refusal patient, including "call 9-1-1 for further problems"		
Properly corrects errors and omissions		
Writes cautiously, avoids jargon, opinions, inferences, or any derogatory/libelous remarks		
Signs run report		
Uses EMS supplement form if needed		
Student exhibits competence with skill		

Any items in the Not Done column should be evaluated with student. Check marks in this column do not necessarily mean student was unsuccessful as all lines are not completed on all patients. Evaluation of each PCR should be based on the scenario given.

Student must be able to write an EMS report with consistency and accuracy.

☐ Successful ☐ Unsuccessful Examiner Initials: _____

©2006 Prentice-Hall Inc.

Overall Scenario Management—Behavioral

Student: _____   Examiner: _____

Date: _____   Scenario: _____

NOTE: This skill sheet is to be done after the student completes a scenario as the TEAM LEADER. It is to let the student know if he or she is beginning to "put it all together" and use critical thinking skills to manage an EMS call. PLEASE notice that it is graded on a different basis than the basic lab skill sheet.

	Done ✓	Needs to Improve
SCENE MANAGEMENT		
Recognized hazards and controlled scene—safety, crowd, and patient issues		
Recognized hazards, but did not control the scene		
Unsuccessfully attempted to manage the scene	*	
Did not evaluate the scene and took no control of the scene	*	
PATIENT ASSESSMENT		
Performed a timely, organized complete patient assessment		
Performed complete initial, focused, and ongoing assessments, but in a disorganized manner		
Performed an incomplete assessment	*	
Did not perform an initial assessment	*	
PATIENT MANAGEMENT		
Evaluated assessment findings to manage all aspects of patient condition		
Managed the patient's presenting signs and symptoms without considering all of assessment		
Inadequately managed the patient	*	
Did not manage life-threatening conditions	*	
COMMUNICATION		
Communicated well with crew, patient, family, bystanders, and assisting agencies		
Communicated well with patient and crew		
Communicated with patient and crew, but poor communication skills	*	
Unable to communicate effectively	*	
REPORT AND TRANSFER OF CARE		
Identified correct destination for patient transport, gave accurate, brief report over radio, and provided full report at bedside demonstrating thorough understanding of patient condition and pathophysiological processes		
Identified correct destination and gave accurate radio and bedside report, but did not demonstrate understanding of patient condition and pathophysiological processes		
Identified correct destination, but provided inadequate radio and bedside report	*	
Identified inappropriate destination or provided no radio or bedside report	*	
Student exhibits competence with skill		

Any items that are marked with an * indicate the student needs to improve and a check mark should be placed in the right-hand column. A check mark in the right-hand column indicates that the student was unsuccessful and must attempt the skill again to assure competency. Examiners should use a different-color ink for the second attempt.

☐ Successful   ☐ Unsuccessful   Examiner Initials: _____

©2006 Prentice-Hall Inc.

Patient Assessment: Medical—Behavioral

Student: _____   Examiner: _____

Date: _____   Scenario: _____

	Done ✓	Not Done
Assesses scene safety and utilizes appropriate PPE		*
OVERALL SCENE EVALUATION		
Medical—determines nature of illness/if trauma involved determines MOI		*
Determines the number of patients, location, obstacles, and requests any additional resources as needed		
Verbalizes general impression of the patient as approaches		*
Considers stabilization/spinal motion restriction of spine if trauma involved		*
INITIAL ASSESSMENT		
Determines responsiveness/level of consciousness/AVPU		*
Opens airway with appropriate technique and assesses airway/ventilation		*
Manages airway/ventilation and applies appropriate oxygen therapy in less than 3 minutes		*
Assesses circulation: radial/carotid pulse, skin color, temperature, condition, and turgor		*
Controls any major bleeding		*
Makes rapid transport decision if indicated		
Initiates IV, **obtains BGL**, GCS, and complete vital signs		*
FOCUSED HISTORY AND PHYSICAL EXAMINATION/RAPID ASSESSMENT		
Obtains SAMPLE history		
Obtains OPQRST for differential diagnosis		
Obtains associated symptoms, pertinent negatives/denials		
Evaluates decision to perform focused exam or completes rapid assessment		*
Vital signs including AVPU (and GCS if trauma)		*
Assesses cardiovascular system including heart sounds, peripheral edema, and peripheral perfusion		*
Assesses pulmonary system including reassessing airway, ventilation, breath sounds, pulse oximetry, chest wall excursion, accessory muscle use, or other signs of distress		*
Assesses neurological system including speech, droop, drift, if applicable, and distal movement and sensation		*
Assesses musculoskeletal and integumentary systems		
Assesses behavioral, psychological, and social aspects of patient and situation		
States field impression of patient—behavioral problem (rules out medical diagnosis)		*
Verbalizes treatment plan for patient and calls for appropriate intervention(s)—IVs, potential safety issues		*
Reevaluates transport decision		
ONGOING ASSESSMENT		
Repeats initial assessment		*
Repeats vital signs and evaluates trends		*
Evaluates response to treatments		*
Repeats focused assessment regarding patient complaint or injuries		
Gives radio report to receiving facility		
Turns over patient care with verbal report		*
Student exhibits competence with skill		

Any items in the Not Done column that are marked with an * are mandatory for the student to complete. A check mark in the Not Done column of an item with an * indicates that the student was unsuccessful and must attempt the skill again to assure competency. Examiners should use a different-color ink for the second attempt.

☐ Successful   ☐ Unsuccessful   Examiner Initials: _____

©2006 Prentice-Hall Inc.

Scenario Intubation—Behavioral

Student: _____   **Examiner:** _____

Date: _____

	Done ✓	Not Done
Assesses scene safety and utilizes appropriate PPE		*
Manually opens the airway with technique appropriate for patient condition		*
Checks mouth for blood or potential airway obstruction		*
Suctions or removes loose teeth or foreign materials as needed		
Inserts simple adjunct (oropharyngeal or nasopharyngeal airway)		
Directs assistant to ventilate patient with bag-valve-mask device (room air)		*
Observes chest rise/fall and auscultates bilaterally over lungs for baseline		*
Obtains effective ventilation in less than 30 seconds		*
Attaches oxygen reservoir to bag-valve-mask device and connects to high-flow oxygen		
Ventilates patient and evaluates chest wall/lung compliance		*
Directs assistant to preoxygenate patient		*
Identifies/selects proper equipment for intubation		
Checks laryngoscope light and cuff of ET tube		
Removes all air from cuff and properly inserts stylet if used		
Removes airway adjunct		
Positions patient's head properly and has assistant perform Sellick's maneuver		*
Opens mouth and gently inserts blade while sweeping tongue to side		*
Has assistant maintain Sellick's pressure		
Gently elevates mandible with laryngoscope and visualizes cords		*
Introduces ET tube to side of blade and visualizes tube passing through cords		*
"Threads" ET tube off stylet (if used), maintaining hold on ET tube as stylet removed		
Inflates cuff to proper pressure and disconnects syringe		*
Disconnects mask from bag-valve device and attaches to ET tube without releasing ET tube		
Directs ventilation of patient while maintaining Sellick's maneuver and holding ET tube in place		
Confirms proper placement by auscultation over epigastrium and bilaterally over each lung		*
Directs assistant to release cricoid pressure		*
Secures ET tube		*
Reassesses bilateral lung sounds and compliance		*
Uses secondary device to confirm tube placement		*
Assesses patient's response to intervention		*
Student exhibits competence with skill		

Any items in the Not Done column that are marked with an * are mandatory for the student to complete. A check mark in the Not Done column of an item with an * indicates that the student was unsuccessful and must attempt the skill again to assure competency. Examiners should use a different-color ink for the second attempt.

☐ Successful   ☐ Unsuccessful   Examiner Initials: _____

©2006 Prentice-Hall Inc.

Scenario IV Insertion—Behavioral

Student: _____   Examiner: _____

Date: _____

	Done ✓	Not Done
Selects appropriate IV fluid, checking clarity, color, and expiration date		*
Selects appropriate catheter		
Selects appropriate administration set		
Properly inserts IV tubing into the IV bag		*
Prepares administration set (fills drip chamber and flushes tubing)		*
Cuts or tears tape (at any time before venipuncture)		*
Applies constricting band (checks distal pulse to assure NOT a tourniquet)		*
Palpates suitable vein		*
Cleanses site appropriately		*
Utilizes appropriate PPE		*
Inserts catheter with sterile technique		*
Verbalizes flash/blood return and advances catheter slightly farther		*
Occludes vein with finger at distal end of catheter and removes stylet		
Immediately disposes (or verbalizes disposal) of needle/sharp in proper container		
Obtains blood sample or connects IV tubing to catheter		
Obtains BGL (blood glucose level)		*
Releases constricting band		*
Runs IV for a brief period to ensure patency and adjusts flow rate as appropriate		*
Checks IV site for signs of infiltration		*
Secures catheter (tapes securely or verbalizes)		*
Attaches label with size of catheter, date, time, and "prehospital"		*
Assesses patient's response to intervention		*
Student exhibits competence with skill		

Any items in the Not Done column that are marked with an * are mandatory for the student to complete. A check mark in the Not Done column of an item with an * indicates that the student was unsuccessful and must attempt the skill again to assure competency. Examiners should use a different-color ink for the second attempt.

☐ Successful   ☐ Unsuccessful   Examiner Initials: _____

©2006 Prentice-Hall Inc.

Scenario Radio Report—Behavioral

Student: _____   **Examiner:** _____

Date: _____

	Done ✓	Not Done
Requests and checks for open channel before speaking		
Presses transmit button 1 second before speaking		
Holds microphone 2–3 in. from mouth		
Speaks slowly and clearly		*
Speaks in a normal voice		
Briefly transmits: Agency, unit designation, identification/name		*
Briefly transmits: Patient's age, sex, weight		*
Briefly transmits: Scene description/mechanism of injury or medical problem		*
Briefly transmits: Chief complaint with brief history of *present* illness		*
Briefly transmits: Associated symptoms (unless able to be deferred to bedside report)		
Briefly transmits: Past medical history (usually deferred to bedside report)		
Briefly transmits: Vital signs		*
Briefly transmits: Level of consciousness/GCS on trauma		*
Briefly transmits: General appearance, distress, cardiac rhythm, blood glucose, and other pertinent findings unable to be deferred to bedside report		
Briefly transmits: Interventions by EMS AND response(s)		*
ETA (the more critical the patient, the earlier you need to notify the receiving facility)		
Does not waste airtime		
Protects privacy of patient		*
Echoes dispatch information and any physician orders		*
Writes down dispatch information or physician orders		
Confirms with facility that message is received and potential safety issues		
Demonstrates/verbalizes ability to troubleshoot basic equipment malfunction		
Student exhibits competence with skill		

Any items in the Not Done column that are marked with an * are mandatory for the student to complete. A check mark in the Not Done column of an item with an * indicates that the student was unsuccessful and must attempt the skill again to assure competency. Examiners should use a different-color ink for the second attempt.

☐ Successful   ☐ Unsuccessful   Examiner Initials: _____

©2006 Prentice-Hall Inc.

Scenario Patient Care Report (PCR)—Behavioral

Student: _____   **Examiner:** _____

Date: _____

	Done ✓	Not Done
Records all pertinent dispatch/scene data, using a consistent format		
Completely identifies all additional resources and personnel		
Documents chief complaint, signs/symptoms, position found, age, sex, and weight		
Identifies and records all pertinent, reportable clinical data for each patient		
Documents SAMPLE and OPQRST if applicable		
Records all pertinent negatives		
Records all pertinent denials		
Records accurate, consistent times and patient information		
Includes relevant oral statements of witnesses, bystanders, and patient in "quotes" when appropriate		
Documents initial assessment findings: airway, breathing, and circulation		
Documents any interventions in initial assessment with patient response		
Documents level of consciousness, GCS (if trauma), and VS		
Documents rapid trauma assessment if applicable		
Documents any interventions in rapid trauma assessment with patient response		
Documents focused history and physical assessment		
Documents any interventions in focused assessment with patient response		
Documents repeat VS (every 5 minutes for critical; every 15 minutes for stable)		
Repeats initial assessment and documents findings		
Records ALL treatments with times and patient response(s) in treatment section		
Documents field impression		
Documents transport to specific facility and transfer of care WITH VERBAL REPORT		
Uses correct grammar, abbreviations, spelling, and terminology		
Writes legibly		
Thoroughly documents refusals, denials of transport, and call cancellations		
Documents patient GCS of 15 PRIOR to signing refusal		
Documents advice given to refusal patient, including "call 9-1-1 for further problems"		
Properly corrects errors and omissions		
Writes cautiously, avoids jargon, opinions, inferences, or any derogatory/libelous remarks		
Signs run report		
Uses EMS supplement form if needed		
Student exhibits competence with skill		

Any items in the Not Done column should be evaluated with student. Check marks in this column do not necessarily mean student was unsuccessful as all lines are not completed on all patients. Evaluation of each PCR should be based on the scenario given.

Student must be able to write an EMS report with consistency and accuracy.

☐ Successful   ☐ Unsuccessful   Examiner Initials: _____

©2006 Prentice-Hall Inc.

Overall Scenario Management—Behavioral

Student: _____   Examiner: _____

Date: _____   Scenario: _____

NOTE: This skill sheet is to be done after the student completes a scenario as the TEAM LEADER. It is to let the student know if he or she is beginning to "put it all together" and use critical thinking skills to manage an EMS call. PLEASE notice that it is graded on a different basis than the basic lab skill sheet.

	Done ✓	Needs to Improve
SCENE MANAGEMENT		
Recognized hazards and controlled scene—safety, crowd, and patient issues		
Recognized hazards, but did not control the scene		
Unsuccessfully attempted to manage the scene	*	
Did not evaluate the scene and took no control of the scene	*	
PATIENT ASSESSMENT		
Performed a timely, organized complete patient assessment		
Performed complete initial, focused, and ongoing assessments, but in a disorganized manner		
Performed an incomplete assessment	*	
Did not perform an initial assessment	*	
PATIENT MANAGEMENT		
Evaluated assessment findings to manage all aspects of patient condition		
Managed the patient's presenting signs and symptoms without considering all of assessment		
Inadequately managed the patient	*	
Did not manage life-threatening conditions	*	
COMMUNICATION		
Communicated well with crew, patient, family, bystanders, and assisting agencies		
Communicated well with patient and crew		
Communicated with patient and crew, but poor communication skills	*	
Unable to communicate effectively	*	
REPORT AND TRANSFER OF CARE		
Identified correct destination for patient transport, gave accurate, brief report over radio, and provided full report at bedside demonstrating thorough understanding of patient condition and pathophysiological processes		
Identified correct destination and gave accurate radio and bedside report, but did not demonstrate understanding of patient condition and pathophysiological processes		
Identified correct destination, but provided inadequate radio and bedside report	*	
Identified inappropriate destination or provided no radio or bedside report	*	
Student exhibits competence with skill		

Any items that are marked with an * indicate the student needs to improve and a check mark should be placed in the right-hand column. A check mark in the right-hand column indicates that the student was unsuccessful and must attempt the skill again to assure competency. Examiners should use a different-color ink for the second attempt.

☐ Successful   ☐ Unsuccessful   Examiner Initials: _____

©2006 Prentice-Hall Inc.

Patient Assessment: Medical—Chest Pain

Student: _____   Examiner:_____

Date: _____   Scenario: _____

	Done ✓	Not Done
Assesses scene safety and utilizes appropriate PPE		*
OVERALL SCENE EVALUATION		
Medical—determines nature of illness/if trauma involved determines MOI		*
Determines the number of patients, location, obstacles, and requests any additional resources as needed		
Verbalizes general impression of the patient as approaches		*
Considers stabilization/spinal motion restriction of spine if trauma involved		*
INITIAL ASSESSMENT		
Determines responsiveness/level of consciousness/AVPU		*
Opens airway with appropriate technique and assesses airway/ventilation		*
Manages airway/ventilation and applies appropriate oxygen therapy in less than 3 minutes		*
Assesses circulation: radial/carotid pulse, skin color, temperature, condition, and turgor		*
Controls any major bleeding		*
Makes rapid transport decision if indicated		
Initiates IV, obtains BGL, GCS, and complete vital signs		
FOCUSED HISTORY AND PHYSICAL EXAMINATION/RAPID ASSESSMENT		
Obtains SAMPLE history		
Obtains OPQRST for differential diagnosis		
Obtains associated symptoms, pertinent negatives/denials		
Evaluates decision to perform focused exam or completes rapid assessment		*
Vital signs including AVPU (and GCS if trauma)		*
Assesses cardiovascular system including heart sounds, peripheral edema, and peripheral perfusion		*
Assesses pulmonary system including reassessing airway, ventilation, breath sounds, pulse oximetry, chest wall excursion, accessory muscle use, or other signs of distress		*
Assesses neurological system including speech, droop, drift, if applicable, and distal movement and sensation		*
Assesses musculoskeletal and integumentary systems		
Assesses behavioral, psychological, and social aspects of patient and situation		
States field impression of patient—chest pain (states suspected differential diagnosis)		*
Verbalizes treatment plan for patient and calls for appropriate intervention(s)—IV, must include cardiac monitor		*
Reevaluates transport decision		
ONGOING ASSESSMENT		
Repeats initial assessment		*
Repeats vital signs and evaluates trends		*
Evaluates response to treatments		*
Repeats focused assessment regarding patient complaint or injuries		
Gives radio report to receiving facility		
Turns over patient care with verbal report		*
Student exhibits competence with skill		

Any items in the Not Done column that are marked with an * are mandatory for the student to complete. A check mark in the Not Done column of an item with an * indicates that the student was unsuccessful and must attempt the skill again to assure competency. Examiners should use a different-color ink for the second attempt.

☐ Successful   ☐ Unsuccessful   Examiner Initials: _____

©2006 Prentice-Hall Inc.

Scenario Radio Report—Chest Pain

Student: _____   **Examiner:** _____

Date: _____

	Done ✓	Not Done
Requests and checks for open channel before speaking		
Presses transmit button 1 second before speaking		
Holds microphone 2–3 in. from mouth		
Speaks slowly and clearly		*
Speaks in a normal voice		
Briefly transmits: Agency, unit designation, identification/name		*
Briefly transmits: Patient's age, sex, weight		*
Briefly transmits: Scene description/mechanism of injury or medical problem		*
Briefly transmits: Chief complaint with brief history of *present* illness		*
Briefly transmits: Associated symptoms (unless able to be deferred to bedside report)		
Briefly transmits: Past medical history (usually deferred to bedside report)		
Briefly transmits: Vital signs		*
Briefly transmits: Level of consciousness/GCS on trauma		*
Briefly transmits: General appearance, distress, cardiac rhythm, blood glucose, and other pertinent findings unable to be deferred to bedside report		
Briefly transmits: Interventions by EMS AND response(s)		*
ETA (the more critical the patient, the earlier you need to notify the receiving facility)		
Does not waste airtime		
Protects privacy of patient		*
Echoes dispatch information and any physician orders		*
Writes down dispatch information or physician orders		
Confirms with facility that message is received		
Demonstrates/verbalizes ability to troubleshoot basic equipment malfunction		
Student exhibits competence with skill		

Any items in the Not Done column that are marked with an * are mandatory for the student to complete. A check mark in the Not Done column of an item with an * indicates that the student was unsuccessful and must attempt the skill again to assure competency. Examiners should use a different-color ink for the second attempt.

☐ Successful   ☐ Unsuccessful   Examiner Initials: _____

Scenario Patient Care Report (PCR)—Chest Pain

Student: _____   Examiner: _____

Date: _____

	Done ✓	Not Done
Records all pertinent dispatch/scene data, using a consistent format		
Completely identifies all additional resources and personnel		
Documents chief complaint, signs/symptoms, position found, age, sex, and weight		
Identifies and records all pertinent, reportable clinical data for each patient		
Documents SAMPLE and OPQRST if applicable		
Records all pertinent negatives		
Records all pertinent denials		
Records accurate, consistent times and patient information		
Includes relevant oral statements of witnesses, bystanders, and patient in "quotes" when appropriate		
Documents initial assessment findings: airway, breathing, and circulation		
Documents any interventions in initial assessment with patient response		
Documents level of consciousness, GCS (if trauma), and VS		
Documents rapid trauma assessment if applicable		
Documents any interventions in rapid trauma assessment with patient response		
Documents focused history and physical assessment		
Documents any interventions in focused assessment with patient response		
Documents repeat VS (every 5 minutes for critical; every 15 minutes for stable)		
Repeats initial assessment and documents findings		
Records ALL treatments with times and patient response(s) in treatment section		
Documents field impression		
Documents transport to specific facility and transfer of care WITH VERBAL REPORT		
Uses correct grammar, abbreviations, spelling, and terminology		
Writes legibly		
Thoroughly documents refusals, denials of transport, and call cancellations		
Documents patient GCS of 15 PRIOR to signing refusal		
Documents advice given to refusal patient, including "call 9-1-1 for further problems"		
Properly corrects errors and omissions		
Writes cautiously, avoids jargon, opinions, inferences, or any derogatory/libelous remarks		
Signs run report		
Uses EMS supplement form if needed		
Student exhibits competence with skill		

Any items in the Not Done column should be evaluated with student. Check marks in this column do not necessarily mean student was unsuccessful as all lines are not completed on all patients. Evaluation of each PCR should be based on the scenario given.

Student must be able to write an EMS report with consistency and accuracy.

☐ Successful   ☐ Unsuccessful   Examiner Initials: _____

©2006 Prentice-Hall Inc.

Overall Scenario Management—Chest Pain

Student: _____   Examiner: _____

Date: _____   Scenario: _____

NOTE: This skill sheet is to be done after the student completes a scenario as the **TEAM LEADER**. It is to let the student know if he or she is beginning to "put it all together" and use critical thinking skills to manage an EMS call. **PLEASE** notice that it is graded on a different basis than the basic lab skill sheet.

	Done ✓	Needs to Improve
SCENE MANAGEMENT		
Recognized hazards and controlled scene—safety, crowd, and patient issues		
Recognized hazards, but did not control the scene		
Unsuccessfully attempted to manage the scene	*	
Did not evaluate the scene and took no control of the scene	*	
PATIENT ASSESSMENT		
Performed a timely, organized complete patient assessment		
Performed complete initial, focused, and ongoing assessments, but in a disorganized manner		
Performed an incomplete assessment	*	
Did not perform an initial assessment	*	
PATIENT MANAGEMENT		
Evaluated assessment findings to manage all aspects of patient condition		
Managed the patient's presenting signs and symptoms without considering all of assessment		
Inadequately managed the patient	*	
Did not manage life-threatening conditions	*	
COMMUNICATION		
Communicated well with crew, patient, family, bystanders, and assisting agencies		
Communicated well with patient and crew		
Communicated with patient and crew, but poor communication skills	*	
Unable to communicate effectively	*	
REPORT AND TRANSFER OF CARE		
Identified correct destination for patient transport, gave accurate, brief report over radio, and provided full report at bedside demonstrating thorough understanding of patient condition and pathophysiological processes		
Identified correct destination and gave accurate radio and bedside report, but did not demonstrate understanding of patient condition and pathophysiological processes		
Identified correct destination, but provided inadequate radio and bedside report	*	
Identified inappropriate destination or provided no radio or bedside report	*	
Student exhibits competence with skill		

Any items that are marked with an * indicate the student needs to improve and a check mark should be placed in the right-hand column. A check mark in the right-hand column indicates that the student was unsuccessful and must attempt the skill again to assure competency. Examiners should use a different-color ink for the second attempt.

☐ Successful   ☐ Unsuccessful   Examiner Initials: _____

©2006 Prentice-Hall Inc.

Patient Assessment: Medical—Diabetic

Student: _____   Examiner: _____

Date: _____   Scenario: _____

	Done ✓	Not Done
Assesses scene safety and utilizes appropriate PPE		*
OVERALL SCENE EVALUATION		
Medical—determines nature of illness/if trauma involved determines MOI		*
Determines the number of patients, location, obstacles, and requests any additional resources as needed		
Verbalizes general impression of the patient as approaches		*
Considers stabilization/spinal motion restriction of spine if trauma involved		*
INITIAL ASSESSMENT		
Determines responsiveness/level of consciousness/AVPU		*
Opens airway with appropriate technique and assesses airway/ventilation		*
Manages airway/ventilation and applies appropriate oxygen therapy in less than 3 minutes		*
Assesses circulation: radial/carotid pulse, skin color, temperature, condition, and turgor		*
Controls any major bleeding		*
Makes rapid transport decision if indicated		
Initiates IV, **obtains BGL,** GCS, and complete vital signs		*
FOCUSED HISTORY AND PHYSICAL EXAMINATION/RAPID ASSESSMENT		
Obtains SAMPLE history		
Obtains OPQRST for differential diagnosis		
Obtains associated symptoms, pertinent negatives/denials		
Evaluates decision to perform focused exam or completes rapid assessment		*
Vital signs including AVPU (and GCS if trauma)		*
Assesses cardiovascular system including heart sounds, peripheral edema, and peripheral perfusion		*
Assesses pulmonary system including reassessing airway, ventilation, breath sounds, pulse oximetry, chest wall excursion, accessory muscle use, or other signs of distress		*
Assesses neurological system including speech, droop, drift, if applicable, and distal movement and sensation		*
Assesses musculoskeletal and integumentary systems		
Assesses behavioral, psychological, and social aspects of patient and situation		
States field impression of patient—insulin shock or diabetic ketoacidosis		*
Verbalizes treatment plan for patient and calls for appropriate intervention(s)—IVs, glucose, fluids, may need to include cardiac monitor due to potential for "silent" MI, etc.		*
Reevaluates transport decision		
ONGOING ASSESSMENT		
Repeats initial assessment		*
Repeats vital signs and evaluates trends		*
Evaluates response to treatments		*
Repeats focused assessment regarding patient complaint or injuries		
Gives radio report to receiving facility		
Turns over patient care with verbal report		*
Student exhibits competence with skill		

Any items in the Not Done column that are marked with an * are mandatory for the student to complete. A check mark in the Not Done column of an item with an * indicates that the student was unsuccessful and must attempt the skill again to assure competency. Examiners should use a different-color ink for the second attempt.

☐ Successful   ☐ Unsuccessful   Examiner Initials: _____

©2006 Prentice-Hall Inc.

Scenario Intubation—Diabetic

Student: _____   **Examiner:** _____

Date: _____

	Done ✓	Not Done
Assesses scene safety and utilizes appropriate PPE		*
Manually opens the airway with technique appropriate for patient condition		*
Checks mouth for blood or potential airway obstruction		*
Suctions or removes loose teeth or foreign materials as needed		
Inserts simple adjunct (oropharyngeal or nasopharyngeal airway)		
Directs assistant to ventilate patient with bag-valve-mask device (room air)		*
Observes chest rise/fall and auscultates bilaterally over lungs for baseline		*
Obtains effective ventilation in less than 30 seconds		*
Attaches oxygen reservoir to bag-valve-mask device and connects to high-flow oxygen		
Ventilates patient and evaluates chest wall/lung compliance		*
Directs assistant to preoxygenate patient		*
Identifies/selects proper equipment for intubation		
Checks laryngoscope light and cuff of ET tube		
Removes all air from cuff and properly inserts stylet if used		
Removes airway adjunct		
Positions patient's head properly and has assistant perform Sellick's maneuver		*
Opens mouth and gently inserts blade while sweeping tongue to side		*
Has assistant maintain Sellick's pressure		
Gently elevates mandible with laryngoscope and visualizes cords		*
Introduces ET tube to side of blade and visualizes tube passing through cords		*
"Threads" ET tube off stylet (if used), maintaining hold on ET tube as stylet removed		
Inflates cuff to proper pressure and disconnects syringe		*
Disconnects mask from bag-valve device and attaches to ET tube without releasing ET tube		
Directs ventilation of patient while maintaining Sellick's maneuver and holding ET tube in place		
Confirms proper placement by auscultation over epigastrium and bilaterally over each lung		*
Directs assistant to release cricoid pressure		*
Secures ET tube		*
Reassesses bilateral lung sounds and compliance		*
Uses secondary device to confirm tube placement		*
Assesses patient's response to intervention		*
Student exhibits competence with skill		

Any items in the Not Done column that are marked with an * are mandatory for the student to complete. A check mark in the Not Done column of an item with an * indicates that the student was unsuccessful and must attempt the skill again to assure competency. Examiners should use a different-color ink for the second attempt.

☐ Successful   ☐ Unsuccessful   Examiner Initials: _____

©2006 Prentice-Hall Inc.

Scenario IV Insertion—Diabetic

Student: _____   **Examiner:** _____

Date: _____

	Done ✓	Not Done
Selects appropriate IV fluid, checking clarity, color, and expiration date		*
Selects appropriate catheter		
Selects appropriate administration set		
Properly inserts IV tubing into the IV bag		*
Prepares administration set (fills drip chamber and flushes tubing)		*
Cuts or tears tape (at any time before venipuncture)		*
Applies constricting band (checks distal pulse to assure NOT a tourniquet)		*
Palpates suitable vein		*
Cleanses site appropriately		*
Utilizes appropriate PPE		*
Inserts catheter with sterile technique		*
Verbalizes flash/blood return and advances catheter slightly farther		*
Occludes vein with finger at distal end of catheter and removes stylet		
Immediately disposes (or verbalizes disposal) of needle/sharp in proper container		
Obtains blood sample or connects IV tubing to catheter		
Obtains BGL (blood glucose level)		*
Releases constricting band		*
Runs IV for a brief period to ensure patency and adjusts flow rate as appropriate		*
Checks IV site for signs of infiltration		*
Secures catheter (tapes securely or verbalizes)		*
Attaches label with size of catheter, date, time, and "prehospital"		*
Assesses patient's response to intervention		*
Student exhibits competence with skill		

Any items in the Not Done column that are marked with an * are mandatory for the student to complete. A check mark in the Not Done column of an item with an * indicates that the student was unsuccessful and must attempt the skill again to assure competency. Examiners should use a different-color ink for the second attempt.

☐ Successful   ☐ Unsuccessful   Examiner Initials: _____

©2006 Prentice-Hall Inc.

Scenario Radio Report—Diabetic

Student: _____   **Examiner:** _____

Date: _____

	Done ✓	Not Done
Requests and checks for open channel before speaking		
Presses transmit button 1 second before speaking		
Holds microphone 2–3 in. from mouth		
Speaks slowly and clearly		*
Speaks in a normal voice		
Briefly transmits: Agency, unit designation, identification/name		*
Briefly transmits: Patient's age, sex, weight		*
Briefly transmits: Scene description/mechanism of injury or medical problem		*
Briefly transmits: Chief complaint with brief history of *present* illness		*
Briefly transmits: Associated symptoms (unless able to be deferred to bedside report)		
Briefly transmits: Past medical history (usually deferred to bedside report)		
Briefly transmits: Vital signs		*
Briefly transmits: Level of consciousness/GCS on trauma		*
Briefly transmits: General appearance, distress, cardiac rhythm, blood glucose, and other pertinent findings unable to be deferred to bedside report		
Briefly transmits: Interventions by EMS AND response(s)		*
ETA (the more critical the patient, the earlier you need to notify the receiving facility)		
Does not waste airtime		
Protects privacy of patient		*
Echoes dispatch information and any physician orders		*
Writes down dispatch information or physician orders		
Confirms with facility that message is received		
Demonstrates/verbalizes ability to troubleshoot basic equipment malfunction		
Student exhibits competence with skill		

Any items in the Not Done column that are marked with an * are mandatory for the student to complete. A check mark in the Not Done column of an item with an * indicates that the student was unsuccessful and must attempt the skill again to assure competency. Examiners should use a different-color ink for the second attempt.

☐ Successful   ☐ Unsuccessful   Examiner Initials:_____

©2006 Prentice-Hall Inc.

Scenario Patient Care Report (PCR)—Diabetic

Student: _____   Examiner:_____

Date: _____

	Done ✓	Not Done
Records all pertinent dispatch/scene data, using a consistent format		
Completely identifies all additional resources and personnel		
Documents chief complaint, signs/symptoms, position found, age, sex, and weight		
Identifies and records all pertinent, reportable clinical data for each patient		
Documents SAMPLE and OPQRST if applicable		
Records all pertinent negatives		
Records all pertinent denials		
Records accurate consistent times and patient information		
Includes relevant oral statements of witnesses, bystanders, and patient in "quotes" when appropriate		
Documents initial assessment findings: airway, breathing, and circulation		
Documents any interventions in initial assessment with patient response		
Documents level of consciousness, GCS (if trauma), and VS		
Documents rapid trauma assessment if applicable		
Documents any interventions in rapid trauma assessment with patient response		
Documents focused history and physical assessment		
Documents any interventions in focused assessment with patient response		
Documents repeat VS (every 5 minutes for critical; every 15 minutes for stable)		
Repeats initial assessment and documents findings		
Records ALL treatments with times and patient response(s) in treatment section		
Documents field impression		
Documents transport to specific facility and transfer of care WITH VERBAL REPORT		
Uses correct grammar, abbreviations, spelling, and terminology		
Writes legibly		
Thoroughly documents refusals, denials of transport, and call cancellations		
Documents patient GCS of 15 PRIOR to signing refusal		
Documents advice given to refusal patient, including "call 9-1-1 for further problems"		
Properly corrects errors and omissions		
Writes cautiously, avoids jargon, opinions, inferences, or any derogatory/libelous remarks		
Signs run report		
Uses EMS supplement form if needed		
Student exhibits competence with skill		

Any items in the Not Done column should be evaluated with student. Check marks in this column do not necessarily mean student was unsuccessful as all lines are not completed on all patients. Evaluation of each PCR should be based on the scenario given.

Student must be able to write an EMS report with consistency and accuracy.

☐ Successful   ☐ Unsuccessful   Examiner Initials: _____

©2006 Prentice-Hall Inc.

Overall Scenario Management—Diabetic

Student: _____   Examiner: _____

Date: _____   Scenario: _____

NOTE: This skill sheet is to be done after the student completes a scenario as the TEAM LEADER. It is to let the student know if he or she is beginning to "put it all together" and use critical thinking skills to manage an EMS call. PLEASE notice that it is graded on a different basis than the basic lab skill sheet.

	Done ✓	Needs to Improve
SCENE MANAGEMENT		
Recognized hazards and controlled scene—safety, crowd, and patient issues		
Recognized hazards, but did not control the scene		
Unsuccessfully attempted to manage the scene	*	
Did not evaluate the scene and took no control of the scene	*	
PATIENT ASSESSMENT		
Performed a timely, organized complete patient assessment		
Performed complete initial, focused, and ongoing assessments, but in a disorganized manner		
Performed an incomplete assessment	*	
Did not perform an initial assessment	*	
PATIENT MANAGEMENT		
Evaluated assessment findings to manage all aspects of patient condition		
Managed the patient's presenting signs and symptoms without considering all of assessment		
Inadequately managed the patient	*	
Did not manage life-threatening conditions	*	
COMMUNICATION		
Communicated well with crew, patient, family, bystanders, and assisting agencies		
Communicated well with patient and crew		
Communicated with patient and crew, but poor communication skills	*	
Unable to communicate effectively	*	
REPORT AND TRANSFER OF CARE		
Identified correct destination for patient transport, gave accurate, brief report over radio, and provided full report at bedside demonstrating thorough understanding of patient condition and pathophysiological processes		
Identified correct destination and gave accurate radio and bedside report, but did not demonstrate understanding of patient condition and pathophysiological processes		
Identified correct destination, but provided inadequate radio and bedside report	*	
Identified inappropriate destination or provided no radio or bedside report	*	
Student exhibits competence with skill		

Any items that are marked with an * indicate the student needs to improve and a check mark should be placed in the right-hand column. A check mark in the right-hand column indicates that the student was unsuccessful and must attempt the skill again to assure competency. Examiners should use a different-color ink for the second attempt.

☐ Successful   ☐ Unsuccessful   Examiner Initials: _____

©2006 Prentice-Hall Inc.

Patient Assessment: Medical—Environmental/Thermal

Student: _____   Examiner: _____

Date: _____   Scenario: _____

	Done ✓	Not Done
Assesses scene safety and utilizes appropriate PPE		*
OVERALL SCENE EVALUATION		
Medical—determines nature of illness/if trauma involved determines MOI		*
Determines the number of patients, location, obstacles, and requests any additional resources as needed		
Verbalizes general impression of the patient as approaches		*
Considers stabilization/spinal motion restriction of spine if trauma involved		*
INITIAL ASSESSMENT		
Determines responsiveness/level of consciousness/AVPU		*
Opens airway with appropriate technique and assesses airway/ventilation		*
Manages airway/ventilation and applies appropriate oxygen therapy in less than 3 minutes		*
Assesses circulation: radial/carotid pulse, skin color, temperature, condition, and turgor		*
Controls any major bleeding		*
Makes rapid transport decision if indicated		
Initiates IV, obtains BGL, GCS, and complete vital signs		
FOCUSED HISTORY AND PHYSICAL EXAMINATION/RAPID ASSESSMENT		
Obtains SAMPLE history		
Obtains OPQRST for differential diagnosis		
Obtains associated symptoms, pertinent negatives/denials		
Evaluates decision to perform focused exam or completes rapid assessment		*
Vital signs including AVPU (and GCS if trauma)		*
Assesses cardiovascular system including heart sounds, peripheral edema, and peripheral perfusion		*
Assesses pulmonary system including reassessing airway, ventilation, breath sounds, pulse oximetry, chest wall excursion, accessory muscle use, or other signs of distress		*
Assesses neurological system including speech, droop, drift, if applicable, and distal movement and sensation		*
Assesses musculoskeletal and integumentary systems		
Assesses behavioral, psychological, and social aspects of patient and situation		
States field impression of patient—environmental and/or thermal emergency (specifies injury/illness suspected)		*
Verbalizes treatment plan for patient and calls for appropriate intervention(s)—IVs, specific treatments		*
Reevaluates transport decision		
ONGOING ASSESSMENT		
Repeats initial assessment		*
Repeats vital signs and evaluates trends		*
Evaluates response to treatments		*
Repeats focused assessment regarding patient complaint or injuries		
Gives radio report to receiving facility		
Turns over patient care with verbal report		*
Student exhibits competence with skill		

Any items in the Not Done column that are marked with an * are mandatory for the student to complete. A check mark in the Not Done column of an item with an * indicates that the student was unsuccessful and must attempt the skill again to assure competency. Examiners should use a different-color ink for the second attempt.

☐ Successful   ☐ Unsuccessful   Examiner Initials: _____

©2006 Prentice-Hall Inc.

Scenario Intubation—Environmental / Thermal

Student: _____   **Examiner:** _____

Date: _____

	Done ✓	Not Done
Assesses scene safety and utilizes appropriate PPE		*
Manually opens the airway with technique appropriate for patient condition		*
Checks mouth for blood or potential airway obstruction		*
Suctions or removes loose teeth or foreign materials as needed		
Inserts simple adjunct (oropharyngeal or nasopharyngeal airway)		
Directs assistant to ventilate patient with bag-valve-mask device (room air)		*
Observes chest rise/fall and auscultates bilaterally over lungs for baseline		*
Obtains effective ventilation in less than 30 seconds		*
Attaches oxygen reservoir to bag-valve-mask device and connects to high-flow oxygen		
Ventilates patient and evaluates chest wall/lung compliance		*
Directs assistant to preoxygenate patient		*
Identifies/selects proper equipment for intubation		
Checks laryngoscope light and cuff of ET tube		
Removes all air from cuff and properly inserts stylet if used		
Removes airway adjunct		
Positions patient's head properly and has assistant perform Sellick's maneuver		*
Opens mouth and gently inserts blade while sweeping tongue to side		*
Has assistant maintain Sellick's pressure		
Gently elevates mandible with laryngoscope and visualizes cords		*
Introduces ET tube to side of blade and visualizes tube passing through cords		*
"Threads" ET tube off stylet (if used), maintaining hold on ET tube as stylet removed		
Inflates cuff to proper pressure and disconnects syringe		*
Disconnects mask from bag-valve device and attaches to ET tube without releasing ET tube		
Directs ventilation of patient while maintaining Sellick's maneuver and holding ET tube in place		
Confirms proper placement by auscultation over epigastrium and bilaterally over each lung		*
Directs assistant to release cricoid pressure		*
Secures ET tube		*
Reassesses bilateral lung sounds and compliance		*
Uses secondary device to confirm tube placement		*
Assesses patient's response to intervention		*
Student exhibits competence with skill		

Any items in the Not Done column that are marked with an * are mandatory for the student to complete. A check mark in the Not Done column of an item with an * indicates that the student was unsuccessful and must attempt the skill again to assure competency. Examiners should use a different-color ink for the second attempt.

☐ Successful   ☐ Unsuccessful   Examiner Initials: _____

©2006 Prentice-Hall Inc.

Scenario IV Insertion—Environmental/Thermal

Student: _____   **Examiner:** _____

Date: _____

	Done ✓	Not Done
Selects appropriate IV fluid, checking clarity, color, and expiration date		*
Selects appropriate catheter		
Selects appropriate administration set		
Properly inserts IV tubing into the IV bag		*
Prepares administration set (fills drip chamber and flushes tubing)		*
Cuts or tears tape (at any time before venipuncture)		*
Applies constricting band (checks distal pulse to assure NOT a tourniquet)		*
Palpates suitable vein		*
Cleanses site appropriately		*
Utilizes appropriate PPE		*
Inserts catheter with sterile technique		*
Verbalizes flash/blood return and advances catheter slightly farther		*
Occludes vein with finger at distal end of catheter and removes stylet		
Immediately disposes (or verbalizes disposal) of needle/sharp in proper container		
Obtains blood sample or connects IV tubing to catheter		
Obtains BGL (blood glucose level)		*
Releases constricting band		*
Runs IV for a brief period to ensure patency and adjusts flow rate as appropriate		*
Checks IV site for signs of infiltration		*
Secures catheter (tapes securely or verbalizes)		*
Attaches label with size of catheter, date, time, and "prehospital"		*
Assesses patient's response to intervention		*
Student exhibits competence with skill		

Any items in the Not Done column that are marked with an * are mandatory for the student to complete. A check mark in the Not Done column of an item with an * indicates that the student was unsuccessful and must attempt the skill again to assure competency. Examiners should use a different-color ink for the second attempt.

☐ Successful   ☐ Unsuccessful   Examiner Initials: _____

©2006 Prentice-Hall Inc.

Scenario Radio Report—Environmental/Thermal

Student: _____   **Examiner:** _____

Date: _____

	Done ✓	Not Done
Requests and checks for open channel before speaking		
Presses transmit button 1 second before speaking		
Holds microphone 2–3 in. from mouth		
Speaks slowly and clearly		*
Speaks in a normal voice		
Briefly transmits: Agency, unit designation, identification/name		*
Briefly transmits: Patient's age, sex, weight		*
Briefly transmits: Scene description/mechanism of injury or medical problem		*
Briefly transmits: Chief complaint with brief history of *present* illness		*
Briefly transmits: Associated symptoms (unless able to be deferred to bedside report)		
Briefly transmits: Past medical history (usually deferred to bedside report)		
Briefly transmits: Vital signs		*
Briefly transmits: Level of consciousness/GCS on trauma		*
Briefly transmits: General appearance, distress, cardiac rhythm, blood glucose, and other pertinent findings unable to be deferred to bedside report		
Briefly transmits: Interventions by EMS AND response(s)		*
ETA (the more critical the patient, the earlier you need to notify the receiving facility)		
Does not waste airtime		
Protects privacy of patient		*
Echoes dispatch information and any physician orders		*
Writes down dispatch information or physician orders		
Confirms with facility that message is received		
Demonstrates/verbalizes ability to troubleshoot basic equipment malfunction		
Student exhibits competence with skill		

Any items in the Not Done column that are marked with an * are mandatory for the student to complete. A check mark in the Not Done column of an item with an * indicates that the student was unsuccessful and must attempt the skill again to assure competency. Examiners should use a different-color ink for the second attempt.

☐ Successful   ☐ Unsuccessful   Examiner Initials: _____

©2006 Prentice-Hall Inc.

Scenario Patient Care Report (PCR)—Environmental/Thermal

Student: _____   Examiner: _____

Date: _____

	Done ✓	Not Done
Records all pertinent dispatch/scene data, using a consistent format		
Completely identifies all additional resources and personnel		
Documents chief complaint, signs/symptoms, position found, age, sex, and weight		
Identifies and records all pertinent, reportable clinical data for each patient		
Documents SAMPLE and OPQRST if applicable		
Records all pertinent negatives		
Records all pertinent denials		
Records accurate, consistent times and patient information		
Includes relevant oral statements of witnesses, bystanders, and patient in "quotes" when appropriate		
Documents initial assessment findings: airway, breathing, and circulation		
Documents any interventions in initial assessment with patient response		
Documents level of consciousness, GCS (if trauma), and VS		
Documents rapid trauma assessment if applicable		
Documents any interventions in rapid trauma assessment with patient response		
Documents focused history and physical assessment		
Documents any interventions in focused assessment with patient response		
Documents repeat VS (every 5 minutes for critical; every 15 minutes for stable)		
Repeats initial assessment and documents findings		
Records ALL treatments with times and patient response(s) in treatment section		
Documents field impression		
Documents transport to specific facility and transfer of care WITH VERBAL REPORT		
Uses correct grammar, abbreviations, spelling, and terminology		
Writes legibly		
Thoroughly documents refusals, denials of transport, and call cancellations		
Documents patient GCS of 15 PRIOR to signing refusal		
Documents advice given to refusal patient, including "call 9-1-1 for further problems"		
Properly corrects errors and omissions		
Writes cautiously, avoids jargon, opinions, inferences, or any derogatory/libelous remarks		
Signs run report		
Uses EMS supplement form if needed		
Student exhibits competence with skill		

Any items in the Not Done column should be evaluated with student. Check marks in this column do not necessarily mean student was unsuccessful as all lines are not completed on all patients. Evaluation of each PCR should be based on the scenario given.

Student must be able to write an EMS report with consistency and accuracy.

☐ Successful   ☐ Unsuccessful   Examiner Initials: _____

©2006 Prentice-Hall Inc.

Overall Scenario Management—Environmental/Thermal

Student: _____   Examiner: _____

Date: _____   Scenario: _____

NOTE: This skill sheet is to be done after the student completes a scenario as the TEAM LEADER. It is to let the student know if he or she is beginning to "put it all together" and use critical thinking skills to manage an EMS call. PLEASE notice that it is graded on a different basis than the basic lab skill sheet.

	Done ✓	Needs to Improve
SCENE MANAGEMENT		
Recognized hazards and controlled scene—safety, crowd, and patient issues		
Recognized hazards, but did not control the scene		
Unsuccessfully attempted to manage the scene	*	
Did not evaluate the scene and took no control of the scene	*	
PATIENT ASSESSMENT		
Performed a timely, organized complete patient assessment		
Performed complete initial, focused, and ongoing assessments, but in a disorganized manner		
Performed an incomplete assessment	*	
Did not perform an initial assessment	*	
PATIENT MANAGEMENT		
Evaluated assessment findings to manage all aspects of patient condition		
Managed the patient's presenting signs and symptoms without considering all of assessment		
Inadequately managed the patient	*	
Did not manage life-threatening conditions	*	
COMMUNICATION		
Communicated well with crew, patient, family, bystanders, and assisting agencies		
Communicated well with patient and crew		
Communicated with patient and crew, but poor communication skills	*	
Unable to communicate effectively	*	
REPORT AND TRANSFER OF CARE		
Identified correct destination for patient transport, gave accurate, brief report over radio, and provided full report at bedside demonstrating thorough understanding of patient condition and pathophysiological processes		
Identified correct destination and gave accurate radio and bedside report, but did not demonstrate understanding of patient condition and pathophysiological processes		
Identified correct destination, but provided inadequate radio and bedside report	*	
Identified inappropriate destination or provided no radio or bedside report	*	
Student exhibits competence with skill		

Any items that are marked with an * indicate the student needs to improve and a check mark should be placed in the right-hand column. A check mark in the right-hand column indicates that the student was unsuccessful and must attempt the skill again to assure competency. Examiners should use a different-color ink for the second attempt.

☐ Successful   ☐ Unsuccessful   Examiner Initials: _____

©2006 Prentice-Hall Inc.

Patient Assessment: Medical—GI Bleeding

Student: _____   **Examiner:** _____

Date: _____   **Scenario:** _____

	Done ✓	Not Done
Assesses scene safety and utilizes appropriate PPE		*
OVERALL SCENE EVALUATION		
Medical—determines nature of illness/if trauma involved determines MOI		*
Determines the number of patients, location, obstacles, and requests any additional resources as needed		
Verbalizes general impression of the patient as approaches		*
Considers stabilization/spinal motion restriction of spine if trauma involved		*
INITIAL ASSESSMENT		
Determines responsiveness/level of consciousness/AVPU		*
Opens airway with appropriate technique and assesses airway/ventilation		*
Manages airway/ventilation and applies appropriate oxygen therapy in less than 3 minutes		*
Assesses circulation: radial/carotid pulse, skin color, temperature, condition, and turgor		*
Controls any major bleeding		*
Makes rapid transport decision if indicated		
Initiates IV (2 if indicated), obtains BGL, GCS, and complete vital signs		
FOCUSED HISTORY AND PHYSICAL EXAMINATION/RAPID ASSESSMENT		
Obtains SAMPLE history		
Obtains OPQRST for differential diagnosis—able to identify upper or lower GI bleed/probable point of origin		*
Obtains associated symptoms, pertinent negatives/denials		
Evaluates decision to perform focused exam or completes rapid assessment		*
Vital signs including AVPU (and GCS if trauma)		*
Assesses cardiovascular system including heart sounds, peripheral edema, and peripheral perfusion		*
Assesses pulmonary system including reassessing airway, ventilation, breath sounds, pulse oximetry, chest wall excursion, accessory muscle use, or other signs of distress		*
Assesses neurological system including speech, droop, drift, if applicable, and distal movement and sensation		*
Assesses musculoskeletal and integumentary systems		
Assesses behavioral, psychological, and social aspects of patient and situation		
States field impression of patient—GI bleed (states above or below Ligament of Treitz)		*
Verbalizes treatment plan for patient and calls for appropriate intervention(s)—IVs, fluids		*
Reevaluates transport decision		
ONGOING ASSESSMENT		
Repeats initial assessment		*
Repeats vital signs and evaluates trends		*
Evaluates response to treatments		*
Repeats focused assessment regarding patient complaint or injuries		
Gives radio report to receiving facility		
Turns over patient care with verbal report		*
Student exhibits competence with skill		

Any items in the Not Done column that are marked with an * are mandatory for the student to complete. A check mark in the Not Done column of an item with an * indicates that the student was unsuccessful and must attempt the skill again to assure competency. Examiners should use a different-color ink for the second attempt.

☐ Successful   ☐ Unsuccessful   Examiner Initials: _____

©2006 Prentice-Hall Inc.

Scenario IV Insertion—GI Bleeding

Student: _____   **Examiner:** _____

Date: _____

	Done ✓	Not Done
Selects appropriate IV fluid, checking clarity, color, and expiration date		*
Selects appropriate catheter		
Selects appropriate administration set		
Properly inserts IV tubing into the IV bag		*
Prepares administration set (fills drip chamber and flushes tubing)		*
Cuts or tears tape (at any time before venipuncture)		*
Applies constricting band (checks distal pulse to assure NOT a tourniquet)		*
Palpates suitable vein		*
Cleanses site appropriately		*
Utilizes appropriate PPE		*
Inserts catheter with sterile technique		*
Verbalizes flash/blood return and advances catheter slightly farther		*
Occludes vein with finger at distal end of catheter and removes stylet		
Immediately disposes (or verbalizes disposal) of needle/sharp in proper container		
Obtains blood sample or connects IV tubing to catheter		
Obtains BGL (blood glucose level)		*
Releases constricting band		*
Runs IV for a brief period to ensure patency and adjusts flow rate as appropriate		*
Checks IV site for signs of infiltration		*
Secures catheter (tapes securely or verbalizes)		*
Attaches label with size of catheter, date, time, and "prehospital"		*
Assesses patient's response to intervention		*
Student exhibits competence with skill		

Any items in the Not Done column that are marked with an * are mandatory for the student to complete. A check mark in the Not Done column of an item with an * indicates that the student was unsuccessful and must attempt the skill again to assure competency. Examiners should use a different-color ink for the second attempt.

☐ Successful   ☐ Unsuccessful   Examiner Initials: _____

Scenario Radio Report—GI Bleeding

Student: _____   **Examiner:** _____

Date: _____

	Done ✓	Not Done
Requests and checks for open channel before speaking		
Presses transmit button 1 second before speaking		
Holds microphone 2–3 in. from mouth		
Speaks slowly and clearly		*
Speaks in a normal voice		
Briefly transmits: Agency, unit designation, identification/name		*
Briefly transmits: Patient's age, sex, weight		*
Briefly transmits: Scene description/mechanism of injury or medical problem		*
Briefly transmits: Chief complaint with brief history of *present* illness		*
Briefly transmits: Associated symptoms (unless able to be deferred to bedside report)		
Briefly transmits: Past medical history (usually deferred to bedside report)		
Briefly transmits: Vital signs		*
Briefly transmits: Level of consciousness/GCS on trauma		*
Briefly transmits: General appearance, distress, cardiac rhythm, blood glucose, and other pertinent findings unable to be deferred to bedside report		
Briefly transmits: Interventions by EMS AND response(s)		*
ETA (the more critical the patient, the earlier you need to notify the receiving facility)		
Does not waste airtime		
Protects privacy of patient		*
Echoes dispatch information and any physician orders		*
Writes down dispatch information or physician orders		
Confirms with facility that message is received		
Demonstrates/verbalizes ability to troubleshoot basic equipment malfunction		
Student exhibits competence with skill		

Any items in the Not Done column that are marked with an * are mandatory for the student to complete. A check mark in the Not Done column of an item with an * indicates that the student was unsuccessful and must attempt the skill again to assure competency. Examiners should use a different-color ink for the second attempt.

☐ Successful   ☐ Unsuccessful   Examiner Initials: _____

©2006 Prentice-Hall Inc.

Overall Scenario Management—GI Bleeding

Student: _____   Examiner: _____

Date: _____   Scenario: _____

NOTE: This skill sheet is to be done after the student completes a scenario as the TEAM LEADER. It is to let the student know if he or she is beginning to "put it all together" and use critical thinking skills to manage an EMS call. PLEASE notice that it is graded on a different basis than the basic lab skill sheet.

	Done ✓	Needs to Improve
SCENE MANAGEMENT		
Recognized hazards and controlled scene—safety, crowd, and patient issues		
Recognized hazards, but did not control the scene		
Unsuccessfully attempted to manage the scene	*	
Did not evaluate the scene and took no control of the scene	*	
PATIENT ASSESSMENT		
Performed a timely, organized complete patient assessment		
Performed complete initial, focused, and ongoing assessments, but in a disorganized manner		
Performed an incomplete assessment	*	
Did not perform an initial assessment	*	
PATIENT MANAGEMENT		
Evaluated assessment findings to manage all aspects of patient condition		
Managed the patient's presenting signs and symptoms without considering all of assessment		
Inadequately managed the patient	*	
Did not manage life-threatening conditions	*	
COMMUNICATION		
Communicated well with crew, patient, family, bystanders, and assisting agencies		
Communicated well with patient and crew		
Communicated with patient and crew, but poor communication skills	*	
Unable to communicate effectively	*	
REPORT AND TRANSFER OF CARE		
Identified correct destination for patient transport, gave accurate, brief report over radio, and provided full report at bedside demonstrating thorough understanding of patient condition and pathophysiological processes		
Identified correct destination and gave accurate radio and bedside report, but did not demonstrate understanding of patient condition and pathophysiological processes		
Identified correct destination, but provided inadequate radio and bedside report	*	
Identified inappropriate destination or provided no radio or bedside report	*	
Student exhibits competence with skill		

Any items that are marked with an * indicate the student needs to improve and a check mark should be placed in the right-hand column. A check mark in the right-hand column indicates that the student was unsuccessful and must attempt the skill again to assure competency. Examiners should use a different-color ink for the second attempt.

☐ Successful   ☐ Unsuccessful   Examiner Initials: _____

©2006 Prentice-Hall Inc.

Patient Assessment: Medical—Seizure

Student: _____   Examiner: _____

Date: _____   Scenario: _____

	Done ✓	Not Done *
Assesses scene safety and utilizes appropriate PPE		*
OVERALL SCENE EVALUATION		
Medical—determines nature of illness/if trauma involved determines MOI		*
Determines the number of patients, location, obstacles, and requests any additional resources as needed		
Verbalizes general impression of the patient as approaches		*
Considers stabilization/spinal motion restriction of spine if trauma involved		*
INITIAL ASSESSMENT		
Determines responsiveness/level of consciousness/AVPU		*
Opens airway with appropriate technique and assesses airway/ventilation		*
Manages airway/ventilation and applies appropriate oxygen therapy in less than 3 minutes		*
Assesses circulation: radial/carotid pulse, skin color, temperature, condition, and turgor		*
Controls any major bleeding		*
Makes rapid transport decision if indicated		
Clears surrounding area and protects actively seizing patient from furthur harm.		
Initiates IV, **obtains BGL,** GCS, and complete vital signs		*
FOCUSED HISTORY AND PHYSICAL EXAMINATION/RAPID ASSESSMENT		
Obtains SAMPLE history		
Obtains OPQRST for differential diagnosis		
Obtains associated symptoms, pertinent negatives/denials		
Evaluates decision to perform focused exam or completes rapid assessment		*
Vital signs including AVPU (and GCS if trauma)		*
Assesses cardiovascular system including heart sounds, peripheral edema, and peripheral perfusion		*
Assesses pulmonary system including reassessing airway, ventilation, breath sounds, pulse oximetry, chest wall excursion, accessory muscle use, or other signs of distress		*
Assesses neurological system including speech, droop, drift, if applicable, and distal movement and sensation		*
Assesses musculoskeletal and integumentary systems		
Assesses behavioral, psychological, and social aspects of patient and situation		
States field impression of patient—seizure (states suspected differential diagnosis—cause)		*
Verbalizes treatment plan for patient and calls for appropriate intervention(s)—IV, Valium (IV or rectal), nasal Versed, Magnesium for eclampsia		*
Reevaluates transport decision		
ONGOING ASSESSMENT		
Repeats initial assessment		*
Repeats vital signs and evaluates trends		*
Evaluates response to treatments		*
Repeats focused assessment regarding patient complaint or injuries		
Gives radio report to receiving facility		
Turns over patient care with verbal report		*
Student exhibits competence with skill		

Any items in the Not Done column that are marked with an * are mandatory for the student to complete. A check mark in the Not Done column of an item with an * indicates that the student was unsuccessful and must attempt the skill again to assure competency. Examiners should use a different-color ink for the second attempt.

☐ Successful   ☐ Unsuccessful   Examiner Initials: _____

©2006 Prentice-Hall Inc.

Scenario Intubation—Seizure

Student: _____   **Examiner:** _____

Date: _____

	Done ✓	Not Done
Assesses scene safety and utilizes appropriate PPE		*
Manually opens the airway with technique appropriate for patient condition/may need RSI		*
Checks mouth for blood or potential airway obstruction		*
Suctions or removes loose teeth or foreign materials as needed		
Inserts simple adjunct (oropharyngeal or nasopharyngeal airway)		
Directs assistant to ventilate patient with bag-valve-mask device (room air)		*
Observes chest rise/fall and auscultates bilaterally over lungs for baseline		*
Obtains effective ventilation in less than 30 seconds		*
Attaches oxygen reservoir to bag-valve-mask device and connects to high-flow oxygen		
Ventilates patient and evaluates chest wall/lung compliance		*
Directs assistant to preoxygenate patient		*
Identifies/selects proper equipment for intubation		
Checks laryngoscope light and cuff of ET tube		
Removes all air from cuff and properly inserts stylet if used		
Removes airway adjunct		
Positions patient's head properly and has assistant perform Sellick's maneuver		*
Opens mouth and gently inserts blade while sweeping tongue to side		*
Has assistant maintain Sellick's pressure		
Gently elevates mandible with laryngoscope and visualizes cords		*
Introduces ET tube to side of blade and visualizes tube passing through cords		*
"Threads" ET tube off stylet (if used), maintaining hold on ET tube as stylet removed		
Inflates cuff to proper pressure and disconnects syringe		*
Disconnects mask from bag-valve device and attaches to ET tube without releasing ET tube		
Directs ventilation of patient while maintaining Sellick's maneuver and holding ET tube in place		
Confirms proper placement by auscultation over epigastrium and bilaterally over each lung		*
Directs assistant to release cricoid pressure		*
Secures ET tube		*
Reassesses bilateral lung sounds and compliance		*
Uses secondary device to confirm tube placement		*
Assesses patient's response to intervention		*
Student exhibits competence with skill		

Any items in the Not Done column that are marked with an * are mandatory for the student to complete. A check mark in the Not Done column of an item with an * indicates that the student was unsuccessful and must attempt the skill again to assure competency. Examiners should use a different-color ink for the second attempt.

☐ Successful   ☐ Unsuccessful   Examiner Initials: _____

©2006 Prentice-Hall Inc.

Scenario IV Insertion—Seizure

Student: _____   Examiner: _____

Date: _____

	Done ✓	Not Done
Selects appropriate IV fluid, checking clarity, color, and expiration date		*
Selects appropriate catheter		
Selects appropriate administration set		
Properly inserts IV tubing into the IV bag		*
Prepares administration set (fills drip chamber and flushes tubing)		*
Cuts or tears tape (at any time before venipuncture)		*
Applies constricting band (checks distal pulse to assure NOT a tourniquet)		*
Palpates suitable vein—does not use forceful restraint that may cause harm during seizure		*
Cleanses site appropriately		*
Utilizes appropriate PPE		*
Inserts catheter with sterile technique		*
Verbalizes flash/blood return and advances catheter slightly farther		*
Occludes vein with finger at distal end of catheter and removes stylet		
Immediately disposes (or verbalizes disposal) of needle/sharp in proper container		
Obtains blood sample or connects IV tubing to catheter		
Obtains BGL (blood glucose level)		*
Releases constricting band		*
Runs IV for a brief period to ensure patency and adjusts flow rate as appropriate		*
Checks IV site for signs of infiltration		*
Secures catheter (tapes securely or verbalizes)		*
Attaches label with size of catheter, date, time, and "prehospital"		*
Assesses patient's response to intervention		*
Student exhibits competence with skill		

Any items in the Not Done column that are marked with an * are mandatory for the student to complete. A check mark in the Not Done column of an item with an * indicates that the student was unsuccessful and must attempt the skill again to assure competency. Examiners should use a different-color ink for the second attempt.

☐ Successful   ☐ Unsuccessful   Examiner Initials: _____

©2006 Prentice-Hall Inc.

Scenario Radio Report—Seizure

Student: _____   Examiner: _____

Date: _____

	Done ✓	Not Done
Requests and checks for open channel before speaking		
Presses transmit button 1 second before speaking		
Holds microphone 2–3 in. from mouth		
Speaks slowly and clearly		*
Speaks in a normal voice		
Briefly transmits: Agency, unit designation, identification/name		*
Briefly transmits: Patient's age, sex, weight		*
Briefly transmits: Scene description/mechanism of injury or medical problem		*
Briefly transmits: Chief complaint with brief history of *present* illness		*
Briefly transmits: Associated symptoms (unless able to be deferred to bedside report)		
Briefly transmits: Past medical history (usually deferred to bedside report)		
Briefly transmits: Vital signs		*
Briefly transmits: Level of consciousness/GCS on trauma		*
Briefly transmits: General appearance, distress, cardiac rhythm, blood glucose, and other pertinent findings unable to be deferred to bedside report		
Briefly transmits: Interventions by EMS AND response(s)		*
ETA (the more critical the patient, the earlier you need to notify the receiving facility)		
Does not waste airtime		
Protects privacy of patient		*
Echoes dispatch information and any physician orders		*
Writes down dispatch information or physician orders		
Confirms with facility that message is received		
Demonstrates/verbalizes ability to troubleshoot basic equipment malfunction		
Student exhibits competence with skill		

Any items in the Not Done column that are marked with an * are mandatory for the student to complete. A check mark in the Not Done column of an item with an * indicates that the student was unsuccessful and must attempt the skill again to assure competency. Examiners should use a different-color ink for the second attempt.

☐ Successful   ☐ Unsuccessful   Examiner Initials: _____

Scenario Patient Care Report (PCR)—Seizure

Student: _____   Examiner:_____

Date: _____

	Done ✓	Not Done
Records all pertinent dispatch/scene data, using a consistent format		
Completely identifies all additional resources and personnel		
Documents chief complaint, signs/symptoms, position found, age, sex, and weight		
Identifies and records all pertinent, reportable clinical data for each patient		
Documents SAMPLE and OPQRST if applicable		
Records all pertinent negatives		
Records all pertinent denials		
Records accurate, consistent times and patient information		
Includes relevant oral statements of witnesses, bystanders, and patient in "quotes" when appropriate		
Documents initial assessment findings: airway, breathing, and circulation		
Documents any interventions in initial assessment with patient response		
Documents level of consciousness, GCS (if trauma), and VS		
Documents rapid trauma assessment if applicable		
Documents any interventions in rapid trauma assessment with patient response		
Documents focused history and physical assessment		
Documents any interventions in focused assessment with patient response		
Documents repeat VS (every 5 minutes for critical; every 15 minutes for stable)		
Repeats initial assessment and documents findings		
Records ALL treatments with times and patient response(s) in treatment section		
Documents field impression		
Documents transport to specific facility and transfer of care WITH VERBAL REPORT		
Uses correct grammar, abbreviations, spelling, and terminology		
Writes legibly		
Thoroughly documents refusals, denials of transport, and call cancellations		
Documents patient GCS of 15 PRIOR to signing refusal		
Documents advice given to refusal patient, including "call 9-1-1 for further problems"		
Properly corrects errors and omissions		
Writes cautiously, avoids jargon, opinions, inferences, or any derogatory/libelous remarks		
Signs run report		
Uses EMS supplement form if needed		
Student exhibits competence with skill		

Any items in the Not Done column should be evaluated with student. Check marks in this column do not necessarily mean student was unsuccessful as all lines are not completed on all patients. Evaluation of each PCR should be based on the scenario given.

Student must be able to write an EMS report with consistency and accuracy.

☐ Successful   ☐ Unsuccessful   Examiner Initials: _____

©2006 Prentice-Hall Inc.

Overall Scenario Management—Seizure

Student: _____   Examiner: _____

Date: _____   Scenario: _____

NOTE: This skill sheet is to be done after the student completes a scenario as the TEAM LEADER. It is to let the student know if he or she is beginning to "put it all together" and use critical thinking skills to manage an EMS call. PLEASE notice that it is graded on a different basis than the basic lab skill sheet.

	Done ✓	Needs to Improve
SCENE MANAGEMENT		
Recognized hazards and controlled scene—safety, crowd, and patient issues		
Recognized hazards, but did not control the scene		
Unsuccessfully attempted to manage the scene	*	
Did not evaluate the scene and took no control of the scene	*	
PATIENT ASSESSMENT		
Performed a timely, organized complete patient assessment		
Performed complete initial, focused, and ongoing assessments, but in a disorganized manner		
Performed an incomplete assessment	*	
Did not perform an initial assessment	*	
PATIENT MANAGEMENT		
Evaluated assessment findings to manage all aspects of patient condition		
Managed the patient's presenting signs and symptoms without considering all of assessment		
Inadequately managed the patient	*	
Did not manage life-threatening conditions	*	
COMMUNICATION		
Communicated well with crew, patient, family, bystanders, and assisting agencies		
Communicated well with patient and crew		
Communicated with patient and crew, but poor communication skills	*	
Unable to communicate effectively	*	
REPORT AND TRANSFER OF CARE		
Identified correct destination for patient transport, gave accurate, brief report over radio, and provided full report at bedside demonstrating thorough understanding of patient condition and pathophysiological processes		
Identified correct destination and gave accurate radio and bedside report, but did not demonstrate understanding of patient condition and pathophysiological processes		
Identified correct destination, but provided inadequate radio and bedside report	*	
Identified inappropriate destination or provided no radio or bedside report	*	
Student exhibits competence with skill		

Any items that are marked with an * indicate the student needs to improve and a check mark should be placed in the right-hand column. A check mark in the right-hand column indicates that the student was unsuccessful and must attempt the skill again to assure competency. Examiners should use a different-color ink for the second attempt.

☐ Successful   ☐ Unsuccessful   Examiner Initials: _____

©2006 Prentice-Hall Inc.

Patient Assessment: Medical—Toxicologic/Hazardous Material

Student: _____   Examiner: _____

Date: _____   Scenario: _____

	Done ✓	Not Done
Assesses scene safety and utilizes appropriate PPE—recognizes if potential hazardous material incident		*
OVERALL SCENE EVALUATION		
Medical—determines nature of illness/if trauma involved determines MOI		*
Determines the number of patients, location, obstacles, and requests any additional resources as needed		
Verbalizes general impression of the patient as approaches		*
Considers stabilization/spinal motion restriction of spine if trauma involved		*
INITIAL ASSESSMENT		
Determines responsiveness/level of consciousness/AVPU		*
Opens airway with appropriate technique and assesses airway/ventilation		*
Manages airway/ventilation and applies appropriate oxygen therapy in less than 3 minutes		*
Assesses circulation: radial/carotid pulse, skin color, temperature, condition, and turgor		*
Controls any major bleeding		*
Makes rapid transport decision if indicated		
Initiates IV, obtains BGL, GCS, and complete vital signs		
FOCUSED HISTORY AND PHYSICAL EXAMINATION/RAPID ASSESSMENT		
Obtains SAMPLE history		
Obtains OPQRST for differential diagnosis		
Obtains associated symptoms, pertinent negatives/denials		
Evaluates decision to perform focused exam or completes rapid assessment		*
Vital signs including AVPU (and GCS if trauma)		*
Assesses cardiovascular system including heart sounds, peripheral edema, and peripheral perfusion		*
Assesses pulmonary system including reassessing airway, ventilation, breath sounds, pulse oximetry, chest wall excursion, accessory muscle use, or other signs of distress		*
Assesses neurological system including speech, droop, drift, if applicable, and distal movement and sensation		*
Assesses musculoskeletal and integumentary systems		
Assesses behavioral, psychological, and social aspects of patient and situation		
States field impression of patient—toxicologic/hazardous material incident		*
Verbalizes treatment plan for patient and calls for appropriate intervention(s)—decontamination, specific antidotes		*
Reevaluates transport decision		
ONGOING ASSESSMENT		
Repeats initial assessment		*
Repeats vital signs and evaluates trends		*
Evaluates response to treatments		*
Repeats focused assessment regarding patient complaint or injuries		
Gives radio report to receiving facility		
Turns over patient care with verbal report		*
Student exhibits competence with skill		

Any items in the Not Done column that are marked with an * are mandatory for the student to complete. A check mark in the Not Done column of an item with an * indicates that the student was unsuccessful and must attempt the skill again to assure competency. Examiners should use a different-color ink for the second attempt.

☐ Successful   ☐ Unsuccessful   Examiner Initials: _____

©2006 Prentice-Hall Inc.

Scenario Intubation—Toxicologic/Hazardous Material

Student: _____   **Examiner:** _____

Date: _____

	Done ✓	Not Done
Assesses scene safety and utilizes appropriate PPE or decontamination procedure if needed		*
Manually opens the airway with technique appropriate for patient condition		*
Checks mouth for blood or potential airway obstruction		*
Suctions or removes loose teeth or foreign materials as needed		
Inserts simple adjunct (oropharyngeal or nasopharyngeal airway)		
Directs assistant to ventilate patient with bag-valve-mask device (room air)		*
Observes chest rise/fall and auscultates bilaterally over lungs for baseline		*
Obtains effective ventilation in less than 30 seconds		*
Attaches oxygen reservoir to bag-valve-mask device and connects to high-flow oxygen		
Ventilates patient and evaluates chest wall/lung compliance		*
Directs assistant to preoxygenate patient		*
Identifies/selects proper equipment for intubation		
Checks laryngoscope light and cuff of ET tube		
Removes all air from cuff and properly inserts stylet if used		
Removes airway adjunct		
Positions patient's head properly and has assistant perform Sellick's maneuver		*
Opens mouth and gently inserts blade while sweeping tongue to side		*
Has assistant maintain Sellick's pressure		
Gently elevates mandible with laryngoscope and visualizes cords		*
Introduces ET tube to side of blade and visualizes tube passing through cords		*
"Threads" ET tube off stylet (if used), maintaining hold on ET tube as stylet removed		
Inflates cuff to proper pressure and disconnects syringe		*
Disconnects mask from bag-valve device and attaches to ET tube without releasing ET tube		
Directs ventilation of patient while maintaining Sellick's maneuver and holding ET tube in place		
Confirms proper placement by auscultation over epigastrium and bilaterally over each lung		*
Directs assistant to release cricoid pressure		*
Secures ET tube		*
Reassesses bilateral lung sounds and compliance		*
Uses secondary device to confirm tube placement		*
Assesses patient's response to intervention		*
Student exhibits competence with skill		

Any items in the Not Done column that are marked with an * are mandatory for the student to complete. A check mark in the Not Done column of an item with an * indicates that the student was unsuccessful and must attempt the skill again to assure competency. Examiners should use a different-color ink for the second attempt.

☐ Successful   ☐ Unsuccessful   Examiner Initials: _____

©2006 Prentice-Hall Inc.

Scenario IV Insertion—Toxicologic/Hazardous Material

Student: _____   **Examiner:** _____

Date: _____

	Done ✓	Not Done
Selects appropriate IV fluid, checking clarity, color, and expiration date		*
Selects appropriate catheter		
Selects appropriate administration set		
Properly inserts IV tubing into the IV bag		*
Prepares administration set (fills drip chamber and flushes tubing)		*
Cuts or tears tape (at any time before venipuncture)		*
Applies constricting band (checks distal pulse to assure NOT a tourniquet)		*
Palpates suitable vein		*
Cleanses site appropriately		*
Utilizes appropriate PPE		*
Inserts catheter with sterile technique		*
Verbalizes flash/blood return and advances catheter slightly farther		*
Occludes vein with finger at distal end of catheter and removes stylet		
Immediately disposes (or verbalizes disposal) of needle/sharp in proper container		
Obtains blood sample or connects IV tubing to catheter		
Obtains BGL (blood glucose level)		*
Releases constricting band		*
Runs IV for a brief period to ensure patency and adjusts flow rate as appropriate		*
Checks IV site for signs of infiltration		*
Secures catheter (tapes securely or verbalizes)		*
Attaches label with size of catheter, date, time, and "prehospital"		*
Assesses patient's response to intervention		*
Student exhibits competence with skill		

Any items in the Not Done column that are marked with an * are mandatory for the student to complete. A check mark in the Not Done column of an item with an * indicates that the student was unsuccessful and must attempt the skill again to assure competency. Examiners should use a different-color ink for the second attempt.

☐ Successful   ☐ Unsuccessful   Examiner Initials: _____

©2006 Prentice-Hall Inc.

Scenario Radio Report—Toxicologic/Hazardous Material

Student: _____   **Examiner:** _____

Date: _____

	Done ✓	Not Done
Requests and checks for open channel before speaking		
Presses transmit button 1 second before speaking		
Holds microphone 2–3 in. from mouth		
Speaks slowly and clearly		*
Speaks in a normal voice		
Briefly transmits: Agency, unit designation, identification/name		*
Briefly transmits: Patient's age, sex, weight		*
Briefly transmits: Scene description/mechanism of injury or medical problem		*
Briefly transmits: Chief complaint with brief history of *present* illness		*
Briefly transmits: Associated symptoms (unless able to be deferred to bedside report)		
Briefly transmits: Past medical history (usually deferred to bedside report)		
Briefly transmits: Vital signs		*
Briefly transmits: Level of consciousness/GCS on trauma		*
Briefly transmits: General appearance, distress, cardiac rhythm, blood glucose, and other pertinent findings unable to be deferred to bedside report		
Briefly transmits: Interventions by EMS AND response(s)		*
ETA (the more critical the patient, the earlier you need to notify the receiving facility)		
Does not waste airtime		
Protects privacy of patient		*
Echoes dispatch information and any physician orders		*
Writes down dispatch information or physician orders		
Confirms with facility that message is received		
Demonstrates/verbalizes ability to troubleshoot basic equipment malfunction		
Student exhibits competence with skill		

Any items in the Not Done column that are marked with an * are mandatory for the student to complete. A check mark in the Not Done column of an item with an * indicates that the student was unsuccessful and must attempt the skill again to assure competency. Examiners should use a different-color ink for the second attempt.

☐ Successful   ☐ Unsuccessful   Examiner Initials: _____

©2006 Prentice-Hall Inc.

Scenario Patient Care Report (PCR)—Toxicologic/Hazardous Material

Student: _____   Examiner: _____

Date: _____

	Done ✓	Not Done
Records all pertinent dispatch/scene data, using a consistent format		
Completely identifies all additional resources and personnel		
Documents chief complaint, signs/symptoms, position found, age, sex, and weight		
Identifies and records all pertinent, reportable clinical data for each patient		
Documents SAMPLE and OPQRST if applicable		
Records all pertinent negatives		
Records all pertinent denials		
Records accurate, consistent times and patient information		
Includes relevant oral statements of witnesses, bystanders, and patient in "quotes" when appropriate		
Documents initial assessment findings: airway, breathing, and circulation		
Documents any interventions in initial assessment with patient response		
Documents level of consciousness, GCS (if trauma), and VS		
Documents rapid trauma assessment if applicable		
Documents any interventions in rapid trauma assessment with patient response		
Documents focused history and physical assessment		
Documents any interventions in focused assessment with patient response		
Documents repeat VS (every 5 minutes for critical; every 15 minutes for stable)		
Repeats initial assessment and documents findings		
Records ALL treatments with times and patient response(s) in treatment section		
Documents field impression		
Documents transport to specific facility and transfer of care WITH VERBAL REPORT		
Uses correct grammar, abbreviations, spelling, and terminology		
Writes legibly		
Thoroughly documents refusals, denials of transport, and call cancellations		
Documents patient GCS of 15 PRIOR to signing refusal		
Documents advice given to refusal patient, including "call 9-1-1 for further problems"		
Properly corrects errors and omissions		
Writes cautiously, avoids jargon, opinions, inferences, or any derogatory/libelous remarks		
Signs run report		
Uses EMS supplement form if needed		
Student exhibits competence with skill		

Any items in the Not Done column should be evaluated with student. Check marks in this column do not necessarily mean student was unsuccessful as all lines are not completed on all patients. Evaluation of each PCR should be based on the scenario given.

Student must be able to write an EMS report with consistency and accuracy.

☐ Successful   ☐ Unsuccessful   Examiner Initials: _____

©2006 Prentice-Hall Inc.

Overall Scenario Management—Toxicologic/Hazardous Material

Student: _____   Examiner: _____

Date: _____   Scenario: _____

NOTE: This skill sheet is to be done after the student completes a scenario as the TEAM LEADER. It is to let the student know if he or she is beginning to "put it all together" and use critical thinking skills to manage an EMS call. PLEASE notice that it is graded on a different basis than the basic lab skill sheet.

	Done ✓	Needs to Improve
SCENE MANAGEMENT		
Recognized hazards and controlled scene—safety, crowd, and patient issues		
Recognized hazards, but did not control the scene		
Unsuccessfully attempted to manage the scene	*	
Did not evaluate the scene and took no control of the scene	*	
PATIENT ASSESSMENT		
Performed a timely, organized complete patient assessment		
Performed complete initial, focused, and ongoing assessments, but in a disorganized manner		
Performed an incomplete assessment	*	
Did not perform an initial assessment	*	
PATIENT MANAGEMENT		
Evaluated assessment findings to manage all aspects of patient condition		
Managed the patient's presenting signs and symptoms without considering all of assessment		
Inadequately managed the patient	*	
Did not manage life-threatening conditions	*	
COMMUNICATION		
Communicated well with crew, patient, family, bystanders, and assisting agencies		
Communicated well with patient and crew		
Communicated with patient and crew, but poor communication skills	*	
Unable to communicate effectively	*	
REPORT AND TRANSFER OF CARE		
Identified correct destination for patient transport, gave accurate, brief report over radio, and provided full report at bedside demonstrating thorough understanding of patient condition and pathophysiological processes		
Identified correct destination and gave accurate radio and bedside report, but did not demonstrate understanding of patient condition and pathophysiological processes		
Identified correct destination, but provided inadequate radio and bedside report	*	
Identified inappropriate destination or provided no radio or bedside report	*	
Student exhibits competence with skill		

Any items that are marked with an * indicate the student needs to improve and a check mark should be placed in the right-hand column. A check mark in the right-hand column indicates that the student was unsuccessful and must attempt the skill again to assure competency. Examiners should use a different-color ink for the second attempt.

☐ Successful   ☐ Unsuccessful   Examiner Initials: _____

DAILY DISCUSSIONS AND PERTINENT POINTS— MEDICAL

Student: _____   **Date:** _____

Instructor: _____

	Instructor Initials
Develop a patient management plan for the behavioral/psychiatric patient, based on scenario field impressions.	
Differentiate strategies a paramedic uses when interviewing a patient who is hostile compared to one who is cooperative.	
Discuss the strategies for interviewing a patient who is unmotivated to talk.	
Describe the use of facilitation, reflection, clarification, sympathetic responses, confrontation, and interpretation.	
Differentiate between facilitation, reflection, clarification, sympathetic responses, confrontation, and interpretation.	
Define the following terms: a. Affect b. Anger c. Anxiety d. Confusion e. Depression f. Fear g. Mental status h. Open-ended question i. Posture	
Advocate for empathetic and respectful treatment of individuals experiencing behavioral emergencies.	
Discuss the effects of hypoglycemia with relation to symptoms of ETOH, trauma, stroke, seizure, etc., and the importance of performing a BGL on all altered level of consciousness patients.	
Discuss possible findings and considerations in assessing the various living environments of elderly patients.	
Discuss society's view of aging and the social, financial, and ethical issues facing the elderly.	
Describe the local resources available to assist the elderly and create strategies to refer at-risk patients to appropriate community services.	
Discuss issues facing society concerning the elderly.	
Discuss common emotional and psychological reactions to aging to include causes and manifestations.	
Demonstrate and advocate appropriate interactions with the elderly that convey respect for their position in life, in both lab and clinical areas.	
Recognize the emotional need for independence in the elderly while simultaneously attending to their apparent acute dependence.	
Recognize and appreciate the many impediments to physical and emotional well-being in the elderly.	
Recognize and appreciate the physical and emotional difficulties associated with being a caretaker of an impaired elderly person, particularly the patient with Alzheimer's disease.	
Identify community resources that are able to assist victims of abuse and assault.	
Discuss the documentation associated with abused and assaulted patients.	
Demonstrate sensitivity to the abused patient in both lab and clinical areas.	
Value the behavior of the abused patient.	
Attend to the emotional state of the abused patient.	
Recognize the value of nonverbal communication with the abused patient.	
Attend to the needs for reassurance, empathy, and compassion with the abused patient.	
Listen to the concerns expressed by the abused patient.	
Listen to and value the concerns expressed by the sexually assaulted patient.	
Discuss signs of financial impairment and accommodations that may be needed to properly manage the patient with a financial impairment.	
Identify local health care agencies and transportation resources for patients with special needs.	
Describe aging as a risk factor for disease.	
Discuss familial diseases and associated risk factors.	
Restate unique interviewing techniques to employ with patients who have special needs.	

    ©2006 Prentice-Hall Inc.

Value the role of the home care professional and understand his or her role in patient care along the life span continuum.	

Define the following terms:
  a. Substance or drug abuse
  b. Substance or drug dependence
  c. Tolerance
  d. Withdrawal
  e. Addiction	

Define *homeostasis* and relate the concept to environmental influences.	
Describe the general process of thermal regulation, including substances used and wastes generated.	
Value the sense of urgency for initial assessment and interventions for patients with hematologic crises.	
Apply the epidemiology to develop prevention strategies for urological emergencies.	
Value the patient's desire to remain in the home setting.	
Value the patient's desire to accept or deny hospice care.	

Value the uses of long-term venous access in the home health setting, including but not limited to:
  a. Chemotherapy
  b. Home pain management
  c. Nutrition therapy
  d. Congestive heart therapy
  e. Antibiotic therapy	

Formulate means of conveying empathy to patients whose ability to communicate is limited by their condition.	
Discuss and observe different types of decubitus dressings.	
Discuss and observe stages of decubiti.	
Discuss different PPE required for various organisms or potential organisms.	
Discuss wound care related to diagnoses (e.g., diabetic, postoperative osteomyelitis, etc.).	
Discuss home oxygen delivery systems including liquid oxygen, compressed air blenders, and oxygen concentrators.	
Discuss PCA pumps, narcotic patches, and other home pain-relief delivery systems and how they may relate to prehospital emergency care.	
Discuss emergency responses to terminally ill/hospice patients with regard to treatment versus resuscitation.	
Value the difference between treating a patient with a valid DNRO who has an emergency situation, and not initiating resuscitation measures for a patient with a valid DNRO.	
Discuss termination of resuscitation measures and circumstances that may be encountered in the prehospital care setting.	
Value the family dynamics of the terminally ill patient and the family response to the terminal event.	
Defend the rights of the family of a terminally ill hospice patient to call 9-1-1 and how this relates to the stages of the grieving process.	
Describe and discuss the rationale for the various types of PPE.	
Discuss different PPE required for various organisms or potential organisms.	
Advocate compliance with standards and guidelines by role modeling adherence to universal/standard precautions and appropriate PPE.	
Value the importance of immunization, especially in children and populations at risk.	
Value the safe management of a patient with an infectious/communicable disease.	
Advocate respect for the feelings of patients, family, and others at the scene of an infectious/communicable disease.	
Advocate empathy for a patient with an infectious/communicable disease.	
Value the importance of infectious/communicable disease control.	
Consistently demonstrate the use of BSI/appropriate PPE.	
Discuss recognition of presenting signs of a patient with a communicable disease.	
Anticipate accommodations that may be needed in order to properly manage a patient with a communicable disease.	

SECTION 7

*

Cardiology

Fabulous Factoids

Skill Sheets

Daily Discussions and Pertinent Points

FABULOUS FACTOIDS—CARDIOLOGY

Remember that the cardiac monitor shows only electrical, not mechanical, activity.

Electrocution from alternating current (AC)—found in homes—results in asystole; DC results in ventricular fibrillation.

Carotid sinus massage frequently causes asystole or embolus to brain causing stroke. Use other vagal maneuvers first.

The main reason artificial hearts cause complications is that their makers still haven't been able to duplicate surfaces as smooth as the endocardium. Clots still form.

Correlate the patient's pulse with the monitor. Treat the patient—NOT the monitor!

The highest average BP in America is in the Orange County area of California.

When treating a pulseless patient, the medic must consider conditions that may be causing decreased cardiac output, as some of these are treatable. A helpful mnemonic for troubleshooting pulselessness in PEA or asystole is also a reminder that pulseless patients need blood sugar checks and epinephrine.

OH Sugar Get THAT EPI

O₂ Hypoxia
Hypovolemia

Sugar

Get someone to check for toxins

Tension pneumothorax
Hypothermia
Acidosis
Tamponade
Embolus
Potassium
Injury/trauma

CONTRIBUTING FACTORS TO PULSELESSNESS (MIMICS OF PEA)			
	Condition	Treatment	Hints that patient may have this
O	O_2/ventilation	Ventilate	slow HR; cyanosis; obstruction
H	Hypovolemia	NS bolus(es)	Hx; ST; flat neck veins; ?P w/CPR
S	Sugar/hypoglycemia	SUGAR - Glucose/Dextrose 50%	Pale, cool, diaphoretic, Hx, Medic Alert
G	OD, toxic exposure	GET the cause, then use antidote	Pill bottles, track marks, containers, plant
T	Tension Pneumo	Decompress	+JVD; ↓Breath Sounds; ↓compliance
H	Hypothermia	Warm	Wet; cold environment
A	Acidosis	Ventilate; HCO_3	Low volt QRS; renal fail/DM; Hx; dialysis
T	Tamponade	Pericardiocentesis	ST; no pulse w/CPR; JVD, Beck's Triad
E	Emboli (coronary, pulmonary) AMI/ACS	Fibrinolytics	ST; Hx (PE); elevated ST
P	Potassium (hypo/hyper kalemia)	HCO_3; Glucose & insulin; CaCl; dialysis	"T" wave = K+ tent; u wave; long QT; wide tachycardia
I	Injuries/trauma	Hemostasis; may need volume	Kehr's, Cullen's, Grey-Turner's; abdominal distention, obvious hemorrhage

Asystole

MY . . . Does TEA Treat A CODE?

My fault—✓ leads, power, gain, monitor
Your fault—✓ asystole in at least two leads

Does—does patient have a valid DNR?

TCP
Epi
Atropine

Treat causes (same as PEA)

A—All ALS done correctly? Consider calling . . . unless special situation (below)

Cold
OD (most likely to respond to Rx)
Drowning
Electrocution

Bradycardia

All PTs Don't Expect Isuprel

Atropine
Pacing/Trancutaneous
Dopamine

©2006 Prentice-Hall Inc.

Epi
Isuprel

Notes:

Electricity
  no rhythm or pulse (VF/VT) 2-3-4 (200 j, 300 j, 360 j)
  + rhythm and pulse; 1-2-3-4 (100 j, 200 j, 300 j, 360 j)

Amiodarone
  NO pulse 300/30/30
  Perfusing—150 over 10 minutes

Epinephrine
  1 mg of drug can be in either 1 cc or 10 cc: it is still ONE mg of Epi
    1:1 (1mg/1cc) is called 1:1000
    1:10 (1 mg/10cc) is called 1:10,000
    Just eliminate the last 3 zeros

Procainamide—20–50 mg/min to max 17 mg/kg

Chest pain—MONA

Block Algorithm

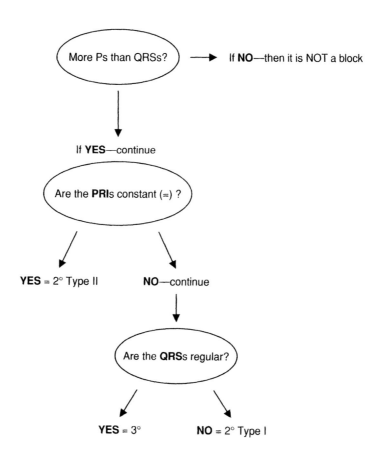

Stroke Volume times Heart Rate = Cardiac Output

$$SV \times HR = CO$$

Cardiac Output times Peripheral Vascular Resistance = Blood Pressure

$$CO \times PVR = BP$$

Treat: Rate—Rhythm—BP
Three components: Pump—Fluid—Container

As a paramedic, you can treat all three. The trick is to find which one you NEED to treat, because the BP has three components: $HR \times SV \times PVR$.

Drugs of the Section (see Emergency Drug Quiz Key, p. xxxiv–xxxv):

ASA
NTG
Adenocard
Cordarone
Procardia
Retavase

Pathophysiologies of the Section: 7.01–7.36 (see Checklist, p. 597–598)

©2006 Prentice-Hall Inc.

SKILL SHEETS

Lead Placement

Student: _____   Examiner:_____

Date: _____

	Done ✓	Not Done
Utilizes appropriate PPE		*
Preps the skin		*
Places electrodes according to manufacturer's recommendations for 3 lead cable		*
Places four limb leads according to manufacturer's recommendations for 12 lead		*
Places lead V1		
Places lead V2		
Places lead V4		
Places lead V3		
Places lead V6		
Places lead V5		
Ensures that all leads are attached		*
Checks quality of tracing being received		*
Can verbalize troubleshooting of poor-quality tracing		*
Records tracing		
Student exhibits competence with skill		

Any items in the Not Done column that are marked with an * are mandatory for the student to complete. A check mark in the Not Done column of an item with an * indicates that the student was unsuccessful and must attempt the skill again to assure competency. Examiners should use a different-color ink for the second attempt.

☐ Successful   ☐ Unsuccessful   Examiner Initials: _____

Automated External Defibrillator (AED)

Student: _____   **Examiner:** _____

Date: _____

	Done ✓	Not Done
Determines scene safety and utilizes appropriate PPE		*
Briefly questions rescuer about arrest events		*
Directs rescuer to stop CPR		*
Verifies absence of spontaneous pulse and advises rescuer to continue CPR		*
Turns on AED power		*
Attaches AED to patient		*
Stops CPR and ensures all individuals are standing clear of patient (visually AND verbally)		*
Initiates analysis of patient		*
Delivers shock if advised		*
Immediately resumes CPR (start with compressions)		*
Gathers additional information on arrest event		
Confirms effectiveness of CPR (ventilation and compression)		*
Directs insertion of simple airway adjunct (OPA/NPA)		
Directs ventilation of patient		*
Assures high concentration of oxygen		*
Assures CPR continues without unnecessary/prolonged interruption		
Reevaluates patient after 5 cycles (2 mins)		*
Repeats AED analysis following advice of AED		*
Prepares patient for transport		
Verbalizes continuing sequence to be followed during transport		
Student exhibits competence with skill		

Any items in the Not Done column that are marked with an * are mandatory for the student to complete. A check mark in the Not Done column of an item with an * indicates that the student was unsuccessful and must attempt the skill again to assure competency. Examiners should use a different-color ink for the second attempt.

☐ Successful   ☐ Unsuccessful   Examiner Initials: _____

©2006 Prentice-Hall Inc.

Defibrillation

Student: _____   **Examiner:** _____

Date: _____

	Done ✓	Not Done
Utilizes appropriate PPE		*
Confirms patient is unresponsive, apneic, and pulseless		*
Assures adequate CPR by auscultation of breath sounds and palpating pulse WITH CPR		*
Applies electrode gel to paddles or places commercial defibrillation pads to patient's exposed thorax		*
Turns on monitor/defibrillator		*
Observes and interprets rhythm		*
Recognizes indications for defibrillation		*
Verbalizes charging to appropriate joules per current ACLS guidelines (uses 25 j on manikin)		*
Places paddles to right of sternum and over apex using 25-lb paddle pressure (or pads)		*
Instructs to "CLEAR to head, CLEAR to feet, CLEAR to me" and visually clears all three		*
Reverifies rhythm		*
Delivers countershock		*
Checks pulse, leads, and monitor		
Interprets rhythm and proceeds to appropriate algorithm per current ACLS guidelines		*
Student exhibits competence with skill		

Any items in the Not Done column that are marked with an * are mandatory for the student to complete. A check mark in the Not Done column of an item with an * indicates that the student was unsuccessful and must attempt the skill again to assure competency. Examiners should use a different-color ink for the second attempt.

☐ Successful   ☐ Unsuccessful   Examiner Initials: _____

Synchronized Cardioversion

Student: _____   **Examiner:** _____

Date: _____

	Done ✓	Not Done
Utilizes appropriate PPE		*
Confirms dysrhythmia and patient condition indicating synchronized cardioversion		*
Explains procedure and sedates patient if vital signs permit		*
Turns on monitor/defibrillator, making sure "synchronized" switch is on		*
Verifies that monitor is "reading" the QRS complexes (marking the R wave)		*
Applies conductive gel to paddles or uses commercial defibrillation pads and places to right of sternum and over apex		*
Charges paddles to appropriate joules for dysrhythmia (uses 25 j on manikin)		*
Instructs to "CLEAR to head, CLEAR to feet, CLEAR to me" and visually clears all three		*
Reverifies rhythm		*
Presses and holds buttons until shock is delivered		*
Rechecks patient—pulse, leads, and monitor		*
Assesses patient's response to intervention		*
If no changes noted, repeats at appropriate joules		
Student exhibits competence with skill		

Any items in the Not Done column that are marked with an * are mandatory for the student to complete. A check mark in the Not Done column of an item with an * indicates that the student was unsuccessful and must attempt the skill again to assure competency. Examiners should use a different-color ink for the second attempt.

☐ Successful   ☐ Unsuccessful   Examiner Initials: _____

©2006 Prentice-Hall Inc.

Transcutaneous Pacing (TCP)

Student: _____   **Examiner:** _____

Date: _____

	Done ✓	Not Done
Utilizes appropriate PPE		*
Confirms patient condition and rhythm indicating need for TCP		*
Applies pacing electrodes per manufacturer's recommendations		*
Connects electrodes		*
Sets desired rate (60–80/min)		*
Turns voltage (mA) setting to zero		*
Turns pacer on		*
Slowly increases voltage until ventricular capture noted		*
Checks patient, pulse, and blood pressure		*
Readjusts rate and voltage as needed		
Monitors patient response to TCP		*
Considers sedation if hemodynamically improved		*
Student exhibits competence with skill		

Any items in the Not Done column that are marked with an * are mandatory for the student to complete. A check mark in the Not Done column of an item with an * indicates that the student was unsuccessful and must attempt the skill again to assure competency. Examiners should use a different-color ink for the second attempt.

☐ Successful   ☐ Unsuccessful   Examiner Initials: _____

Vagal Maneuvers

Student: _____   **Examiner:** _____

Date: _____

	Done ✓	Not Done
Utilizes appropriate PPE		*
Explains procedure(s) to patient		*
Places patient on cardiac monitor		*
Initiates IV		*
Properly directs patient to perform any of the following: 　1. Has patient hold breath and "bear down" for count of 5 　2. Has patient place his or her own finger in his or her own mouth and "blow" 　3. Has patient submerge face in ice water		*
Does NOT perform carotid massage as a vagal maneuver		*
Observes patient for response		*
Reassesses patient and repeats as needed		*
Continuously monitors for change from stable status to unstable		*
Documents procedure (verbalizes documentation) correctly		
Student exhibits competence with skill		

Any items in the Not Done column that are marked with an * are mandatory for the student to complete. A check mark in the Not Done column of an item with an * indicates that the student was unsuccessful and must attempt the skill again to assure competency. Examiners should use a different-color ink for the second attempt.

☐ Successful   ☐ Unsuccessful   Examiner Initials: _____

©2006 Prentice-Hall Inc.

Carotid Sinus Massage

Student: _____   Examiner: _____

Date: _____

	Done ✓	Not Done
Utilizes appropriate PPE		*
Assesses patient for indications for carotid sinus massage (CSM)		*
Initiates IV line		*
Attempts other vagal maneuvers first		*
Listens to both carotids for the presence of bruits		*
If bruits present, verbalizes CSM is NOT indicated		*
If carotids clear, gently rubs ONE carotid artery		*
Monitors EKG continuously for desired response or undesired complication		*
Verbalizes asystole is a potential complication of CSM		
If unsuccessful, tries other carotid		
Reassesses patient		*
Student exhibits competence with skill		

Any items in the Not Done column that are marked with an * are mandatory for the student to complete. A check mark in the Not Done column of an item with an * indicates that the student was unsuccessful and must attempt the skill again to assure competency. Examiners should use a different-color ink for the second attempt.

☐ Successful   ☐ Unsuccessful   Examiner Initials: _____

Pleural Decompression

Student: _____   **Examiner:** _____

Date: _____

	Done ✓	Not Done
Utilizes appropriate PPE		*
Evaluates patient for indications and obtains baseline lung sounds and assessment		*
Prepares equipment (14 gauge 2¼-in. catheter-over-needle) and explains procedure to patient		*
Palpates at 2nd intercostal space/midclavicular line		*
Cleanses site appropriately		*
Inserts needle at superior border of 3rd rib, avoiding artery, vein, and nerve		*
Advances until feels "pop" and rush of air released		*
Checks patient for improvement in clinical status		*
Removes needle from catheter, disposes of needle properly, and applies flutter valve		*
Secures in place		
Reassesses patient for improvement		*
Assesses patient's response to intervention		*
Documents procedure and response correctly		
Student exhibits competence with skill		

Any items in the Not Done column that are marked with an * are mandatory for the student to complete. A check mark in the Not Done column of an item with an * indicates that the student was unsuccessful and must attempt the skill again to assure competency. Examiners should use a different-color ink for the second attempt.

☐ Successful   ☐ Unsuccessful   Examiner Initials: _____

©2006 Prentice-Hall Inc.

Static Cardiology

Student: _____   Examiner: _____

Date: _____

NOTE: Examiner to show a mounted strip and written scenario to student. Student interprets strip and verbalizes treatment. Examiner records answers. If treatment all correct, check box; if incorrect, check the incorrect ITEM. Examiner can then evaluate student's success based on criticality of incorrect items checked.

	Correct	Incorrect
STRIP 1 Interpretation:		
Treatment:		
STRIP 2 Interpretation:		
Treatment:		
STRIP 3 Interpretation:		
Treatment:		
STRIP 4 Interpretation:		
Treatment:		
Student exhibits competence with skill		

Student may miss interpretation (call 2° Type II a 3°)—but MUST treat patient correctly (bradycardia).

☐ Successful   ☐ Unsuccessful   Examiner Initials: _____

Dynamic Cardiology

Student: _____   **Examiner:** _____

When recording scenario you are to circle any errors or omissions you catch. You may use abbreviations such as ABC or PLM (pulse, leads, monitor), CPR, ET, ↑, ↓, ✓, →, shk, part of drug names (epi), BBS (bilateral breath sounds), or abbreviate rhythms (ST, SVT, VF, VT, AFib, etc.). If an intervention is done in the wrong order or late, draw an arrow to where it should have been done.

Scenario: _____

Successful? (Please circle)   YES   NO   **Examiner Initials:** _____   **Date:** _____

©2006 Prentice-Hall Inc.

Asystole Flow Sheet (must verbalize treatable causes)

Student: _____   **Examiner:** _____

When recording scenario you are to circle any errors or omissions you catch. You may use abbreviations such as ABC or PLM (pulse, leads, monitor), CPR, ET, ↑, ↓, ✓, →, shk, part of drug names (epi), BBS (bilateral breath sounds), or abbreviate rhythms (ST, SVT, VF, VT, AFib, etc.). If an intervention is done in the wrong order or late, draw an arrow to where it should have been done.

Scenario:

Successful? (Please circle)   YES   NO   Examiner Initials: _____   Date: _____

Scenario Intubation—Asystole

Student: _____   Examiner: _____

Date: _____

	Done ✓	Not Done
Assesses scene safety and utilizes appropriate PPE		*
Manually opens the airway with technique appropriate for patient condition		*
Checks mouth for blood or potential airway obstruction		*
Suctions or removes loose teeth or foreign materials as needed		
Inserts simple adjunct (oropharyngeal or nasopharyngeal airway)		
Directs assistant to ventilate patient with bag-valve-mask device (room air)		*
Observes chest rise/fall and auscultates bilaterally over lungs for baseline		*
Obtains effective ventilation in less than 30 seconds		*
Attaches oxygen reservoir to bag-valve-mask device and connects to high-flow oxygen		
Ventilates patient and evaluates chest wall/lung compliance		*
Directs assistant to preoxygenate patient		*
Identifies/selects proper equipment for intubation		
Checks laryngoscope light and cuff of ET tube		
Removes all air from cuff and properly inserts stylet if used		
Removes airway adjunct		
Positions patient's head properly and has assistant perform Sellick's maneuver		*
Opens mouth and gently inserts blade while sweeping tongue to side		*
Has assistant maintain Sellick's pressure		
Gently elevates mandible with laryngoscope and visualizes cords		*
Introduces ET tube to side of blade and visualizes tube passing through cords		*
"Threads" ET tube off stylet (if used), maintaining hold on ET tube as stylet removed		
Inflates cuff to proper pressure and disconnects syringe		*
Disconnects mask from bag-valve device and attaches to ET tube without releasing ET tube		
Directs ventilation of patient while maintaining Sellick's maneuver and holding ET tube in place		
Confirms proper placement by auscultation over epigastrium and bilaterally over each lung		*
Directs assistant to release cricoid pressure		*
Secures ET tube		*
Reassesses bilateral lung sounds and compliance		*
Uses secondary device to confirm tube placement		*
Assesses patient's response to intervention		*
Verbalizes medications that can be administered via the ET tube according to ACLS		*
Student exhibits competence with skill		

Any items in the Not Done column that are marked with an * are mandatory for the student to complete. A check mark in the Not Done column of an item with an * indicates that the student was unsuccessful and must attempt the skill again to assure competency. Examiners should use a different-color ink for the second attempt.

☐ Successful   ☐ Unsuccessful   Examiner Initials: _____

©2006 Prentice-Hall Inc.

Scenario Radio Report—Asystole

Student: _____   Examiner: _____

Date: _____

	Done ✓	Not Done
Requests and checks for open channel before speaking		
Presses transmit button 1 second before speaking		
Holds microphone 2–3 in. from mouth		
Speaks slowly and clearly		*
Speaks in a normal voice		
Briefly transmits: Agency, unit designation, identification/name		*
Briefly transmits: Patient's age, sex, weight		*
Briefly transmits: Scene description/mechanism of injury or medical problem		*
Briefly transmits: Chief complaint with brief history of *present* illness		*
Briefly transmits: Associated symptoms (unless able to be deferred to bedside report)		
Briefly transmits: Past medical history (usually deferred to bedside report)		
Briefly transmits: Vital signs		*
Briefly transmits: Level of consciousness/GCS on trauma		*
Briefly transmits: General appearance, distress, cardiac rhythm, blood glucose, and other pertinent findings unable to be deferred to bedside report		
Briefly transmits: Interventions by EMS AND response(s)		*
ETA (the more critical the patient, the earlier you need to notify the receiving facility)		
Does not waste airtime		
Protects privacy of patient		*
Echoes dispatch information and any physician orders		*
Writes down dispatch information or physician orders		
Confirms with facility that message is received		
Demonstrates/verbalizes ability to troubleshoot basic equipment malfunction		
Student exhibits competence with skill		

Any items in the Not Done column that are marked with an * are mandatory for the student to complete. A check mark in the Not Done column of an item with an * indicates that the student was unsuccessful and must attempt the skill again to assure competency. Examiners should use a different-color ink for the second attempt.

☐ Successful   ☐ Unsuccessful   Examiner Initials: _____

©2006 Prentice-Hall Inc.

Scenario Patient Care Report (PCR)—Asystole

Student: _____   **Examiner:** _____

Date: _____

	Done ✓	Not Done
Records all pertinent dispatch/scene data, using a consistent format		
Completely identifies all additional resources and personnel		
Documents chief complaint, signs/symptoms, position found, age, sex, and weight		
Identifies and records all pertinent, reportable clinical data for each patient		
Documents SAMPLE and OPQRST if applicable		
Records all pertinent negatives		
Records all pertinent denials		
Records accurate, consistent times and patient information		
Includes relevant oral statements of witnesses, bystanders, and patient in "quotes" when appropriate		
Documents initial assessment findings: airway, breathing, and circulation		
Documents any interventions in initial assessment with patient response		
Documents level of consciousness, GCS (if trauma), and VS		
Documents rapid trauma assessment if applicable		
Documents any interventions in rapid trauma assessment with patient response		
Documents focused history and physical assessment		
Documents any interventions in focused assessment with patient response		
Documents repeat VS (every 5 minutes for critical; every 15 minutes for stable)		
Repeats initial assessment and documents findings		
Records ALL treatments with times and patient response(s) in treatment section		
Documents field impression		
Documents transport to specific facility and transfer of care WITH VERBAL REPORT		
Uses correct grammar, abbreviations, spelling, and terminology		
Writes legibly		
Thoroughly documents refusals, denials of transport, and call cancellations		
Documents patient GCS of 15 PRIOR to signing refusal		
Documents advice given to refusal patient, including "call 9-1-1 for further problems"		
Properly corrects errors and omissions		
Writes cautiously, avoids jargon, opinions, inferences, or any derogatory/libelous remarks		
Signs run report		
Uses EMS supplement form if needed		
Student exhibits competence with skill		

Any items in the Not Done column should be evaluated with student. Check marks in this column do not necessarily mean student was unsuccessful as all lines are not completed on all patients. Evaluation of each PCR should be based on the scenario given.

Student must be able to write an EMS report with consistency and accuracy.

☐ Successful   ☐ Unsuccessful   Examiner Initials: _____

©2006 Prentice-Hall Inc.

Overall Scenario Management—Asystole

Student: _____   Examiner: _____

Date: _____   Scenario: _____

NOTE: This skill sheet is to be done after the student completes a scenario as the TEAM LEADER. It is to let the student know if he or she is beginning to "put it all together" and use critical thinking skills to manage an EMS call. PLEASE notice that it is graded on a different basis than the basic lab skill sheet.

	Done ✓	Needs to Improve
SCENE MANAGEMENT		
Recognized hazards and controlled scene—safety, crowd, and patient issues		
Recognized hazards, but did not control the scene		
Unsuccessfully attempted to manage the scene	*	
Did not evaluate the scene and took no control of the scene	*	
PATIENT ASSESSMENT		
Performed a timely, organized complete patient assessment		
Performed complete initial, focused, and ongoing assessments, but in a disorganized manner		
Performed an incomplete assessment	*	
Did not perform an initial assessment	*	
PATIENT MANAGEMENT		
Evaluated assessment findings to manage all aspects of patient condition		
Managed the patient's presenting signs and symptoms without considering all of assessment		
Inadequately managed the patient	*	
Did not manage life-threatening conditions	*	
COMMUNICATION		
Communicated well with crew, patient, family, bystanders, and assisting agencies		
Communicated well with patient and crew		
Communicated with patient and crew, but poor communication skills	*	
Unable to communicate effectively	*	
REPORT AND TRANSFER OF CARE		
Identified correct destination for patient transport, gave accurate, brief report over radio, and provided full report at bedside demonstrating thorough understanding of patient condition and pathophysiological processes		
Identified correct destination and gave accurate radio and bedside report, but did not demonstrate understanding of patient condition and pathophysiological processes		
Identified correct destination, but provided inadequate radio and bedside report	*	
Identified inappropriate destination or provided no radio or bedside report	*	
Student exhibits competence with skill		

Any items that are marked with an * indicate the student needs to improve and a check mark should be placed in the right-hand column. A check mark in the right-hand column indicates that the student was unsuccessful and must attempt the skill again to assure competency. Examiners should use a different-color ink for the second attempt.

☐ Successful   ☐ Unsuccessful   Examiner Initials: _____

Ventricular Fibrillation (VF) Flow Sheet

Student: _____   **Examiner:** _____

When recording scenario you are to circle any errors or omissions you catch. You may use abbreviations such as ABC or PLM (pulse, leads, monitor), CPR, ET, ↑, ↓, ✓, →, shk, part of drug names (epi), BBS (bilateral breath sounds), or abbreviate rhythms (ST, SVT, VF, VT, AFib, etc.). If an intervention is done in the wrong order or late, draw an arrow to where it should have been done.

Scenario:

Successful? (Please circle)   YES   NO   **Examiner Initials:** _____   **Date:** _____

©2006 Prentice-Hall Inc.

Scenario Intubation—Ventricular Fibrillation

Student: _____   **Examiner:** _____

Date: _____

	Done ✓	Not Done
Assesses scene safety and utilizes appropriate PPE		*
Manually opens the airway with technique appropriate for patient condition		*
Checks mouth for blood or potential airway obstruction		*
Suctions or removes loose teeth or foreign materials as needed		
Inserts simple adjunct (oropharyngeal or nasopharyngeal airway)		
Directs assistant to ventilate patient with bag-valve-mask device (room air)		*
Observes chest rise/fall and auscultates bilaterally over lungs for baseline		*
Obtains effective ventilation in less than 30 seconds		*
Attaches oxygen reservoir to bag-valve-mask device and connects to high-flow oxygen		
Ventilates patient and evaluates chest wall/lung compliance		*
Directs assistant to preoxygenate patient		*
Identifies/selects proper equipment for intubation		
Checks laryngoscope light and cuff of ET tube		
Removes all air from cuff and properly inserts stylet if used		
Removes airway adjunct		
Positions patient's head properly and has assistant perform Sellick's maneuver		*
Opens mouth and gently inserts blade while sweeping tongue to side		*
Has assistant maintain Sellick's pressure		
Gently elevates mandible with laryngoscope and visualizes cords		*
Introduces ET tube to side of blade and visualizes tube passing through cords		*
"Threads" ET tube off stylet (if used), maintaining hold on ET tube as stylet removed		
Inflates cuff to proper pressure and disconnects syringe		*
Disconnects mask from bag-valve device and attaches to ET tube without releasing ET tube		
Directs ventilation of patient while maintaining Sellick's maneuver and holding ET tube in place		
Confirms proper placement by auscultation over epigastrium and bilaterally over each lung		*
Directs assistant to release cricoid pressure		*
Secures ET tube		*
Reassesses bilateral lung sounds and compliance		*
Uses secondary device to confirm tube placement		*
Assesses patient's response to intervention		*
Student exhibits competence with skill		

Any items in the Not Done column that are marked with an * are mandatory for the student to complete. A check mark in the Not Done column of an item with an * indicates that the student was unsuccessful and must attempt the skill again to assure competency. Examiners should use a different-color ink for the second attempt.

☐ Successful   ☐ Unsuccessful   Examiner Initials: _____

Scenario Radio Report—Ventricular Fibrillation

Student: _____   **Examiner:** _____

Date: _____

	Done ✓	Not Done
Requests and checks for open channel before speaking		
Presses transmit button 1 second before speaking		
Holds microphone 2–3 in. from mouth		
Speaks slowly and clearly		*
Speaks in a normal voice		
Briefly transmits: Agency, unit designation, identification/name		*
Briefly transmits: Patient's age, sex, weight		*
Briefly transmits: Scene description/mechanism of injury or medical problem		*
Briefly transmits: Chief complaint with brief history of *present* illness		*
Briefly transmits: Associated symptoms (unless able to be deferred to bedside report)		
Briefly transmits: Past medical history (usually deferred to bedside report)		
Briefly transmits: Vital signs		*
Briefly transmits: Level of consciousness/GCS on trauma		*
Briefly transmits: General appearance, distress, cardiac rhythm, blood glucose, and other pertinent findings unable to be deferred to bedside report		
Briefly transmits: Interventions by EMS AND response(s)		*
ETA (the more critical the patient, the earlier you need to notify the receiving facility)		
Does not waste airtime		
Protects privacy of patient		*
Echoes dispatch information and any physician orders		*
Writes down dispatch information or physician orders		
Confirms with facility that message is received		
Demonstrates/verbalizes ability to troubleshoot basic equipment malfunction		
Student exhibits competence with skill		

Any items in the Not Done column that are marked with an * are mandatory for the student to complete. A check mark in the Not Done column of an item with an * indicates that the student was unsuccessful and must attempt the skill again to assure competency. Examiners should use a different-color ink for the second attempt.

☐ Successful   ☐ Unsuccessful   Examiner Initials: _____

©2006 Prentice-Hall Inc.

Scenario Patient Care Report (PCR)—Ventricular Fibrillation

Student: _____   Examiner: _____

Date: _____

	Done ✓	Not Done
Records all pertinent dispatch/scene data, using a consistent format		
Completely identifies all additional resources and personnel		
Documents chief complaint, signs/symptoms, position found, age, sex, and weight		
Identifies and records all pertinent, reportable clinical data for each patient		
Documents SAMPLE and OPQRST if applicable		
Records all pertinent negatives		
Records all pertinent denials		
Records accurate, consistent times and patient information		
Includes relevant oral statements of witnesses, bystanders, and patient in "quotes" when appropriate		
Documents initial assessment findings: airway, breathing, and circulation		
Documents any interventions in initial assessment with patient response		
Documents level of consciousness, GCS (if trauma), and VS		
Documents rapid trauma assessment if applicable		
Documents any interventions in rapid trauma assessment with patient response		
Documents focused history and physical assessment		
Documents any interventions in focused assessment with patient response		
Documents repeat VS (every 5 minutes for critical; every 15 minutes for stable)		
Repeats initial assessment and documents findings		
Records ALL treatments with times and patient response(s) in treatment section		
Documents field impression		
Documents transport to specific facility and transfer of care WITH VERBAL REPORT		
Uses correct grammar, abbreviations, spelling, and terminology		
Writes legibly		
Thoroughly documents refusals, denials of transport, and call cancellations		
Documents patient GCS of 15 PRIOR to signing refusal		
Documents advice given to refusal patient, including "call 9-1-1 for further problems"		
Properly corrects errors and omissions		
Writes cautiously, avoids jargon, opinions, inferences, or any derogatory/libelous remarks		
Signs run report		
Uses EMS supplement form if needed		
Student exhibits competence with skill		

Any items in the Not Done column should be evaluated with student. Check marks in this column do not necessarily mean student was unsuccessful as all lines are not completed on all patients. Evaluation of each PCR should be based on the scenario given.

Student must be able to write an EMS report with consistency and accuracy.

☐ Successful   ☐ Unsuccessful   Examiner Initials: _____

©2006 Prentice-Hall Inc.

Overall Scenario Management—Ventricular Fibrillation

Student: _____   Examiner: _____

Date: _____   Scenario: _____

NOTE: This skill sheet is to be done after the student completes a scenario as the **TEAM LEADER**. It is to let the student know if he or she is beginning to "put it all together" and use critical thinking skills to manage an EMS call. PLEASE notice that it is graded on a different basis than the basic lab skill sheet.

	Done ✓	Needs to Improve
SCENE MANAGEMENT		
Recognized hazards and controlled scene—safety, crowd, and patient issues		
Recognized hazards, but did not control the scene		
Unsuccessfully attempted to manage the scene	*	
Did not evaluate the scene and took no control of the scene	*	
PATIENT ASSESSMENT		
Performed a timely, organized complete patient assessment		
Performed complete initial, focused, and ongoing assessments, but in a disorganized manner		
Performed an incomplete assessment	*	
Did not perform an initial assessment	*	
PATIENT MANAGEMENT		
Evaluated assessment findings to manage all aspects of patient condition		
Managed the patient's presenting signs and symptoms without considering all of assessment		
Inadequately managed the patient	*	
Did not manage life-threatening conditions	*	
COMMUNICATION		
Communicated well with crew, patient, family, bystanders, and assisting agencies		
Communicated well with patient and crew		
Communicated with patient and crew, but poor communication skills	*	
Unable to communicate effectively	*	
REPORT AND TRANSFER OF CARE		
Identified correct destination for patient transport, gave accurate, brief report over radio, and provided full report at bedside demonstrating thorough understanding of patient condition and pathophysiological processes		
Identified correct destination and gave accurate radio and bedside report, but did not demonstrate understanding of patient condition and pathophysiological processes		
Identified correct destination, but provided inadequate radio and bedside report	*	
Identified inappropriate destination or provided no radio or bedside report	*	
Student exhibits competence with skill		

Any items that are marked with an * indicate the student needs to improve and a check mark should be placed in the right-hand column. A check mark in the right-hand column indicates that the student was unsuccessful and must attempt the skill again to assure competency. Examiners should use a different-color ink for the second attempt.

☐ Successful   ☐ Unsuccessful   Examiner Initials: _____

©2006 Prentice-Hall Inc.

Ventricular Tachycardia (VT) Flow Sheet

Student: _____   Examiner:_____

When recording scenario you are to circle any errors or omissions you catch. You may use abbreviations such as ABC or PLM (pulse, leads, monitor), CPR, ET, ↑, ↓, ✓, →, shk, part of drug names (epi), BBS (bilateral breath sounds), or abbreviate rhythms (ST, SVT, VF, VT, AFib, etc.). If an intervention is done in the wrong order or late, draw an arrow to where it should have been done.

Scenario:

Successful? (Please circle)   YES   NO   Examiner Initials: _____   Date: _____

©2006 Prentice-Hall Inc.

Scenario Intubation—Ventricular Tachycardia

Student: _____   Examiner: _____

Date: _____

	Done ✓	Not Done
Assesses scene safety and utilizes appropriate PPE		*
Manually opens the airway with technique appropriate for patient condition		*
Checks mouth for blood or potential airway obstruction		*
Suctions or removes loose teeth or foreign materials as needed		
Inserts simple adjunct (oropharyngeal or nasopharyngeal airway)		
Directs assistant to ventilate patient with bag-valve-mask device (room air)		*
Observes chest rise/fall and auscultates bilaterally over lungs for baseline		*
Obtains effective ventilation in less than 30 seconds		*
Attaches oxygen reservoir to bag-valve-mask device and connects to high-flow oxygen		
Ventilates patient and evaluates chest wall/lung compliance		*
Directs assistant to preoxygenate patient		*
Identifies/selects proper equipment for intubation		
Checks laryngoscope light and cuff of ET tube		
Removes all air from cuff and properly inserts stylet if used		
Removes airway adjunct		
Positions patient's head properly and has assistant perform Sellick's maneuver		*
Opens mouth and gently inserts blade while sweeping tongue to side		*
Has assistant maintain Sellick's pressure		
Gently elevates mandible with laryngoscope and visualizes cords		*
Introduces ET tube to side of blade and visualizes tube passing through cords		*
"Threads" ET tube off stylet (if used), maintaining hold on ET tube as stylet removed		
Inflates cuff to proper pressure and disconnects syringe		*
Disconnects mask from bag-valve device and attaches to ET tube without releasing ET tube		
Directs ventilation of patient while maintaining Sellick's maneuver and holding ET tube in place		
Confirms proper placement by auscultation over epigastrium and bilaterally over each lung		*
Directs assistant to release cricoid pressure		*
Secures ET tube		*
Reassesses bilateral lung sounds and compliance		*
Uses secondary device to confirm tube placement		*
Assesses patient's response to intervention		*
Student exhibits competence with skill		

Any items in the Not Done column that are marked with an * are mandatory for the student to complete. A check mark in the Not Done column of an item with an * indicates that the student was unsuccessful and must attempt the skill again to assure competency. Examiners should use a different-color ink for the second attempt.

☐ Successful   ☐ Unsuccessful   Examiner Initials: _____

©2006 Prentice-Hall Inc.

Scenario Radio Report—Ventricular Tachycardia

Student: _____   Examiner: _____

Date: _____

	Done ✓	Not Done
Requests and checks for open channel before speaking		
Presses transmit button 1 second before speaking		
Holds microphone 2–3 in. from mouth		
Speaks slowly and clearly		*
Speaks in a normal voice		
Briefly transmits: Agency, unit designation, identification/name		*
Briefly transmits: Patient's age, sex, weight		*
Briefly transmits: Scene description/mechanism of injury or medical problem		*
Briefly transmits: Chief complaint with brief history of *present* illness		*
Briefly transmits: Associated symptoms (unless able to be deferred to bedside report)		
Briefly transmits: Past medical history (usually deferred to bedside report)		
Briefly transmits: Vital signs		*
Briefly transmits: Level of consciousness/GCS on trauma		*
Briefly transmits: General appearance, distress, cardiac rhythm, blood glucose, and other pertinent findings unable to be deferred to bedside report		
Briefly transmits: Interventions by EMS AND response(s)		*
ETA (the more critical the patient, the earlier you need to notify the receiving facility)		
Does not waste airtime		
Protects privacy of patient		*
Echoes dispatch information and any physician orders		*
Writes down dispatch information or physician orders		
Confirms with facility that message is received		
Demonstrates/verbalizes ability to troubleshoot basic equipment malfunction		
Student exhibits competence with skill		

Any items in the Not Done column that are marked with an * are mandatory for the student to complete. A check mark in the Not Done column of an item with an * indicates that the student was unsuccessful and must attempt the skill again to assure competency. Examiners should use a different-color ink for the second attempt.

☐ Successful   ☐ Unsuccessful   Examiner Initials: _____

©2006 Prentice-Hall Inc.

Scenario Patient Care Report (PCR)—Ventricular Tachycardia

Student: _____   Examiner: _____

Date: _____

	Done ✓	Not Done
Records all pertinent dispatch/scene data, using a consistent format		
Completely identifies all additional resources and personnel		
Documents chief complaint, signs/symptoms, position found, age, sex, and weight		
Identifies and records all pertinent, reportable clinical data for each patient		
Documents SAMPLE and OPQRST if applicable		
Records all pertinent negatives		
Records all pertinent denials		
Records accurate, consistent times and patient information		
Includes relevant oral statements of witnesses, bystanders, and patient in "quotes" when appropriate		
Documents initial assessment findings: airway, breathing, and circulation		
Documents any interventions in initial assessment with patient response		
Documents level of consciousness, GCS (if trauma), and VS		
Documents rapid trauma assessment if applicable		
Documents any interventions in rapid trauma assessment with patient response		
Documents focused history and physical assessment		
Documents any interventions in focused assessment with patient response		
Documents repeat VS (every 5 minutes for critical; every 15 minutes for stable)		
Repeats initial assessment and documents findings		
Records ALL treatments with times and patient response(s) in treatment section		
Documents field impression		
Documents transport to specific facility and transfer of care WITH VERBAL REPORT		
Uses correct grammar, abbreviations, spelling, and terminology		
Writes legibly		
Thoroughly documents refusals, denials of transport, and call cancellations		
Documents patient GCS of 15 PRIOR to signing refusal		
Documents advice given to refusal patient, including "call 9-1-1 for further problems"		
Properly corrects errors and omissions		
Writes cautiously, avoids jargon, opinions, inferences, or any derogatory/libelous remarks		
Signs run report		
Uses EMS supplement form if needed		
Student exhibits competence with skill		

Any items in the Not Done column should be evaluated with student. Check marks in this column do not necessarily mean student was unsuccessful as all lines are not completed on all patients. Evaluation of each PCR should be based on the scenario given.

Student must be able to write an EMS report with consistency and accuracy.

☐ Successful   ☐ Unsuccessful   Examiner Initials: _____

©2006 Prentice-Hall Inc.

Overall Scenario Management—Ventricular Tachycardia

Student: _____   Examiner: _____

Date: _____   Scenario: _____

NOTE: This skill sheet is to be done after the student completes a scenario as the TEAM LEADER. It is to let the student know if he or she is beginning to "put it all together" and use critical thinking skills to manage an EMS call. PLEASE notice that it is graded on a different basis than the basic lab skill sheet.

	Done ✓	Needs to Improve
SCENE MANAGEMENT		
Recognized hazards and controlled scene—safety, crowd, and patient issues		
Recognized hazards, but did not control the scene		
Unsuccessfully attempted to manage the scene	*	
Did not evaluate the scene and took no control of the scene	*	
PATIENT ASSESSMENT		
Performed a timely, organized complete patient assessment		
Performed complete initial, focused, and ongoing assessments, but in a disorganized manner		
Performed an incomplete assessment	*	
Did not perform an initial assessment	*	
PATIENT MANAGEMENT		
Evaluated assessment findings to manage all aspects of patient condition		
Managed the patient's presenting signs and symptoms without considering all of assessment		
Inadequately managed the patient	*	
Did not manage life-threatening conditions	*	
COMMUNICATION		
Communicated well with crew, patient, family, bystanders, and assisting agencies		
Communicated well with patient and crew		
Communicated with patient and crew, but poor communication skills	*	
Unable to communicate effectively	*	
REPORT AND TRANSFER OF CARE		
Identified correct destination for patient transport, gave accurate, brief report over radio, and provided full report at bedside demonstrating thorough understanding of patient condition and pathophysiological processes		
Identified correct destination and gave accurate radio and bedside report, but did not demonstrate understanding of patient condition and pathophysiological processes		
Identified correct destination, but provided inadequate radio and bedside report	*	
Identified inappropriate destination or provided no radio or bedside report	*	
Student exhibits competence with skill		

Any items that are marked with an * indicate the student needs to improve and a check mark should be placed in the right-hand column. A check mark in the right-hand column indicates that the student was unsuccessful and must attempt the skill again to assure competency. Examiners should use a different-color ink for the second attempt.

☐ Successful   ☐ Unsuccessful   Examiner Initials: _____

Pulseless Electrical Activity (PEA) Flow Sheet (must verbalize treatable causes)

Student: _____   Examiner: _____

When recording scenario you are to circle any errors or omissions you catch. You may use abbreviations such as ABC or PLM (pulse, leads, monitor), CPR, ET, ↑, ↓, ✓, →, shk, part of drug names (epi), BBS (bilateral breath sounds), or abbreviate rhythms (ST, SVT, VF, VT, AFib, etc.). If an intervention is done in the wrong order or late, draw an arrow to where it should have been done.

Scenario:

Successful? (Please circle)   YES   NO   Examiner Initials: _____   Date: _____

©2006 Prentice-Hall Inc.

Scenario Intubation—Pulseless Electrical Activity (PEA)

Student: _____   Examiner: _____

Date: _____

	Done ✓	Not Done
Assesses scene safety and utilizes appropriate PPE		*
Manually opens the airway with technique appropriate for patient condition		*
Checks mouth for blood or potential airway obstruction		*
Suctions or removes loose teeth or foreign materials as needed		
Inserts simple adjunct (oropharyngeal or nasopharyngeal airway)		
Directs assistant to ventilate patient with bag-valve-mask device (room air)		*
Observes chest rise/fall and auscultates bilaterally over lungs for baseline		*
Obtains effective ventilation in less than 30 seconds		*
Attaches oxygen reservoir to bag-valve-mask device and connects to high-flow oxygen		
Ventilates patient and evaluates chest wall/lung compliance		*
Directs assistant to preoxygenate patient		*
Identifies/selects proper equipment for intubation		
Checks laryngoscope light and cuff of ET tube		
Removes all air from cuff and properly inserts stylet if used		
Removes airway adjunct		
Positions patient's head properly and has assistant perform Sellick's maneuver		*
Opens mouth and gently inserts blade while sweeping tongue to side		*
Has assistant maintain Sellick's pressure		
Gently elevates mandible with laryngoscope and visualizes cords		*
Introduces ET tube to side of blade and visualizes tube passing through cords		*
"Threads" ET tube off stylet (if used), maintaining hold on ET tube as stylet removed		
Inflates cuff to proper pressure and disconnects syringe		*
Disconnects mask from bag-valve device and attaches to ET tube without releasing ET tube		
Directs ventilation of patient while maintaining Sellick's maneuver and holding ET tube in place		
Confirms proper placement by auscultation over epigastrium and bilaterally over each lung		*
Directs assistant to release cricoid pressure		*
Secures ET tube		*
Reassesses bilateral lung sounds and compliance		*
Uses secondary device to confirm tube placement		*
Assesses patient's response to intervention		*
Student exhibits competence with skill		

Any items in the Not Done column that are marked with an * are mandatory for the student to complete. A check mark in the Not Done column of an item with an * indicates that the student was unsuccessful and must attempt the skill again to assure competency. Examiners should use a different-color ink for the second attempt.

☐ Successful   ☐ Unsuccessful   Examiner Initials: _____

©2006 Prentice-Hall Inc.

Scenario Radio Report—Pulseless Electrical Activity (PEA)

Student: _____   Examiner: _____

Date: _____

	Done ✓	Not Done
Requests and checks for open channel before speaking		
Presses transmit button 1 second before speaking		
Holds microphone 2–3 in. from mouth		
Speaks slowly and clearly		*
Speaks in a normal voice		
Briefly transmits: Agency, unit designation, identification/name		*
Briefly transmits: Patient's age, sex, weight		*
Briefly transmits: Scene description/mechanism of injury or medical problem		*
Briefly transmits: Chief complaint with brief history of *present* illness		*
Briefly transmits: Associated symptoms (unless able to be deferred to bedside report)		
Briefly transmits: Past medical history (usually deferred to bedside report)		
Briefly transmits: Vital signs		*
Briefly transmits: Level of consciousness/GCS on trauma		*
Briefly transmits: General appearance, distress, cardiac rhythm, blood glucose, and other pertinent findings unable to be deferred to bedside report		
Briefly transmits: Interventions by EMS AND response(s)		*
ETA (the more critical the patient, the earlier you need to notify the receiving facility)		
Does not waste airtime		
Protects privacy of patient		*
Echoes dispatch information and any physician orders		*
Writes down dispatch information or physician orders		
Confirms with facility that message is received		
Demonstrates/verbalizes ability to troubleshoot basic equipment malfunction		
Student exhibits competence with skill		

Any items in the Not Done column that are marked with an * are mandatory for the student to complete. A check mark in the Not Done column of an item with an * indicates that the student was unsuccessful and must attempt the skill again to assure competency. Examiners should use a different-color ink for the second attempt.

☐ Successful   ☐ Unsuccessful   Examiner Initials: _____

©2006 Prentice-Hall Inc.

Scenario Patient Care Report (PCR)—Pulseless Electrical Activity (PEA)

Student: _____   Examiner: _____

Date: _____

	Done ✓	Not Done
Records all pertinent dispatch/scene data, using a consistent format		
Completely identifies all additional resources and personnel		
Documents chief complaint, signs/symptoms, position found, age, sex, and weight		
Identifies and records all pertinent, reportable clinical data for each patient		
Documents SAMPLE and OPQRST if applicable		
Records all pertinent negatives		
Records all pertinent denials		
Records accurate, consistent times and patient information		
Includes relevant oral statements of witnesses, bystanders, and patient in "quotes" when appropriate		
Documents initial assessment findings: airway, breathing, and circulation		
Documents any interventions in initial assessment with patient response		
Documents level of consciousness, GCS (if trauma), and VS		
Documents rapid trauma assessment if applicable		
Documents any interventions in rapid trauma assessment with patient response		
Documents focused history and physical assessment		
Documents any interventions in focused assessment with patient response		
Documents repeat VS (every 5 minutes for critical; every 15 minutes for stable)		
Repeats initial assessment and documents findings		
Records ALL treatments with times and patient response(s) in treatment section		
Documents field impression		
Documents transport to specific facility and transfer of care WITH VERBAL REPORT		
Uses correct grammar, abbreviations, spelling, and terminology		
Writes legibly		
Thoroughly documents refusals, denials of transport, and call cancellations		
Documents patient GCS of 15 PRIOR to signing refusal		
Documents advice given to refusal patient, including "call 9-1-1 for further problems"		
Properly corrects errors and omissions		
Writes cautiously, avoids jargon, opinions, inferences, or any derogatory/libelous remarks		
Signs run report		
Uses EMS supplement form if needed		
Student exhibits competence with skill		

Any items in the Not Done column should be evaluated with student. Check marks in this column do not necessarily mean student was unsuccessful as all lines are not completed on all patients. Evaluation of each PCR should be based on the scenario given.

Student must be able to write an EMS report with consistency and accuracy.

☐ Successful   ☐ Unsuccessful   Examiner Initials: _____

Overall Scenario Management—Pulseless Electrical Activity (PEA)

Student: _____   Examiner: _____

Date: _____   Scenario: _____

NOTE: This skill sheet is to be done after the student completes a scenario as the TEAM LEADER. It is to let the student know if he or she is beginning to "put it all together" and use critical thinking skills to manage an EMS call. PLEASE notice that it is graded on a different basis than the basic lab skill sheet.

	Done ✓	Needs to Improve
SCENE MANAGEMENT		
Recognized hazards and controlled scene—safety, crowd, and patient issues		
Recognized hazards, but did not control the scene		
Unsuccessfully attempted to manage the scene	*	
Did not evaluate the scene and took no control of the scene	*	
PATIENT ASSESSMENT		
Performed a timely, organized complete patient assessment		
Performed complete initial, focused, and ongoing assessments, but in a disorganized manner		
Performed an incomplete assessment	*	
Did not perform an initial assessment	*	
PATIENT MANAGEMENT		
Evaluated assessment findings to manage all aspects of patient condition		
Managed the patient's presenting signs and symptoms without considering all of assessment		
Inadequately managed the patient	*	
Did not manage life-threatening conditions	*	
COMMUNICATION		
Communicated well with crew, patient, family, bystanders, and assisting agencies		
Communicated well with patient and crew		
Communicated with patient and crew, but poor communication skills	*	
Unable to communicate effectively	*	
REPORT AND TRANSFER OF CARE		
Identified correct destination for patient transport, gave accurate, brief report over radio, and provided full report at bedside demonstrating thorough understanding of patient condition and pathophysiological processes		
Identified correct destination and gave accurate radio and bedside report, but did not demonstrate understanding of patient condition and pathophysiological processes		
Identified correct destination, but provided inadequate radio and bedside report	*	
Identified inappropriate destination or provided no radio or bedside report	*	
Student exhibits competence with skill		

Any items that are marked with an * indicate the student needs to improve and a check mark should be placed in the right-hand column. A check mark in the right-hand column indicates that the student was unsuccessful and must attempt the skill again to assure competency. Examiners should use a different-color ink for the second attempt.

☐ Successful   ☐ Unsuccessful   Examiner Initials: _____

©2006 Prentice-Hall Inc.

Patient Assessment: Cardiology—Acute Myocardial Infarction (AMI)

Student: _____   **Examiner:** _____

Date: _____   **Scenario:** _____

	Done ✓	Not Done
Assesses scene safety and utilizes appropriate PPE		*
OVERALL SCENE EVALUATION		
Medical—determines nature of illness/if trauma involved determines MOI		*
Determines the number of patients, location, obstacles, and requests any additional resources as needed		
Verbalizes general impression of the patient as approaches		*
Considers stabilization/spinal motion restriction of spine if trauma involved		*
INITIAL ASSESSMENT		
Determines responsiveness/level of consciousness/AVPU		*
Opens airway with appropriate technique and assesses airway/ventilation		*
Manages airway/ventilation and applies appropriate oxygen therapy in less than 3 minutes		*
Assesses circulation: radial/carotid pulse, skin color, temperature, condition, and turgor		*
Controls any major bleeding		*
Makes rapid transport decision if indicated		
Initiates IV, obtains BGL, GCS, **12-Lead EKG**, and complete vital signs		
FOCUSED HISTORY AND PHYSICAL EXAMINATION/RAPID ASSESSMENT		
Obtains SAMPLE history		
Obtains OPQRST for differential diagnosis		
Obtains associated symptoms, pertinent negatives/denials		
Evaluates decision to perform focused exam or completes rapid assessment		*
Vital signs including AVPU (and GCS if trauma)		*
Assesses cardiovascular system including heart sounds, peripheral edema, and peripheral perfusion		*
Assesses pulmonary system including reassessing airway, ventilation, breath sounds, pulse oximetry, chest wall excursion, accessory muscle use, or other signs of distress		*
Assesses neurological system including speech, droop, drift, if applicable, and distal movement and sensation		*
Assesses musculoskeletal and integumentary systems		
Assesses behavioral, psychological, and social aspects of patient and situation		
States field impression of patient—AMI		*
Verbalizes treatment plan for patient and calls for appropriate intervention(s)—IVs, NTG, ASA, Morphine		*
Reevaluates transport decision		
ONGOING ASSESSMENT		
Repeats initial assessment		*
Repeats vital signs and evaluates trends		*
Evaluates response to treatments		*
Repeats focused assessment regarding patient complaint or injuries and evaluates for fibrinolytic exclusion criteria		
Gives radio report to receiving facility		
Turns over patient care with verbal report		*
Student exhibits competence with skill		

Any items in the Not Done column that are marked with an * are mandatory for the student to complete. A check mark in the Not Done column of an item with an * indicates that the student was unsuccessful and must attempt the skill again to assure competency. Examiners should use a different-color ink for the second attempt.

☐ Successful   ☐ Unsuccessful   Examiner Initials: _____

Scenario Intubation—Acute Myocardial Infarction (AMI)

Student: _____   Examiner: _____

Date: _____

	Done ✓	Not Done
Assesses scene safety and utilizes appropriate PPE		*
Manually opens the airway with technique appropriate for patient condition		*
Checks mouth for blood or potential airway obstruction		*
Suctions or removes loose teeth or foreign materials as needed		
Inserts simple adjunct (oropharyngeal or nasopharyngeal airway)		
Directs assistant to ventilate patient with bag-valve-mask device (room air)		*
Observes chest rise/fall and auscultates bilaterally over lungs for baseline		*
Obtains effective ventilation in less than 30 seconds		*
Attaches oxygen reservoir to bag-valve-mask device and connects to high-flow oxygen		
Ventilates patient and evaluates chest wall/lung compliance		*
Directs assistant to preoxygenate patient		*
Identifies/selects proper equipment for intubation		
Checks laryngoscope light and cuff of ET tube		
Removes all air from cuff and properly inserts stylet if used		
Removes airway adjunct		
Positions patient's head properly and has assistant perform Sellick's maneuver		*
Opens mouth and gently inserts blade while sweeping tongue to side		*
Has assistant maintain Sellick's pressure		
Gently elevates mandible with laryngoscope and visualizes cords		*
Introduces ET tube to side of blade and visualizes tube passing through cords		*
"Threads" ET tube off stylet (if used), maintaining hold on ET tube as stylet removed		
Inflates cuff to proper pressure and disconnects syringe		*
Disconnects mask from bag-valve device and attaches to ET tube without releasing ET tube		
Directs ventilation of patient while maintaining Sellick's maneuver and holding ET tube in place		
Confirms proper placement by auscultation over epigastrium and bilaterally over each lung		*
Directs assistant to release cricoid pressure		*
Secures ET tube		*
Reassesses bilateral lung sounds and compliance		*
Uses secondary device to confirm tube placement		*
Assesses patient's response to intervention		*
Student exhibits competence with skill		

Any items in the Not Done column that are marked with an * are mandatory for the student to complete. A check mark in the Not Done column of an item with an * indicates that the student was unsuccessful and must attempt the skill again to assure competency. Examiners should use a different-color ink for the second attempt.

☐ Successful   ☐ Unsuccessful   Examiner Initials: _____

©2006 Prentice-Hall Inc.

Scenario Radio Report—Acute Myocardial Infarction (AMI)

Student: _____   **Examiner:** _____

Date: _____

	Done ✓	Not Done
Requests and checks for open channel before speaking		
Presses transmit button 1 second before speaking		
Holds microphone 2–3 in. from mouth		
Speaks slowly and clearly		*
Speaks in a normal voice		
Briefly transmits: Agency, unit designation, identification/name		*
Briefly transmits: Patient's age, sex, weight		*
Briefly transmits: Scene description/mechanism of injury or medical problem		*
Briefly transmits: Chief complaint with brief history of *present* illness		*
Briefly transmits: Associated symptoms (unless able to be deferred to bedside report)		
Briefly transmits: Past medical history (usually deferred to bedside report)		
Briefly transmits: Vital signs		*
Briefly transmits: Level of consciousness/GCS on trauma		*
Briefly transmits: General appearance, distress, cardiac rhythm, blood glucose, and other pertinent findings unable to be deferred to bedside report		
Briefly transmits: Interventions by EMS AND response(s)		*
ETA (the more critical the patient, the earlier you need to notify the receiving facility)		
Does not waste airtime		
Protects privacy of patient		*
Echoes dispatch information and any physician orders		*
Writes down dispatch information or physician orders		
Confirms with facility that message is received		
Demonstrates/verbalizes ability to troubleshoot basic equipment malfunction		
Student exhibits competence with skill		

Any items in the Not Done column that are marked with an * are mandatory for the student to complete. A check mark in the Not Done column of an item with an * indicates that the student was unsuccessful and must attempt the skill again to assure competency. Examiners should use a different-color ink for the second attempt.

☐ Successful   ☐ Unsuccessful   Examiner Initials: _____

©2006 Prentice-Hall Inc.

Scenario Patient Care Report (PCR)—Acute Myocardial Infarction (AMI)

Student: _____   Examiner: _____

Date: _____

	Done ✓	Not Done
Records all pertinent dispatch/scene data, using a consistent format		
Completely identifies all additional resources and personnel		
Documents chief complaint, signs/symptoms, position found, age, sex, and weight		
Identifies and records all pertinent, reportable clinical data for each patient		
Documents SAMPLE and OPQRST if applicable		
Records all pertinent negatives		
Records all pertinent denials		
Records accurate, consistent times and patient information		
Includes relevant oral statements of witnesses, bystanders, and patient in "quotes" when appropriate		
Documents initial assessment findings: airway, breathing, and circulation		
Documents any interventions in initial assessment with patient response		
Documents level of consciousness, GCS (if trauma), and VS		
Documents rapid trauma assessment if applicable		
Documents any interventions in rapid trauma assessment with patient response		
Documents focused history and physical assessment		
Documents any interventions in focused assessment with patient response		
Documents repeat VS (every 5 minutes for critical; every 15 minutes for stable)		
Repeats initial assessment and documents findings		
Records ALL treatments with times and patient response(s) in treatment section		
Documents field impression		
Documents transport to specific facility and transfer of care WITH VERBAL REPORT		
Uses correct grammar, abbreviations, spelling, and terminology		
Writes legibly		
Thoroughly documents refusals, denials of transport, and call cancellations		
Documents patient GCS of 15 PRIOR to signing refusal		
Documents advice given to refusal patient, including "call 9-1-1 for further problems"		
Properly corrects errors and omissions		
Writes cautiously, avoids jargon, opinions, inferences, or any derogatory/libelous remarks		
Signs run report		
Uses EMS supplement form if needed		
Student exhibits competence with skill		

Any items in the Not Done column should be evaluated with student. Check marks in this column do not necessarily mean student was unsuccessful as all lines are not completed on all patients. Evaluation of each PCR should be based on the scenario given.

Student must be able to write an EMS report with consistency and accuracy.

☐ Successful   ☐ Unsuccessful   Examiner Initials: _____

©2006 Prentice-Hall Inc.

Overall Scenario Management—Acute Myocardial Infarction (AMI)

Student: _____   Examiner: _____

Date: _____   Scenario: _____

NOTE: This skill sheet is to be done after the student completes a scenario as the TEAM LEADER. It is to let the student know if he or she is beginning to "put it all together" and use critical thinking skills to manage an EMS call. PLEASE notice that it is graded on a different basis than the basic lab skill sheet.

	Done ✓	Needs to Improve
SCENE MANAGEMENT		
Recognized hazards and controlled scene—safety, crowd, and patient issues		
Recognized hazards, but did not control the scene		
Unsuccessfully attempted to manage the scene	*	
Did not evaluate the scene and took no control of the scene	*	
PATIENT ASSESSMENT		
Performed a timely, organized complete patient assessment		
Performed complete initial, focused, and ongoing assessments, but in a disorganized manner		
Performed an incomplete assessment	*	
Did not perform an initial assessment	*	
PATIENT MANAGEMENT		
Evaluated assessment findings to manage all aspects of patient condition		
Managed the patient's presenting signs and symptoms without considering all of assessment		
Inadequately managed the patient	*	
Did not manage life-threatening conditions	*	
COMMUNICATION		
Communicated well with crew, patient, family, bystanders, and assisting agencies		
Communicated well with patient and crew		
Communicated with patient and crew, but poor communication skills	*	
Unable to communicate effectively	*	
REPORT AND TRANSFER OF CARE		
Identified correct destination for patient transport, gave accurate, brief report over radio, and provided full report at bedside demonstrating thorough understanding of patient condition and pathophysiological processes		
Identified correct destination and gave accurate radio and bedside report, but did not demonstrate understanding of patient condition and pathophysiological processes		
Identified correct destination, but provided inadequate radio and bedside report	*	
Identified inappropriate destination or provided no radio or bedside report	*	
Student exhibits competence with skill		

Any items that are marked with an * indicate the student needs to improve and a check mark should be placed in the right-hand column. A check mark in the right-hand column indicates that the student was unsuccessful and must attempt the skill again to assure competency. Examiners should use a different-color ink for the second attempt.

☐ Successful   ☐ Unsuccessful   Examiner Initials: _____

Patient Assessment: Cardiology—Bradycardia

Student: _____   Examiner: _____

Date: _____   Scenario: _____

	Done ✓	Not Done
Assesses scene safety and utilizes appropriate PPE		*
OVERALL SCENE EVALUATION		
Medical—determines nature of illness/if trauma involved determines MOI		*
Determines the number of patients, location, obstacles, and requests any additional resources as needed		
Verbalizes general impression of the patient as approaches		*
Considers stabilization/spinal motion restriction of spine if trauma involved		*
INITIAL ASSESSMENT		
Determines responsiveness/level of consciousness/AVPU		*
Opens airway with appropriate technique and assesses airway/ventilation		*
Manages airway/ventilation and applies appropriate oxygen therapy in less than 3 minutes		*
Assesses circulation: radial/carotid pulse, skin color, temperature, condition, and turgor		*
Controls any major bleeding		*
Makes rapid transport decision if indicated		
Initiates IV, obtains BGL, GCS, **12-Lead EKG,** and complete vital signs		
FOCUSED HISTORY AND PHYSICAL EXAMINATION/RAPID ASSESSMENT		
Obtains SAMPLE history		
Obtains OPQRST for differential diagnosis		
Obtains associated symptoms, pertinent negatives/denials		
Evaluates decision to perform focused exam or completes rapid assessment		*
Vital signs including AVPU (and GCS if trauma)		*
Assesses cardiovascular system including heart sounds, peripheral edema, and peripheral perfusion		*
Assesses pulmonary system including reassessing airway, ventilation, breath sounds, pulse oximetry, chest wall excursion, accessory muscle use, or other signs of distress		*
Assesses neurological system including speech, droop, drift, if applicable, and distal movement and sensation		*
Assesses musculoskeletal and integumentary systems		
Assesses behavioral, psychological, and social aspects of patient and situation		
States field impression of patient—bradycardia (identifies if patient stable or unstable)—TREAT PATIENT		*
Verbalizes treatment plan for patient and calls for appropriate intervention(s)—IVs, TCP, current ACLS, or none		*
Reevaluates transport decision		
ONGOING ASSESSMENT		
Repeats initial assessment		*
Repeats vital signs and evaluates trends		*
Evaluates response to treatments		*
Repeats focused assessment regarding patient complaint or injuries		
Gives radio report to receiving facility		
Turns over patient care with verbal report		*
Student exhibits competence with skill		

Any items in the Not Done column that are marked with an * are mandatory for the student to complete. A check mark in the Not Done column of an item with an * indicates that the student was unsuccessful and must attempt the skill again to assure competency. Examiners should use a different-color ink for the second attempt.

☐ Successful   ☐ Unsuccessful   Examiner Initials: _____

     ©2006 Prentice-Hall Inc.

Scenario Radio Report—Bradycardia

Student: _____   **Examiner:** _____

Date: _____

	Done ✓	Not Done
Requests and checks for open channel before speaking		
Presses transmit button 1 second before speaking		
Holds microphone 2–3 in. from mouth		
Speaks slowly and clearly		*
Speaks in a normal voice		
Briefly transmits: Agency, unit designation, identification/name		*
Briefly transmits: Patient's age, sex, weight		*
Briefly transmits: Scene description/mechanism of injury or medical problem		*
Briefly transmits: Chief complaint with brief history of *present* illness		*
Briefly transmits: Associated symptoms (unless able to be deferred to bedside report)		
Briefly transmits: Past medical history (usually deferred to bedside report)		
Briefly transmits: Vital signs		*
Briefly transmits: Level of consciousness/GCS on trauma		*
Briefly transmits: General appearance, distress, cardiac rhythm, blood glucose, and other pertinent findings unable to be deferred to bedside report		
Briefly transmits: Interventions by EMS AND response(s)		*
ETA (the more critical the patient, the earlier you need to notify the receiving facility)		
Does not waste airtime		
Protects privacy of patient		*
Echoes dispatch information and any physician orders		*
Writes down dispatch information or physician orders		
Confirms with facility that message is received		
Demonstrates/verbalizes ability to troubleshoot basic equipment malfunction		
Student exhibits competence with skill		

Any items in the Not Done column that are marked with an * are mandatory for the student to complete. A check mark in the Not Done column of an item with an * indicates that the student was unsuccessful and must attempt the skill again to assure competency. Examiners should use a different-color ink for the second attempt.

☐ Successful   ☐ Unsuccessful   Examiner Initials: _____

Scenario Patient Care Report (PCR)—Bradycardia

Student: _____   Examiner: _____

Date: _____

	Done ✓	Not Done
Records all pertinent dispatch/scene data, using a consistent format		
Completely identifies all additional resources and personnel		
Documents chief complaint, signs/symptoms, position found, age, sex, and weight		
Identifies and records all pertinent, reportable clinical data for each patient		
Documents SAMPLE and OPQRST if applicable		
Records all pertinent negatives		
Records all pertinent denials		
Records accurate, consistent times and patient information		
Includes relevant oral statements of witnesses, bystanders, and patient in "quotes" when appropriate		
Documents initial assessment findings: airway, breathing, and circulation		
Documents any interventions in initial assessment with patient response		
Documents level of consciousness, GCS (if trauma), and VS		
Documents rapid trauma assessment if applicable		
Documents any interventions in rapid trauma assessment with patient response		
Documents focused history and physical assessment		
Documents any interventions in focused assessment with patient response		
Documents repeat VS (every 5 minutes for critical; every 15 minutes for stable)		
Repeats initial assessment and documents findings		
Records ALL treatments with times and patient response(s) in treatment section		
Documents field impression		
Documents transport to specific facility and transfer of care WITH VERBAL REPORT		
Uses correct grammar, abbreviations, spelling, and terminology		
Writes legibly		
Thoroughly documents refusals, denials of transport, and call cancellations		
Documents patient GCS of 15 PRIOR to signing refusal		
Documents advice given to refusal patient, including "call 9-1-1 for further problems"		
Properly corrects errors and omissions		
Writes cautiously, avoids jargon, opinions, inferences, or any derogatory/libelous remarks		
Signs run report		
Uses EMS supplement form if needed		
Student exhibits competence with skill		

Any items in the Not Done column should be evaluated with student. Check marks in this column do not necessarily mean student was unsuccessful as all lines are not completed on all patients. Evaluation of each PCR should be based on the scenario given.

Student must be able to write an EMS report with consistency and accuracy.

☐ Successful   ☐ Unsuccessful   Examiner Initials: _____

©2006 Prentice-Hall Inc.

Overall Scenario Management—Bradycardia

Student: _____   Examiner: _____

Date: _____   Scenario: _____

NOTE: This skill sheet is to be done after the student completes a scenario as the TEAM LEADER. It is to let the student know if he or she is beginning to "put it all together" and use critical thinking skills to manage an EMS call. PLEASE notice that it is graded on a different basis than the basic lab skill sheet.

	Done ✓	Needs to Improve
SCENE MANAGEMENT		
Recognized hazards and controlled scene—safety, crowd, and patient issues		
Recognized hazards, but did not control the scene		
Unsuccessfully attempted to manage the scene	*	
Did not evaluate the scene and took no control of the scene	*	
PATIENT ASSESSMENT		
Performed a timely, organized complete patient assessment		
Performed complete initial, focused, and ongoing assessments, but in a disorganized manner		
Performed an incomplete assessment	*	
Did not perform an initial assessment	*	
PATIENT MANAGEMENT		
Evaluated assessment findings to manage all aspects of patient condition		
Managed the patient's presenting signs and symptoms without considering all of assessment		
Inadequately managed the patient	*	
Did not manage life-threatening conditions	*	
COMMUNICATION		
Communicated well with crew, patient, family, bystanders, and assisting agencies		
Communicated well with patient and crew		
Communicated with patient and crew, but poor communication skills	*	
Unable to communicate effectively	*	
REPORT AND TRANSFER OF CARE		
Identified correct destination for patient transport, gave accurate, brief report over radio, and provided full report at bedside demonstrating thorough understanding of patient condition and pathophysiological processes		
Identified correct destination and gave accurate radio and bedside report, but did not demonstrate understanding of patient condition and pathophysiological processes		
Identified correct destination, but provided inadequate radio and bedside report	*	
Identified inappropriate destination or provided no radio or bedside report	*	
Student exhibits competence with skill		

Any items that are marked with an * indicate the student needs to improve and a check mark should be placed in the right-hand column. A check mark in the right-hand column indicates that the student was unsuccessful and must attempt the skill again to assure competency. Examiners should use a different-color ink for the second attempt.

☐ Successful   ☐ Unsuccessful   Examiner Initials: _____

Patient Assessment: Cardiology—Cardiogenic Shock

Student: _____   Examiner: _____

Date: _____   Scenario: _____

	Done ✓	Not Done
Assesses scene safety and utilizes appropriate PPE		*
OVERALL SCENE EVALUATION		
Medical—determines nature of illness/if trauma involved determines MOI		*
Determines the number of patients, location, obstacles, and requests any additional resources as needed		
Verbalizes general impression of the patient as approaches		*
Considers stabilization/spinal motion restriction of spine if trauma involved		*
INITIAL ASSESSMENT		
Determines responsiveness/level of consciousness/AVPU		*
Opens airway with appropriate technique and assesses airway/ventilation—BREATH SOUNDS		*
Manages airway/ventilation and applies appropriate oxygen therapy in less than 3 minutes		*
Assesses circulation: radial/carotid pulse, skin color, temperature, condition, and turgor		*
Controls any major bleeding		*
Makes rapid transport decision if indicated		
Initiates IV, obtains BGL, GCS, **12-Lead EKG,** and complete vital signs		
FOCUSED HISTORY AND PHYSICAL EXAMINATION/RAPID ASSESSMENT		
Obtains SAMPLE history		
Obtains OPQRST for differential diagnosis		
Obtains associated symptoms, pertinent negatives/denials		
Evaluates decision to perform focused exam or completes rapid assessment		*
Vital signs including AVPU (and GCS if trauma)		*
Assesses cardiovascular system including heart sounds, peripheral edema, and peripheral perfusion		*
Assesses pulmonary system including reassessing airway, ventilation, breath sounds, pulse oximetry, chest wall excursion, accessory muscle use, or other signs of distress		*
Assesses neurological system including speech, droop, drift, if applicable, and distal movement and sensation		*
Assesses musculoskeletal and integumentary systems		
Assesses behavioral, psychological, and social aspects of patient and situation		
States field impression of patient—cardiogenic shock (pathophysiology of left versus right ventricular failure)		*
Verbalizes treatment plan for patient and calls for appropriate intervention(s)—IVs, dopamine, ACLS guidelines		*
Reevaluates transport decision		
ONGOING ASSESSMENT		
Repeats initial assessment		*
Repeats vital signs and evaluates trends		*
Evaluates response to treatments		*
Repeats focused assessment regarding patient complaint or injuries		
Gives radio report to receiving facility		
Turns over patient care with verbal report		*
Student exhibits competence with skill		

Any items in the Not Done column that are marked with an * are mandatory for the student to complete. A check mark in the Not Done column of an item with an * indicates that the student was unsuccessful and must attempt the skill again to assure competency. Examiners should use a different-color ink for the second attempt.

☐ Successful   ☐ Unsuccessful   Examiner Initials: _____

©2006 Prentice-Hall Inc.

Scenario Intubation—Cardiogenic Shock

Student: _____   Examiner: _____

Date: _____

	Done ✓	Not Done
Assesses scene safety and utilizes appropriate PPE		*
Manually opens the airway with technique appropriate for patient condition		*
Checks mouth for blood or potential airway obstruction		*
Suctions or removes loose teeth or foreign materials as needed		
Inserts simple adjunct (oropharyngeal or nasopharyngeal airway)		
Directs assistant to ventilate patient with bag-valve-mask device (room air)		*
Observes chest rise/fall and auscultates bilaterally over lungs for baseline		*
Obtains effective ventilation in less than 30 seconds		*
Attaches oxygen reservoir to bag-valve-mask device and connects to high-flow oxygen		
Ventilates patient and evaluates chest wall/lung compliance		*
Directs assistant to preoxygenate patient		*
Identifies/selects proper equipment for intubation		
Checks laryngoscope light and cuff of ET tube		
Removes all air from cuff and properly inserts stylet if used		
Removes airway adjunct		
Positions patient's head properly and has assistant perform Sellick's maneuver		*
Opens mouth and gently inserts blade while sweeping tongue to side		*
Has assistant maintain Sellick's pressure		
Gently elevates mandible with laryngoscope and visualizes cords		*
Introduces ET tube to side of blade and visualizes tube passing through cords		*
"Threads" ET tube off stylet (if used), maintaining hold on ET tube as stylet removed		
Inflates cuff to proper pressure and disconnects syringe		*
Disconnects mask from bag-valve device and attaches to ET tube without releasing ET tube		
Directs ventilation of patient while maintaining Sellick's maneuver and holding ET tube in place		
Confirms proper placement by auscultation over epigastrium and bilaterally over each lung		*
Directs assistant to release cricoid pressure		*
Secures ET tube		*
Reassesses bilateral lung sounds and compliance		*
Uses secondary device to confirm tube placement		*
Assesses patient's response to intervention		*
Student exhibits competence with skill		

Any items in the Not Done column that are marked with an * are mandatory for the student to complete. A check mark in the Not Done column of an item with an * indicates that the student was unsuccessful and must attempt the skill again to assure competency. Examiners should use a different-color ink for the second attempt.

☐ Successful   ☐ Unsuccessful   Examiner Initials: _____

©2006 Prentice-Hall Inc.

Scenario Radio Report—Cardiogenic Shock

Student: _____   Examiner: _____

Date: _____

	Done ✓	Not Done
Requests and checks for open channel before speaking		
Presses transmit button 1 second before speaking		
Holds microphone 2–3 in. from mouth		
Speaks slowly and clearly		*
Speaks in a normal voice		
Briefly transmits: Agency, unit designation, identification/name		*
Briefly transmits: Patient's age, sex, weight		*
Briefly transmits: Scene description/mechanism of injury or medical problem		*
Briefly transmits: Chief complaint with brief history of *present* illness		*
Briefly transmits: Associated symptoms (unless able to be deferred to bedside report)		
Briefly transmits: Past medical history (usually deferred to bedside report)		
Briefly transmits: Vital signs		*
Briefly transmits: Level of consciousness/GCS on trauma		*
Briefly transmits: General appearance, distress, cardiac rhythm, blood glucose, and other pertinent findings unable to be deferred to bedside report		
Briefly transmits: Interventions by EMS AND response(s)		*
ETA (the more critical the patient, the earlier you need to notify the receiving facility)		
Does not waste airtime		
Protects privacy of patient		*
Echoes dispatch information and any physician orders		*
Writes down dispatch information or physician orders		
Confirms with facility that message is received		
Demonstrates/verbalizes ability to troubleshoot basic equipment malfunction		
Student exhibits competence with skill		

Any items in the Not Done column that are marked with an * are mandatory for the student to complete. A check mark in the Not Done column of an item with an * indicates that the student was unsuccessful and must attempt the skill again to assure competency. Examiners should use a different-color ink for the second attempt.

☐ Successful   ☐ Unsuccessful   Examiner Initials: _____

©2006 Prentice-Hall Inc.

Scenario Patient Care Report (PCR)—Cardiogenic Shock

Student: _____   Examiner: _____

Date: _____

	Done ✓	Not Done
Records all pertinent dispatch/scene data, using a consistent format		
Completely identifies all additional resources and personnel		
Documents chief complaint, signs/symptoms, position found, age, sex, and weight		
Identifies and records all pertinent, reportable clinical data for each patient		
Documents SAMPLE and OPQRST if applicable		
Records all pertinent negatives		
Records all pertinent denials		
Records accurate, consistent times and patient information		
Includes relevant oral statements of witnesses, bystanders, and patient in "quotes" when appropriate		
Documents initial assessment findings: airway, breathing, and circulation		
Documents any interventions in initial assessment with patient response		
Documents level of consciousness, GCS (if trauma), and VS		
Documents rapid trauma assessment if applicable		
Documents any interventions in rapid trauma assessment with patient response		
Documents focused history and physical assessment		
Documents any interventions in focused assessment with patient response		
Documents repeat VS (every 5 minutes for critical; every 15 minutes for stable)		
Repeats initial assessment and documents findings		
Records ALL treatments with times and patient response(s) in treatment section		
Documents field impression		
Documents transport to specific facility and transfer of care WITH VERBAL REPORT		
Uses correct grammar, abbreviations, spelling, and terminology		
Writes legibly		
Thoroughly documents refusals, denials of transport, and call cancellations		
Documents patient GCS of 15 PRIOR to signing refusal		
Documents advice given to refusal patient, including "call 9-1-1 for further problems"		
Properly corrects errors and omissions		
Writes cautiously, avoids jargon, opinions, inferences, or any derogatory/libelous remarks		
Signs run report		
Uses EMS supplement form if needed		
Student exhibits competence with skill		

Any items in the Not Done column should be evaluated with student. Check marks in this column do not necessarily mean student was unsuccessful as all lines are not completed on all patients. Evaluation of each PCR should be based on the scenario given.

Student must be able to write an EMS report with consistency and accuracy.

☐ Successful   ☐ Unsuccessful   Examiner Initials: _____

Overall Scenario Management—Cardiogenic Shock

Student: _____   Examiner: _____

Date: _____   Scenario: _____

NOTE: This skill sheet is to be done after the student completes a scenario as the **TEAM LEADER**. It is to let the student know if he or she is beginning to "put it all together" and use critical thinking skills to manage an EMS call. PLEASE notice that it is graded on a different basis than the basic lab skill sheet.

	Done ✓	Needs to Improve
SCENE MANAGEMENT		
Recognized hazards and controlled scene—safety, crowd, and patient issues		
Recognized hazards, but did not control the scene		
Unsuccessfully attempted to manage the scene	*	
Did not evaluate the scene and took no control of the scene	*	
PATIENT ASSESSMENT		
Performed a timely, organized complete patient assessment		
Performed complete initial, focused, and ongoing assessments, but in a disorganized manner		
Performed an incomplete assessment	*	
Did not perform an initial assessment	*	
PATIENT MANAGEMENT		
Evaluated assessment findings to manage all aspects of patient condition		
Managed the patient's presenting signs and symptoms without considering all of assessment		
Inadequately managed the patient	*	
Did not manage life-threatening conditions	*	
COMMUNICATION		
Communicated well with crew, patient, family, bystanders, and assisting agencies		
Communicated well with patient and crew		
Communicated with patient and crew, but poor communication skills	*	
Unable to communicate effectively	*	
REPORT AND TRANSFER OF CARE		
Identified correct destination for patient transport, gave accurate, brief report over radio, and provided full report at bedside demonstrating thorough understanding of patient condition and pathophysiological processes		
Identified correct destination and gave accurate radio and bedside report, but did not demonstrate understanding of patient condition and pathophysiological processes		
Identified correct destination, but provided inadequate radio and bedside report	*	
Identified inappropriate destination or provided no radio or bedside report	*	
Student exhibits competence with skill		

Any items that are marked with an * indicate the student needs to improve and a check mark should be placed in the right-hand column. A check mark in the right-hand column indicates that the student was unsuccessful and must attempt the skill again to assure competency. Examiners should use a different-color ink for the second attempt.

☐ Successful   ☐ Unsuccessful   Examiner Initials: _____

©2006 Prentice-Hall Inc.

Patient Assessment: Cardiology—Medical Arrest

Student: _____   Examiner: _____

Date: _____   Scenario: _____

	Done ✓	Not Done
Assesses scene safety and utilizes appropriate PPE		*
OVERALL SCENE EVALUATION		
Medical—determines nature of illness/if trauma involved determines MOI		*
Determines the number of patients, location, obstacles, and requests any additional resources as needed		
Verbalizes general impression of the patient as approaches		*
Considers stabilization/spinal motion restriction of spine if trauma involved		*
INITIAL ASSESSMENT		
Determines responsiveness/level of consciousness/AVPU		*
Opens airway with appropriate technique and assesses airway/ventilation		*
Manages airway/ventilation and applies appropriate oxygen therapy in less than 3 minutes		*
Assesses circulation: radial/carotid pulse, skin color, temperature, condition, and turgor		*
Controls any major bleeding		*
Makes rapid transport decision if indicated		
Initiates IV, obtains BGL, GCS, **12-Lead EKG if not initially in arrest,** and complete vital signs		
FOCUSED HISTORY AND PHYSICAL EXAMINATION/RAPID ASSESSMENT		
Obtains SAMPLE history		
Obtains OPQRST for differential diagnosis		
Obtains associated symptoms, pertinent negatives/denials		
Evaluates decision to perform focused exam or completes rapid assessment		*
Vital signs including AVPU (and GCS if trauma)		*
Assesses cardiovascular system including heart sounds, peripheral edema, and peripheral perfusion		*
Assesses pulmonary system including reassessing airway, ventilation, breath sounds, pulse oximetry, chest wall excursion, accessory muscle use, or other signs of distress		*
Assesses neurological system including speech, droop, drift, if applicable, and distal movement and sensation		*
Assesses musculoskeletal and integumentary systems		
Assesses behavioral, psychological, and social aspects of patient and situation		
States field impression of patient—cardiac arrest due to medical (rules out low BGL, drugs, etc.)		*
Verbalizes treatment plan for patient and calls for appropriate intervention(s)—current ACLS guidelines		*
Reevaluates transport decision		
ONGOING ASSESSMENT		
Repeats initial assessment		*
Repeats vital signs and evaluates trends		*
Evaluates response to treatments		*
Repeats focused assessment regarding patient complaint or injuries		
Gives radio report to receiving facility		
Turns over patient care with verbal report		*
Student exhibits competence with skill		

Any items in the Not Done column that are marked with an * are mandatory for the student to complete. A check mark in the Not Done column of an item with an * indicates that the student was unsuccessful and must attempt the skill again to assure competency. Examiners should use a different-color ink for the second attempt.

☐ Successful   ☐ Unsuccessful   Examiner Initials: _____

Scenario Intubation—Medical Arrest

Student: _____   Examiner: _____

Date: _____

	Done ✓	Not Done
Assesses scene safety and utilizes appropriate PPE		*
Manually opens the airway with technique appropriate for patient condition		*
Checks mouth for blood or potential airway obstruction		*
Suctions or removes loose teeth or foreign materials as needed		
Inserts simple adjunct (oropharyngeal or nasopharyngeal airway)		
Directs assistant to ventilate patient with bag-valve-mask device (room air)		*
Observes chest rise/fall and auscultates bilaterally over lungs for baseline		*
Obtains effective ventilation in less than 30 seconds		*
Attaches oxygen reservoir to bag-valve-mask device and connects to high-flow oxygen		
Ventilates patient and evaluates chest wall/lung compliance		*
Directs assistant to preoxygenate patient		*
Identifies/selects proper equipment for intubation		
Checks laryngoscope light and cuff of ET tube		
Removes all air from cuff and properly inserts stylet if used		
Removes airway adjunct		
Positions patient's head properly and has assistant perform Sellick's maneuver		*
Opens mouth and gently inserts blade while sweeping tongue to side		*
Has assistant maintain Sellick's pressure		
Gently elevates mandible with laryngoscope and visualizes cords		*
Introduces ET tube to side of blade and visualizes tube passing through cords		*
"Threads" ET tube off stylet (if used), maintaining hold on ET tube as stylet removed		
Inflates cuff to proper pressure and disconnects syringe		*
Disconnects mask from bag-valve device and attaches to ET tube without releasing ET tube		
Directs ventilation of patient while maintaining Sellick's maneuver and holding ET tube in place		
Confirms proper placement by auscultation over epigastrium and bilaterally over each lung		*
Directs assistant to release cricoid pressure		*
Secures ET tube		*
Reassesses bilateral lung sounds and compliance		*
Uses secondary device to confirm tube placement		*
Assesses patient's response to intervention		*
Verbalizes medications that can be administered via the ET tube according to ACLS guidelines		
Student exhibits competence with skill		

Any items in the Not Done column that are marked with an * are mandatory for the student to complete. A check mark in the Not Done column of an item with an * indicates that the student was unsuccessful and must attempt the skill again to assure competency. Examiners should use a different-color ink for the second attempt.

☐ Successful   ☐ Unsuccessful   Examiner Initials: _____

©2006 Prentice-Hall Inc.

Scenario Radio Report—Medical Arrest

Student: _____   **Examiner:** _____

Date: _____

	Done ✓	Not Done
Requests and checks for open channel before speaking		
Presses transmit button 1 second before speaking		
Holds microphone 2–3 in. from mouth		
Speaks slowly and clearly		*
Speaks in a normal voice		
Briefly transmits: Agency, unit designation, identification/name		*
Briefly transmits: Patient's age, sex, weight		*
Briefly transmits: Scene description/mechanism of injury or medical problem		*
Briefly transmits: Chief complaint with brief history of *present* illness		*
Briefly transmits: Associated symptoms (unless able to be deferred to bedside report)		
Briefly transmits: Past medical history (usually deferred to bedside report)		
Briefly transmits: Vital signs		*
Briefly transmits: Level of consciousness/GCS on trauma		*
Briefly transmits: General appearance, distress, cardiac rhythm, blood glucose, and other pertinent findings unable to be deferred to bedside report		
Briefly transmits: Interventions by EMS AND response(s)		*
ETA (the more critical the patient, the earlier you need to notify the receiving facility)		
Does not waste airtime		
Protects privacy of patient		*
Echoes dispatch information and any physician orders		*
Writes down dispatch information or physician orders		
Confirms with facility that message is received		
Demonstrates/verbalizes ability to troubleshoot basic equipment malfunction		
Student exhibits competence with skill		

Any items in the Not Done column that are marked with an * are mandatory for the student to complete. A check mark in the Not Done column of an item with an * indicates that the student was unsuccessful and must attempt the skill again to assure competency. Examiners should use a different-color ink for the second attempt.

☐ Successful   ☐ Unsuccessful   Examiner Initials: _____

Scenario Patient Care Report (PCR)—Medical Arrest

Student: _____   Examiner: _____

Date: _____

	Done ✓	Not Done
Records all pertinent dispatch/scene data, using a consistent format		
Completely identifies all additional resources and personnel		
Documents chief complaint, signs/symptoms, position found, age, sex, and weight		
Identifies and records all pertinent, reportable clinical data for each patient		
Documents SAMPLE and OPQRST if applicable		
Records all pertinent negatives		
Records all pertinent denials		
Records accurate, consistent times and patient information		
Includes relevant oral statements of witnesses, bystanders, and patient in "quotes" when appropriate		
Documents initial assessment findings: airway, breathing, and circulation		
Documents any interventions in initial assessment with patient response		
Documents level of consciousness, GCS (if trauma), and VS		
Documents rapid trauma assessment if applicable		
Documents any interventions in rapid trauma assessment with patient response		
Documents focused history and physical assessment		
Documents any interventions in focused assessment with patient response		
Documents repeat VS (every 5 minutes for critical; every 15 minutes for stable)		
Repeats initial assessment and documents findings		
Records ALL treatments with times and patient response(s) in treatment section		
Documents field impression		
Documents transport to specific facility and transfer of care WITH VERBAL REPORT		
Uses correct grammar, abbreviations, spelling, and terminology		
Writes legibly		
Thoroughly documents refusals, denials of transport, and call cancellations		
Documents patient GCS of 15 PRIOR to signing refusal		
Documents advice given to refusal patient, including "call 9-1-1 for further problems"		
Properly corrects errors and omissions		
Writes cautiously, avoids jargon, opinions, inferences, or any derogatory/libelous remarks		
Signs run report		
Uses EMS supplement form if needed		
Student exhibits competence with skill		

Any items in the Not Done column should be evaluated with student. Check marks in this column do not necessarily mean student was unsuccessful as all lines are not completed on all patients. Evaluation of each PCR should be based on the scenario given.

Student must be able to write an EMS report with consistency and accuracy.

☐ Successful   ☐ Unsuccessful   Examiner Initials: _____

                         ©2006 Prentice-Hall Inc.

Overall Scenario Management—Medical Arrest

Student: _____   Examiner: _____

Date: _____   Scenario: _____

NOTE: This skill sheet is to be done after the student completes a scenario as the TEAM LEADER. It is to let the student know if he or she is beginning to "put it all together" and use critical thinking skills to manage an EMS call. PLEASE notice that it is graded on a different basis than the basic lab skill sheet.

	Done ✓	Needs to Improve
SCENE MANAGEMENT		
Recognized hazards and controlled scene—safety, crowd, and patient issues		
Recognized hazards, but did not control the scene		
Unsuccessfully attempted to manage the scene	*	
Did not evaluate the scene and took no control of the scene	*	
PATIENT ASSESSMENT		
Performed a timely, organized complete patient assessment		
Performed complete initial, focused, and ongoing assessments, but in a disorganized manner		
Performed an incomplete assessment	*	
Did not perform an initial assessment	*	
PATIENT MANAGEMENT		
Evaluated assessment findings to manage all aspects of patient condition		
Managed the patient's presenting signs and symptoms without considering all of assessment		
Inadequately managed the patient	*	
Did not manage life-threatening conditions	*	
COMMUNICATION		
Communicated well with crew, patient, family, bystanders, and assisting agencies		
Communicated well with patient and crew		
Communicated with patient and crew, but poor communication skills	*	
Unable to communicate effectively	*	
REPORT AND TRANSFER OF CARE		
Identified correct destination for patient transport, gave accurate, brief report over radio, and provided full report at bedside demonstrating thorough understanding of patient condition and pathophysiological processes		
Identified correct destination and gave accurate radio and bedside report, but did not demonstrate understanding of patient condition and pathophysiological processes		
Identified correct destination, but provided inadequate radio and bedside report	*	
Identified inappropriate destination or provided no radio or bedside report	*	
Student exhibits competence with skill		

Any items that are marked with an * indicate the student needs to improve and a check mark should be placed in the right-hand column. A check mark in the right-hand column indicates that the student was unsuccessful and must attempt the skill again to assure competency. Examiners should use a different-color ink for the second attempt.

☐ Successful   ☐ Unsuccessful   Examiner Initials: _____

©2006 Prentice-Hall Inc.

Patient Assessment: Cardiology—Pulmonary Edema

Student: _____   Examiner: _____

Date: _____   Scenario: _____

	Done ✓	Not Done
Assesses scene safety and utilizes appropriate PPE		*
OVERALL SCENE EVALUATION		
Medical—determines nature of illness/if trauma involved determines MOI		*
Determines the number of patients, location, obstacles, and requests any additional resources as needed		
Verbalizes general impression of the patient as approaches		*
Considers stabilization/spinal motion restriction of spine if trauma involved		*
INITIAL ASSESSMENT		
Determines responsiveness/level of consciousness/AVPU		*
Opens airway with appropriate technique and assesses airway/ventilation		*
Manages airway/ventilation and applies appropriate oxygen therapy in less than 3 minutes		*
Assesses circulation: radial/carotid pulse, skin color, temperature, condition, and turgor		*
Controls any major bleeding		*
Makes rapid transport decision if indicated		
Initiates IV, obtains BGL, GCS, **12-Lead EKG,** and complete vital signs		
FOCUSED HISTORY AND PHYSICAL EXAMINATION/RAPID ASSESSMENT		
Obtains SAMPLE history		
Obtains OPQRST for differential diagnosis		
Obtains associated symptoms, pertinent negatives/denials		
Evaluates decision to perform focused exam or completes rapid assessment		*
Vital signs including AVPU (and GCS if trauma)		*
Assesses cardiovascular system including heart sounds, peripheral edema, and peripheral perfusion		*
Assesses pulmonary system including reassessing airway, ventilation, breath sounds, pulse oximetry, chest wall excursion, accessory muscle use, or other signs of distress		*
Assesses neurological system including speech, droop, drift, if applicable, and distal movement and sensation		*
Assesses musculoskeletal and integumentary systems		
Assesses behavioral, psychological, and social aspects of patient and situation		
States field impression of patient—pulmonary edema (verbalizes common cause of pulmonary edema is AMI)		*
Verbalizes treatment plan for patient and calls for appropriate intervention(s)—NTG, Lasix, Morphine, CPAP, PPV		*
Reevaluates transport decision		
ONGOING ASSESSMENT		
Repeats initial assessment		*
Repeats vital signs and evaluates trends		*
Evaluates response to treatments		*
Repeats focused assessment regarding patient complaint or injuries		
Gives radio report to receiving facility		
Turns over patient care with verbal report		*
Student exhibits competence with skill		

Any items in the Not Done column that are marked with an * are mandatory for the student to complete. A check mark in the Not Done column of an item with an * indicates that the student was unsuccessful and must attempt the skill again to assure competency. Examiners should use a different-color ink for the second attempt.

☐ Successful   ☐ Unsuccessful   Examiner Initials: _____

Scenario Intubation—Pulmonary Edema

Student: _____   Examiner: _____

Date: _____

	Done ✓	Not Done
Assesses scene safety and utilizes appropriate PPE		*
Manually opens the airway with technique appropriate for patient condition		*
Checks mouth for blood or potential airway obstruction		*
Suctions or removes loose teeth or foreign materials as needed		
Inserts simple adjunct (oropharyngeal or nasopharyngeal airway)		
Directs assistant to ventilate patient with bag-valve-mask device (room air)		*
Observes chest rise/fall and auscultates bilaterally over lungs for baseline		*
Obtains effective ventilation in less than 30 seconds		*
Attaches oxygen reservoir to bag-valve-mask device and connects to high-flow oxygen		
Ventilates patient and evaluates chest wall/lung compliance		*
Directs assistant to preoxygenate patient		*
Identifies/selects proper equipment for intubation		
Checks laryngoscope light and cuff of ET tube		
Removes all air from cuff and properly inserts stylet if used		
Removes airway adjunct		
Positions patient's head properly and has assistant perform Sellick's maneuver		*
Opens mouth and gently inserts blade while sweeping tongue to side		*
Has assistant maintain Sellick's pressure		
Gently elevates mandible with laryngoscope and visualizes cords		*
Introduces ET tube to side of blade and visualizes tube passing through cords		*
"Threads" ET tube off stylet (if used), maintaining hold on ET tube as stylet removed		
Inflates cuff to proper pressure and disconnects syringe		*
Disconnects mask from bag-valve device and attaches to ET tube without releasing ET tube		
Directs ventilation of patient while maintaining Sellick's maneuver and holding ET tube in place		
Confirms proper placement by auscultation over epigastrium and bilaterally over each lung		*
Directs assistant to release cricoid pressure		*
Secures ET tube		*
Reassesses bilateral lung sounds and compliance		*
Uses secondary device to confirm tube placement		*
Assesses patient's response to intervention		*
Student exhibits competence with skill		

Any items in the Not Done column that are marked with an * are mandatory for the student to complete. A check mark in the Not Done column of an item with an * indicates that the student was unsuccessful and must attempt the skill again to assure competency. Examiners should use a different-color ink for the second attempt.

☐ Successful   ☐ Unsuccessful   Examiner Initials: _____

©2006 Prentice-Hall Inc.

Scenario Radio Report—Pulmonary Edema

Student: _____   **Examiner:** _____

Date: _____

	Done ✓	Not Done
Requests and checks for open channel before speaking		
Presses transmit button 1 second before speaking		
Holds microphone 2–3 in. from mouth		
Speaks slowly and clearly		*
Speaks in a normal voice		
Briefly transmits: Agency, unit designation, identification/name		*
Briefly transmits: Patient's age, sex, weight		*
Briefly transmits: Scene description/mechanism of injury or medical problem		*
Briefly transmits: Chief complaint with brief history of *present* illness		*
Briefly transmits: Associated symptoms (unless able to be deferred to bedside report)		
Briefly transmits: Past medical history (usually deferred to bedside report)		
Briefly transmits: Vital signs	*	*
Briefly transmits: Level of consciousness/GCS on trauma		*
Briefly transmits: General appearance, distress, cardiac rhythm, blood glucose, and other pertinent findings unable to be deferred to bedside report		
Briefly transmits: Interventions by EMS AND response(s)		*
ETA (the more critical the patient, the earlier you need to notify the receiving facility)		
Does not waste airtime		
Protects privacy of patient		*
Echoes dispatch information and any physician orders		*
Writes down dispatch information or physician orders		
Confirms with facility that message is received		
Demonstrates/verbalizes ability to troubleshoot basic equipment malfunction		
Student exhibits competence with skill		

Any items in the Not Done column that are marked with an * are mandatory for the student to complete. A check mark in the Not Done column of an item with an * indicates that the student was unsuccessful and must attempt the skill again to assure competency. Examiners should use a different-color ink for the second attempt.

☐ Successful   ☐ Unsuccessful   Examiner Initials: _____

©2006 Prentice-Hall Inc.

Scenario Patient Care Report (PCR)—Pulmonary Edema

Student: _____   Examiner: _____

Date: _____

	Done ✓	Not Done
Records all pertinent dispatch/scene data, using a consistent format		
Completely identifies all additional resources and personnel		
Documents chief complaint, signs/symptoms, position found, age, sex, and weight		
Identifies and records all pertinent, reportable clinical data for each patient		
Documents SAMPLE and OPQRST if applicable		
Records all pertinent negatives		
Records all pertinent denials		
Records accurate, consistent times and patient information		
Includes relevant oral statements of witnesses, bystanders, and patient in "quotes" when appropriate		
Documents initial assessment findings: airway, breathing, and circulation		
Documents any interventions in initial assessment with patient response		
Documents level of consciousness, GCS (if trauma), and VS		
Documents rapid trauma assessment if applicable		
Documents any interventions in rapid trauma assessment with patient response		
Documents focused history and physical assessment		
Documents any interventions in focused assessment with patient response		
Documents repeat VS (every 5 minutes for critical; every 15 minutes for stable)		
Repeats initial assessment and documents findings		
Records ALL treatments with times and patient response(s) in treatment section		
Documents field impression		
Documents transport to specific facility and transfer of care WITH VERBAL REPORT		
Uses correct grammar, abbreviations, spelling, and terminology		
Writes legibly		
Thoroughly documents refusals, denials of transport, and call cancellations		
Documents patient GCS of 15 PRIOR to signing refusal		
Documents advice given to refusal patient, including "call 9-1-1 for further problems"		
Properly corrects errors and omissions		
Writes cautiously, avoids jargon, opinions, inferences, or any derogatory/libelous remarks		
Signs run report		
Uses EMS supplement form if needed		
Student exhibits competence with skill		

Any items in the Not Done column should be evaluated with student. Check marks in this column do not necessarily mean student was unsuccessful as all lines are not completed on all patients. Evaluation of each PCR should be based on the scenario given.

Student must be able to write an EMS report with consistency and accuracy.

☐ Successful   ☐ Unsuccessful   Examiner Initials: _____

Overall Scenario Management—Pulmonary Edema

Student: _____   Examiner: _____

Date: _____   Scenario: _____

NOTE: This skill sheet is to be done after the student completes a scenario as the **TEAM LEADER.** It is to let the student know if he or she is beginning to "put it all together" and use critical thinking skills to manage an EMS call. PLEASE notice that it is graded on a different basis than the basic lab skill sheet.

	Done ✓	Needs to Improve
SCENE MANAGEMENT		
Recognized hazards and controlled scene—safety, crowd, and patient issues		
Recognized hazards, but did not control the scene		
Unsuccessfully attempted to manage the scene	*	
Did not evaluate the scene and took no control of the scene	*	
PATIENT ASSESSMENT		
Performed a timely, organized complete patient assessment		
Performed complete initial, focused, and ongoing assessments, but in a disorganized manner		
Performed an incomplete assessment	*	
Did not perform an initial assessment	*	
PATIENT MANAGEMENT		
Evaluated assessment findings to manage all aspects of patient condition		
Managed the patient's presenting signs and symptoms without considering all of assessment		
Inadequately managed the patient	*	
Did not manage life-threatening conditions	*	
COMMUNICATION		
Communicated well with crew, patient, family, bystanders, and assisting agencies		
Communicated well with patient and crew		
Communicated with patient and crew, but poor communication skills	*	
Unable to communicate effectively	*	
REPORT AND TRANSFER OF CARE		
Identified correct destination for patient transport, gave accurate, brief report over radio, and provided full report at bedside demonstrating thorough understanding of patient condition and pathophysiological processes		
Identified correct destination and gave accurate radio and bedside report, but did not demonstrate understanding of patient condition and pathophysiological processes		
Identified correct destination, but provided inadequate radio and bedside report	*	
Identified inappropriate destination or provided no radio or bedside report	*	
Student exhibits competence with skill		

Any items that are marked with an * indicate the student needs to improve and a check mark should be placed in the right-hand column. A check mark in the right-hand column indicates that the student was unsuccessful and must attempt the skill again to assure competency. Examiners should use a different-color ink for the second attempt.

☐ Successful   ☐ Unsuccessful   Examiner Initials: _____

©2006 Prentice-Hall Inc.

Patient Assessment: Cardiology—Renal Dialysis Code

Student: _____   Examiner: _____

Date: _____   Scenario: _____

	Done ✓	Not Done
Assesses scene safety and utilizes appropriate PPE		*
OVERALL SCENE EVALUATION		
Medical—determines nature of illness/if trauma involved determines MOI		*
Determines the number of patients, location, obstacles, and requests any additional resources as needed		
Verbalizes general impression of the patient as approaches		*
Considers stabilization/spinal motion restriction of spine if trauma involved		*
INITIAL ASSESSMENT		
Determines responsiveness/level of consciousness/AVPU		*
Opens airway with appropriate technique and assesses airway/ventilation		*
Manages airway/ventilation and applies appropriate oxygen therapy in less than 3 minutes		*
Assesses circulation: radial/carotid pulse, skin color, temperature, condition, and turgor		*
Controls any major bleeding		*
Makes rapid transport decision if indicated		
Initiates IV, obtains BGL, GCS, **12-Lead EKG if not initially in arrest,** and complete vital signs		
FOCUSED HISTORY AND PHYSICAL EXAMINATION/RAPID ASSESSMENT		
Obtains SAMPLE history		
Obtains OPQRST for differential diagnosis		
Obtains associated symptoms, pertinent negatives/denials		
Evaluates decision to perform focused exam or completes rapid assessment		*
Vital signs including AVPU (and GCS if trauma)		*
Assesses cardiovascular system including heart sounds, peripheral edema, and peripheral perfusion		*
Assesses pulmonary system including reassessing airway, ventilation, breath sounds, pulse oximetry, chest wall excursion, accessory muscle use, or other signs of distress		*
Assesses neurological system including speech, droop, drift, if applicable, and distal movement and sensation		*
Assesses musculoskeletal and integumentary systems		
Assesses behavioral, psychological, and social aspects of patient and situation		
States field impression of patient—recognizes RENAL DIALYSIS patient and pathophysiology		*
Verbalizes treatment plan for patient and calls for appropriate intervention(s)—IV, CALCIUM and BICARB, ACLS		*
Reevaluates transport decision		
ONGOING ASSESSMENT		
Repeats initial assessment		*
Repeats vital signs and evaluates trends		*
Evaluates response to treatments		*
Repeats focused assessment regarding patient complaint or injuries		
Gives radio report to receiving facility		
Turns over patient care with verbal report		*
Student exhibits competence with skill		

Any items in the Not Done column that are marked with an * are mandatory for the student to complete. A check mark in the Not Done column of an item with an * indicates that the student was unsuccessful and must attempt the skill again to assure competency. Examiners should use a different-color ink for the second attempt.

☐ Successful   ☐ Unsuccessful   Examiner Initials: _____

Scenario Intubation—Renal Dialysis Code

Student: _____   Examiner: _____

Date: _____

	Done ✓	Not Done
Assesses scene safety and utilizes appropriate PPE		*
Manually opens the airway with technique appropriate for patient condition		*
Checks mouth for blood or potential airway obstruction		*
Suctions or removes loose teeth or foreign materials as needed		
Inserts simple adjunct (oropharyngeal or nasopharyngeal airway)		
Directs assistant to ventilate patient with bag-valve-mask device (room air)		*
Observes chest rise/fall and auscultates bilaterally over lungs for baseline		*
Obtains effective ventilation in less than 30 seconds		*
Attaches oxygen reservoir to bag-valve-mask device and connects to high-flow oxygen		
Ventilates patient and evaluates chest wall/lung compliance		*
Directs assistant to preoxygenate patient		*
Identifies/selects proper equipment for intubation		
Checks laryngoscope light and cuff of ET tube		
Removes all air from cuff and properly inserts stylet if used		
Removes airway adjunct		
Positions patient's head properly and has assistant perform Sellick's maneuver		*
Opens mouth and gently inserts blade while sweeping tongue to side		*
Has assistant maintain Sellick's pressure		
Gently elevates mandible with laryngoscope and visualizes cords		*
Introduces ET tube to side of blade and visualizes tube passing through cords		*
"Threads" ET tube off stylet (if used), maintaining hold on ET tube as stylet removed		
Inflates cuff to proper pressure and disconnects syringe		*
Disconnects mask from bag-valve device and attaches to ET tube without releasing ET tube		
Directs ventilation of patient while maintaining Sellick's maneuver and holding ET tube in place		
Confirms proper placement by auscultation over epigastrium and bilaterally over each lung		*
Directs assistant to release cricoid pressure		*
Secures ET tube		*
Reassesses bilateral lung sounds and compliance		*
Uses secondary device to confirm tube placement		*
Assesses patient's response to intervention		*
Student exhibits competence with skill		

Any items in the Not Done column that are marked with an * are mandatory for the student to complete. A check mark in the Not Done column of an item with an * indicates that the student was unsuccessful and must attempt the skill again to assure competency. Examiners should use a different-color ink for the second attempt.

☐ Successful   ☐ Unsuccessful   Examiner Initials: _____

©2006 Prentice-Hall Inc.

Scenario Radio Report—Renal Dialysis Code

Student: _____   Examiner: _____

Date: _____

	Done ✓	Not Done
Requests and checks for open channel before speaking		
Presses transmit button 1 second before speaking		
Holds microphone 2–3 in. from mouth		
Speaks slowly and clearly		*
Speaks in a normal voice		
Briefly transmits: Agency, unit designation, identification/name		*
Briefly transmits: Patient's age, sex, weight		*
Briefly transmits: Scene description/mechanism of injury or medical problem		*
Briefly transmits: Chief complaint with brief history of *present* illness		*
Briefly transmits: Associated symptoms (unless able to be deferred to bedside report)		
Briefly transmits: Past medical history (usually deferred to bedside report)		
Briefly transmits: Vital signs		*
Briefly transmits: Level of consciousness/GCS on trauma		*
Briefly transmits: General appearance, distress, cardiac rhythm, blood glucose, and other pertinent findings unable to be deferred to bedside report		
Briefly transmits: Interventions by EMS AND response(s)		*
ETA (the more critical the patient, the earlier you need to notify the receiving facility)		
Does not waste airtime		
Protects privacy of patient		*
Echoes dispatch information and any physician orders		*
Writes down dispatch information or physician orders		
Confirms with facility that message is received		
Demonstrates/verbalizes ability to troubleshoot basic equipment malfunction		
Student exhibits competence with skill		

Any items in the Not Done column that are marked with an * are mandatory for the student to complete. A check mark in the Not Done column of an item with an * indicates that the student was unsuccessful and must attempt the skill again to assure competency. Examiners should use a different-color ink for the second attempt.

☐ Successful   ☐ Unsuccessful   Examiner Initials: _____

Scenario Patient Care Report (PCR)—Renal Dialysis Code

Student: _____   Examiner: _____

Date: _____

	Done ✓	Not Done
Records all pertinent dispatch/scene data, using a consistent format		
Completely identifies all additional resources and personnel		
Documents chief complaint, signs/symptoms, position found, age, sex, and weight		
Identifies and records all pertinent, reportable clinical data for each patient		
Documents SAMPLE and OPQRST if applicable		
Records all pertinent negatives		
Records all pertinent denials		
Records accurate, consistent times and patient information		
Includes relevant oral statements of witnesses, bystanders, and patient in "quotes" when appropriate		
Documents initial assessment findings: airway, breathing, and circulation		
Documents any interventions in initial assessment with patient response		
Documents level of consciousness, GCS (if trauma), and VS		
Documents rapid trauma assessment if applicable		
Documents any interventions in rapid trauma assessment with patient response		
Documents focused history and physical assessment		
Documents any interventions in focused assessment with patient response		
Documents repeat VS (every 5 minutes for critical; every 15 minutes for stable)		
Repeats initial assessment and documents findings		
Records ALL treatments with times and patient response(s) in treatment section		
Documents field impression		
Documents transport to specific facility and transfer of care WITH VERBAL REPORT		
Uses correct grammar, abbreviations, spelling, and terminology		
Writes legibly		
Thoroughly documents refusals, denials of transport, and call cancellations		
Documents patient GCS of 15 PRIOR to signing refusal		
Documents advice given to refusal patient, including "call 9-1-1 for further problems"		
Properly corrects errors and omissions		
Writes cautiously, avoids jargon, opinions, inferences, or any derogatory/libelous remarks		
Signs run report		
Uses EMS supplement form if needed		
Student exhibits competence with skill		

Any items in the Not Done column should be evaluated with student. Check marks in this column do not necessarily mean student was unsuccessful as all lines are not completed on all patients. Evaluation of each PCR should be based on the scenario given.

Student must be able to write an EMS report with consistency and accuracy.

☐ Successful   ☐ Unsuccessful   Examiner Initials: _____

©2006 Prentice-Hall Inc.

Overall Scenario Management—Renal Dialysis Code

Student: _____   Examiner: _____

Date: _____   Scenario: _____

NOTE: This skill sheet is to be done after the student completes a scenario as the **TEAM LEADER**. It is to let the student know if he or she is beginning to "put it all together" and use critical thinking skills to manage an EMS call. PLEASE notice that it is graded on a different basis than the basic lab skill sheet.

	Done ✓	Needs to Improve
SCENE MANAGEMENT		
Recognized hazards and controlled scene—safety, crowd, and patient issues		
Recognized hazards, but did not control the scene		
Unsuccessfully attempted to manage the scene	*	
Did not evaluate the scene and took no control of the scene	*	
PATIENT ASSESSMENT		
Performed a timely, organized complete patient assessment		
Performed complete initial, focused, and ongoing assessments, but in a disorganized manner		
Performed an incomplete assessment	*	
Did not perform an initial assessment	*	
PATIENT MANAGEMENT		
Evaluated assessment findings to manage all aspects of patient condition		
Managed the patient's presenting signs and symptoms without considering all of assessment		
Inadequately managed the patient	*	
Did not manage life-threatening conditions	*	
COMMUNICATION		
Communicated well with crew, patient, family, bystanders, and assisting agencies		
Communicated well with patient and crew		
Communicated with patient and crew, but poor communication skills	*	
Unable to communicate effectively	*	
REPORT AND TRANSFER OF CARE		
Identified correct destination for patient transport, gave accurate, brief report over radio, and provided full report at bedside demonstrating thorough understanding of patient condition and pathophysiological processes		
Identified correct destination and gave accurate radio and bedside report, but did not demonstrate understanding of patient condition and pathophysiological processes		
Identified correct destination, but provided inadequate radio and bedside report	*	
Identified inappropriate destination or provided no radio or bedside report	*	
Student exhibits competence with skill		

Any items that are marked with an * indicate the student needs to improve and a check mark should be placed in the right-hand column. A check mark in the right-hand column indicates that the student was unsuccessful and must attempt the skill again to assure competency. Examiners
should use a different-color ink for the second attempt.

☐ Successful   ☐ Unsuccessful   Examiner Initials: _____

©2006 Prentice-Hall Inc.

Patient Assessment: Cardiology—Stable Tachycardia

Student: _____   Examiner: _____

Date: _____   Scenario: _____

	Done ✓	Not Done
Assesses scene safety and utilizes appropriate PPE		*
OVERALL SCENE EVALUATION		
Medical—determines nature of illness/if trauma involved determines MOI		*
Determines the number of patients, location, obstacles, and requests any additional resources as needed		
Verbalizes general impression of the patient as approaches		*
Considers stabilization/spinal motion restriction of spine if trauma involved		*
INITIAL ASSESSMENT		
Determines responsiveness/level of consciousness/AVPU		*
Opens airway with appropriate technique and assesses airway/ventilation		*
Manages airway/ventilation and applies appropriate oxygen therapy in less than 3 minutes		*
Assesses circulation: radial/carotid pulse, skin color, temperature, condition, and turgor		*
Controls any major bleeding		*
Makes rapid transport decision if indicated		
Initiates IV, obtains BGL, GCS, **12-Lead EKG,** and complete vital signs		
FOCUSED HISTORY AND PHYSICAL EXAMINATION/RAPID ASSESSMENT		
Obtains SAMPLE history		
Obtains OPQRST for differential diagnosis		
Obtains associated symptoms, pertinent negatives/denials		
Evaluates decision to perform focused exam or completes rapid assessment		*
Vital signs including AVPU (and GCS if trauma)		*
Assesses cardiovascular system including heart sounds, peripheral edema, and peripheral perfusion		*
Assesses pulmonary system including reassessing airway, ventilation, breath sounds, pulse oximetry, chest wall excursion, accessory muscle use, or other signs of distress		*
Assesses neurological system including speech, droop, drift, if applicable, and distal movement and sensation		*
Assesses musculoskeletal and integumentary systems		
Assesses behavioral, psychological, and social aspects of patient and situation		
States field impression of patient—STABLE tachycardia		*
Verbalizes treatment plan for patient and calls for appropriate intervention(s)—IV, vagal, look for cause, follow ACLS		*
Reevaluates transport decision		
ONGOING ASSESSMENT		
Repeats initial assessment		*
Repeats vital signs and evaluates trends		*
Evaluates response to treatments		*
Repeats focused assessment regarding patient complaint or injuries		
Gives radio report to receiving facility		
Turns over patient care with verbal report		*
Student exhibits competence with skill		

Any items in the Not Done column that are marked with an * are mandatory for the student to complete. A check mark in the Not Done column of an item with an * indicates that the student was unsuccessful and must attempt the skill again to assure competency. Examiners should use a different-color ink for the second attempt.

☐ Successful   ☐ Unsuccessful   Examiner Initials: _____

©2006 Prentice-Hall Inc.

Scenario Radio Report—Stable Tachycardia

Student: _____   **Examiner:** _____

Date: _____

	Done ✓	Not Done
Requests and checks for open channel before speaking		
Presses transmit button 1 second before speaking		
Holds microphone 2–3 in. from mouth		
Speaks slowly and clearly		*
Speaks in a normal voice		
Briefly transmits: Agency, unit designation, identification/name		*
Briefly transmits: Patient's age, sex, weight		*
Briefly transmits: Scene description/mechanism of injury or medical problem		*
Briefly transmits: Chief complaint with brief history of *present* illness		*
Briefly transmits: Associated symptoms (unless able to be deferred to bedside report)		
Briefly transmits: Past medical history (usually deferred to bedside report)		
Briefly transmits: Vital signs		*
Briefly transmits: Level of consciousness/GCS on trauma		*
Briefly transmits: General appearance, distress, cardiac rhythm, blood glucose, and other pertinent findings unable to be deferred to bedside report		
Briefly transmits: Interventions by EMS AND response(s)		*
ETA (the more critical the patient, the earlier you need to notify the receiving facility)		
Does not waste airtime		
Protects privacy of patient		*
Echoes dispatch information and any physician orders		*
Writes down dispatch information or physician orders		
Confirms with facility that message is received		
Demonstrates/verbalizes ability to troubleshoot basic equipment malfunction		
Student exhibits competence with skill		

Any items in the Not Done column that are marked with an * are mandatory for the student to complete. A check mark in the Not Done column of an item with an * indicates that the student was unsuccessful and must attempt the skill again to assure competency. Examiners should use a different-color ink for the second attempt.

☐ Successful   ☐ Unsuccessful   Examiner Initials: _____

Scenario Patient Care Report (PCR)—Stable Tachycardia

Student: _____   Examiner: _____

Date: _____

	Done ✓	Not Done
Records all pertinent dispatch/scene data, using a consistent format		
Completely identifies all additional resources and personnel		
Documents chief complaint, signs/symptoms, position found, age, sex, and weight		
Identifies and records all pertinent, reportable clinical data for each patient		
Documents SAMPLE and OPQRST if applicable		
Records all pertinent negatives		
Records all pertinent denials		
Records accurate, consistent times and patient information		
Includes relevant oral statements of witnesses, bystanders, and patient in "quotes" when appropriate		
Documents initial assessment findings: airway, breathing, and circulation		
Documents any interventions in initial assessment with patient response		
Documents level of consciousness, GCS (if trauma), and VS		
Documents rapid trauma assessment if applicable		
Documents any interventions in rapid trauma assessment with patient response		
Documents focused history and physical assessment		
Documents any interventions in focused assessment with patient response		
Documents repeat VS (every 5 minutes for critical; every 15 minutes for stable)		
Repeats initial assessment and documents findings		
Records ALL treatments with times and patient response(s) in treatment section		
Documents field impression		
Documents transport to specific facility and transfer of care WITH VERBAL REPORT		
Uses correct grammar, abbreviations, spelling, and terminology		
Writes legibly		
Thoroughly documents refusals, denials of transport, and call cancellations		
Documents patient GCS of 15 PRIOR to signing refusal		
Documents advice given to refusal patient, including "call 9-1-1 for further problems"		
Properly corrects errors and omissions		
Writes cautiously, avoids jargon, opinions, inferences, or any derogatory/libelous remarks		
Signs run report		
Uses EMS supplement form if needed		
Student exhibits competence with skill		

Any items in the Not Done column should be evaluated with student. Check marks in this column do not necessarily mean student was unsuccessful as all lines are not completed on all patients. Evaluation of each PCR should be based on the scenario given.

Student must be able to write an EMS report with consistency and accuracy.

☐ Successful   ☐ Unsuccessful   Examiner Initials: _____

©2006 Prentice-Hall Inc.

Overall Scenario Management—Stable Tachycardia

Student: _____   Examiner: _____

Date: _____   Scenario: _____

NOTE: This skill sheet is to be done after the student completes a scenario as the **TEAM LEADER.** It is to let the student know if he or she is beginning to "put it all together" and use critical thinking skills to manage an EMS call. PLEASE notice that it is graded on a different basis than the basic lab skill sheet.

	Done ✓	Needs to Improve
SCENE MANAGEMENT		
Recognized hazards and controlled scene—safety, crowd, and patient issues		
Recognized hazards, but did not control the scene		
Unsuccessfully attempted to manage the scene	*	
Did not evaluate the scene and took no control of the scene	*	
PATIENT ASSESSMENT		
Performed a timely, organized complete patient assessment		
Performed complete initial, focused, and ongoing assessments, but in a disorganized manner		
Performed an incomplete assessment	*	
Did not perform an initial assessment	*	
PATIENT MANAGEMENT		
Evaluated assessment findings to manage all aspects of patient condition		
Managed the patient's presenting signs and symptoms without considering all of assessment		
Inadequately managed the patient	*	
Did not manage life-threatening conditions	*	
COMMUNICATION		
Communicated well with crew, patient, family, bystanders, and assisting agencies		
Communicated well with patient and crew		
Communicated with patient and crew, but poor communication skills	*	
Unable to communicate effectively	*	
REPORT AND TRANSFER OF CARE		
Identified correct destination for patient transport, gave accurate, brief report over radio, and provided full report at bedside demonstrating thorough understanding of patient condition and pathophysiological processes		
Identified correct destination and gave accurate radio and bedside report, but did not demonstrate understanding of patient condition and pathophysiological processes		
Identified correct destination, but provided inadequate radio and bedside report	*	
Identified inappropriate destination or provided no radio or bedside report	*	
Student exhibits competence with skill		

Any items that are marked with an * indicate the student needs to improve and a check mark should be placed in the right-hand column. A check mark in the right-hand column indicates that the student was unsuccessful and must attempt the skill again to assure competency. Examiners should use a different-color ink for the second attempt.

☐ Successful   ☐ Unsuccessful   Examiner Initials: _____

Patient Assessment: Cardiology—Syncope

Student: _____   Examiner: _____

Date: _____   Scenario: _____

	Done ✓	Not Done
Assesses scene safety and utilizes appropriate PPE		*
OVERALL SCENE EVALUATION		
Medical—determines nature of illness/if trauma involved determines MOI		*
Determines the number of patients, location, obstacles, and requests any additional resources as needed		
Verbalizes general impression of the patient as approaches		*
Considers stabilization/spinal motion restriction of spine if trauma involved		*
INITIAL ASSESSMENT		
Determines responsiveness/level of consciousness/AVPU		*
Opens airway with appropriate technique and assesses airway/ventilation		*
Manages airway/ventilation and applies appropriate oxygen therapy in less than 3 minutes		*
Assesses circulation: radial/carotid pulse, skin color, temperature, condition, and turgor		*
Controls any major bleeding		*
Makes rapid transport decision if indicated		
Initiates IV, obtains BGL, GCS, **12-Lead EKG,** and complete vital signs		
FOCUSED HISTORY AND PHYSICAL EXAMINATION/RAPID ASSESSMENT		
Obtains SAMPLE history		
Obtains OPQRST for differential diagnosis		
Obtains associated symptoms, pertinent negatives/denials		
Evaluates decision to perform focused exam or completes rapid assessment		*
Vital signs including AVPU (and GCS if trauma)		*
Assesses cardiovascular system including heart sounds, peripheral edema, and peripheral perfusion		*
Assesses pulmonary system including reassessing airway, ventilation, breath sounds, pulse oximetry, chest wall excursion, accessory muscle use, or other signs of distress		*
Assesses neurological system including speech, droop, drift, if applicable, and distal movement and sensation		*
Assesses musculoskeletal and integumentary systems		
Assesses behavioral, psychological, and social aspects of patient and situation		
States field impression of patient—syncope (must consider cardiac origin until proven otherwise)		*
Verbalizes treatment plan for patient and calls for appropriate intervention(s)—IV, monitor, treat patient per ACLS		*
Reevaluates transport decision		
ONGOING ASSESSMENT		
Repeats initial assessment		*
Repeats vital signs and evaluates trends		*
Evaluates response to treatments		*
Repeats focused assessment regarding patient complaint or injuries		
Gives radio report to receiving facility		
Turns over patient care with verbal report		*
Student exhibits competence with skill		

Any items in the Not Done column that are marked with an * are mandatory for the student to complete. A check mark in the Not Done column of an item with an * indicates that the student was unsuccessful and must attempt the skill again to assure competency. Examiners should use a different-color ink for the second attempt.

☐ Successful   ☐ Unsuccessful   Examiner Initials: _____

©2006 Prentice-Hall Inc.

Scenario Radio Report—Syncope

Student: _____   **Examiner:** _____

Date: _____

	Done ✓	Not Done
Requests and checks for open channel before speaking		
Presses transmit button 1 second before speaking		
Holds microphone 2–3 in. from mouth		
Speaks slowly and clearly		*
Speaks in a normal voice		
Briefly transmits: Agency, unit designation, identification/name		*
Briefly transmits: Patient's age, sex, weight		*
Briefly transmits: Scene description/mechanism of injury or medical problem		*
Briefly transmits: Chief complaint with brief history of *present* illness		*
Briefly transmits: Associated symptoms (unless able to be deferred to bedside report)		
Briefly transmits: Past medical history (usually deferred to bedside report)		
Briefly transmits: Vital signs		*
Briefly transmits: Level of consciousness/GCS on trauma		*
Briefly transmits: General appearance, distress, cardiac rhythm, blood glucose, and other pertinent findings unable to be deferred to bedside report		
Briefly transmits: Interventions by EMS AND response(s)		*
ETA (the more critical the patient, the earlier you need to notify the receiving facility)		
Does not waste airtime		
Protects privacy of patient		*
Echoes dispatch information and any physician orders		*
Writes down dispatch information or physician orders		
Confirms with facility that message is received		
Demonstrates/verbalizes ability to troubleshoot basic equipment malfunction		
Student exhibits competence with skill		

Any items in the Not Done column that are marked with an * are mandatory for the student to complete. A check mark in the Not Done column of an item with an * indicates that the student was unsuccessful and must attempt the skill again to assure competency. Examiners should use a different-color ink for the second attempt.

☐ Successful   ☐ Unsuccessful   Examiner Initials: _____

Scenario Patient Care Report (PCR)—Syncope

Student: _____   Examiner: _____

Date: _____

	Done ✓	Not Done
Records all pertinent dispatch/scene data, using a consistent format		
Completely identifies all additional resources and personnel		
Documents chief complaint, signs/symptoms, position found, age, sex, and weight		
Identifies and records all pertinent, reportable clinical data for each patient		
Documents SAMPLE and OPQRST if applicable		
Records all pertinent negatives		
Records all pertinent denials		
Records accurate, consistent times and patient information		
Includes relevant oral statements of witnesses, bystanders, and patient in "quotes" when appropriate		
Documents initial assessment findings: airway, breathing, and circulation		
Documents any interventions in initial assessment with patient response		
Documents level of consciousness, GCS (if trauma), and VS		
Documents rapid trauma assessment if applicable		
Documents any interventions in rapid trauma assessment with patient response		
Documents focused history and physical assessment		
Documents any interventions in focused assessment with patient response		
Documents repeat VS (every 5 minutes for critical; every 15 minutes for stable)		
Repeats initial assessment and documents findings		
Records ALL treatments with times and patient response(s) in treatment section		
Documents field impression		
Documents transport to specific facility and transfer of care WITH VERBAL REPORT		
Uses correct grammar, abbreviations, spelling, and terminology		
Writes legibly		
Thoroughly documents refusals, denials of transport, and call cancellations		
Documents patient GCS of 15 PRIOR to signing refusal		
Documents advice given to refusal patient, including "call 9-1-1 for further problems"		
Properly corrects errors and omissions		
Writes cautiously, avoids jargon, opinions, inferences, or any derogatory/libelous remarks		
Signs run report		
Uses EMS supplement form if needed		
Student exhibits competence with skill		

Any items in the Not Done column should be evaluated with student. Check marks in this column do not necessarily mean student was unsuccessful as all lines are not completed on all patients. Evaluation of each PCR should be based on the scenario given.

Student must be able to write an EMS report with consistency and accuracy.

☐ Successful   ☐ Unsuccessful   Examiner Initials: _____

©2006 Prentice-Hall Inc.

Overall Scenario Management—Syncope

Student: _____ Examiner: _____

Date: _____ Scenario: _____

NOTE: This skill sheet is to be done after the student completes a scenario as the TEAM LEADER. It is to let the student know if he or she is beginning to "put it all together" and use critical thinking skills to manage an EMS call. PLEASE notice that it is graded on a different basis than the basic lab skill sheet.

	Done ✓	Needs to Improve
SCENE MANAGEMENT		
Recognized hazards and controlled scene—safety, crowd, and patient issues		
Recognized hazards, but did not control the scene		
Unsuccessfully attempted to manage the scene	*	
Did not evaluate the scene and took no control of the scene	*	
PATIENT ASSESSMENT		
Performed a timely, organized complete patient assessment		
Performed complete initial, focused, and ongoing assessments, but in a disorganized manner		
Performed an incomplete assessment	*	
Did not perform an initial assessment	*	
PATIENT MANAGEMENT		
Evaluated assessment findings to manage all aspects of patient condition		
Managed the patient's presenting signs and symptoms without considering all of assessment		
Inadequately managed the patient	*	
Did not manage life-threatening conditions	*	
COMMUNICATION		
Communicated well with crew, patient, family, bystanders, and assisting agencies		
Communicated well with patient and crew		
Communicated with patient and crew, but poor communication skills	*	
Unable to communicate effectively	*	
REPORT AND TRANSFER OF CARE		
Identified correct destination for patient transport, gave accurate, brief report over radio, and provided full report at bedside demonstrating thorough understanding of patient condition and pathophysiological processes		
Identified correct destination and gave accurate radio and bedside report, but did not demonstrate understanding of patient condition and pathophysiological processes		
Identified correct destination, but provided inadequate radio and bedside report	*	
Identified inappropriate destination or provided no radio or bedside report	*	
Student exhibits competence with skill		

Any items that are marked with an * indicate the student needs to improve and a check mark should be placed in the right-hand column. A check mark in the right-hand column indicates that the student was unsuccessful and must attempt the skill again to assure competency. Examiners should use a different-color ink for the second attempt.

☐ Successful ☐ Unsuccessful Examiner Initials: _____

©2006 Prentice-Hall Inc.

Patient Assessment: Cardiology—Unstable Tachycardia

Student: _____   Examiner: _____

Date: _____   Scenario: _____

	Done ✓	Not Done *
Assesses scene safety and utilizes appropriate PPE		*
OVERALL SCENE EVALUATION		
Medical—determines nature of illness/if trauma involved determines MOI		*
Determines the number of patients, location, obstacles, and requests any additional resources as needed		
Verbalizes general impression of the patient as approaches		*
Considers stabilization/spinal motion restriction of spine if trauma involved		*
INITIAL ASSESSMENT		
Determines responsiveness/level of consciousness/AVPU		*
Opens airway with appropriate technique and assesses airway/ventilation		*
Manages airway/ventilation and applies appropriate oxygen therapy in less than 3 minutes		*
Assesses circulation: radial/carotid pulse, skin color, temperature, condition, and turgor		*
Controls any major bleeding		*
Makes rapid transport decision if indicated		
Initiates IV, obtains BGL, GCS, **12-Lead EKG,** and complete vital signs		
FOCUSED HISTORY AND PHYSICAL EXAMINATION/RAPID ASSESSMENT		
Obtains SAMPLE history		
Obtains OPQRST for differential diagnosis		
Obtains associated symptoms, pertinent negatives/denials		
Evaluates decision to perform focused exam or completes rapid assessment		*
Vital signs including AVPU (and GCS if trauma)		*
Assesses cardiovascular system including heart sounds, peripheral edema, and peripheral perfusion		*
Assesses pulmonary system including reassessing airway, ventilation, breath sounds, pulse oximetry, chest wall excursion, accessory muscle use, or other signs of distress		*
Assesses neurological system including speech, droop, drift, if applicable, and distal movement and sensation		*
Assesses musculoskeletal and integumentary systems		
Assesses behavioral, psychological, and social aspects of patient and situation		
States field impression of patient—UNSTABLE tachycardia		*
Verbalizes treatment plan for patient and calls for appropriate intervention(s)—IV, treat per current ACLS		*
Reevaluates transport decision		
ONGOING ASSESSMENT		
Repeats initial assessment		*
Repeats vital signs and evaluates trends		*
Evaluates response to treatments		*
Repeats focused assessment regarding patient complaint or injuries		
Gives radio report to receiving facility		
Turns over patient care with verbal report		*
Student exhibits competence with skill		

Any items in the Not Done column that are marked with an * are mandatory for the student to complete. A check mark in the Not Done column of an item with an * indicates that the student was unsuccessful and must attempt the skill again to assure competency. Examiners should use a different-color ink for the second attempt.

☐ Successful   ☐ Unsuccessful   Examiner Initials: _____

©2006 Prentice-Hall Inc.

Scenario Radio Report—Unstable Tachycardia

Student: _____   Examiner: _____

Date: _____

	Done ✓	Not Done
Requests and checks for open channel before speaking		
Presses transmit button 1 second before speaking		
Holds microphone 2–3 in. from mouth		
Speaks slowly and clearly		*
Speaks in a normal voice		
Briefly transmits: Agency, unit designation, identification/name		*
Briefly transmits: Patient's age, sex, weight		*
Briefly transmits: Scene description/mechanism of injury or medical problem		*
Briefly transmits: Chief complaint with brief history of *present* illness		*
Briefly transmits: Associated symptoms (unless able to be deferred to bedside report)		
Briefly transmits: Past medical history (usually deferred to bedside report)		
Briefly transmits: Vital signs		*
Briefly transmits: Level of consciousness/GCS on trauma		*
Briefly transmits: General appearance, distress, cardiac rhythm, blood glucose, and other pertinent findings unable to be deferred to bedside report		
Briefly transmits: Interventions by EMS AND response(s)		*
ETA (the more critical the patient, the earlier you need to notify the receiving facility)		
Does not waste airtime		
Protects privacy of patient		*
Echoes dispatch information and any physician orders		*
Writes down dispatch information or physician orders		
Confirms with facility that message is received		
Demonstrates/verbalizes ability to troubleshoot basic equipment malfunction		
Student exhibits competence with skill		

Any items in the Not Done column that are marked with an * are mandatory for the student to complete. A check mark in the Not Done column of an item with an * indicates that the student was unsuccessful and must attempt the skill again to assure competency. Examiners should use a different-color ink for the second attempt.

☐ Successful   ☐ Unsuccessful   Examiner Initials: _____

Scenario Patient Care Report (PCR)—Unstable Tachycardia

Student: _____   Examiner: _____

Date: _____

	Done ✓	Not Done
Records all pertinent dispatch/scene data, using a consistent format		
Completely identifies all additional resources and personnel		
Documents chief complaint, signs/symptoms, position found, age, sex, and weight		
Identifies and records all pertinent, reportable clinical data for each patient		
Documents SAMPLE and OPQRST if applicable		
Records all pertinent negatives		
Records all pertinent denials		
Records accurate, consistent times and patient information		
Includes relevant oral statements of witnesses, bystanders, and patient in "quotes" when appropriate		
Documents initial assessment findings: airway, breathing, and circulation		
Documents any interventions in initial assessment with patient response		
Documents level of consciousness, GCS (if trauma), and VS		
Documents rapid trauma assessment if applicable		
Documents any interventions in rapid trauma assessment with patient response		
Documents focused history and physical assessment		
Documents any interventions in focused assessment with patient response		
Documents repeat VS (every 5 minutes for critical; every 15 minutes for stable)		
Repeats initial assessment and documents findings		
Records ALL treatments with times and patient response(s) in treatment section		
Documents field impression		
Documents transport to specific facility and transfer of care WITH VERBAL REPORT		
Uses correct grammar, abbreviations, spelling, and terminology		
Writes legibly		
Thoroughly documents refusals, denials of transport, and call cancellations		
Documents patient GCS of 15 PRIOR to signing refusal		
Documents advice given to refusal patient, including "call 9-1-1 for further problems"		
Properly corrects errors and omissions		
Writes cautiously, avoids jargon, opinions, inferences, or any derogatory/libelous remarks		
Signs run report		
Uses EMS supplement form if needed		
Student exhibits competence with skill		

Any items in the Not Done column should be evaluated with student. Check marks in this column do not necessarily mean student was unsuccessful as all lines are not completed on all patients. Evaluation of each PCR should be based on the scenario given.

Student must be able to write an EMS report with consistency and accuracy.

☐ Successful   ☐ Unsuccessful   Examiner Initials: _____

©2006 Prentice-Hall Inc.

Overall Scenario Management—Unstable Tachycardia

Student: _____   Examiner: _____

Date: _____   Scenario: _____

NOTE: This skill sheet is to be done after the student completes a scenario as the TEAM LEADER. It is to let the student know if he or she is beginning to "put it all together" and use critical thinking skills to manage an EMS call. PLEASE notice that it is graded on a different basis than the basic lab skill sheet.

	Done ✓	Needs to Improve
SCENE MANAGEMENT		
Recognized hazards and controlled scene—safety, crowd, and patient issues		
Recognized hazards, but did not control the scene		
Unsuccessfully attempted to manage the scene	*	
Did not evaluate the scene and took no control of the scene	*	
PATIENT ASSESSMENT		
Performed a timely, organized complete patient assessment		
Performed complete initial, focused, and ongoing assessments, but in a disorganized manner		
Performed an incomplete assessment	*	
Did not perform an initial assessment	*	
PATIENT MANAGEMENT		
Evaluated assessment findings to manage all aspects of patient condition		
Managed the patient's presenting signs and symptoms without considering all of assessment		
Inadequately managed the patient	*	
Did not manage life-threatening conditions	*	
COMMUNICATION		
Communicated well with crew, patient, family, bystanders, and assisting agencies		
Communicated well with patient and crew		
Communicated with patient and crew, but poor communication skills	*	
Unable to communicate effectively	*	
REPORT AND TRANSFER OF CARE		
Identified correct destination for patient transport, gave accurate, brief report over radio, and provided full report at bedside demonstrating thorough understanding of patient condition and pathophysiological processes		
Identified correct destination and gave accurate radio and bedside report, but did not demonstrate understanding of patient condition and pathophysiological processes		
Identified correct destination, but provided inadequate radio and bedside report	*	
Identified inappropriate destination or provided no radio or bedside report	*	
Student exhibits competence with skill		

Any items that are marked with an * indicate the student needs to improve and a check mark should be placed in the right-hand column. A check mark in the right-hand column indicates that the student was unsuccessful and must attempt the skill again to assure competency. Examiners should use a different-color ink for the second attempt.

☐ Successful   ☐ Unsuccessful   Examiner Initials: _____

©2006 Prentice-Hall Inc.

DAILY DISCUSSIONS AND PERTINENT POINTS—CARDIOLOGY

Student: _____   **Date:** _____

Instructor: _____

	Instructor Initials
Discuss how periodic risk assessments and knowledge of warning signs contribute to cancer and cardiovascular disease prevention.	
Based on the pathophysiology and clinical evaluation of the patient with chest pain, characterize the clinical problems according to their life-threatening potential.	
Apply knowledge of the epidemiology of cardiovascular disease to develop prevention strategies.	
Value the sense of urgency for initial assessment and intervention in the patient with cardiac compromise.	
Value and defend the sense of urgency necessary to protect the window of opportunity for reperfusion in the patient with suspected myocardial infarction.	
Defend patient situations in which EKG rhythm analysis is indicated.	
Value and defend the application of a transcutaneous pacing system.	
Value and defend the urgency in identifying pacemaker malfunction.	
Explain the purpose of advance directives relative to patient care and how the paramedic should care for a patient who is covered by an advance directive.	
Discuss the responsibilities of the paramedic relative to resuscitation efforts for patients who are potential organ donors.	
Value and defend the urgency in rapid determination of and rapid intervention of patients in cardiac arrest.	
Value and defend the possibility of termination of resuscitation efforts in the out-of-hospital setting.	
Based on the pathophysiology and clinical evaluation of the patient with acute MI, characterize the clinical problems according to their life-threatening potential.	
Defend the measures that may be taken to prevent or minimize complications in the patient with a suspected MI.	
Identify the characteristics of the patient population at risk for developing a hypertensive emergency.	
Identify the progressive vascular changes associated with sustained hypertension.	
Describe the clinical features of the patient in a hypertensive emergency.	
Rank the clinical problems of patients in hypertensive emergencies according to their sense of urgency.	
From the priority of clinical problems identified, state the management responsibilities for the patient with a hypertensive emergency.	
Defend the urgency based on the severity of the patient's clinical problems in a hypertensive emergency.	
Describe the epidemiology, morbidity, and mortality of heart failure.	
Define the principal causes and terminology associated with heart failure.	
Identify the factors that may precipitate or aggravate heart failure.	
Describe the physiological effects of heart failure.	
Based on the pathophysiology and clinical evaluation of the patient with vascular disorders, characterize the clinical problems according to their life-threatening potential.	
Value and defend the sense of urgency in identifying peripheral vascular occlusion.	
Value and defend the sense of urgency in recognizing signs of aortic aneurysm.	
Describe the characteristics of patients most likely to develop cardiogenic shock.	
Describe the most commonly used pharmacological agents in the management of cardiogenic shock in terms of therapeutic effects, dosages, routes of administration, side effects, and toxic effects.	
Demonstrate intubation techniques on a manikin during ACLS scenario practice.	
Discuss the special considerations of renal dialysis codes with regard to pathophysiology of hyperkalemia and metabolic acidosis.	
Describe the pathophysiological principles behind renal dialysis.	
Discuss different pharmacological considerations in treatment of renal dialysis arrests based on pathophysiology.	
Discuss WHY drugs are in the ACLS algorithms in the order/place that they are.	

©2006 Prentice-Hall Inc.

SECTION 8

*

Specialty

Part 1: Gyn/OB/Neonatal/Peds

Fabulous Factoids

Skill Sheets

Patient Assessment: Gyn—Vaginal Bleeding
Scenario Radio Report—Vaginal Bleeding
Scenario Patient Care Report (PCR)—Vaginal Bleeding
Overall Scenario Management—Vaginal Bleeding
Infant/Child Car Seat Spinal Motion Restriction (SMR)
Pregnant Patient to LBB (Supine Patient)
Prolapsed Cord Presentation
Breech Presentation
APGAR Score
Childbirth
Neonatal Resuscitation Equipment
Meconium Aspiration
Neonatal Ventilatory Management
Neonatal Resuscitation
Umbilical Vein Cannulation
Neonatal Orogastric Tube Insertion
Neonatal Pleural Decompression
Postpartum Hemorrhage Management
Pediatric Manual Airway Maneuvers
Pediatric Nasopharyngeal/Oropharyngeal Airways
Pediatric Ventilatory Management
Pediatric Pleural Decompression
Pediatric Handheld Nebulizer Medication Administration
Pediatric Nebulizer via Mask
Pediatric Intraosseus Insertion
Childbirth Scenario
Overall Scenario Management—Childbirth Scenario
Patient Assessment: Medical—Pediatric
Scenario Radio Report—Pediatric Medical
Scenario Patient Care Report (PCR)—Pediatric Medical

Daily Discussions and Pertinent Points

FABULOUS FACTOIDS—SPECIALTY: GYN/OB/NEONATAL/PEDS/CHRONIC CARE/ HOME HEALTH

Gynecology is from the Greek *gynaik* meaning woman.

Sixteenth-century French physicians prescribed chocolate as a treatment for venereal disease.

The classic Chandelier sign indicates PID. Jiggling the stretcher jiggles the cervix, causing pain.

Ectopic pregnancy kills women. Consider it as possible in every woman of childbearing age with abdominal pain and vaginal bleeding.

Jimmy Carter was the first president born in a hospital.

At 12–13 weeks, you should need a Doppler device to detect FHT; at 18–20 weeks, you should need only a stethoscope. Expect a rate of 140–200.

There are 13,000 babies born in motor vehicles every year.

A mother's pregnancy history is normally described as follows: G4P2-2022. Translated, this is Gravida 4 (4 times pregnant), Para 2 (2 viable deliveries), number of full-term pregnancies (2), number of preemies (0), number of abortions (2), number of viable children (2).

Some 99% of bleeding in pregnancy occurs in the first trimester (20:1).

If a pregnant woman contracts rubella during the first trimester, fetal infection occurs in 80%.

About 10% of abortions are spontaneous. Patients usually complain of crampy lower abdominal pain or back pain.

When the mother is in shock, the body's compensatory mechanism considers the fetus an unnecessary appendage and shunts blood from it to mom's heart, brain, and lungs. This means the baby may be in distress long before the mother shows signs of trouble.

Life-threatening vaginal bleeding occurs with a ruptured ectopic pregnancy/placenta previa/abruptio placenta.

Leopold's maneuver is the use of four steps in palpating the uterus in order to determine the position and presentation of the fetus.

What differentiates eclampsia from preeclampsia? (the seizures)

The highest number of children ever produced from a multiple birth is 10!

Mouth before Nose (alphabetical)—good to remember neonatal order of suction.

The time of a neonate's first breath is unrelated to cutting the cord.

Prenatal history = 4T history (*twins, term, tinge, tracks*)

   Twins—reminds you to find out if patient has multiple gestation

   Term—patient's due date

   Tinge—if her membranes have ruptured, need to know the COLOR of the amniotic fluid

   Tracks—any history of substance abuse or pain medication during labor

©2006 Prentice-Hall Inc.

One in 270 pregnancies will result in identical twins.

Twins are born an average 24 days earlier than single babies.

Always consider apnea in a newborn as secondary apnea and rapidly treat with ventilatory assistance.

If a newborn is not breathing, DO NOT withhold resuscitation until determining APGAR.

Cold infants quickly become distressed infants.

If a neonate does not cry immediately, stimulate by gently rubbing back or flicking feet—do not spank or vigorously rub.

Do not milk or strip the umbilical cord.

Of the vital signs, fetal heart rate is the most reliable indicator of neonatal distress.

Suction a neonate no longer than 10 seconds.

Never deprive a newborn of oxygen in the field for fear of oxygen toxicity.

Naloxone may induce a withdrawal reaction in an infant born to a narcotic-addicted mother.

If you suspect a diaphragmatic hernia, do not use a BVM—it will worsen the condition by causing gastric distension.

Prematurity should not be a factor in short-term resuscitation.

In treating hypovolemia in newborns, do not use solutions containing dextrose. They can produce hypokalemia or worsen ischemic brain injury.

Neonate with a fever has meningitis until proven otherwise.

In assessing a neonate with a fever, remember that infants have a limited ability to control their body temperature—fever can be serious.

Warm your hands before touching a neonate.

Because hypoglycemia can have a catastrophic effect on a neonate's brain, you should determine the blood glucose on all sick infants.

A newborn's brain triples in weight the first year.

Examine/assess infants and toddlers from toe to head.

In assessing infants, pay special attention to the fontanelles—especially the anterior.

Do not trick or lie to child—explain everything.

Why are infants nose breathers? (designed to breast-feed)

Alternative airways (EOA, PTL, biluminal, etc.) cannot be used in children. Properly sized LMA can be used, but it does not protect the airway from aspiration.

Count pediatric respiratory rates for 1 minute.

Infant, toddler, or child in arrest has an airway obstruction until proven otherwise.

Children with pneumonia often present with abdominal pain instead of chest pain.

Febrile seizure diagnosis is NOT made in field.

The more invasive the procedure, the later in the exam of the child you should perform it.

Tachycardia and bradycardia can both be the result of hypoxia in infants and children.

Septic shock kills.

Trauma is the leading cause of death in children.

Children develop pulmonary contusions following blunt trauma to the chest—without any fractures.

Burns are the second leading cause of death in children.

At ALL points in a SIDS case, use the baby's name.

Elderly patients often suffer from more than one illness.

The average American senior citizen takes 14 prescription drugs.

In taking a medical history, remember to ask if the patient is taking a prescribed med as directed.

Multiple meds MAY mean multiple doctors—check the names. Drug interactions may be the root of your diagnosis.

In treating incontinence, remember to respect the patient's modesty and dignity.

Because initial hearing loss frequently involves high-frequency sounds, some elderly patients may have problems understanding female medics.

©2006 Prentice-Hall Inc.

DO NOT assume that a confused, disoriented patient is "just senile." This constitutes failure to assess for a serious underlying problem or hearing loss.

In treating respiratory disorders in the elderly, DO NOT FLUID OVERLOAD.

DO NOT transmit a disease to the elderly—even a minor cold.

Heart sounds are generally softer in the elderly because of a thickening of lung tissues between the heart and the chest wall.

In the elderly patient, exercise intolerance (fatigue) is a key symptom of angina (CHF).

Elderly patients with AMI are less likely to have classic symptoms; they are usually dyspneic (may also have weakness).

Elderly patients with gastrointestinal complaints should be aggressively managed.

Elderly hypothermic patients may not shiver.

Drugs of the Section (see Emergency Drug Quiz Key, p. xxxi):

Magnesium sulfate
Pitocin

Pathophysiologies of the Section: 8.01–8.20 (see Checklist, p. 598)

©2006 Prentice-Hall Inc.

SKILL SHEETS

Patient Assessment: Gyn—Vaginal Bleeding

Student: _____ **Examiner:** _____

Date: _____ **Scenario:** _____

	Done ✓	Not Done
Assesses scene safety and utilizes appropriate PPE		*
OVERALL SCENE EVALUATION		
Medical—determines nature of illness/if trauma involved determines MOI		*
Determines the number of patients, location, obstacles, and requests any additional resources as needed		
Verbalizes general impression of the patient as approaches		*
Considers stabilization/spinal motion restriction of spine if trauma involved		*
INITIAL ASSESSMENT		
Determines responsiveness/level of consciousness/AVPU		*
Opens airway with appropriate technique and assesses airway/ventilation		*
Manages airway/ventilation and applies appropriate oxygen therapy in less than 3 minutes		*
Assesses circulation: radial/carotid pulse, skin color, temperature, condition, and turgor		*
Controls any major bleeding		*
Makes rapid transport decision if indicated		
Initiates IV, obtains BGL, GCS, and complete vital signs		
FOCUSED HISTORY AND PHYSICAL EXAMINATION/RAPID ASSESSMENT		
Obtains SAMPLE history		
Obtains OPQRST for differential diagnosis		
Obtains associated symptoms, pertinent negatives/denials		
Evaluates decision to perform focused exam or completes rapid assessment		*
Vital signs including AVPU (and GCS if trauma)		*
Assesses cardiovascular system including heart sounds, peripheral edema, and peripheral perfusion		*
Assesses pulmonary system including reassessing airway, ventilation, breath sounds, pulse oximetry, chest wall excursion, accessory muscle use, or other signs of distress		*
Assesses neurological system including speech, droop, drift, if applicable, and distal movement and sensation		*
Assesses musculoskeletal and integumentary systems		
Assesses behavioral, psychological, and social aspects of patient and situation		
States field impression of patient—vaginal bleeding, states possible causes		*
Verbalizes treatment plan for patient and calls for appropriate intervention(s)—2 large-bore IVs		*
Reevaluates transport decision		
ONGOING ASSESSMENT		
Repeats initial assessment		*
Repeats vital signs and evaluates trends		*
Evaluates response to treatments		*
Repeats focused assessment regarding patient complaint or injuries		
Gives radio report to receiving facility		
Turns over patient care with verbal report		*
Student exhibits competence with skill		

Any items in the Not Done column that are marked with an * are mandatory for the student to complete. A check mark in the Not Done column of an item with an * indicates that the student was unsuccessful and must attempt the skill again to assure competency. Examiners should use a different-color ink for the second attempt.

☐ Successful   ☐ Unsuccessful   Examiner Initials: _____

Scenario Radio Report—Vaginal Bleeding

Student: _____   **Examiner:** _____

Date: _____

	Done ✓	Not Done
Requests and checks for open channel before speaking		
Presses transmit button 1 second before speaking		
Holds microphone 2–3 in. from mouth		
Speaks slowly and clearly		*
Speaks in a normal voice		
Briefly transmits: Agency, unit designation, identification/name		*
Briefly transmits: Patient's age, sex, weight		*
Briefly transmits: Scene description/mechanism of injury or medical problem		*
Briefly transmits: Chief complaint with brief history of *present* illness		*
Briefly transmits: Associated symptoms (unless able to be deferred to bedside report)		
Briefly transmits: Past medical history (usually deferred to bedside report)		
Briefly transmits: Vital signs		*
Briefly transmits: Level of consciousness/GCS on trauma		*
Briefly transmits: General appearance, distress, cardiac rhythm, blood glucose, and other pertinent findings unable to be deferred to bedside report		
Briefly transmits: Interventions by EMS AND response(s)		*
ETA (the more critical the patient, the earlier you need to notify the receiving facility)		
Does not waste airtime		
Protects privacy of patient		*
Echoes dispatch information and any physician orders		*
Writes down dispatch information or physician orders		
Confirms with facility that message is received		
Demonstrates/verbalizes ability to troubleshoot basic equipment malfunction		
Student exhibits competence with skill		

Any items in the Not Done column that are marked with an * are mandatory for the student to complete. A check mark in the Not Done column of an item with an * indicates that the student was unsuccessful and must attempt the skill again to assure competency. Examiners should use a different-color ink for the second attempt.

☐ Successful   ☐ Unsuccessful   Examiner Initials: _____

Scenario Patient Care Report (PCR)—Vaginal Bleeding

Student: _____   **Examiner:** _____

Date: _____

	Done ✓	Not Done
Records all pertinent dispatch/scene data, using a consistent format		
Completely identifies all additional resources and personnel		
Documents chief complaint, signs/symptoms, position found, age, sex, and weight		
Identifies and records all pertinent, reportable clinical data for each patient		
Documents SAMPLE and OPQRST if applicable		
Records all pertinent negatives		
Records all pertinent denials		
Records accurate, consistent times and patient information		
Includes relevant oral statements of witnesses, bystanders, and patient in "quotes" when appropriate		
Documents initial assessment findings: airway, breathing, and circulation		
Documents any interventions in initial assessment with patient response		
Documents level of consciousness, GCS (if trauma), and VS		
Documents rapid trauma assessment if applicable		
Documents any interventions in rapid trauma assessment with patient response		
Documents focused history and physical assessment		
Documents any interventions in focused assessment with patient response		
Documents repeat VS (every 5 minutes for critical; every 15 minutes for stable)		
Repeats initial assessment and documents findings		
Records ALL treatments with times and patient response(s) in treatment section		
Documents field impression		
Documents transport to specific facility and transfer of care WITH VERBAL REPORT		
Uses correct grammar, abbreviations, spelling, and terminology		
Writes legibly		
Thoroughly documents refusals, denials of transport, and call cancellations		
Documents patient GCS of 15 PRIOR to signing refusal		
Documents advice given to refusal patient, including "call 9-1-1 for further problems"		
Properly corrects errors and omissions		
Writes cautiously, avoids jargon, opinions, inferences, or any derogatory/libelous remarks		
Signs run report		
Uses EMS supplement form if needed		
Student exhibits competence with skill		

Any items in the Not Done column should be evaluated with student. Check marks in this column do not necessarily mean student was unsuccessful as all lines are not completed on all patients. Evaluation of each PCR should be based on the scenario given.

Student must be able to write an EMS report with consistency and accuracy.

☐ Successful   ☐ Unsuccessful   Examiner Initials: _____

©2006 Prentice-Hall Inc.

Overall Scenario Management—Vaginal Bleeding

Student: _____   Examiner: _____

Date: _____   Scenario: _____

NOTE: This skill sheet is to be done after the student completes a scenario as the **TEAM LEADER**. It is to let the student know if he or she is beginning to "put it all together" and use critical thinking skills to manage an EMS call. **PLEASE** notice that it is graded on a different basis than the basic lab skill sheet.

	Done ✓	Needs to Improve
SCENE MANAGEMENT		
Recognized hazards and controlled scene—safety, crowd, and patient issues		
Recognized hazards, but did not control the scene		
Unsuccessfully attempted to manage the scene	*	
Did not evaluate the scene and took no control of the scene	*	
PATIENT ASSESSMENT		
Performed a timely, organized complete patient assessment		
Performed complete initial, focused, and ongoing assessments, but in a disorganized manner		
Performed an incomplete assessment	*	
Did not perform an initial assessment	*	
PATIENT MANAGEMENT		
Evaluated assessment findings to manage all aspects of patient condition		
Managed the patient's presenting signs and symptoms without considering all of assessment		
Inadequately managed the patient	*	
Did not manage life-threatening conditions	*	
COMMUNICATION		
Communicated well with crew, patient, family, bystanders, and assisting agencies		
Communicated well with patient and crew		
Communicated with patient and crew, but poor communication skills	*	
Unable to communicate effectively	*	
REPORT AND TRANSFER OF CARE		
Identified correct destination for patient transport, gave accurate, brief report over radio, and provided full report at bedside demonstrating thorough understanding of patient condition and pathophysiological processes		
Identified correct destination and gave accurate radio and bedside report, but did not demonstrate understanding of patient condition and pathophysiological processes		
Identified correct destination, but provided inadequate radio and bedside report	*	
Identified inappropriate destination or provided no radio or bedside report	*	
Student exhibits competence with skill		

Any items that are marked with an * indicate the student needs to improve and a check mark should be placed in the right-hand column. A check mark in the right-hand column indicates that the student was unsuccessful and must attempt the skill again to assure competency. Examiners should use a different-color ink for the second attempt.

☐ Successful   ☐ Unsuccessful   Examiner Initials: _____

     ©2006 Prentice-Hall Inc.

Infant/Child Car Seat Spinal Motion Restriction (SMR)

Student: _____   Examiner: _____

Date: _____

	Done ✓	Not Done
Assesses scene safety and utilizes appropriate PPE		*
Takes or directs manual cervical SMR		*
Performs ABCD, including distal PMS		*
Checks car seat integrity		*
Performs visual and palpation body survey for glass and DCAP-BLS-TIC/DCAP-BTLS		*
Resecures restraining straps		
Restricts motion of head and shoulders with towel roll or blanket roll as appropriate		*
Reassesses ABCD and distal PMS		*
Secures car seat to rescue unit		*
Monitors infant/child at all times		*
Student exhibits competence with skill		

Any items in the Not Done column that are marked with an * are mandatory for the student to complete. A check mark in the Not Done column of an item with an * indicates that the student was unsuccessful and must attempt the skill again to assure competency. Examiners should use a different-color ink for the second attempt.

☐ Successful   ☐ Unsuccessful   Examiner Initials: _____

©2006 Prentice-Hall Inc.

Pregnant Patient to LBB (Supine Patient)

Student: _____   Examiner: _____

Date: _____

	Done ✓	Not Done
Assesses scene safety and utilizes appropriate PPE		*
Directs assistant to place/maintain head in neutral in-line position		*
Performs initial assessment		
Checks perfusion status, manually displacing gravid uterus to left if compromised		*
Assesses distal PMS (pulse/movement/sensation) in each extremity		*
Applies appropriately sized extrication collar		*
Positions the motion restriction device (LBB) appropriately		
Log rolls patient and checks back/buttocks		
Directs movement of the patient onto the device without compromising the integrity of the spine		*
Applies padding to voids between the torso and the device as necessary		*
Secures the patient's torso to the device		*
Evaluates and pads behind the patient's head as necessary		
Secures the patient's head to the device		*
Secures the patient's legs to the device		
Secures the patient's arms to the device		
Reassesses distal PMS in each extremity		*
Recognizes potential for SHS (supine hypotensive syndrome)		*
Tilts board to left, relieving pressure of gravid uterus on vena cava		*
Reassesses perfusion status, SMR, and distal PMS		*
Assesses patient's response to intervention		*
Student exhibits competence with skill		

Any items in the Not Done column that are marked with an * are mandatory for the student to complete. A check mark in the Not Done column of an item with an * indicates that the student was unsuccessful and must attempt the skill again to assure competency. Examiners should use a different-color ink for the second attempt.

☐ Successful   ☐ Unsuccessful   Examiner Initials: _____

©2006 Prentice-Hall Inc.

Prolapsed Cord Presentation

Student: _____   **Examiner:** _____

Date: _____

	Done ✓	Not Done
Utilizes appropriate PPE		*
Checks perineum and evaluates cord for pulsation		*
Places mother in knee-chest position		*
Places sterile hand into vagina to relieve pressure on cord by gently pressing against presenting part and elevating part off the cord		*
Administers high-flow oxygen to mother		*
Directs second paramedic to initiate IV and provides IV fluid bolus to slow contractions		*
Assesses patient's response to intervention		*
Rapid transport		*
If baby begins to deliver, provides airway for neonate while in birth canal		*
Student exhibits competence with skill		

Any items in the Not Done column that are marked with an * are mandatory for the student to complete. A check mark in the Not Done column of an item with an * indicates that the student was unsuccessful and must attempt the skill again to assure competency. Examiners should use a different-color ink for the second attempt.

☐ Successful   ☐ Unsuccessful   Examiner Initials: _____

Breech Presentation

Student: _____

Examiner: _____

Date: _____

	Done ✓	Not Done
Utilizes appropriate PPE		*
Checks perineum for imminent delivery		*
Suspects breech presentation from presenting part and pregnancy history		*
Positions mother and prepares for delivery during rapid transport		*
Inserts hand beside torso of neonate and attempts to extract BOTH legs, enabling sterile hand to provide airway for neonate while still in birth canal (fingers in V framing nose)		*
Directs second paramedic to initiate IV at wide open rate to slow contractions		*
Assesses patient's response to intervention		*
Maintains airway throughout transport if infant does not deliver		*
Student exhibits competence with skill		

Any items in the Not Done column that are marked with an * are mandatory for the student to complete. A check mark in the Not Done column of an item with an * indicates that the student was unsuccessful and must attempt the skill again to assure competency. Examiners should use a different-color ink for the second attempt.

☐ Successful   ☐ Unsuccessful   Examiner Initials: _____

©2006 Prentice-Hall Inc.

APGAR Score

Student: _____   **Examiner:** _____

Date: _____

	Done ✓	Not Done
Utilizes appropriate PPE		*
Scores neonate using APGAR criteria below at 1 minute after birth		*
Appropriately cares for neonate		*
Scores neonate using APGAR criteria below at 5 minutes		*
Student exhibits competence with skill		

Sign	0	1	2
Appearance (skin color)	Blue, pale	Body pink, extremities blue	Completely pink
Pulse (heart rate)	Absent	Less than 100/minute	Greater than 100/minute
Grimace (irritability)	No response	Grimace	Cough, sneeze, cry
Activity (muscle tone)	Limp	Some flexion	Active motion
Respirations (effort)	Absent	Slow, irregular	Good, crying

Any items in the Not Done column that are marked with an * are mandatory for the student to complete. A check mark in the Not Done column of an item with an * indicates that the student was unsuccessful and must attempt the skill again to assure competency. Examiners should use a different-color ink for the second attempt.

☐ Successful   ☐ Unsuccessful   Examiner Initials: _____

©2006 Prentice-Hall Inc.

Childbirth

Student: _____   **Examiner:** _____

Date: _____

	Done ✓	Not Done
Determines scene safety and utilizes appropriate PPE		*
Obtains prenatal history		
Examines for crowning (present) and prepares for imminent delivery		*
Explains to patient and family both situation and expectations, takes appropriate PPE		
Positions the patient		
Takes/verbalizes sterile technique, opens OB Kit, and drapes patient		
Supports perineum to prevent tearing, gentle pressure to head to prevent explosive delivery		*
As head delivers, feels for nuchal cord, gently removing if necessary		*
After head delivers, suctions mouth, then nose of infant until clear		*
Rotates shoulder as body delivers, tips as necessary to ease baby out		*
Dries, warms, and wraps infant, then places on firm surface at level of mother		*
Notes time of birth		
Evaluates infant's airway status if not briskly crying, suction PRN		*
Evaluates infant's breathing and circulatory status		*
Feels cord for absence of pulsations		
Places umbilical clamps at approximately 6 and 10 in. from infant		
Cuts or directs father to cut cord with scalpel between the clamps		
Checks cord ends for bleeding		
Evaluates infant for 1-minute APGAR		*
Allows placenta to deliver spontaneously, bags all tissue, and takes to hospital		*
Massages fundus/puts baby to breast to control bleeding		
Examines mother for hemorrhage and places sterile pad to perineum		*
Evaluates infant for 5-minute APGAR		*
Reassesses mother and infant en route to hospital		*
Student exhibits competence with skill		

Any items in the Not Done column that are marked with an * are mandatory for the student to complete. A check mark in the Not Done column of an item with an * indicates that the student was unsuccessful and must attempt the skill again to assure competency. Examiners should use a different-color ink for the second attempt.

☐ Successful   ☐ Unsuccessful   Examiner Initials: _____

     ©2006 Prentice-Hall Inc.

Neonatal Resuscitation Equipment

Student: _____

Date: _____

Examiner: _____

	Done ✓	Not Done
Demonstrates familiarity with neonatal BVM		*
Demonstrates familiarity with neonatal EKG monitoring		
Demonstrates familiarity with neonatal diapering		*
Demonstrates familiarity with neonatal Broselow (or other brand) tape use		*
Demonstrates familiarity with neonatal blood glucose level		*
Demonstrates familiarity with dilution for neonatal glucose and bicarbonate administration		*
Demonstrates familiarity with neonatal umbilical clamp and tape		*
Demonstrates familiarity with neonatal intubation equipment		*
Student exhibits competence with skill		

Any items in the Not Done column that are marked with an * are mandatory for the student to complete. A check mark in the Not Done column of an item with an * indicates that the student was unsuccessful and must attempt the skill again to assure competency. Examiners should use a different-color ink for the second attempt.

☐ Successful   ☐ Unsuccessful   Examiner Initials: _____

©2006 Prentice-Hall Inc.

Meconium Aspiration

Student: _____   **Examiner:** _____

Date: _____

	Done ✓	Not Done
Utilizes appropriate PPE		*
Evaluates presence of particulate meconium in thick amniotic fluid		*
Evaluates that neonate is depressed		*
Intubates neonate and uses ET as suction catheter, applying suction as removed		*
Rinses ET tube with saline		*
Intubates and suctions while withdrawing ET tube		*
Repeats until clear or infant improves		*
Continues with neonatal resuscitation		*
Student exhibits competence with skill		

Any items in the Not Done column that are marked with an * are mandatory for the student to complete. A check mark in the Not Done column of an item with an * indicates that the student was unsuccessful and must attempt the skill again to assure competency. Examiners should use a different-color ink for the second attempt.

☐ Successful   ☐ Unsuccessful   Examiner Initials: _____

©2006 Prentice-Hall Inc.

Neonatal Ventilatory Management

Student: _____   Examiner: _____

Date: _____

	Done ✓	Not Done
Recognizes neonatal resuscitation in progress and utilizes appropriate PPE		*
Manually opens the airway, using towel under shoulders for positioning		*
Checks mouth for potential airway obstruction		*
Gently ventilates infant with BVM device attached to high-flow oxygen at respiratory rate 30–60/minute		*
Observes chest rise/fall and feels compliance for baseline		*
Obtains effective ventilation in less than 20 seconds		*
Directs assistant to take over ventilation		
Auscultates bilateral lung sounds for baseline		*
Directs assistant to preoxygenate patient		*
Identifies/selects proper equipment for intubation including suction and cardiac monitor		
Checks laryngoscope light and selects appropriate uncuffed tube (size of little finger)		
Adjusts infant's head position if needed		*
Places infant on cardiac monitor with audible tone for monitoring heart rate during intubation		
Opens mouth and gently inserts blade while sweeping tongue to side		*
Uses pediatric handle and holds with only two fingers and thumb—light pressure		
Gently elevates mandible with laryngoscope and visualizes cords		*
Introduces ET tube to side of blade and visualizes tube passing through cords		*
"Threads" ET tube off stylet (if used), maintaining hold on ET tube as stylet removed		
Inflates cuff to proper pressure and disconnects syringe		*
Disconnects mask from bag-valve device and attaches to ET tube without releasing ET tube		
Directs ventilation of patient while maintains holding ET tube in place		
Confirms proper placement by auscultation over epigastrium and bilaterally over each lung		*
Secures ET tube		*
Restricts cervical spine motion to prevent ET tube dislodgement		*
Reassesses bilateral lung sounds, compliance, and infant's heart rate		*
Uses secondary device to confirm tube placement		*
Assesses infant's response to intervention		*
Verbalizes medications that may be given to neonate via ET tube if further resuscitation needed		
Student exhibits competence with skill		

Any items in the Not Done column that are marked with an * are mandatory for the student to complete. A check mark in the Not Done column of an item with an * indicates that the student was unsuccessful and must attempt the skill again to assure competency. Examiners should use a different-color ink for the second attempt.

☐ Successful   ☐ Unsuccessful   Examiner Initials: _____

©2006 Prentice-Hall Inc.

Neonatal Resuscitation

Student: _____   Examiner: _____

Date: _____

	Done ✓	Not Done
Utilizes appropriate PPE		*
Suctions **M**outh then **N**ose while infant "on the perineum"		
Suctions neonate immediately upon delivery		*
Briskly dries neonate and uses new towel/blanket to wrap neonate		*
Notes time of birth		
Places infant supine with head slightly below body, neck slightly extended using 3/4-in. thickness towel under shoulders		
Stimulates infant by rubbing back or flicking feet		*
Assesses APGAR at 1 minute if neonate does not need resuscitation		*
If neonate inadequately ventilating, central cyanosis is present, depressed, or decreased heart rate present (less than 100), initiates resuscitation with BVM ventilation 30–60/minute		*
CHECKS BLOOD GLUCOSE—treats if hypoglycemia present (with only 10–12.5% dextrose)		*
Reevaluates after 30 seconds of oxygen		*
If neonate apneic, heart rate less than 60 and not improving, or central cyanosis is still present, initiates chest compressions (3 compressions [90/min]:1 ventilation [30/min])		*
Reevaluates in 30 seconds		*
If not responding to BVM, tracheal suction is required, prolonged ventilation is required, diaphragmatic hernia suspected, or inadequate respiratory effort found—intubates neonate		*
Reevaluates in 30 seconds		*
If infant not improving, initiates UVC and gives 10 ml/kg of crystalloid		*
Rapidly transports with continued resuscitation and medications		*
Considers prenatal drug use—CALLS for Narcan (after obtaining good history/no addiction)		
Continues to reassess neonate minimum of every 30 seconds		*
If infant responds to resuscitation at any point, obtains APGAR (5 minutes)		*
Student exhibits competence with skill		

Any items in the Not Done column that are marked with an * are mandatory for the student to complete. A check mark in the Not Done column of an item with an * indicates that the student was unsuccessful and must attempt the skill again to assure competency. Examiners should use a different-color ink for the second attempt.

☐ Successful   ☐ Unsuccessful   Examiner Initials: _____

©2006 Prentice-Hall Inc.

Umbilical Vein Cannulation

Student: _____   **Examiner:** _____

Date: _____

	Done ✓	Not Done
Utilizes appropriate PPE		*
Verifies cord end has good hemostasis		*
Prepares equipment (Umbilical Vein Catheter [UVC] or STERILE 5 Fr feeding tube), umbilical tape, IV fluid, tubing, sterile cloth/field, sterile gloves, 4 × 4s, and tape		*
Sets out sterile field with scalpel, UVC/feeding tube, and sterile gauze sponges		
Sets up IV fluid of choice with minidrip tubing and primes line with **NO** AIR BUBBLES		*
Puts on 2 pairs of sterile gloves (in case of contamination during procedure assistant can remove the contaminated glove, leaving your hand sterile)		*
With left hand grasps umbilical clamp and with right hand uses scalpel to cut cord immediately proximal to clamp, realizing left hand now unsterile		*
With right hand places sterile 4 × 4 around outside of umbilical cord		
With left hand grasps OUTSIDE of 4 × 4 wrapping umbilical cord and visualizes umbilical vein and two umbilical arteries (may use right hand to blot end of cord with sterile 4 × 4)		*
With sterile right hand takes UVC/feeding tube and holds end out for **assistant** to hook up nonsterile IV tubing and PRIMES THE UVC/feeding tube, then **DISCONNECTS**		*
Keeps the UVC/feeding tube sterile in sterile right hand and advances into umbilical vein		*
Palpating the cord through left hand 4 × 4, advances until catheter is felt at level of abdomen		*
Advances catheter to "feel" tip passing through abdominal wall and STOPS		*
Verbalizes that advancing catheter too far into abdomen may enter neonate's liver		*
Visualizes blood return and has assistant start IV running slowly PRIOR to hooking up		*
Verifying NO AIR in UVC/feeding tube, has assistant hook IV tubing to end of UVC/feeding tube		*
Has assistant continue IV infusion at TKO rate, verifying rate visually		
"Purse strings" catheter to umbilical cord being certain to monitor for any change in drip rate		*
Secures IV tubing and connection with small amount of tape		*
Pads abdomen around cord and covers neonate to maintain warmth		*
Assesses infant's response to intervention		*
Exposes site only when using for meds or when moving neonate, to prevent dislodging		
Documents procedure including rate maintained, MAINTENANCE OF STERILE TECHNIQUE, and VISUALIZATION OF BLOOD RETURN		
Student exhibits competence with skill		

Any items in the Not Done column that are marked with an * are mandatory for the student to complete. A check mark in the Not Done column of an item with an * indicates that the student was unsuccessful and must attempt the skill again to assure competency. Examiners should use a different-color ink for the second attempt.

☐ Successful   ☐ Unsuccessful   Examiner Initials: _____

©2006 Prentice-Hall Inc.

Neonatal Orogastric Tube Insertion

Student: _____   **Examiner:** _____

Date: _____

	Done ✓	Not Done
Utilizes appropriate PPE		*
Obtains equipment (suction, OG/feeding tube, lubricant, tape, irrigating syringe, water)		*
Verifies secure airway in unresponsive infant		*
Positions infant supine		*
Measures tube from xiphoid process to earlobe to mouth and tapes depth marking		*
Lubricates tube		
Passes tip through oral cavity to posterior pharynx (along tongue side of ET tube)		
Passes tube slowly and posteriorly, checking mouth for curling		*
Determines proper tube placement by auscultation over epigastrium of injected AIR		*
Aspirates stomach contents for secondary verification		*
Secures tube in place		*
Places to suction (continuous only for emptying initial contents, then intermittent)		
Saves gastric contents		
Assesses infant's response to intervention		*
Documents procedure correctly		
Student exhibits competence with skill		

Any items in the Not Done column that are marked with an * are mandatory for the student to complete. A check mark in the Not Done column of an item with an * indicates that the student was unsuccessful and must attempt the skill again to assure competency. Examiners should use a different-color ink for the second attempt.

☐ Successful   ☐ Unsuccessful   Examiner Initials: _____

©2006 Prentice-Hall Inc.

Neonatal Pleural Decompression

Student: _____   **Examiner:** _____

Date: _____

	Done ✓	Not Done
Utilizes appropriate PPE		*
Evaluates neonate for indications and obtains baseline lung sounds and assessment		*
Prepares equipment		
Palpates at 4th intercostal space/anterior axillary line (usually nipple line)		*
Cleanses site appropriately		*
Inserts 22 gauge catheter at superior border of 5th rib, avoiding artery, vein, and nerve		*
Advances until feels "pop" and rush of air released		*
Checks neonate for improvement in clinical status		*
Removes needle from catheter, disposes of needle properly, and applies flutter valve		*
Secures in place		
Reassesses neonate for improvement		*
Documents procedure and response correctly		
Student exhibits competence with skill		

Any items in the Not Done column that are marked with an * are mandatory for the student to complete. A check mark in the Not Done column of an item with an * indicates that the student was unsuccessful and must attempt the skill again to assure competency. Examiners should use a different-color ink for the second attempt.

☐ Successful   ☐ Unsuccessful   Examiner Initials: _____

Postpartum Hemorrhage Management

Student: _____   Examiner: _____

Date: _____

	Done ✓	Not Done
Utilizes appropriate PPE		*
Administers high-flow oxygen		*
Massages fundus		*
Places patient in Trendelenberg		*
Keeps patient warm		*
Initiates peripheral IV (2 large-bore IVs if possible) of crystalloid at wide open rate		*
Replaces perineal pads as needed to evaluate blood loss		
Verifies placenta has delivered		*
Starts Pitocin drip or administers IM Pitocin (IM=10 units/IV=20 units/1,000 cc to run at 20–40 microunits per minute—1–2 **cc** per minute or per local protocol)		*
Assesses patient's response to interventions		*
Rapid transport		*
Monitors for blood loss		
Student exhibits competence with skill		

Any items in the Not Done column that are marked with an * are mandatory for the student to complete. A check mark in the Not Done column of an item with an * indicates that the student was unsuccessful and must attempt the skill again to assure competency. Examiners should use a different-color ink for the second attempt.

☐ Successful   ☐ Unsuccessful   Examiner Initials: _____

©2006 Prentice-Hall Inc.

Pediatric Manual Airway Maneuvers

Student: _____   **Examiner:** _____

Date: _____

Head-Tilt/Chin Lift	Done ✓	Not Done
Utilizes appropriate PPE		*
Places patient supine and positions self at side of patient's head		
Places one hand on forehead—uses soft hand pressure to forehead, tilts the head back **slightly**		*
Puts two fingers under bony part of chin and lifts jaw anteriorly to open airway		*
Assesses patient's response to intervention		*
Student exhibits competence with skill		

Any items in the Not Done column that are marked with an * are mandatory for the student to complete. A check mark in the Not Done column of an item with an * indicates that the student was unsuccessful and must attempt the skill again to assure competency. Examiners should use a different-color ink for the second attempt.

☐ Successful   ☐ Unsuccessful   Examiner Initials: _____

Trauma Jaw-Thrust	Done ✓	Not Done
Utilizes appropriate PPE		*
Places patient supine and positions self at top of patient's head		
Applies fingers to each side of jaw at the mandibular angles		*
Elevates jaw anteriorly without tilting head		*
Assesses patient's response to intervention		*
Student exhibits competence with skill		

Any items in the Not Done column that are marked with an * are mandatory for the student to complete. A check mark in the Not Done column of an item with an * indicates that the student was unsuccessful and must attempt the skill again to assure competency. Examiners should use a different-color ink for the second attempt.

☐ Successful   ☐ Unsuccessful   Examiner Initials: _____

©2006 Prentice-Hall Inc.

Pediatric Nasopharyngeal/Oropharyngeal Airways

Student: _____   Examiner: _____

Date: _____

Nasopharyngeal Airway	Done ✓	Not Done
Utilizes appropriate PPE		*
Adjusts patient's head slightly to place in sniffing position if no history of trauma		*
Directs preoxygenation with 100% oxygen if indicated		
Measures NPA from tip of nose to angle of jaw and diameter of nostril		*
Lubricates exterior of tube with water-soluble jelly		
Pushes gently upward on tip of nose and passes NPA into nostril, bevel toward septum		*
Verifies appropriate position of airway, breath sounds, chest rise, and airflow		*
Ventilates with 100% oxygen		
Assesses patient's response to intervention		*
Student exhibits competence with skill		

Any items in the Not Done column that are marked with an * are mandatory for the student to complete. A check mark in the Not Done column of an item with an * indicates that the student was unsuccessful and must attempt the skill again to assure competency. Examiners should use a different-color ink for the second attempt.

☐ Successful   ☐ Unsuccessful   Examiner Initials: _____

Oropharyngeal Airway (unresponsive)	Done ✓	Not Done
Utilizes appropriate PPE		*
Verifies unresponsiveness and absence of gag reflex		*
Adjusts patient's head slightly to place it in sniffing position if no history of trauma		*
Opens mouth and removes any visible obstructions		*
Directs preoxygenation with 100% oxygen if indicated		
Measures OPA from corner of mouth to earlobe		*
Grasps patient's jaw and lifts anteriorly		*
With other hand, holds OPA at proximal end and inserts into patient's mouth with curve reversed and tip pointing to roof of mouth **OR** uses tongue blade correctly to assist insertion		*
As tip reaches level of soft palate, gently rotates 180° as advances to proper depth		*
Verifies appropriate position of airway, breath sounds, and chest rise		*
Ventilates with 100% oxygen		
Assesses patient's response to intervention		*
Student exhibits competence with skill		

Any items in the Not Done column that are marked with an * are mandatory for the student to complete. A check mark in the Not Done column of an item with an * indicates that the student was unsuccessful and must attempt the skill again to assure competency. Examiners should use a different-color ink for the second attempt.

☐ Successful   ☐ Unsuccessful   Examiner Initials: _____

     ©2006 Prentice-Hall Inc.

Pediatric Ventilatory Management

Student: _____   **Examiner:** _____

Date: _____

	Done ✓	Not Done
Assesses scene safety and utilizes appropriate PPE		*
Manually opens the airway with technique appropriate for patient condition		*
Checks mouth for blood or potential airway obstruction		*
Suctions or removes loose teeth or foreign materials as needed		
Inserts simple adjunct (oropharyngeal or nasopharyngeal airway)		
Directs assistant to ventilate patient with bag-valve-mask device (room air)		*
Observes chest rise/fall and auscultates bilaterally over lungs for baseline		*
Obtains effective ventilation in less than 20 seconds		*
Attaches oxygen reservoir to bag-valve-mask device and connects to high-flow oxygen		
Ventilates patient and evaluates chest wall/lung compliance		*
Directs assistant to preoxygenate patient		*
Identifies/selects proper equipment for intubation—uncuffed tube/size of little finger		
Checks laryngoscope light and properly inserts stylet if used		
Places patient on cardiac monitor to continuously observe heart rate during intubation (audible)		
Positions patient in neutral or sniffing position and removes airway adjunct		
Opens mouth and gently inserts blade while sweeping tongue to side		*
Uses small laryngoscope handle and holds gently with only two fingers and thumb		
Gently elevates mandible with laryngoscope and visualizes cords		*
Introduces ET tube to side of blade and visualizes tube passing through cords		*
"Threads" ET tube off stylet (if used), maintaining hold on ET tube as stylet removed		
Verbalizes smallest portion of pediatric airway is the cricothyroid ring		*
Disconnects mask from bag-valve device and attaches to ET tube without releasing ET tube		
Directs ventilation of patient while continuing to hold ET tube in place		
Confirms proper placement by auscultation over epigastrium and bilaterally over each lung		*
Secures ET tube		*
Restricts cervical spine motion to prevent dislodging ET tube		*
Reassesses heart rate, bilateral lung sounds, and compliance		*
Uses secondary device to confirm tube placement		*
Assesses patient's response to intervention		*
Considers OGT to decrease any abdominal distension that may compromise ventilation		
Student exhibits competence with skill		

Any items in the Not Done column that are marked with an * are mandatory for the student to complete. A check mark in the Not Done column of an item with an * indicates that the student was unsuccessful and must attempt the skill again to assure competency. Examiners should use a different-color ink for the second attempt.

☐ Successful   ☐ Unsuccessful   Examiner Initials: _____

©2006 Prentice-Hall Inc.

Pediatric Pleural Decompression

Student: _____   **Examiner:** _____

Date: _____

	Done ✓	Not Done
Utilizes appropriate PPE		*
Evaluates patient for indications and obtains baseline lung sounds and assessment		*
Prepares equipment and explains procedure		
Palpates at 2nd intercostal space / midclavicular line		*
Cleanses site appropriately		*
Inserts 20 gauge catheter at superior border of 3rd rib, avoiding artery, vein, and nerve		*
Advances until feels "pop" and rush of air released		*
Checks patient for improvement in clinical status		*
Removes needle from catheter, disposes of needle properly, and applies flutter valve		*
Secures in place		
Reassesses patient for improvement		*
Documents procedure and response correctly		
Student exhibits competence with skill		

Any items in the Not Done column that are marked with an * are mandatory for the student to complete. A check mark in the Not Done column of an item with an * indicates that the student was unsuccessful and must attempt the skill again to assure competency. Examiners should use a different-color ink for the second attempt.

☐ Successful   ☐ Unsuccessful   Examiner Initials: _____

©2006 Prentice-Hall Inc.

Pediatric Handheld Nebulizer Medication Administration

Student: _____   **Examiner:** _____

Date: _____

	Done ✓	Not Done
Utilizes appropriate PPE		*
Ensures that patient has adequate tidal volume for procedure		*
Elicits allergy history from and explains procedure to parent/guardian and child		*
Selects correct medication		*
Inspects medication for clarity, discoloration, and expiration date		*
Obtains baseline lung sounds		*
Places patient on cardiac monitor/pulse oximetry		*
Places medication into nebulizer reservoir and tightly closes		
Hooks appropriate end of nebulizer tubing to oxygen source		
Secures mask to reservoir end		
Turns on oxygen until mist flows from mouthpiece of nebulizer		
Explains mouthpiece to patient/appropriate terminology for age (may use *snorkel*, *scuba*, etc.)		*
Encourages patient to breathe slowly with adequate tidal volume		*
Adjusts oxygen flow so medicated mist is inhaled with each breath, not flowing throughout		*
Monitors patient throughout administration		*
Reassesses patient for change in condition—both desired and undesired effects		*
Correctly documents administration and patient response		
Student exhibits competence with skill		

Any items in the Not Done column that are marked with an * are mandatory for the student to complete. A check mark in the Not Done column of an item with an * indicates that the student was unsuccessful and must attempt the skill again to assure competency. Examiners should use a different-color ink for the second attempt.

☐ Successful   ☐ Unsuccessful   Examiner Initials: _____

©2006 Prentice-Hall Inc.

Pediatric Nebulizer via Mask

Student: _____   Examiner: _____

Date: _____

	Done ✓	Not Done
Utilizes appropriate PPE		*
Ensures that patient has adequate tidal volume for procedure		*
Elicits allergy history from and explains procedure to parent/guardian		*
Explains procedure to patient		
Selects correct medication		*
Inspects medication for clarity, discoloration, and expiration date		*
Obtains baseline lung sounds		*
Places patient on cardiac monitor		*
Places medication into nebulizer reservoir and tightly closes		
Hooks appropriate end of nebulizer tubing to oxygen source		
Hooks up patient circuit to nebulizer reservoir		
Turns on oxygen until mist flows from patient end of nebulizer		
Places nebulizer circuit to pediatric mask (or paper cup)		
Explains as space mask, scuba mask, or other creative, interesting breathing apparatus depending on age of child		*
Encourages patient to breathe slowly with adequate tidal volume		*
Adjusts oxygen flow so medicated mist is inhaled with each breath		*
Monitors patient throughout administration		*
Reassesses patient for change in condition—both desired and undesired effects		*
Correctly documents administration and patient response		
Student exhibits competence with skill		

Any items in the Not Done column that are marked with an * are mandatory for the student to complete. A check mark in the Not Done column of an item with an * indicates that the student was unsuccessful and must attempt the skill again to assure competency. Examiners should use a different-color ink for the second attempt.

☐ Successful   ☐ Unsuccessful   Examiner Initials: _____

©2006 Prentice-Hall Inc.

Pediatric Intraosseus Insertion

Student: _____   **Examiner:** _____

Date: _____

	Done ✓	Not Done
Verbalizes indications for fluid administration and peripheral line is unable to be obtained		*
Selects correct IV fluid, proper size of bag, and checks clarity and expiration date		*
Prepares appropriate equipment to include IO needle, syringe, 10 cc sterile saline		
Selects extension set and minidrip administration set or Volutrol/Buretrol		
Attaches administration set to bag		*
Prepares administration set (fills drip chamber and flushes tubing)		*
Draws saline into syringe and attaches to extension tubing		*
Primes extension tubing until NO air is in tubing or fluid		*
Cuts or tears tape (at any time before IO puncture)		*
Utilizes appropriate PPE (prior to IO puncture)		*
Identifies proper anatomical site for IO puncture		*
Checks distal PMS (pulse, movement, sensation) in extremity		*
Cleanses site appropriately		*
Firmly grasps tibia and inserts needle at 90° angle to tibial plateau		*
With controlled pressure, "twists" needle into bone until feel "pop"		*
Unscrews cap and removes stylet from needle		*
Properly disposes of stylet		*
Attaches syringe and extension set to IO needle and aspirates		*
Slowly injects saline to assure proper placement of needle		*
Connects administration set and adjusts flow rate as appropriate		*
Secures needle with tape and supports with bulky dressing		*
Assesses patient's response to intervention		*
Student exhibits competence with skill		

Any items in the Not Done column that are marked with an * are mandatory for the student to complete. A check mark in the Not Done column of an item with an * indicates that the student was unsuccessful and must attempt the skill again to assure competency. Examiners should use a different-color ink for the second attempt.

☐ Successful   ☐ Unsuccessful   Examiner Initials: _____

©2006 Prentice-Hall Inc.

Childbirth Scenario

Student: _____

Examiner: _____

Date: _____

	Done ✓	Not Done
Determines scene safety and utilizes appropriate PPE		*
Obtains prenatal history		*
Examines for crowning (present) and prepares for imminent delivery		*
Explains to patient and family both situation and expectations, takes appropriate extra PPE		*
Positions the patient and times contractions		
Initiates IV of crystalloid if time permits		
Takes/verbalizes sterile technique, opens OB Kit, and drapes patient		*
Encourages mother to breathe and push during contraction		
Supports perineum to prevent tearing, gentle pressure to head to prevent explosive delivery		*
As head delivers, feels for nuchal cord, gently removing if necessary		*
After head delivers, suctions mouth, then nose of infant until clear		*
Rotates shoulder as body delivers, tips as necessary to ease baby out		
Dries, warms, and wraps infant, then places on firm surface at level of mother		*
Notes time of birth		
Evaluates infant's airway status if not briskly crying, suction PRN		*
Evaluates infant's breathing and circulatory status		*
Feels cord for absence of pulsations		*
Places umbilical clamps at approximately 6 and 10 in. from infant		*
Cuts or directs father to cut cord with scalpel between the clamps		*
Checks cord ends for bleeding, if still bleeding, utilizes another clamp		*
Evaluates infant for 1-minute APGAR		*
Allows placenta to deliver spontaneously, bags all tissue, and takes to hospital		*
Massages fundus/puts baby to breast to control bleeding		*
Examines mother for hemorrhage and places sterile pad to perineum		*
Evaluates infant for 5-minute APGAR		*
Reassesses mother and infant en route to hospital		*
Student exhibits competence with skill		

Any items in the Not Done column that are marked with an * are mandatory for the student to complete. A check mark in the Not Done column of an item with an * indicates that the student was unsuccessful and must attempt the skill again to assure competency. Examiners should use a different-color ink for the second attempt.

☐ Successful   ☐ Unsuccessful   Examiner Initials: _____

©2006 Prentice-Hall Inc.

Overall Scenario Management—Childbirth Scenario

Student: _____   Examiner: _____

Date: _____   Scenario: _____

NOTE: This skill sheet is to be done after the student completes a scenario as the TEAM LEADER. It is to let the student know if he or she is beginning to "put it all together" and use critical thinking skills to manage an EMS call. PLEASE notice that it is graded on a different basis than the basic lab skill sheet.

	Done ✓	Needs to Improve
SCENE MANAGEMENT		
Recognized hazards and controlled scene—safety, crowd, and patient issues		
Recognized hazards, but did not control the scene		
Unsuccessfully attempted to manage the scene	*	
Did not evaluate the scene and took no control of the scene	*	
PATIENT ASSESSMENT		
Performed a timely, organized complete patient assessment		
Performed complete initial, focused, and ongoing assessments, but in a disorganized manner		
Performed an incomplete assessment	*	
Did not perform an initial assessment	*	
PATIENT MANAGEMENT		
Evaluated assessment findings to manage all aspects of patient condition		
Managed the patient's presenting signs and symptoms without considering all of assessment		
Inadequately managed the patient	*	
Did not manage life-threatening conditions	*	
COMMUNICATION		
Communicated well with crew, patient, family, bystanders, and assisting agencies		
Communicated well with patient and crew		
Communicated with patient and crew, but poor communication skills	*	
Unable to communicate effectively	*	
REPORT AND TRANSFER OF CARE		
Identified correct destination for patient transport, gave accurate, brief report over radio, and provided full report at bedside demonstrating thorough understanding of patient condition and pathophysiological processes		
Identified correct destination and gave accurate radio and bedside report, but did not demonstrate understanding of patient condition and pathophysiological processes		
Identified correct destination, but provided inadequate radio and bedside report	*	
Identified inappropriate destination or provided no radio or bedside report	*	
Student exhibits competence with skill		

Any items that are marked with an * indicate the student needs to improve and a check mark should be placed in the right-hand column. A check mark in the right-hand column indicates that the student was unsuccessful and must attempt the skill again to assure competency. Examiners should use a different-color ink for the second attempt.

☐ Successful   ☐ Unsuccessful   Examiner Initials: _____

Patient Assessment: Medical—Pediatric

Student: _____   Examiner: _____

Date: _____   Scenario: _____

	Done ✓	Not Done
Assesses scene safety and utilizes appropriate PPE		*
OVERALL SCENE EVALUATION		
Medical—determines nature of illness/if trauma involved determines MOI		*
Determines the number of patients, location, obstacles, and requests any additional resources as needed		
Verbalizes general impression of the patient as approaches		*
Considers stabilization/spinal motion restriction of spine if trauma involved		*
INITIAL ASSESSMENT		
Determines responsiveness/level of consciousness/AVPU		*
Opens airway with appropriate technique and assesses airway/ventilation		*
Manages airway/ventilation and applies appropriate oxygen therapy in less than 3 minutes		*
Assesses circulation: radial/carotid pulse, skin color, temperature, condition, and turgor		*
Controls any major bleeding		*
Makes rapid transport decision if indicated, to appropriate facility		*
Obtains Broselow (or other brand) tape weight/dosage area for reference if needed		*
Initiates IV or IO if critical, obtains BGL, GCS, and complete vital signs		*
FOCUSED HISTORY AND PHYSICAL EXAMINATION/RAPID ASSESSMENT		
Obtains SAMPLE history from patient or caregiver		*
Obtains OPQRST from patient or caregiver for differential diagnosis		
Obtains associated symptoms, pertinent negatives/denials		
Evaluates decision to perform focused exam or completes rapid assessment (toe-to-head exam for younger child)		*
Vital signs including AVPU (and GCS if trauma)		*
Assesses cardiovascular system including heart sounds, peripheral perfusion (capillary refill)		*
Assesses pulmonary system including reassessing airway, ventilation, breath sounds, pulse oximetry, chest wall excursion, accessory muscle use, nasal flaring, sternal retractions, or other signs of distress		*
Assesses neurological system and distal movement and sensation		*
Assesses musculoskeletal and integumentary systems		
Assesses behavioral, psychological, and social aspects of patient and situation for possible abuse/neglect		
States field impression of patient—pediatric medical (states suspected differential diagnosis)		*
Verbalizes treatment plan for patient and calls for appropriate intervention(s)—IV unless suspected epiglottitis		*
Reevaluates transport decision		
ONGOING ASSESSMENT		
Repeats initial assessment		*
Repeats vital signs and evaluates trends		*
Evaluates response to treatments		*
Repeats focused assessment regarding patient complaint or injuries		
Gives radio report to appropriate receiving facility		
Turns over patient care with verbal report		*
Student exhibits competence with skill		

Any items in the Not Done column that are marked with an * are mandatory for the student to complete. A check mark in the Not Done column of an item with an * indicates that the student was unsuccessful and must attempt the skill again to assure competency. Examiners should use a different-color ink for the second attempt.

☐ Successful   ☐ Unsuccessful   Examiner Initials: _____

©2006 Prentice-Hall Inc.

Scenario Radio Report—Pediatric Medical

Student: _____   **Examiner:** _____

Date: _____

	Done ✓	Not Done
Requests and checks for open channel before speaking		
Presses transmit button 1 second before speaking		
Holds microphone 2–3 in. from mouth		
Speaks slowly and clearly		*
Speaks in a normal voice		
Briefly transmits: Agency, unit designation, identification/name		*
Briefly transmits: Patient's age, sex, weight		*
Briefly transmits: Scene description/mechanism of injury or medical problem		*
Briefly transmits: Chief complaint with brief history of *present* illness		*
Briefly transmits: Associated symptoms (unless able to be deferred to bedside report)		
Briefly transmits: Past medical history (usually deferred to bedside report)		
Briefly transmits: Vital signs		*
Briefly transmits: Level of consciousness/GCS on trauma		*
Briefly transmits: General appearance, distress, cardiac rhythm, blood glucose, and other pertinent findings unable to be deferred to bedside report		
Briefly transmits: Interventions by EMS AND response(s)		*
ETA (the more critical the patient, the earlier you need to notify the receiving facility)		
Does not waste airtime		
Protects privacy of patient		*
Echoes dispatch information and any physician orders		*
Writes down dispatch information or physician orders		
Confirms with facility that message is received		
Demonstrates/verbalizes ability to troubleshoot basic equipment malfunction		
Student exhibits competence with skill		

Any items in the Not Done column that are marked with an * are mandatory for the student to complete. A check mark in the Not Done column of an item with an * indicates that the student was unsuccessful and must attempt the skill again to assure competency. Examiners should use a different-color ink for the second attempt.

☐ Successful   ☐ Unsuccessful   Examiner Initials: _____

©2006 Prentice-Hall Inc.

Scenario Patient Care Report (PCR)—Pediatric Medical

Student: _____   Examiner: _____

Date: _____

	Done ✓	Not Done
Records all pertinent dispatch/scene data, using a consistent format		
Completely identifies all additional resources and personnel		
Documents chief complaint, signs/symptoms, position found, age, sex, and weight		
Identifies and records all pertinent, reportable clinical data for each patient		
Documents SAMPLE and OPQRST if applicable		
Records all pertinent negatives		
Records all pertinent denials		
Records accurate, consistent times and patient information		
Includes relevant oral statements of witnesses, bystanders, and patient in "quotes" when appropriate		
Documents initial assessment findings: airway, breathing, and circulation		
Documents any interventions in initial assessment with patient response		
Documents level of consciousness, GCS (if trauma), and VS		
Documents rapid trauma assessment if applicable		
Documents any interventions in rapid trauma assessment with patient response		
Documents focused history and physical assessment		
Documents any interventions in focused assessment with patient response		
Documents repeat VS (every 5 minutes for critical; every 15 minutes for stable)		
Repeats initial assessment and documents findings		
Records ALL treatments with times and patient response(s) in treatment section		
Documents field impression and person suspected abuse/neglect reported to if applicable		
Documents transport to specific facility and transfer of care WITH VERBAL REPORT		
Uses correct grammar, abbreviations, spelling, and terminology		
Writes legibly		
Thoroughly documents refusals, denials of transport, and call cancellations		
Documents parent/legal guardian understanding of possible complications to signing refusal		
Documents advice given to refusing parent, including "call 9-1-1 for further problems"		
Properly corrects errors and omissions		
Writes cautiously, avoids jargon, opinions, inferences, or any derogatory/libelous remarks		
Signs run report		
Uses EMS supplement form if needed		
Student exhibits competence with skill		

Any items in the Not Done column should be evaluated with student. Check marks in this column do not necessarily mean student was unsuccessful as all lines are not completed on all patients. Evaluation of each PCR should be based on the scenario given.

Student must be able to write an EMS report with consistency and accuracy.

☐ Successful   ☐ Unsuccessful   Examiner Initials: _____

                    ©2006 Prentice-Hall Inc.

Overall Scenario Management—Pediatric Medical

Student: _____   Examiner: _____

Date: _____   Scenario: _____

NOTE: This skill sheet is to be done after the student completes a scenario as the TEAM LEADER. It is to let the student know if he or she is beginning to "put it all together" and use critical thinking skills to manage an EMS call. PLEASE notice that it is graded on a different basis than the basic lab skill sheet.

	Done ✓	Needs to Improve
SCENE MANAGEMENT		
Recognized hazards and controlled scene—safety, crowd, and patient issues		
Recognized hazards, but did not control the scene		
Unsuccessfully attempted to manage the scene	*	
Did not evaluate the scene and took no control of the scene	*	
PATIENT ASSESSMENT		
Performed a timely, organized complete patient assessment		
Performed complete initial, focused, and ongoing assessments, but in a disorganized manner		
Performed an incomplete assessment	*	
Did not perform an initial assessment	*	
PATIENT MANAGEMENT		
Evaluated assessment findings to manage all aspects of patient condition		
Managed the patient's presenting signs and symptoms without considering all of assessment		
Inadequately managed the patient	*	
Did not manage life-threatening conditions	*	
COMMUNICATION		
Communicated well with crew, patient, family, bystanders, and assisting agencies		
Communicated well with patient and crew		
Communicated with patient and crew, but poor communication skills	*	
Unable to communicate effectively	*	
REPORT AND TRANSFER OF CARE		
Identified correct destination for patient transport, gave accurate, brief report over radio, and provided full report at bedside demonstrating thorough understanding of patient condition and pathophysiological processes		
Identified correct destination and gave accurate radio and bedside report, but did not demonstrate understanding of patient condition and pathophysiological processes		
Identified correct destination, but provided inadequate radio and bedside report	*	
Identified inappropriate destination or provided no radio or bedside report	*	
Student exhibits competence with skill		

Any items that are marked with an * indicate the student needs to improve and a check mark should be placed in the right-hand column. A check mark in the right-hand column indicates that the student was unsuccessful and must attempt the skill again to assure competency. Examiners should use a different-color ink for the second attempt.

☐ Successful   ☐ Unsuccessful   Examiner Initials: _____

Patient Assessment: Medical—Pediatric

Student: _____   Examiner: _____

Date: _____   Scenario: _____

	Done ✓	Not Done
Assesses scene safety and utilizes appropriate PPE		*
OVERALL SCENE EVALUATION		
Medical—determines nature of illness/if trauma involved determines MOI		*
Determines the number of patients, location, obstacles, and requests any additional resources as needed		
Verbalizes general impression of the patient as approaches		*
Considers stabilization/spinal motion restriction of spine if trauma involved		*
INITIAL ASSESSMENT		
Determines responsiveness/level of consciousness/AVPU		*
Opens airway with appropriate technique and assesses airway/ventilation		*
Manages airway/ventilation and applies appropriate oxygen therapy in less than 3 minutes		*
Assesses circulation: radial/carotid pulse, skin color, temperature, condition, and turgor		*
Controls any major bleeding		*
Makes rapid transport decision if indicated, to appropriate facility		*
Obtains Broselow (or other brand) tape weight/dosage area for reference if needed		*
Initiates IV or IO if critical, obtains BGL, GCS, and complete vital signs		*
FOCUSED HISTORY AND PHYSICAL EXAMINATION/RAPID ASSESSMENT		
Obtains SAMPLE history from patient or caregiver		*
Obtains OPQRST from patient or caregiver for differential diagnosis		
Obtains associated symptoms, pertinent negatives/denials		
Evaluates decision to perform focused exam or completes rapid assessment (toe-to-head exam for younger child)		*
Vital signs including AVPU (and GCS if trauma)		*
Assesses cardiovascular system including heart sounds, peripheral perfusion (capillary refill)		*
Assesses pulmonary system including reassessing airway, ventilation, breath sounds, pulse oximetry, chest wall excursion, accessory muscle use, nasal flaring, sternal retractions, or other signs of distress		*
Assesses neurological system and distal movement and sensation		*
Assesses musculoskeletal and integumentary systems		
Assesses behavioral, psychological, and social aspects of patient and situation for possible abuse/neglect		
States field impression of patient—pediatric medical (states suspected differential diagnosis)		*
Verbalizes treatment plan for patient and calls for appropriate intervention(s)—IV unless suspected epiglottitis		*
Reevaluates transport decision		
ONGOING ASSESSMENT		
Repeats initial assessment		*
Repeats vital signs and evaluates trends		*
Evaluates response to treatments		*
Repeats focused assessment regarding patient complaint or injuries		
Gives radio report to appropriate receiving facility		
Turns over patient care with verbal report		*
Student exhibits competence with skill		

Any items in the Not Done column that are marked with an * are mandatory for the student to complete. A check mark in the Not Done column of an item with an * indicates that the student was unsuccessful and must attempt the skill again to assure competency. Examiners should use a different-color ink for the second attempt.

☐ Successful   ☐ Unsuccessful   Examiner Initials: _____

©2006 Prentice-Hall Inc.

Scenario Radio Report—Pediatric Medical

Student: _____   **Examiner:** _____

Date: _____

	Done ✓	Not Done
Requests and checks for open channel before speaking		
Presses transmit button 1 second before speaking		
Holds microphone 2–3 in. from mouth		
Speaks slowly and clearly		*
Speaks in a normal voice		
Briefly transmits: Agency, unit designation, identification/name		*
Briefly transmits: Patient's age, sex, weight		*
Briefly transmits: Scene description/mechanism of injury or medical problem		*
Briefly transmits: Chief complaint with brief history of *present* illness		*
Briefly transmits: Associated symptoms (unless able to be deferred to bedside report)		
Briefly transmits: Past medical history (usually deferred to bedside report)		
Briefly transmits: Vital signs		*
Briefly transmits: Level of consciousness/GCS on trauma		*
Briefly transmits: General appearance, distress, cardiac rhythm, blood glucose, and other pertinent findings unable to be deferred to bedside report		
Briefly transmits: Interventions by EMS AND response(s)		*
ETA (the more critical the patient, the earlier you need to notify the receiving facility)		
Does not waste airtime		
Protects privacy of patient		*
Echoes dispatch information and any physician orders		*
Writes down dispatch information or physician orders		
Confirms with facility that message is received		
Demonstrates/verbalizes ability to troubleshoot basic equipment malfunction		
Student exhibits competence with skill		

Any items in the Not Done column that are marked with an * are mandatory for the student to complete. A check mark in the Not Done column of an item with an * indicates that the student was unsuccessful and must attempt the skill again to assure competency. Examiners should use a different-color ink for the second attempt.

☐ Successful   ☐ Unsuccessful   Examiner Initials: _____

©2006 Prentice-Hall Inc.

Scenario Patient Care Report (PCR)—Pediatric Medical

Student: _____   Examiner: _____

Date: _____

	Done ✓	Not Done
Records all pertinent dispatch/scene data, using a consistent format		
Completely identifies all additional resources and personnel		
Documents chief complaint, signs/symptoms, position found, age, sex, and weight		
Identifies and records all pertinent, reportable clinical data for each patient		
Documents SAMPLE and OPQRST if applicable		
Records all pertinent negatives		
Records all pertinent denials		
Records accurate, consistent times and patient information		
Includes relevant oral statements of witnesses, bystanders, and patient in "quotes" when appropriate		
Documents initial assessment findings: airway, breathing, and circulation		
Documents any interventions in initial assessment with patient response		
Documents level of consciousness, GCS (if trauma), and VS		
Documents rapid trauma assessment if applicable		
Documents any interventions in rapid trauma assessment with patient response		
Documents focused history and physical assessment		
Documents any interventions in focused assessment with patient response		
Documents repeat VS (every 5 minutes for critical; every 15 minutes for stable)		
Repeats initial assessment and documents findings		
Records ALL treatments with times and patient response(s) in treatment section		
Documents field impression and person suspected abuse/neglect reported to if applicable		
Documents transport to specific facility and transfer of care WITH VERBAL REPORT		
Uses correct grammar, abbreviations, spelling, and terminology		
Writes legibly		
Thoroughly documents refusals, denials of transport, and call cancellations		
Documents parent/legal guardian understanding of possible complications to signing refusal		
Documents advice given to refusing parent, including "call 9-1-1 for further problems"		
Properly corrects errors and omissions		
Writes cautiously, avoids jargon, opinions, inferences, or any derogatory/libelous remarks		
Signs run report		
Uses EMS supplement form if needed		
Student exhibits competence with skill		

Any items in the Not Done column should be evaluated with student. Check marks in this column do not necessarily mean student was unsuccessful as all lines are not completed on all patients. Evaluation of each PCR should be based on the scenario given.

Student must be able to write an EMS report with consistency and accuracy.

☐ Successful   ☐ Unsuccessful   Examiner Initials: _____

                    ©2006 Prentice-Hall Inc.

Overall Scenario Management—Pediatric Medical

Student: _____   Examiner: _____

Date: _____   Scenario: _____

NOTE: This skill sheet is to be done after the student completes a scenario as the TEAM LEADER. It is to let the student know if he or she is beginning to "put it all together" and use critical thinking skills to manage an EMS call. PLEASE notice that it is graded on a different basis than the basic lab skill sheet.

	Done ✓	Needs to Improve
SCENE MANAGEMENT		
Recognized hazards and controlled scene—safety, crowd, and patient issues		
Recognized hazards, but did not control the scene		
Unsuccessfully attempted to manage the scene	*	
Did not evaluate the scene and took no control of the scene	*	
PATIENT ASSESSMENT		
Performed a timely, organized complete patient assessment		
Performed complete initial, focused, and ongoing assessments, but in a disorganized manner		
Performed an incomplete assessment	*	
Did not perform an initial assessment	*	
PATIENT MANAGEMENT		
Evaluated assessment findings to manage all aspects of patient condition		
Managed the patient's presenting signs and symptoms without considering all of assessment		
Inadequately managed the patient	*	
Did not manage life-threatening conditions	*	
COMMUNICATION		
Communicated well with crew, patient, family, bystanders, and assisting agencies		
Communicated well with patient and crew		
Communicated with patient and crew, but poor communication skills	*	
Unable to communicate effectively	*	
REPORT AND TRANSFER OF CARE		
Identified correct destination for patient transport, gave accurate, brief report over radio, and provided full report at bedside demonstrating thorough understanding of patient condition and pathophysiological processes		
Identified correct destination and gave accurate radio and bedside report, but did not demonstrate understanding of patient condition and pathophysiological processes		
Identified correct destination, but provided inadequate radio and bedside report	*	
Identified inappropriate destination or provided no radio or bedside report	*	
Student exhibits competence with skill		

Any items that are marked with an * indicate the student needs to improve and a check mark should be placed in the right-hand column. A check mark in the right-hand column indicates that the student was unsuccessful and must attempt the skill again to assure competency. Examiners should use a different-color ink for the second attempt.

☐ Successful   ☐ Unsuccessful   Examiner Initials: _____

Patient Assessment: Trauma—Pediatric

Student: _____   Examiner: _____

Date: _____

	Done ✓	Not Done
Assesses scene safety and utilizes appropriate PPE		*
OVERALL SCENE EVALUATION		
Trauma—assesses mechanism of injury/if medical component determines nature of illness		*
Determines the number of patients, location, obstacles, and requests any additional resources as needed		
Verbalizes general impression of the patient as approaches		*
Stabilizes C-spine/spinal motion restriction (SMR) of spine		*
INITIAL ASSESSMENT/RESUSCITATION		
Determines responsiveness/level of consciousness/AVPU		*
Opens airway with appropriate technique and assesses airway/ventilation		*
Manages airway/ventilation and applies appropriate oxygen therapy in less than 3 minutes		*
Assesses circulation: radial/carotid pulse, skin color, temperature, condition, and turgor		*
Controls any major bleeding and makes rapid transport decision		*
Obtains Broselow (or other brand) tape weight/dosage area for reference if needed		*
Obtains IV or IO if critical, obtains BGL, GCS, and complete vital signs		*
RAPID TRAUMA ASSESSMENT (If patient is Trauma Alert or Load and Go)		
Assesses abdomen		
Rapidly palpates each extremity assessing for obvious injuries and distal PMS		
Provides spinal motion restriction (SMR) on LBB or pediatric immobilizer, checking posterior torso and legs		
Secures head LAST		
Identifies patient problem: pediatric trauma—verbalizes consideration of possible abuse		*
Loads patient/initiates transport (to appropriate LZ or to appropriate facility) in less than 10 minutes		*
Reassesses ABCs and interventions		*
FOCUSED HISTORY AND PHYSICAL ASSESSMENT		
Reassesses interventions and further assesses injuries found		
Obtains vital signs and GCS (Glasgow Coma Score)		
Obtains SAMPLE history from patient/caregiver		
Inspects and palpates head, facial, and neck regions		
Inspects, palpates, and auscultates chest/thorax		
Inspects and palpates abdomen and pelvis		
Inspects and palpates upper and lower extremities checking distal PMS		
Inspects and palpates posterior torso		
Manages all injuries/wounds appropriately—verbalizes awareness of common signs of child abuse		*
Repeats initial assessment, vital signs, and evaluates trends		*
Evaluates response to interventions/treatments		*
Performs ongoing assessment (VS every 5 minutes for critical patient/every 15 minutes for stable patient)		*
Gives radio report to appropriate receiving facility and flight team if applicable		
Turns over patient care with verbal report		*
Student exhibits competence with skill		

Any items in the Not Done column that are marked with an * are mandatory for the student to complete. A check mark in the Not Done column of an item with an * indicates that the student was unsuccessful and must attempt the skill again to assure competency. Examiners should use a different-color ink for the second attempt.

☐ Successful   ☐ Unsuccessful   Examiner Initials: _____

©2006 Prentice-Hall Inc.

Scenario Radio Report—Pediatric Trauma

Student: _____   **Examiner:** _____

Date: _____

	Done ✓	Not Done
Requests and checks for open channel before speaking		
Presses transmit button 1 second before speaking		
Holds microphone 2–3 in. from mouth		
Speaks slowly and clearly		*
Speaks in a normal voice		
Briefly transmits: Agency, unit designation, identification/name		*
Briefly transmits: Patient's age, sex, weight		*
Briefly transmits: Scene description/mechanism of injury or medical problem		*
Briefly transmits: Chief complaint with brief history of *present* illness		*
Briefly transmits: Associated symptoms (unless able to be deferred to bedside report)		
Briefly transmits: Past medical history (usually deferred to bedside report)		
Briefly transmits: Vital signs		*
Briefly transmits: Level of consciousness/GCS on trauma		*
Briefly transmits: General appearance, distress, cardiac rhythm, blood glucose, and other pertinent findings unable to be deferred to bedside report		
Briefly transmits: Interventions by EMS AND response(s)		*
ETA (the more critical the patient, the earlier you need to notify the receiving facility)		
Does not waste airtime		
Protects privacy of patient		*
Echoes dispatch information and any physician orders		*
Writes down dispatch information or physician orders		
Confirms with facility that message is received		
Demonstrates/verbalizes ability to troubleshoot basic equipment malfunction		
Student exhibits competence with skill		

Any items in the Not Done column that are marked with an * are mandatory for the student to complete. A check mark in the Not Done column of an item with an * indicates that the student was unsuccessful and must attempt the skill again to assure competency. Examiners should use a different-color ink for the second attempt.

☐ Successful   ☐ Unsuccessful   Examiner Initials: _____

Scenario Patient Care Report (PCR)—Pediatric Trauma

Student: _____   Examiner: _____

Date: _____

	Done ✓	Not Done
Records all pertinent dispatch/scene data, using a consistent format		
Completely identifies all additional resources and personnel		
Documents chief complaint, signs/symptoms, position found, age, sex, and weight		
Identifies and records all pertinent, reportable clinical data for each patient		
Documents SAMPLE and OPQRST if applicable		
Records all pertinent negatives		
Records all pertinent denials		
Records accurate, consistent times and patient information		
Includes relevant oral statements of witnesses, bystanders, and patient in "quotes" when appropriate		
Documents initial assessment findings: airway, breathing, and circulation		
Documents any interventions in initial assessment with patient response		
Documents level of consciousness, GCS (if trauma), and VS		
Documents rapid trauma assessment if applicable		
Documents any interventions in rapid trauma assessment with patient response		
Documents focused history and physical assessment		
Documents any interventions in focused assessment with patient response		
Documents repeat VS (every 5 minutes for critical; every 15 minutes for stable)		
Repeats initial assessment and documents findings		
Records ALL treatments with times and patient response(s) in treatment section		
Documents field impression and person suspected abuse/neglect reported to if applicable		
Documents transport to specific facility and transfer of care WITH VERBAL REPORT		
Uses correct grammar, abbreviations, spelling, and terminology		
Writes legibly		
Thoroughly documents refusals, denials of transport, and call cancellations		
Documents parent/legal guardian understanding of possible complications to signing refusal		
Documents advice given to refusing parent, including "call 9-1-1 for further problems"		
Properly corrects errors and omissions		
Writes cautiously, avoids jargon, opinions, inferences, or any derogatory/libelous remarks		
Signs run report		
Uses EMS supplement form if needed		
Student exhibits competence with skill		

Any items in the Not Done column should be evaluated with student. Check marks in this column do not necessarily mean student was unsuccessful as all lines are not completed on all patients. Evaluation of each PCR should be based on the scenario given.

Student must be able to write an EMS report with consistency and accuracy.

☐ Successful   ☐ Unsuccessful   Examiner Initials: _____

    ©2006 Prentice-Hall Inc.

Overall Scenario Management—Pediatric Trauma

Student: _____   Examiner: _____

Date: _____   Scenario: _____

NOTE: This skill sheet is to be done after the student completes a scenario as the TEAM LEADER. It is to let the student know if he or she is beginning to "put it all together" and use critical thinking skills to manage an EMS call. PLEASE notice that it is graded on a different basis than the basic lab skill sheet.

	Done ✓	Needs to Improve
SCENE MANAGEMENT		
Recognized hazards and controlled scene—safety, crowd, and patient issues		
Recognized hazards, but did not control the scene		
Unsuccessfully attempted to manage the scene	*	
Did not evaluate the scene and took no control of the scene	*	
PATIENT ASSESSMENT		
Performed a timely, organized complete patient assessment		
Performed complete initial, focused, and ongoing assessments, but in a disorganized manner		
Performed an incomplete assessment	*	
Did not perform an initial assessment	*	
PATIENT MANAGEMENT		
Evaluated assessment findings to manage all aspects of patient condition		
Managed the patient's presenting signs and symptoms without considering all of assessment		
Inadequately managed the patient	*	
Did not manage life-threatening conditions	*	
COMMUNICATION		
Communicated well with crew, patient, family, bystanders, and assisting agencies		
Communicated well with patient and crew		
Communicated with patient and crew, but poor communication skills	*	
Unable to communicate effectively	*	
REPORT AND TRANSFER OF CARE		
Identified correct destination for patient transport, gave accurate, brief report over radio, and provided full report at bedside demonstrating thorough understanding of patient condition and pathophysiological processes		
Identified correct destination and gave accurate radio and bedside report, but did not demonstrate understanding of patient condition and pathophysiological processes		
Identified correct destination, but provided inadequate radio and bedside report	*	
Identified inappropriate destination or provided no radio or bedside report	*	
Student exhibits competence with skill		

Any items that are marked with an * indicate the student needs to improve and a check mark should be placed in the right-hand column. A check mark in the right-hand column indicates that the student was unsuccessful and must attempt the skill again to assure competency. Examiners should use a different-color ink for the second attempt.

☐ Successful   ☐ Unsuccessful   Examiner Initials: _____

DAILY DISCUSSIONS AND PERTINENT POINTS—
SPECIALTY: GYN/OB/NEONATAL/PEDS

Student: _____   **Date:** _____

Instructor: _____

	Instructor Initials
Value the importance of maintaining a patient's modesty and privacy while still being able to obtain necessary information.	
Defend the need to provide care for a patient of sexual assault, while still preventing destruction of crime scene information.	
Serve as a role model for other EMS providers when discussing or caring for patients with gynecological emergencies, in both lab and clinical areas.	
Advocate the need for treating two patients (mother and baby).	
Value the importance of maintaining a patient's modesty and privacy during assessment and management.	
Serve as a role model for other EMS providers when discussing or performing the steps of childbirth in classroom, lab, and clinical areas.	
Recognize the emotional impact of newborn/neonate injuries/illnesses on parents/guardians.	
Recognize and appreciate the physical and emotional difficulties associated with separation of the parent/guardian and a newborn/neonate.	
Listen to the concerns expressed by parents/guardians.	
Identify methods/mechanisms that prevent injuries to infants and children.	
Outline differences in adult and childhood anatomy and physiology.	
Discuss the parent/caregiver responses to the death of an infant or child.	
In both lab and clinical areas, demonstrate and advocate appropriate interaction with a neonate/newborn that conveys respect for their position in life.	
Demonstrate and advocate appropriate interactions with the infant/child that convey an understanding of his or her developmental stage, in both lab and clinical areas.	
Recognize the emotional dependence of the infant/child to his or her parent/guardian.	
Recognize the emotional impact of the infant/child injuries and illnesses on the parent/guardian.	
Recognize and appreciate the physical and emotional difficulties associated with separation of the parent/guardian of a special needs child.	
Demonstrate the ability to provide reassurance, empathy, and compassion for the parent/guardian in both lab and clinical areas.	
Attend to/discuss the need for reassurance, empathy, and compassion for the parent/guardian.	
Explain the differences between adult and pediatric airway anatomy.	
Discuss the paramedic's role in the reduction of infant and childhood morbidity and mortality from acute illness and injury.	
Value the importance of immunization, especially in children and populations at risk.	
Defend personal beliefs about withholding or stopping patient care.	
Defend the value of advance medical directives.	

©2006 Prentice-Hall Inc.

Part 2: Chronic Care/Home Health

Skill Sheets

Using an Implantable Venous Access Device (VAD)
Drawing Blood from a Central Venous Catheter (CVC)
Hemodialysis Site Care
Inserting Nasogastric/Nasointestinal Tube for Suction and Enteral Feeding
Administering Enteral Tube Feedings
Nasopharyngeal/Oropharyngeal Suction in Chronic Care
Performing Tracheostomy Suction
Performing Tracheostomy Care
Changing Tracheostomy Inner Cannula
Wound Irrigation
Wound Culture
Changing a Dry Sterile Dressing
Changing a Wet-to-Dry Dressing
Performing Urinary Catheterization—Male
Performing Urinary Catheterization—Female
Irrigating an Open Catheter
Changing a Colostomy Pouch

SKILL SHEETS

Using an Implantable Venous Access Device (VAD)

Student: _____   Examiner: _____

Date: _____

	Done ✓	Not Done
Contacts Medical Control or receives physician order to access VAD		*
Cleanses hands and utilizes appropriate PPE		*
Explains procedure to conscious patient		*
Assembles appropriate equipment, including blood tubes and Huber needle		
Exposes skin and palpates VAD		
Examines VAD area for redness, swelling, pain, or other complication		*
Turns patient's head away from the insertion site		
Puts on sterile gloves and cleanses area with alcohol		
Gathers appropriate equipment, including correct needle (Huber)		
Primes needle and extension set with saline		*
Changes sterile gloves, stabilizes VAD, and inserts needle through skin and septum		*
Feels resistance of needle touching back of port to avoid subQ placement		*
Aspirates blood to verify needle placement and port function		*
Draws blood and wastes first 10 cc, then obtains blood samples		*
Flushes line with saline solution to clear blood and establish patency of line		*
Proceeds with medication administration or fluid infusion		*
Secures needle with sterile dressing		*
Observes area for signs of infiltration		*
If necessary to remove needle, flushes with saline maintaining positive pressure, and clamps		*
Stabilizes VAD and removes needle, applies pressure dressing over insertion site		*
Assesses patient's response to intervention		*
Cleanses hands and documents VAD site appearance and access technique		*
Documents physician giving permission to access port		
Student exhibits competence with skill		

Any items in the Not Done column that are marked with an * are mandatory for the student to complete. A check mark in the Not Done column of an item with an * indicates that the student was unsuccessful and must attempt the skill again to assure competency. Examiners should use a different-color ink for the second attempt.

☐ Successful   ☐ Unsuccessful   Examiner Initials: _____

©2006 Prentice-Hall Inc.

Drawing Blood from a Central Venous Catheter (CVC)

Student: _____   Examiner: _____

Date: _____

	Done ✓	Not Done
Contacts Medical Control or receives physician order to access CVC		*
Cleanses hands and utilizes appropriate PPE		*
Assesses the function and patency of the catheter		*
Explains procedure to conscious patient and checks allergies (to iodine)		*
Prepares syringe of 10 cc sterile saline, empty syringes, blood tubes, and transfer needle		*
Turns patient's head away from the insertion site		
Swabs insertion site with Betadine solution and lets dry		*
Shuts off any IV solutions infusing through other ports of the central line		*
Clamps BROWN (distal) catheter and removes cap, keeping cap sterile		*
Unclamps catheter and aspirates 10 cc of solution/blood, reclamps catheter		*
Discards first blood draw		*
Unclamps catheter and obtains blood sample, reclamps catheter		*
Unclamps catheter and flushes with sterile saline solution, reclamps catheter under pressure		*
Replaces cap on catheter		*
Checks that all clamps are secure and tapes all connections		*
Restarts and adjusts any IV solutions previously infusing through other ports		*
Transfers blood to tubes		*
Labels all blood samples correctly and sends to lab		*
Reassesses patient and documents procedure and physician giving permission		
Correctly disposes of equipment used and cleanses hands		*
Assesses patient's response to intervention		*
Student exhibits competence with skill		

Any items in the Not Done column that are marked with an * are mandatory for the student to complete. A check mark in the Not Done column of an item with an * indicates that the student was unsuccessful and must attempt the skill again to assure competency. Examiners should use a different-color ink for the second attempt.

☐ Successful   ☐ Unsuccessful   Examiner Initials: _____

Hemodialysis Site Care

Student: _____   **Examiner:** _____

Date: _____

	Done ✓	Not Done
Contacts Medical Control or receives physician order to perform dialysis site care		*
Cleanses hands and utilizes appropriate PPE		*
Explains procedure to patient and elicits allergies (to iodine)		*
Evaluates type of hemodialysis access device		*
AV Fistula: Shunt or Graft: Positions extremity for easy access and palpates fistula		*
Palpates over area for thrill (vibration)		*
Auscultates over area for bruit (swishing noise)		*
Palpates pulse and observes capillary refill distal to the fistula		*
Assesses for signs of infection in the area around fistula and the entire extremity		*
Avoids taking BP or initiating IV in arm with shunt/fistula		*
Double-Lumen Catheter: Fills 2 syringes with 10 cc sterile saline		*
If changing caps, primes with sterile saline		*
Opens care kit and places on sterile field		*
Puts on mask and gloves		*
Removes old dressing and gloves, rolling soiled dressing into gloves		*
Puts on sterile gloves and cleanses site with alcohol, assessing site for signs of infection		*
Cleanses surrounding area with Betadine (if no allergy to iodine) and lets dry		*
Applies transparent dressing		*
Closes clamp to both lumens, removes and discards both old caps		*
Cleanses ends of catheter with alcohol and attaches new PRIMED caps		*
Unclamps lumens and flushes with sterile saline per protocol/MD order		*
Properly removes and disposes of PPE		*
Reassesses patient and cleanses hands		*
Documents procedure correctly and physician giving permission		*
Student exhibits competence with skill		

Any items in the Not Done column that are marked with an * are mandatory for the student to complete. A check mark in the Not Done column of an item with an * indicates that the student was unsuccessful and must attempt the skill again to assure competency. Examiners should use a different-color ink for the second attempt.

☐ Successful   ☐ Unsuccessful   Examiner Initials: _____

     ©2006 Prentice-Hall Inc.

Inserting Nasogastric/Nasointestinal Tube for Suction and Enteral Feeding

Student: _____   **Examiner:** _____

Date: _____

	Done ✓	Not Done
Cleanses hands		*
Utilizes appropriate PPE		*
Obtains equipment (suction, tube, lubricant, tape, irrigating syringe, water, straw, basin)		*
Explains procedure to conscious patient or verifies secure airway in unresponsive patient		*
Positions patient (supine for unresponsive, high Fowler's for conscious)		*
Places towel over chest and tissues within reach—provides privacy		
Examines nostrils and assesses as patient breathes through each nostril		
Measures tube from xiphoid process to earlobe to nose and tapes depth marking		*
Adds 15–20 cm if tube is to go below stomach (nasoduodenal or nasojejunal)		
Lubricates 4 in. of tube		*
Small-bore feeding tube: Opens adapter cap on tube and injects water into adapter		
Closes adapter cap		
If equipped with flexi-stylet, checks that stylet does not protrude through holes in feeding tube		*
Passes tip through nostril anterior to posterior along floor of nasal passage		*
Guides tube to nasopharynx		*
Advises conscious patient to continue drinking as tube is passed to measured depth		*
Passes tube slowly and posteriorly in unresponsive patient, checking mouth for curling		*
Determines proper tube placement by auscultation over epigastrium of injected AIR		*
Secures tube in place		*
Places to suction (continuous only for emptying initial contents, then intermittent)		*
Saves gastric contents		*
Reassesses patient and cleanses hands		*
Documents procedure correctly		
Student exhibits competence with skill		

Any items in the Not Done column that are marked with an * are mandatory for the student to complete. A check mark in the Not Done column of an item with an * indicates that the student was unsuccessful and must attempt the skill again to assure competency. Examiners should use a different-color ink for the second attempt.

☐ Successful   ☐ Unsuccessful   Examiner Initials: _____

Administering Enteral Tube Feedings

Student: _____   Examiner: _____

Date: _____

	Done ✓	Not Done
Cleanses hands		*
Utilizes appropriate PPE		*
Gathers supplies and explains procedure to patient if conscious		*
If using bag, adds formula to bag		
Observes oral cavity for sores, abnormalities, or gastric contents (possible aspiration)		*
Auscultates breath sounds for any adventitious sounds indicating possible aspiration		*
Places patient on right side in high Fowler's position and provides privacy		
Auscultates for bowel sounds and observes for abdominal distension		*
Observes insertion site for any signs of infection		*
Checks feeding tube placement by aspirating stomach contents		*
Reinstills aspirated contents		
Primes tubing to remove air and administers tube feeding		
Intermittent bolus: Pinches tubing, removes plunger, attaches barrel to adapter		
Fills with formula and allows to infuse slowly		*
Flushes with 30–60 ml water		
Intermittent gavage: Hangs bag 18 in. above patient's head		
Removes air from tubing and attaches tubing to feeding tube adapter		*
When bag of fluid empty, adds 30–60 ml of water to flush		*
Clamps feeding tube after either of above methods		*
If **continuous gavage:** Adds amount of formula to bag for 4-hour period		*
Labels with date and time, hangs on pole, and primes tubing		*
Threads tubing through pump and attaches to feeding tube adapter		*
Checks tube placement at least every 4 hours, checks residual at least every 4 hours		*
Flushes tube every 4 hours or following any medication administration		
Changes feeding bag every 24 hours (may wash with soap and water)		
Provides oral hygiene every 2–4 hours		
Administers water as prescribed		
Reassesses patient during and after feeding, and cleanses hands		*
Documents procedure correctly		
Student exhibits competence with skill		

Any items in the Not Done column that are marked with an * are mandatory for the student to complete. A check mark in the Not Done column of an item with an * indicates that the student was unsuccessful and must attempt the skill again to assure competency. Examiners should use a different-color ink for the second attempt.

☐ Successful   ☐ Unsuccessful   Examiner Initials: _____

          ©2006 Prentice-Hall Inc.

Nasopharyngeal/Oropharyngeal Suction in Chronic Care

Student: _____   **Examiner:** _____

Date: _____

	Done ✓	Not Done
Cleanses hands		*
Utilizes appropriate PPE (goggles, gown, mask, gloves)		*
Gathers supplies and explains procedure to conscious patient		*
Positions patient in high or semi-Fowler's		
Adjusts suction control to between 110 and 120 mmHg		*
Opens suction kit, using inside of wrapper as sterile field		*
Puts sterile lubricant on field and sterile solution into container		
Carefully lifts wrapped gloves from kit without contaminating field or gloves		*
Opens wrapper and dons sterile gloves		*
Designates one hand clean and one sterile		
Uses sterile hand to pick up catheter and coils tip around fingers		*
Picks up extension tubing and connects to catheter		
Asks patient if prefers to perform suction on him or herself or proceeds as below		
Positions thumb of clean hand over port and dips catheter into sterile solution to check suction		
Oropharyngeal: Asks patient to open mouth and advances catheter, suctioning as withdraws		
Nasopharyngeal: Lubricates catheter and measures from nose to earlobe		*
Inserts and advances with downward tilt and slight rotation		*
Occludes port and suctions while withdrawing—NO LONGER than 15 seconds		*
Repeats both as needed		
Assesses patient's response to intervention		*
Dips catheter into solution to clean and disconnects from extension tubing		*
Removes glove by pulling over catheter		*
Disposes of soiled items appropriately		*
Reassesses patient and cleanses hands		*
Documents procedure correctly		
Student exhibits competence with skill		

Any items in the Not Done column that are marked with an * are mandatory for the student to complete. A check mark in the Not Done column of an item with an * indicates that the student was unsuccessful and must attempt the skill again to assure competency. Examiners should use a different-color ink for the second attempt.

☐ Successful   ☐ Unsuccessful   Examiner Initials: _____

©2006 Prentice-Hall Inc.

Performing Tracheostomy Suction

Student: _____   Examiner: _____

Date: _____

	Done ✓	Not Done
Cleanses hands		*
Utilizes appropriate PPE (gown, mask, goggles/face shield precautions—gown only if patient on contact isolation)		*
Gathers equipment and explains procedure to patient		*
Positions patient in high or semi-Fowler's		
Adjusts suction control between 80 and 100 mmHg		
Opens suction kit, using inside of wrapper as sterile field		*
If sterile solution not included, pours sterile saline solution into sterile container in kit		*
Carefully lifts wrapped gloves from kit without contaminating field or gloves		*
Opens wrapper and dons sterile gloves		*
If sterile solution in kit, opens it		*
Designates one hand sterile and one hand clean		
Uses sterile hand to pick up catheter and coils tip around fingers		*
Picks up extension tubing with clean hand and connects to suction catheter		
Instructs patient to take several slow, deep breaths (to preoxygenate)		*
Uses clean hand to remove oxygen		
Positions thumb of clean hand over suction port		
Dips catheter into sterile solution, activates suction, and observes suction working		
Releases thumb from port, inserts catheter into trach until patient coughs		*
Occludes port and applies intermittent suction while rotating and withdrawing catheter		*
Suctions NO LONGER than 15 seconds		*
Repeats as needed		
Suctions oropharynx well		
Cleans suction catheter tubing by suctioning sterile solution		
Reapplies oxygen		*
Assesses patient's response to intervention		*
Discards equipment appropriately		*
Reassesses patient and cleanses hands		*
Documents procedure correctly		
Student exhibits competence with skill		

Any items in the Not Done column that are marked with an * are mandatory for the student to complete. A check mark in the Not Done column of an item with an * indicates that the student was unsuccessful and must attempt the skill again to assure competency. Examiners should use a different-color ink for the second attempt.

☐ Successful   ☐ Unsuccessful   Examiner Initials: _____

©2006 Prentice-Hall Inc.

Performing Tracheostomy Care

Student: _____

Examiner: _____

Date: _____

	Done ✓	Not Done
Cleanses hands		
Utilizes appropriate PPE (including mask, shield, gown, goggles)		*
Explains procedure to patient and gathers/opens supplies		*
Puts on sterile gloves and suctions tracheostomy tube, removes soiled dressing		*
Notes drainage on dressing and removes gloves by pulling over soiled dressing		*
Opens trach care kit, dons sterile gloves, and opens inner kit with sterile technique		*
Lays out sterile supplies on sterile field and drapes patient's chest		*
Designates one hand sterile and one hand clean		
Uses clean hand to open saline and peroxide (caps outside field), pours into containers		*
Uses sterile hand to clean periostomal skin and under faceplate with sterile cotton tip and H_2O_2		*
Uses clean hand to loosen inner cannula by twisting outer ring counterclockwise		*
Places inner cannula in basin of peroxide, soaks, and cleans with brush and peroxide (if not disposable)—if disposable, disposes of properly		*
Places inner cannula in sterile saline and agitates		*
Inspects cannula for cleanliness, removes excess saline, and replaces (rotate clockwise) or inserts new disposable inner cannula		*
Places new DSD (precut) around stoma		*
If ties damp, removes ties and has assistant hold trach in place		*
Cleanses and dries skin under tie area		*
Applies clean twill tape or Velcro ties and replaces on oxygen		*
Verifies bilateral breath sounds after procedure		*
Assesses patient's response to intervention		*
Removes and correctly disposes of soiled items		*
Reassesses patient and washes hands		*
Documents procedure correctly		
Student exhibits competence with skill		

Any items in the Not Done column that are marked with an * are mandatory for the student to complete. A check mark in the Not Done column of an item with an * indicates that the student was unsuccessful and must attempt the skill again to assure competency. Examiners should use a different-color ink for the second attempt.

☐ Successful   ☐ Unsuccessful   Examiner Initials: _____

©2006 Prentice-Hall Inc.

Changing Tracheostomy Inner Cannula

Student: _____   **Examiner:** _____

Date: _____

	Done ✓	Not Done
Cleanses hands		*
Utilizes appropriate PPE		*
Removes inner cannula (deflates cuff if present)		*
Assists patient to expectorate as needed		*
Suctions through outer cannula as needed		*
Cleanses inner cannula with hydrogen peroxide and saline		*
Cleanses outside of tracheostomy tube with hydrogen peroxide and saline		*
Replaces inner cannula with clean cannula		*
Removes trach tape keeping tube secured and cleans area around stoma and under tape		*
Secures tube with clean tracheostomy (twill) tape		*
Verifies bilateral breath sounds after procedure		*
Assesses patient's response to intervention		*
Cleanses hands		
Documents procedure correctly		
Student exhibits competence with skill		

Any items in the Not Done column that are marked with an * are mandatory for the student to complete. A check mark in the Not Done column of an item with an * indicates that the student was unsuccessful and must attempt the skill again to assure competency. Examiners should use a different-color ink for the second attempt.

☐ Successful   ☐ Unsuccessful   Examiner Initials: _____

©2006 Prentice-Hall Inc.

Wound Irrigation

Student: _____   **Examiner:** _____

Date: _____

	Done ✓	Not Done
Cleanses hands		*
Utilizes appropriate PPE		*
Gathers equipment and explains procedure to conscious patient		*
Assesses patient for pain level and medicates as needed		*
Places waterproof pad on bed and positions patient to allow irrigant to flow into basin		*
Removes old dressing by pulling gloves over it and discards appropriately		*
Assesses wound appearance and drainage (color, quantity, quality, and odor)		*
Cleanses hands and prepares irrigation tray, dressing supplies, and adds irrigation solution		*
Dons sterile gloves and positions basin to "catch" irrigant		*
Fills syringe with irrigant and gently flushes wound until solution is clear		*
Dries wound edges and assesses appearance and drainage		*
Applies sterile dressing, removes gloves, and cleanses hands		*
Assesses patient's response to intervention		*
Reassesses patient and cleanses hands		*
Documents procedure correctly		
Student exhibits competence with skill		

Any items in the Not Done column that are marked with an * are mandatory for the student to complete. A check mark in the Not Done column of an item with an * indicates that the student was unsuccessful and must attempt the skill again to assure competency. Examiners should use a different-color ink for the second attempt.

☐ Successful   ☐ Unsuccessful   Examiner Initials: _____

©2006 Prentice-Hall Inc.

Wound Culture

Student: _____   **Examiner:** _____

Date: _____

	Done ✓	Not Done
Cleanses hands		*
Utilizes appropriate PPE		*
Gathers equipment and explains procedure to patient		*
Removes old dressing, notes drainage, and removes gloves by pulling over dressing to discard		*
Opens sterile supplies and dons sterile gloves		*
Assesses wound's appearance noting quality, quantity, color, and odor of drainage		*
Irrigates wound with sterile saline and dries with sterile gauze		*
Rotates culture swab over granulation tissue without touching inner part of swab stick		*
Replaces culture swab in culture tube and crushes ampule of medium in bottom of tube, if applicable		*
Removes gloves, cleanses hands, dons sterile gloves, and dresses wound		*
Reassesses patient		*
Labels specimen correctly (area cultured, time, date, patient name, name of person obtaining culture) and arranges transport to lab		*
Cleanses hands		*
Assesses patient's response to intervention		*
Documents procedure correctly		
Student exhibits competence with skill		

Any items in the Not Done column that are marked with an * are mandatory for the student to complete. A check mark in the Not Done column of an item with an * indicates that the student was unsuccessful and must attempt the skill again to assure competency. Examiners should use a different-color ink for the second attempt.

☐ Successful   ☐ Unsuccessful   Examiner Initials: _____

©2006 Prentice-Hall Inc.

Changing a Dry Sterile Dressing (home health care only)

Student: _____   Examiner: _____

Date: _____

	Done ✓	Not Done
Cleanses hands		*
Utilizes appropriate PPE		*
Assesses patient's pain level and medicates as needed		*
Gathers supplies and explains procedure to patient		*
Drapes patient, exposing wound area only		
Places moisture-proof bag within reach and makes cuff on bag		*
Unties abdominal binder or removes tape		*
Removes and disposes of old dressing, pulling gloves over dressing and discarding in bag		*
Assesses wound, noting quality, quantity, color, and odor of drainage		*
Sets up sterile supplies and solution		*
Dons sterile gloves		*
Cleanses wound from least contaminated to most contaminated area		*
If drain is present, cleanses dried matter from drain and applies precut dressing		*
Applies sterile dressing and covers with surgipad (5 × 9)		*
Secures with tape or abdominal binder		*
Assesses patient's response to intervention		*
Removes gloves and disposes of soiled items appropriately		*
Reassesses patient and cleanses hands		*
Documents procedure correctly		
Student exhibits competence with skill		

Any items in the Not Done column that are marked with an * are mandatory for the student to complete. A check mark in the Not Done column of an item with an * indicates that the student was unsuccessful and must attempt the skill again to assure competency. Examiners should use a different-color ink for the second attempt.

☐ Successful   ☐ Unsuccessful   Examiner Initials: _____

Changing a Wet-to-Dry Dressing

Student: _____   Examiner: _____

Date: _____

	Done ✓	Not Done
Cleanses hands		*
Utilizes appropriate PPE		*
Assesses patient's pain level and medicates as needed		*
Gathers supplies and explains procedure to patient		*
Drapes patient, exposing wound area only		
Places moisture-proof bag within reach and makes cuff on bag		*
Removes and disposes of old dressing, pulling gloves over dressing and discarding in bag		*
Assesses wound, noting quality, quantity, color, and odor of drainage		*
Sets up sterile supplies and places gauzes in sterile container and adds cleansing solution		*
Dons sterile gloves		*
Squeezes out solution until gauze is fairly moist		*
Cleanses wound from least contaminated to most contaminated areas		*
Opens EACH gauze and gently packs into wound until all wound surfaces within gauze contact		*
Verifies moistened gauze on wound surfaces only—not wound edges		*
Applies dry sterile gauze over wound area		*
Covers with surgipads (5 x 9)		*
Secures with tape or abdominal binder		*
Assesses patient's response to intervention		*
Removes gloves and disposes of soiled items appropriately		*
Reassesses patient and cleanses hands		*
Documents procedure correctly		
Student exhibits competence with skill		

Any items in the Not Done column that are marked with an * are mandatory for the student to complete. A check mark in the Not Done column of an item with an * indicates that the student was unsuccessful and must attempt the skill again to assure competency. Examiners should use a different-color ink for the second attempt.

☐ Successful   ☐ Unsuccessful   Examiner Initials: _____

©2006 Prentice-Hall Inc.

Performing Urinary Catheterization—Male

Student: _____   Examiner: _____

Date: _____

	Done ✓	Not Done
Cleanses hands		*
Utilizes appropriate PPE		*
Checks patient allergies for LATEX—most Foleys are latex, but silicone is available		*
Gathers equipment (selecting appropriately sized catheter) and explains procedure to patient		*
Places patient in supine position with legs spread slightly apart		
Drapes abdomen and thighs, places penis over thighs		
Prepares sterile field, applies sterile gloves, and connects catheter and drainage system		*
Inserts sterile water into balloon to check and removes all water from balloon		*
Checks meatus for blood (contraindication for Foley insertion)		*
Gently retracts foreskin (if present) and, using forceps, cleanses glans penis in circular motion: in to out		*
Injects 10 cc water-soluble lubricant into urethra and/or lubricates distal catheter		*
Holds penis perpendicular to body and pulls up gently		*
Steadily inserts catheter until urine noted; inserts 1 cm further		*
Inflates balloon with sterile water and removes syringe (per catheter recommendations)		*
Gently pulls on catheter until inflation balloon is snuggled against bladder neck		
Rinses Betadine from head of penis and replaces foreskin if retracted earlier		*
Secures catheter to upper thigh, minimizing movement (decreases chance of UTI)		*
Places drainage bag below level of bladder		*
Secures tubing		
Removes gloves, disposes of soiled items appropriately, and cleanses hands		*
Assesses patient and catheter function (including urine color, odor, and amount)		*
Assesses patient's response to intervention		*
Documents size of catheter, balloon amount, and assessment		*
Student exhibits competence with skill		

Any items in the Not Done column that are marked with an * are mandatory for the student to complete. A check mark in the Not Done column of an item with an * indicates that the student was unsuccessful and must attempt the skill again to assure competency. Examiners should use a different-color ink for the second attempt.

☐ Successful   ☐ Unsuccessful   Examiner Initials: _____

Performing Urinary Catheterization—Female

Student: _____   Examiner: _____

Date: _____

	Done ✓	Not Done
Cleanses hands		*
Utilizes appropriate PPE		*
Checks patient allergies for LATEX—most Foleys are latex, but silicone is available		*
Gathers equipment (selecting appropriately sized catheter) and explains procedure to patient		*
Places patient in supine position with legs flexed and spread, feet together		
Prepares sterile field, applies sterile gloves, and connects catheter and drainage system		*
Inserts sterile water into balloon to check integrity and removes all water from balloon		*
Separates labia and, using forceps, cleanses periurethral mucosa; separating hand is now unsterile, must maintain separation of labia		*
Checks for blood at meatus (contraindication for Foley insertion)		*
Generously coats distal catheter with water-soluble lubricant		*
Gently inserts catheter into meatus until urine is noted		*
Inserts 1 cm further		*
Inflates balloon with sterile water and removes syringe (per catheter recommendations)		*
Gently pulls on catheter until inflation balloon is snuggled against bladder neck		
Secures catheter to upper thigh (in a manner that minimizes movement to ↓ chance of UTI)		*
Places drainage bag below level of bladder and secures		*
Removes gloves, disposes of soiled items appropriately, and cleanses hands		*
Assesses patient and catheter function (including urine color, odor, and amount)		*
Assesses patient's response to intervention		*
Documents size of catheter, balloon amount, and assessment		
Student exhibits competence with skill		

Any items in the Not Done column that are marked with an * are mandatory for the student to complete. A check mark in the Not Done column of an item with an * indicates that the student was unsuccessful and must attempt the skill again to assure competency. Examiners should use a different-color ink for the second attempt.

☐ Successful   ☐ Unsuccessful   Examiner Initials: _____

©2006 Prentice-Hall Inc.

Irrigating an Open Catheter

Student: _____   **Examiner:** _____

Date: _____

	Done ✓	Not Done
Cleanses hands		*
Utilizes appropriate PPE		*
Gathers supplies and explains procedure to patient		*
Provides privacy		
Opens sterile drape and forms sterile field		*
Adds basin to field using sterile technique and adds sterile solution		*
Opens syringe, removes tip, fills with solution, and places at end of field (away from basin)		*
Opens alcohol wipes, exposing only half a wipe (does not touch wipe)		*
Dons sterile gloves		*
Cleans junction between catheter and drainage tube with alcohol wipes		*
Simultaneously twists and pulls catheter and drainage tube apart		*
Holds drainage tube and catheter in nondominant hand		*
Places syringe in catheter opening and gently pushes in solution, using plunger		*
Cleans both tips and reconnects catheter and drainage tube		*
Drains solution using gravity (notes results)		*
Cleans area and appropriately disposes of soiled items		*
Evaluates function of catheter		
Reassesses patient and cleanses hands		*
Assesses patient's response to intervention		*
Documents procedure correctly		
Student exhibits competence with skill		

Any items in the Not Done column that are marked with an * are mandatory for the student to complete. A check mark in the Not Done column of an item with an * indicates that the student was unsuccessful and must attempt the skill again to assure competency. Examiners should use a different-color ink for the second attempt.

☐ Successful   ☐ Unsuccessful   Examiner Initials: _____

©2006 Prentice-Hall Inc.

Changing a Colostomy Pouch

Student: _____   **Examiner:** _____

Date: _____

	Done ✓	Not Done
Cleanses hands		*
Utilizes appropriate PPE		*
Gathers equipment and explains procedure to patient		*
Provides privacy and assists patient to sitting position		
Removes soiled pouch, removes clip, and disposes of pouch properly		*
Cleanses skin with soap and water		*
Inspects skin for redness, altered skin integrity, and/or rashes		*
Inspects pouch opening and ensures it fits stoma (uses pouch pattern, if necessary)		*
Applies sealant or paste, if indicated, and applies skin barrier		*
Gently applies pouch and seals inferior opening with clip		*
Removes gloves and cleanses hands		*
Reassesses patient and washes hands		*
Assesses patient's response to intervention		*
Documents procedure correctly		
Student exhibits competence with skill		

Any items in the Not Done column that are marked with an * are mandatory for the student to complete. A check mark in the Not Done column of an item with an * indicates that the student was unsuccessful and must attempt the skill again to assure competency. Examiners should use a different-color ink for the second attempt.

☐ Successful   ☐ Unsuccessful   Examiner Initials: _____

©2006 Prentice-Hall Inc.

SECTION 9

*

Pertinent Points for Paramedic Review

Pay close attention to the *items, facts, and points when reviewing for boards. These indicate the most common knowledge facts needed for boards.

Paramedic Review Section
- *Shock/Fluid Therapy*
- *Trauma*
- *Geriatric*
- *Communicable/Infectious Diseases*
- *Toxicology/Substance Abuse*
- *Environmental*
- *Allergic Reaction/Anaphylaxis*
- *Diabetic Emergencies*
- *CNS Emergencies*
- *Cardiovascular Emergencies*
- *Behavioral/Psych*
- *Xtras*

Scene safety
BSI/PPE
Assess responsiveness
    Airway—ensure the patient has a patent airway.
    Breathing—ensure good rate and quality of respirations.
    Circulation—ensure a pulse; check for hemorrhage. A rapid weak pulse may indicate that a decrease in perfusion is already occurring.
The location of the pulse may also be helpful in determining the B/P—if you have a radial 80 mm Hg, femoral 70 mm Hg, carotid 60 mmHg (minimum systolic).
Shock should be recognized in the initial assessment.

Contraindications for Use of PASG (MAST)

A. The only true contraindication is pulmonary edema.
   1. PASG increases the preload to the heart, thereby increasing the severity of pulmonary edema.

Relative Contraindications of PASG

A. Head injury
   1. An increase in blood supply to the brain will increase ICP.
B. An evisceration or an impaled object in the abdomen
   1. PASG may serve to push the abdominal organs out of the body.
      a. Leg section can still be used.
C. Pregnancy beyond the 1st trimester
   1. PASG may compromise the fetus.
      a. Leg section can still be used.
D. Bleeding above the level of PASG
   1. PASG will serve to increase the blood loss if the bleeding can't be controlled.

Application of PASG (3 Methods)

   1. By placing the PASG over the rescuer's arms, grasping the patient's legs, and sliding them on
   2. By unfolding the PASG, sliding them under the patient, then securing them
   3. Having the PASG on the backboard before putting the patient on the LBB

©2006 Prentice-Hall Inc.

Parkland Formula for Fluid Replacement in Burns

$$\frac{4 \text{ ml} \times \text{Percent of BSA} \times \text{Patient weight in kg}}{2} = \text{Fluid replacement in the first 8 hours}$$

Example: A 70 kg patient with 50% burns will require 7,000 ml (7 L) in the first 8 hours.

$$\frac{4 \times 50 \times 70}{2} = 7,000 \text{ ml} = 7 \text{ L}$$

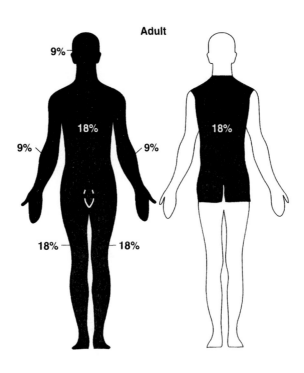

Adult

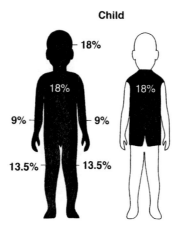

Child

Rule of Nines

Head Injury
Cushing's Reflex = ↑ ICP
- Hypertension
- Bradycardia
- Irregular Respirations

Shock
Opposite of ↑ ICP
- Tachycardia (early sign)
- Tachypnea
- Hypotension (late sign)

Pericardial Tamponade
Beck's Triad
- Muffled heart sounds
- JVD; ↑ venous pressure
- Hypotension; ↓ arterial pressure

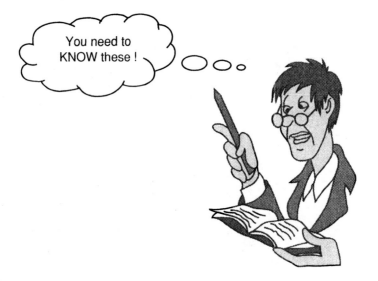

You need to KNOW these !

©2006 Prentice-Hall Inc.

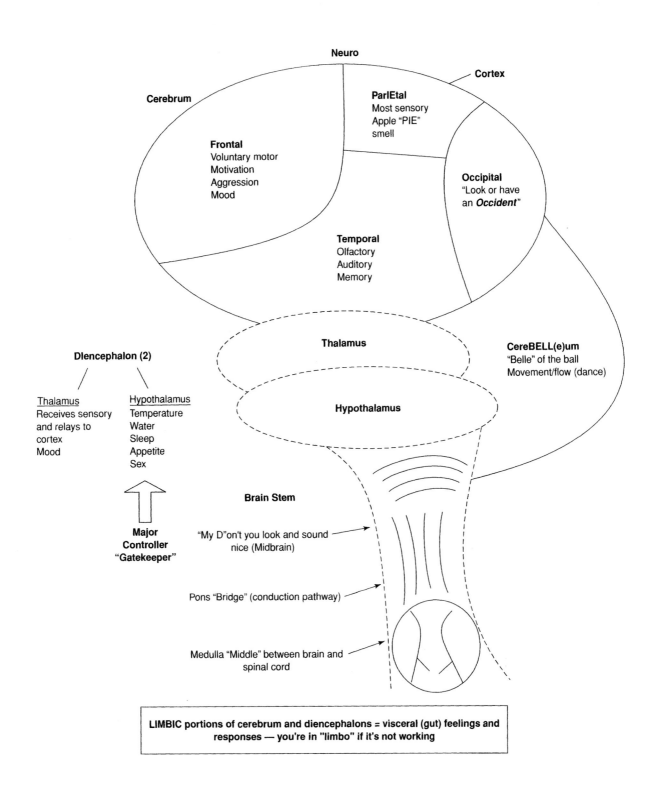

Neuro

Cerebrum

ParlEtal
Most sensory
Apple "PIE"
smell

Cortex

Frontal
Voluntary motor
Motivation
Aggression
Mood

Occipital
"Look or have
an *Occident*"

Temporal
Olfactory
Auditory
Memory

Thalamus

CereBELL(e)um
"Belle" of the ball
Movement/flow (dance)

Dlencephalon (2)

Hypothalamus

Thalamus
Receives sensory
and relays to
cortex
Mood

Hypothalamus
Temperature
Water
Sleep
Appetite
Sex

**Major
Controller
"Gatekeeper"**

Brain Stem

"My D"on't you look and sound
nice (Midbrain)

Pons "Bridge" (conduction pathway)

Medulla "Middle" between brain and
spinal cord

LIMBIC portions of cerebrum and diencephalons = visceral (gut) feelings and
responses — you're in "limbo" if it's not working

Shock/Fluid Therapy

$$\frac{\text{Volume (to be infused)} \times \text{Tubing (drops per cc)}}{\text{Time (in minutes)}} = \text{gtts/min (drops per minute)}$$

- KVO = 10 cc/hr or ml/hr or gtts/min with minidrip tubing
- Complications
  - Local
    - hematoma
    - infiltration (most common)
    - cellulitis
    - thrombophlebitis (inflammation of vein)
  - Systemic
    - air embolus
    - catheter shear (more common in through-the-needle)
    - sepsis
    - pulmonary embolus
- Transfusion Reaction and Pyrogenic Reaction
  - Fever
  - Back pain
  - Chest pain
  - Shock
  - From blood and contaminated IV fluids
- Fluids
  - Crystalloid—does not contain large particles (D_5W, NS, LR)
  - Colloid—large particles or proteins (Albumin, Hespan), draws fluid INTO vessels
  - Hypertonic—50% dextrose, 10% dextrose—fluid drawn INTO vessels (cells to blood vessels)
  - Hypotonic—$\frac{1}{2}$ NS—fluid moves from blood vessels INTO cells (blood vessel to cells)
  - Isotonic—equal (no fluid shift)
  - LR—"buffer"—most like plasma (has K^+)
  - D_5W may be used for cardiac and CHF; used for drips
- Hypovolemic Shock
  - Fluid problem
  - Compensatory—BP ↑ or normal
  - Decompensated—BP ↓
  - Irreversible
  - Signs/symptoms
    - cool, clammy skin
    - anxiety
    - tachypnea
    - tachycardia
  - Replace 3:1 (3 cc for every 1 cc loss)
    - 20 cc/kg fluid replacement for hypovolemia or unknown blood loss
- Cardiogenic Shock
  - Pump problem
  - MI, CHF
  - Use Dopamine
- Neurogenic Shock
  - Container problem (vascular distribution)
  - Spinal cord injury
  - Use
    - dopamine

©2006 Prentice-Hall Inc.

- fluids
  - PASG (can cause metabolic acidosis)
- No sympathetic response, no tachycardia, no pallor, no sweating
- *Never use PASG with pulmonary edema/CHF
- Mechanical Shock
  - Cardiac tamponade
  - Tension pneumothorax

Trauma

- Mechanism of Injury—Steering Wheel, Dashboard, Rear End, T-Bone, etc.
  - Treat while in vehicle (C-collar, IV); SMR before moving, use long axis of body; airway and C-spine at same time
  - Most common rural accident is head-on collision
  - Most deaths on ejection (25% greater chance for death)
- Head, Neck, Spine Trauma
  - A & P of CNS—brain and spinal cord
    *atlas and axis = C-1 and C-2 (Atlas holds the world on his shoulders/nod)
  - CSF, meninges—PAD (pia, arachnoid, dura—from brain out) halo test
- Brain
  - Cerebrum—"finer things in life"
    - personality
    - intelligence
    - judgment
    - sight (in occipital)
  - Cerebellum
    - balance
    - coordination
  - Brain stem
    - vital functions
    - breathing
- Peripheral Nervous System (31 sets of nerves)
  - Afferent = sensory nerves (ascending) body to brain
  - Efferent = motor (descending) brain to body

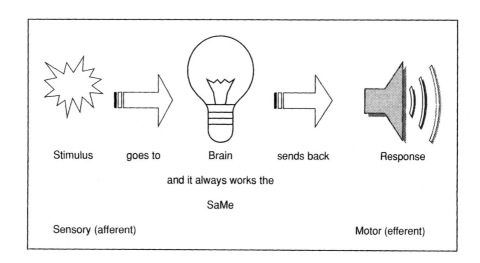

Stimulus   goes to   Brain   sends back   Response

and it always works the

SaMe

Sensory (afferent)   Motor (efferent)

©2006 Prentice-Hall Inc.

- Vertebral Column (33; 7 cervical, 12 thoracic, 5 lumbar, 5 sacrum, 4 coccyx)
  - Times of meals (7 breakfast, 12 lunch, 5 dinner, 9 bedtime snack)
    *cervical and lumbar most often injured
- Dermatomes
  - C-1 and C-2 = respirations (respiratory arrest)
  - C-3 through C-5 = intercostal muscles
  - T-4 = nipple line
  - T-10 = umbilicus
- Facial Injuries—Eye, Nose, Ear
  - Care of eyes of unresponsive patient = tape down to preserve moisture
  - Paralysis of eye muscle from "blow-out" fracture of orbit
  - Impaled object may be removed from cheek if airway problem
    (may remove impaled object in chest if interferes with CPR)
  - Always patch BOTH eyes if patch needed for one
- Cerebral Injuries
  - Subdural—below dura; venous *slow bleed
  - Epidural—above dura; arterial (middle meningeal); alternating LOCs; *fast bleed
  - Coup/contracoup—injury to opposite side of brain from impact; *contracoup is worse
  - Increasing ICP = Cushing's response
  - Neuro exam—LOC, pupils, VS, PMS, GCS, posturing
  - Decorticate—arms flexed
  - Decerebrate—extension (worse) indicates brain stem
- Treatment of Head and Spinal Injuries
  - Maintain adequate ventilation
  - Allow fluid to drain from ears/nose
  - Prevent pressure buildup—do not pack ears or nose
  - Mannitol
  - Solu-Medrol (spinal)
  - Decadron (head)
  - *Most important is how level of consciousness is changing
  - Brain Trauma Foundation recommends hyperventilation (20 breaths/min) for patients with signs
    of impending herniation ONLY
- Chest Injuries
  - Rib fractures—underlying structures
    - anterior lower left = spleen
    - anterior lower right = liver
    - lower posterior = kidneys
  - Traumatic asphyxia
    - crush injury to chest and abdomen
    - bulging eyes and tongue
    - cyanosis
    - JVD
  - Simple pneumothorax—spontaneous
    - tall, young male more prone
    - sudden onset pain and SOB with ↓ breath sounds
  - Tension pneumothorax
    - JVD, tracheal deviation *away* (late)
    - hyperresonant
    - shock
    - asymmetrical chest rise

   ©2006 Prentice-Hall Inc.

- Pleural decompression (adult)
  - 2nd or 3rd ICS in MCL (midclavicular line)
  - 5th or 6th ICS in MAL (midaxillary line)
  - over TOP of rib
- Hemothorax
  - dull (hyporesonant)
  - flat neck veins
  - shock
- Cardiac tamponade
  - Beck's Triad
  - treatment—pericardiocentesis
- Sucking chest wound
  - opening into chest wall allowing air entrance
  - occlusive dressing taped on three sides
- Flail chest
  - three or more ribs fractured in two or more places
  - paradoxical movement
  - splint
  - definitive treatment = positive pressure ventilation
- Thoracic aorta injury
  - chest pain and pain between shoulder blades
  - unequal radial pulses
  - fracture of 2nd rib on the left = diagnostic sign
  - head-on collision
  - often tear at ligamentum arteriosum
- Abdominal Injuries
  - Solid—kidney, liver, spleen, pancreas
  - Hollow—stomach, bladder(s), bowel
  - Peritoneum—lining of abdominal cavity
  - Signs
    - Cullen's—bruising around umbilicus = intra-abdominal bleed
    - Grey-Turner's—bruising to flank = kidney trauma/retro-peritoneal
    - Kehr's—left shoulder pain = ruptured spleen
  - Evisceration
    - moist sterile saline dressing
    - occlusive dressing layer
    - keep warm
- Pelvic Injuries
  - May have multiple fractures
  - Multiple underlying organs
  - May lose 2 liters of blood volume
  - 2 large-bore IVs
  - PASG
- Musculoskeletal Injuries
  - Note: With musculoskeletal trauma you usually place patient on a long backboard (splint)—easy to remember LBB = Ligament Bone to Bone
  - Ligaments attach Bone to Bone (LBB)
  - Tendons attach muscle to bone
  - Sprain = injury to ligament
  - Strain = injury to muscle

- Fractures—greenstick, transverse, spiral, comminuted, oblique, compound (open)
  - pain
  - swelling
  - deformity
  - crepitus
- Splint to prevent complications
  - nerve
  - vascular *worse
- Positions
  - hip—leg shortened and externally rotated
  - posterior hip dislocation—flexed with internal rotation
  - anterior hip dislocation—lateral rotation with prominence in hip/groin
  - anterior shoulder—leaning forward, head of humerus may be seen anteriorly, arm close to chest
  - posterior shoulder—"hollow" shoulder, elbow internally rotated and away from chest
- Splints
  - pillow = ankle and foot
  - sling and swathe = shoulder, clavicle, humerus
  - traction = femur (NOT hip), traction until pain relief (being studied as to efficacy of traction splint use prehospital)
- Soft Tissue and Burns
  - Abrasion, laceration, incision, puncture, avulsion, amputation
    - amputated part in plastic bag (dry), set in/on iced or cool water
  - Impaled—stabilize in place except airway compromise (cheek)
  - Burns—thermal, electrical, chemical, radiation
    - 1°—partial thickness, pain, red, no blisters (sunburn)
    - 2°—partial thickness, pain, red, blisters
    - 3°—full thickness, no pain, dry, white, gray, yellow, black
  - BSA
    - Rule of nines
    - Palmar—surface of patient's hand = 1% BSA
  - Major burns
    - 3°—10%
    - 2°—30–40%
    - respiratory
    - face/neck
    - genitalia
    - circumferential
    - burns with eschar formation
  - Complications
    - hypovolemia (immediate)
    - hypothermia (immediate)
    - infection (delayed)
  - Treatment—STOP the burning process
    - Parkland (4 cc × % BSA × kg—give $\frac{1}{2}$ in first 8 hr)
    - remove jewelry
    - cool burns less than 10% BSA
    - cool burns only 1 minute or less (unless need to stop burning process)
    - moderate to severe—dry sterile dressing/sterile burn sheet
    - keep warm
  - Inhalation injury
    - carbon monoxide (*most common cause of death at fire)

 ©2006 Prentice-Hall Inc.

- toxic fumes
- airway burns—INTUBATE STAT!
- Chemical—acids and alkalis flush with water EXCEPT
  - dry lime—brush off
  - phenol—remove with alcohol
  - sodium metal—cover with oil
  - "solution to pollution is dilution"

Geriatric

- Normal Changes in Body Functions and Systems (functions ↓)
  - Osteoporosis, especially in women
  - Difficulty or frequency in urination
  - Lower total body water
  - Lower thirst, vision, hearing, temperature regulation, lung capacity
  - Silent MI
  - Decreased pain response
- Assessment—Be Patient, Give Them Time
- Meds—Lower Doses of Some Drugs (such as decreased drip for Lidocaine)
- Abuse/Neglect—Must Be Reported (may also be financial abuse)
- Regression—Take on Childlike Behavior

Communicable/Infectious Diseases

- Meningitis
  - Viral
  - Bacterial—one EMS gets from patient most often
  - Fever, nuchal rigidity, high-pitched cry, neuro symptoms, headache, backache, bulging fontanelles in infant
  - Opisthotonos
- Hepatitis
  - Fever, RUQ pain, nausea/vomiting, jaundice, icteric sclera, coke-colored urine, clay-colored stools
  - Hep B has vaccine
  - Hep A is fecal-oral contamination
- TB
  - Night sweats, hemoptysis, cough, weight loss
  - Airborne
  - More common in HIV patients
  - Antibiotic resistant strains
- STDs
  - Syphilis—treponema pallidum, chancre, tabes dorsalis (slap feet)
  - Gonorrhea
    - female may not have symptoms, male—dysuria and discharge
    - most common cause of PID (female)
  - Herpes—female with active herpes in labor MUST have C-section
  - Condyloma accumulata—genital warts very common
- HIV/AIDS
  - Main cause unprotected sex
  - Complications; Kaposi's sarcoma, pneumocystis carinii, monilia (thrush), TB, CMV
- Scabies/Lice—Contagious "Critters"
- Measles, Mumps, Varicella Zoster (chickenpox)
  - Vaccines

- Viral
- Airborne droplets

Toxicology/Substance Abuse

- Inhalation, Injection, Ingestion, Absorption
- Poison Control Center—General Treatment for Poisonings
- Do Not Induce Emesis unless Advised by Poison Control/Medical Control
- If Soon after Ingestion, Charcoal Can Help Absorb the Poison
- Tricyclics (mellaril, elavil, tofranil, amytriptyline)—Give $NaHCO_3$
  - S/sx; bradycardia, hypotension, seizures, resp. arrest, torsades
  - TCA/tricyclic antidepressant—3 Cs and an A (Coma, Convulsions, Cardiac arrhythmias, and Acidosis)
- ASA—Salicylates
  - Causes metabolic acidosis and respiratory alkalosis (to compensate)
  - Hyperventilation, fever, sweating, tachycardia, tinnitus
  - Bicarb
- Drugs
  - Ipecac—not used in many parts of the country now in the prehospital setting
  - Charcoal—absorbs, 1 g/kg or 50 g
  - Specific antidotes
- Insect Stings
  - Brown recluse (fiddleback)—necrotoxic tissue damage (no antivenin)
  - Black widow (red hourglass)—neurotoxic, abdominal cramps/spasms, antidote is calcium *gluconate* (also is an antivenin)
  - Stingers—scrape off (sac attached keeps pumping)—honeybee
- Snakes
  - Pit vipers—necrotoxic (hemolytic)
    - swelling, pain → bleeding (mark the involved area)
    - rattlesnake, copperhead, cottonmouth (water moccasin)
    - NO TK, no ice or cold
    - elliptical eyes, hinged fangs, neurosensory pits, triangular head
    - antivenin available—dose depends on grade envenomation
    - 25% of bites are dry bites (no envenomation)
  - Coral snake
    - round pupils, small fixed fangs toward back of mouth
    - "red touch black—venom lack, red touch yellow—kill a fellow"
    - reaction may be delayed up to 24 hours
    - s/sx; numbness, dyspnea to respiratory paralysis (fatal)
    - antivenin available
- Marine Animals
  - Man-o-war; remove with sand, meat tenderizer, then ammonia
  - Catfish; hot soapy water
- Opiate OD
  - Pinpoint pupils, ↓ respirations, ↓ LOC, ? track marks
  - Narcan (be sure to rule out hypoglycemia)
  - Withdrawal—shaking, sweating, piloerections, seizures
- Hallucinogenics
  - LSD, Angel Trumpet, psilocybins, etc.
  - Can be dangerous—affect respirations
  - Talk down in excitement stage

   ©2006 Prentice-Hall Inc.

- May need Haldol
- No lights, siren
- Stimulants
  - Cocaine, speed
  - Sympathetic stimulation (sympathomimetic)
  - Dilated pupils, tachycardia, tachypnea, VT, seizures, agitation
  - Treat with Valium
- ETOH
  - Like to drink alone, secretly
  - Pancreatitis, ulcer, bleeding, cirrhosis, subdural hematoma, ascites
  - "DT" delerium tremens—48–72 hours after last intake ETOH
  - Hallucinations
  - Shaking tremors, seizures, death
- Organophosphates (cholinergic poisoning)
  - Suspect around fertilizers/bradycardia
  - SLUDGEM—salivation, lacrimation, urination, diarrhea, GI sx, emesis, meiosis
  - Pupils constricted
  - LARGE doses Atropine—control symptoms
  - Workers in agriculture, farmers, migrant workers
  - Paraquat—the only exposure that oxygen is contraindicated

Environmental

Heat

- Heat Cramps—Abdomen/Leg Cramps
  - Working or playing in heat
  - Sweating
  - Cool down, fluids if not nauseated
  - Salt and water loss—water follows sodium
- Heat Exhaustion
  - Tachycardia, sweating, hypotension, headache, weak, vasodilation
  - IV of NS, cool down, Trendelenberg
  - Temp may be normal or elevated
- Heatstroke—Medical Emergency* Brain Is Frying
  - High temps 105°–106°
  - Classic heatstroke = brain problem not fluid loss
    *malfunction of hypothalamus, decreased LOC, NO sweating
  - Exertional—loss of fluid and electrolytes
    *working outside, decreased LOC, tachycardia, NO sweating
  - Failure of heat regulating mechanism after above
  - Treatment: IV, RAPID cooling—true life threat

Cold

- Hypothermia—drugs do not work in severe hypothermia (<90°) delayed/no absorption
  - May try first line ACLS drugs
  - Then adapt much longer time intervals
  - Rough handling causes VF (refer to current ACLS)
- Frostbite
  - Red, then white or gray
  - Only thaw if no chance of refreezing, cover with dry dressing
  - Thaw in warm water <110°

- No alcohol or nicotine
- No massaging of frozen parts
- Drowning (near drowning)
  - Salt water—pulmonary edema (salt pulls fluid into lungs)
  - Fresh water—hemodilution/electrolyte imbalance/surfactant loss
  - "Dry" drowning due to laryngospasm
  - ALL drownings have respiratory and metabolic acidosis and hypoxia
- Radiation
  - Time, distance, shielding
  - Alpha (paper), beta (aluminum), gamma rays (lead)
- Barotrauma—Most Accidents Occur While Ascending
  - Diving—barotrauma to ears or chest (lungs) "squeeze"—on descent
  - Decompression sickness—"bends" (pain in joints, chest pain, spine)—on ascent
- Nitrogen Narcosis—They Don't Come Up—"Happy"—Need to Ascend
- Air Embolus—Position on Left Side Trendelenberg (put air to big toe)

Allergic Reaction/Anaphylaxis

- Food, Meds, Stings
- Airway Problems
  - Bronchoconstriction, laryngeal edema
- Hemodynamics
  - Hypotension due to vasodilation
  - Capillary leakage
- S/sx—Swelling
  - 3rd space shift causing shock, urticaria, pruritis, hoarseness, wheezing, "silent" chest ominous, swollen lips/tongue
- Release of Histamine and Heparin from Mast Cells (vasodilates, increases capillary permeability to get antigen out of bloodstream, bronchoconstriction)
- ABCs of anaphylaxis
  - Adrenalin (Epi)
  - Benadryl
  - Corticosteroids
- Treatment for Simple Allergic Reaction = Albuterol (if wheezing), Benadryl

Diabetic Emergencies

- DKA—Hyperglycemia
  - Insulin produced in Islets of Langerhans (beta cells) in the pancreas
  - Hyperglycemia—too much sugar/no insulin
  - Metabolic acidosis/respiratory alkalosis—Kussmaul (rapid, deep respirations)
  - Polydipsia (thirst), polyuria, polyphagia (hungry)
  - Nausea/vomiting, dehydration, acetone breath, warm, dry skin, fever, flushed
  - Gradual onset—slow fix
  - Causes: not taking insulin, infection, pregnancy
  - Treatment: fluids (IV open), insulin (in hospital), bicarb
  - Type I = Insulin dependent (IDDM)
- Insulin Shock—Hypoglycemia
  - Not enough sugar/too much insulin
  - Sudden onset—rapid fix
  - Cool, clammy, headache, weakness, dizzy, bizarre behavior, violent

©2006 Prentice-Hall Inc.

- 50% dextrose, Thiamine if needed (oral sugar if able)
- Causes: too much insulin, not eating, infection, MI, surgery, too much exercise

CNS Emergencies

- Coma—Oxygen, Narcan, 50% Dextrose if Hypoglycemic
  - Causes of unresponsiveness = AEIOU TIPS
    - *acidosis, alcohol
    - *epilepsy
    - *infection
    - *OD
    - *uremia (kidney)
    - *trauma, tumor
    - *insulin (either diabetic emergency)
    - *psychosis
    - *stroke
- Seizures
  - Grand mal (tonic-clonic)
    - aura, loss of consciousness, tonic (conTraction), clonic (reLaxation), post ictal
    - protect patient—nothing in mouth, position, suction
    - check sugar
    - treatment: Valium
  - Status epilepticus—prolonged or two or more seizures without regaining consciousness
  - Focal motor
    - localized (e.g., one leg)
    - may progress to grand mal
    - treatment: Valium
  - Psychomotor
    - temporal lobe
    - bizarre behavior, may act intoxicated
  - Petit mal
    - common in children
    - many per day
    - may or may not lose consciousness
  - Febrile
    - most common cause of seizures in child <6 years old
    - caused by sudden spike, not amount of degrees
- Stroke/TIA
  - TIA—temporary (<24 hr)
  - Infarct/permanent = stroke
    *Embolus or bleed
  - Visual problems, speech slurring, altered LOC, hemiparesis or hemiplegia, dizzy, other neuro s/sx
  - Make sure problem not glucose or drug related
  - Position supine with head elevated 15°
  - If transport—on side to protect airway, place affected side down
  - CPHSS, LAPSS, or MEND stroke exams
  - Three-hour window for fibrinolytic
  - Pupil may "blow" (3rd cranial nerve pressure from bleeding)
- Subarachnoid Hemorrhage (SAH)
  - Usually caused by aneurysm (Berry)
  - Sudden onset SEVERE headache

- Neuro symptoms to unconscious
- Rapid progression
- Females in 20s or 30s more prone

Cardiovascular Emergencies

- Know A & P Including Valves
  - Pulmonic and aortic also called semilunar
  - Trace the path of a drop of blood
  - Layers of arteries
    - tunica intima (inside)
    - tunica (means coat) media (middle)
    - tunica adventitia (outer)
- Trace Conduction System
- Intrinsic Rates
  - SA 60–100
  - AV 40–60
  - V <40
- Layers of Heart
  - Endometrium—inner
  - Myometrium (most likely for MI* and LV most likely site*) middle/muscle
  - Epicardium—outer
- CO = SV × HR
  - Normal SV 80–100 cc adult male
- Definitions: Preload, Afterload, Starling's Law Regarding Heart
- Electrode Placement I, II*, III
- Poor EKG Tracing/60 cycle; Disconnect Electrical Devices
- Extrasystole = Extra Beat (e.g., PVC)
- Causes of Dysrhythmias
  - Hypoxia
  - Conduction defect
  - Drugs
- Causes of pulselessness (OH Sugar Get THAT EPI) and treatment
  - Oxygen (hypoxia)
  - Hypovolemia
  - Sugar (hypoglycemia)
  - Get the toxins/drugs, OD
  - Tension pneumothorax
  - Hypothermia
  - Acidosis
  - Emboli (coronary, pulmonart, AMI/ACS)
  - Potassium
  - Injuries/trauma
- MI—Nausea, Chest Pain with Radiation, Impending Doom, Cool, Clammy
  - Elevated ST 3 mm
  - Absence of ST elevation does NOT rule out MI
- Angina—Stable (acts the same, relief with rest or rest and NTG) versus Unstable (at rest, no relief, different)
- Treatment MI/Angina—(MONA) Oxygen, ASA, NTG, Morphine (*most effective pain med for MI)
- Pulmonary Edema—LEFT Heart Failure
  - Fluid backup into lungs (LEFT=Lungs)

          ©2006 Prentice-Hall Inc.

- Respiratory distress, rales, tachycardia, HTN (eventual hypotension), tripod position
- Oxygen, NTG, MS, Lasix, PPV
- Morphine decreases preload and afterload
- Right Heart Failure
  - + JVD at 45° angle
  - Pedal or sacral edema
  - Cor pulmonale/RVH
- CPR Guidelines
- Defibrillation and Cardioversion
  - Safety and procedure
  - Successive shocks *decrease* transthoracic resistance (so does conductive medium)
  - Joules for VF, VT, SVT, etc.
  - Caution in patient on Digoxin
  - Peds = 2 j/kg (first shock) then 4 j/kg successive shocks, cardioversion 0.5–1 j/kg
- AAA
  - Abdominal/back pain (may be in groin if dissecting)
  - "Tearing" pain (usually dissecting)
  - Pulsatile mass
  - Unequal pulses to lower extremities
  - Thoracic = HTN
  - Abdominal = hypotension
  - May use PASG/don't inflate unless ruptures
- HTN
  - Hypertensive crisis (200/100 with symptoms or rapid increase of diastolic usually to >130)–neuro sx, headache, epistaxis
  - NTG on physician order but must rule out stroke first

Behavioral/Psych

- Assessment
  - Rule out metabolic causes such as drugs, seizure, hypoglycemia
  - Continuous scene safety
- Psychotic versus Neurotic (psychotic not in touch with reality)
  - Neurotic builds castles in the air
  - Psychotic lives in them
  - Baker Act—danger to self or others; police must initiate
- Interview
  - Ask "open-ended" questions
  - Active listening
  - Paranoid—don't talk with relatives in another room
- Psychiatric Disorders
  - Depression/suicidal
    - helplessness/hopelessness
    - more females try, more males succeed
    - guns number-one successful method
    - OD number-one attempted method
    - suicidal characteristics—single/divorced/separated; drugs or ETOH; chronic or terminal illness; means; history (self or family)
    - contact police—may be homicidal also
    - severe depression patients don't attempt suicide, do that when feeling "better"
  - Anxiety
    - Normal response to stress

- GI sx, dizzy, hyperventilation, SOB
- In MCI/stress give person simple task
- BPD (manic/depressive)
  - Lithium, Haldol, Thorazine
  - Highs—hyperactive
  - Lows may be suicidal
- Schizophrenia
  - Hallucinations—auditory or visual
  - Delusions—false belief (grandeur or paranoid)
  - Thorazine, Lithium, Haldol
- Violent Patient—if Not Suspected in Scene Survey
  - Move fast, one in front and one in back
  - Restrain on back or side
  - Release restraints only at hospital unless impeding circulation or compromising airway
  - Check (and document) very frequently
  - Protect airway and breathing
  - BEST way to deal with violence = avoid contact and call police
- Psych Drugs
  - Haldol
  - TCA—Elavil, Tofranil, Mellaril
  - Extra-pyramidal (reaction) syndrome (EPS) treat with Benadryl
    *also called dystonic reaction

Xtras

"**Jambalaya**" style—tidbits of information added by students after boards on certain facts they had questions about or thought they should have studied

- Hot zone is accident/spill
- Warm zone is for decontamination
- Cold zone is for EMS (no containment suits)
- Localize pain on GCS = will directly make pain stop/purposeful/cross midline
- Withdraw pain on GCS = body moves away from pain
- Decorticate = brain stem
- Decerebrate = bleed out (critical)
- Nervous system disorder is change in mental status
- Abdominal flexion is guarding
- ↑ICP is Cushing's Triad = ↑BP, ↓HR, ↓ or irregular respirations
- Blown pupil from pressure on 3rd CN (oculomotor)
- Intubate head injury, BVM at 1 every 5 seconds; if patient decerebrate go to 1 breath every 3 seconds (this is a last-ditch effort before patient herniates)
- Ascites is loss of fluid into abdomen (with alcoholics)
- Pallor is caused by vasoconstriction
- Cerebellum is for balance and coordination
- ADH and oxytocin from pituitary gland
- Visceral is covering of organ
- Ch-401 is EMS Act/Law: Scope of Practice (FL only)—know your state
- 64E-2 = rules and regulations (FL only)—know your state
- "Trunking" channels a phone call to the next line
- Incident control and command directs scenes
- Wheezes = lower airway (a/w) = asthma

    ©2006 Prentice-Hall Inc.

- Rales/crackles = lower a/w = pulmonary edema = fluid in small a/w
- Rhonchi = lower a/w = pneumonia = fluid in large a/w (rhonchi in the bronchi)
- Cheyne-Stokes = fast/slow/apnea/repeat = head injury ↑ ICP
- Biot's = apnea/hyperventilation/repeat = head injury ↑ ICP
- Kussmaul's = deep and rapid = DKA
- Asthma treatment = (1) albuterol, (2) epi 1:1,000, (3) Solu-Medrol
- Pleural Effusion = fluid in pleural space
- You can hear, touch, see, and smell a sign
- Cricothyrotomy = cut cricothyroid membrane
- Peds glottis at C-1/C-2
- Hypotonic solution moves fluid from blood vessels into the cells—for example, $\frac{1}{2}$ NS
- LR—buffer most like plasma
- ↓ pH = more acid
- ↑ CO_2 = more acid
- **NO PASG ON CHF
- Dopamine receptors dilate renal, mesenteric (cerebral and coronary) vessels
- Remember SaMe (sensory-afferent, motor-efferent)
- Tendons = muscle to bone
- Vascular complication worst problem in fracture/dislocation
- Rule of nines
- Psychomotor seizure: temporal lobe, act drunk with bizarre behavior
- Appendicitis = RLQ pain (McBurney's point), N/V, no appetite
- Cholecystitis = 5 Fs (fair, fat, female, forty, fertile) with right shoulder pain
- Hepatitis = coke-colored urine
- Postural syncope = orthostatic hypotension
- Cholecystitis vomit yellow/green
- Myocardial ischemia = prolonged PRI
- Constipated and no appetite × 2 days = appendicitis
- AMI deaths within 1–2 hours
- Common UTI = cystitis (bladder infection)
- Coronary arteries supply cardiac muscle
- Coronary arteries fed during diastole
- Heart blocks and symptomatic sinus brady get Atropine
- Avoid T wave on cardioversion—hit the R wave
- regular R to R and variable PRI = 3rd degree
- LV most likely to become irritable or excitable
- 40% increase in blood volume during pregnancy
- Neonates lose heat by evaporation
- Amenorrhea is early sign of pregnancy
- Croup is viral
- Epiglottitis is bacterial
- Alkalines (Drano, oven cleaner, etc.) burn more than acids
- Joint injury problem is blood vessel clamping
- Definitive treatment for flail chest = PPV
- Dementia is deterioration of mental status associated with neuro disease/slow onset
- Drug used in field for TCA OD is bicarb
- Do not induce emesis TCA OD
- Croup: viral, fall/winter, night, low fever, treatment = Racemic Epi
- ↓ HR = hypoxia of infant
- TCAs end in "il"
- Sellick's maneuver closes off esophagus via cricoid ring pressure

- Called to scene of possible OD, patient awake and talking a lot, dilated pupils = patient taking amphetamines
- Federal Food, Drug and Cosmetic Act assures safe manufacture and distribution
- Lido does NOT ↓ cardiac function
- Benadryl is NOT used in treatment of COPD and asthma
- Mellaril and Thorazine are tranquilizers/antipsychotics
- Isuprel is mixed drip @ 2–10 mcg/min
- Glucagon acts on releasing glycogen from liver
- On the way to a possible drowning, you notice you are clammy and tachycardic because Epinephrine released by adrenal glands
- Morphine and Valium could mean death when taken with alcohol
- When β (beta) receptors stimulated, HR increases
- Verapamil is contraindicated in WPW
- Albuterol 2.5 mg indicated in treatment of asthma
- Trade name of verapamil = Calan, Isoptin
- Hyperkalemia is NOT a side effect of Lasix
- Epi IV in cardiac arrest does NOT decrease PVR
- Atropine works by blocking vagus nerve to ↑ HR
- Isuprel contraindicated in SVT, PVCs, VT—use Isuprel in blocks
- Drug with + inotropic effect will cause ↑ force of contraction
- NTG works to reduce workload of heart by ↓ preload and afterload
- Atropine is NOT a vasopressor
- Nipride used for hypertensive crisis
- Epi SQ used to treat mild allergic reactions
- NO Verapamil in rapid A Fib
- Deltoid common for IM in adult
- Lido dose 1-1.5 mg/kg up to 3 mg/kg
- Verapamil does NOT cause tachycardia
- NO Lido for PVCs if bradycardic
- HTN is NOT side effect of Lasix
- Mannitol will ↓ ICP—osmotic diuretic
- Isuprel is used in symptomatic bradycardia
- Do not give flumazenil (Romazicon) to Valium OD if mixed with TCAs
- Epi does NOT cause ↓ SVR
- Side effect of diuretic therapy is hypokalemia
- Side effects of Epi are palpitations and HTN
- Valium dose for seizure = 5–10 mg
- Isuprel is pure β—used for symptomatic bradycardia
- No IM or SQ in shock—they are not absorbed
- SQ into connective tissue at 45° angle
- Inderal (propranolol), Atenolol, Metoprolol = β blockers
- β blockers: ↓ HR, force of contraction and automaticity—do NOT give to asthma
- Solu-Medrol (steroid) = spinal cord injury and severe allergic reaction
- Decadron (steroid) = head injury
- Side effects:
  - Epinephrine: HTN, ↑ HR, ischemia, headache, palpitations, shaky
  - Atropine: ↑ HR, VF, VT, flushed skin, blurred vision, dry mouth
  - Lidocaine: convulsions, anxiety, N/V, dizziness, numb lips
  - Morphine: hypotension, respiratory and CNS depression
  - Lasix: hypokalemia, hypotension, transient deafness if pushed too fast
- Magnesium sulfate = CNS depressant and respiratory depressant

©2006 Prentice-Hall Inc.

- Do NOT give digitalis in blocks (use in A Fib and CHF)
- Do NOT give Verapamil to patient on β blockers
- Epi 1:10,000 IV for codes, anaphylaxis with hypotension (0.3–0.5 mg)
- Epi 1:1,000 SQ asthma, allergic reaction (0.3–0.5 mg)
- Vasopressors ↑ BP and ↑ PVR (dopamine/Intropin, Levophed, NE)
- D_{50} = 50 cc/25 g—give SLOW IVP
- Vagus nerve neurotransmitter = ACh
- Carpopedal spasm = hyperventilation
- Hyperkalemia causes peaked T waves
- Bronchoconstriction is NOT a β effect
- 17 lb peds Lido dose = 8 mg
- JVD, clear lungs, narrow pulse pressure = cardiac tamponade
- Talk down LSD
- Chest pain number-one pain reliever Morphine
- 110 lb Lido dose = 50 mg then 2–4 mg/min drip
- Aminophylline dose = 5–6 mg/kg—use for COPD patient
- 21 y.o. asthma = albuterol 2.5 mg via nebulizer
- 81 y.o. VT cardiovert, now pulseless—next action = defibrillate 200 j
- 60 y.o. twisted ankle, HR 54, BP 140/80, treat = splint and transport
- Spontaneous pneumothorax s/sx = knife-like pain, cough
- Verapamil = ↓ vasoconstriction, ↓ conductivity
- You clamped and cut umbilical cord, now bleeding = clamp it again
- Mother bleeding after delivery = massage fundus
- After oxygen, monitor, IV in pulmonary edema = NTG 0.4 mg
- A/W problem with stridor critical
- 3 y.o. with barking cough = croup
- Peds patient with flu "not acting right" = Reyes syndrome
- Wide QRS, regular, no P before QRS = idioventricular
- Intrinsic rate of ventricle = 20–40
- EOA WILL cause vomiting when removed
- MVC patient HR 120, BP 40/palp = hypovolemic shock
- Number-one side effect of Bretylol = hypotension
- Side effect of Lido = seizures
- Contraindication for Verapamil = pulmonary edema, cardiogenic shock
- Pain in chest, "tearing and shearing pain toward neck" with no pedal pulses = dissecting aortic aneurysm
- When palpating the abdomen you should do quadrant that hurts LAST
- Cribbing is used to stabilize vehicle
- Electrical burns cause damage = superficial and deep
- Perform cricothyrotomy for laryngeal edema and facial trauma
- Do a glucose check BEFORE giving D_{50}
- Patient fell thru glass door and has piece of glass in neck = C-spine/a/w, occlusive dressing, stabilize glass, transport
- Complications from IV = phlebitis and emboli
- Routes for Epi = IV, ET, SQ
- Air embolism possible side effect of IV therapy
- Visceral pleura around lungs
- β agonist = stimulates β receptors
- Encoder = person sending message
- Decoder = person receiving message
- Oscilloscope "decodes" EKG

- Lithobid = Lithium
- Remove toxins through semipermeable membranes (like hemodialysis)
- Spleen in LUQ
- Baby should double birth weight in 6–8 months; triple in 1 year
- Loss of consciousness for 3–5 minutes then return = concussion
- Concussion now falls under diffuse axonal injury
- 20 drop set running at 50 gtts in 30 minute infuses = 75 ml
- 60 drop set at 20 gtts in 30 minute infuses = 10 ml
- Amount of RL you give for EBL of 300 cc = 900 cc
- Movement of water from high concentration to low = osmosis
- Tourniquet restricts arterial and venous flow
- First thing occurring in blast injury = compression of air-filled organs
- 65 kg patient—how much Epi for allergic reaction = 0.3–0.5 mg (1:1,000) SQ
- Muscular structure below or behind cervix = fundus
- Mini base stations for telemetry and communication = repeaters
- Group of radio frequencies = bands
- Prolapsed cord = gloved hand, hold baby off cord, transport
- 17 y.o. in transport c/o severe headache = aneurysm
- 21 y.o. with C.P. after coughing = spontaneous pneumothorax
- DTs 48–72 hours after cessation of ETOH
- Ligamentum arteriosum attaches to aorta—causes weak area in trauma
- Size-up begins at time call received
- First link begins when EMS activated
- FDA ensures safety of drugs
- D_5W main use is cardiac and medication administration
- Placenta previa—placenta covers part or all of os
- Most important information for ER doc = c/c, patient condition, treatment
- Most important for trauma = MOI
- Most severe complication of IV = air embolism
- Best treatment for postincident stress = give specific task to complete (check for CISM necessity)
- Unresponsive baby with frantic mother = never use restraint
- Disability act protects people with communicable disease
- No eating or food in ambulance
- IV for COPD at KVO = D_5W
- Treatment for prehospital fever = remove clothing
- Old lady thinks neighbors out to get her = remove from situation and keep her talking
- Infant not breathing, after 1–2 minutes begins spontaneous respirations = assist ventilations (think BLS)
- Bright-red bleeding with cramping in 1st trimester = spontaneous abortion
- Adult asthma attack = treatment aim is to stop bronchial spasms
- Pregnant with seizures = Valium 5–10 mg IV (magnesium sulfate 2–5 g IV)
- BVM most common side effect = vomiting (face seal = number-one problem)
- Common cause of aspiration = removal of EOA
- Most common place for IO = proximal tibia
- NOT a sign of infant dehydration = polyuria
- Sign of infant dehydration = sunken fontanelle(s)
- Lidocaine side effect = muscle twitching, seizures
- Antipsychotics = Haldol, Thorazine
- Antidepressants = Elavil (amitriptylline), Tofranil (imipramine)
- Benadryl is NOT a bronchodilator; it blocks further histamine response
- Ambulance in left lane so traffic will move right in natural fashion

©2006 Prentice-Hall Inc.

- Writing something derogatory = libel (library)
- Saying something derogatory = slander
- Verapamil side effect = bradycardia
- Patient with history WPW in SVT, no s/sx = adenosine 6 mg rapid IVP
- VT = wide bizarre regular
- A Fib = irregularly irregular with NO discernible uniform P
- No pupil reaction in GCS
- APGAR
- Headache, stiff neck, fever = meningitis
- Patient drooling with epiglottitis = transport sitting up
- T-4 = nipple line down
- T-10 = umbilicus down
- Abdominal bleed can take up to several hours to occur
- MCI last to go = stable spinal cord injury
- Lady sitting up with pink, frothy sputum = left heart failure
- Cavitation = object penetration
- Dopamine dosage and drip rate
- Shingles are NOT contagious
- Contraindications for EOA = <16 years old, <5 ft, over 6 ft 8 in., caustic ingestion, esophageal varices, + gag reflex
- Lung compliance = elasticity or stiffness of lungs
- One of first signs of shock = anxiety or tachycardia
- One of first to go in MCI = anxiety and thirst
- Ventilation by other means done before ET insertion
- Primary blast injury causes compression of hollow organs and eardrum problems
- Do NOT hold portable radio horizontal for better reception
- 10 y.o. "not himself," has had flu, sudden onset of N/V, personality changes and irrational behavior = Reyes syndrome
- Status epilepticus—doesn't regain consciousness between seizures
- Neurogenic, anaphylactic, and septic shock—low BP due to vasodilation
- Max amount crystalloid given to adult trauma patient = 2,000–3,000 ml (needs blood)
- Universal recipient = AB+
- Best place for IV cannulation to avoid joints = forearm
- Minidrop set = 60 gtts/ml
- Patient taking 10 mg Valium normally may need 20–30 mg for effect = tolerance
- Severing spinal cord at C-4 = total paralysis including respiratory muscles
- Preferred IM site in field = deltoid first, then gluteus
- COPD mild respiratory distress = nasal cannula
- Intubating peds patient put mild pressure on larynx to assist visualization
- R on T PVC can cause VT or VF
- S/sx asthma = anxiety, hypoxia, wheezing, silent chest deadly
- Transport 3rd trimester pregnant left lateral recumbent
- Lung sounds due to bronchoconstriction = wheezing
- Gallop heart sound (S_3) due to CHF
- How to restrain behavioral emergency = one arm above head, one arm behind side, lying prone with feet tied at end of stretcher (hog tie NOT to be used—prone—due to positional asphyxia deaths)
- Use Mannitol (osmotic diuretic) for ↑ ICP
- Lidocaine suppresses ventricular irritability and automaticity
- Epi vasoconstricts, but ↑ cerebral and coronary blood flow
- First to balance acidosis is bicarb buffer system
- Atropine blocks ACh

- Too low dose Atropine = paradoxical bradycardia
- Too slow push Atropine = paradoxical bradycardia
- CHF if hypotensive use dopamine
- Epi comes from adrenal gland
- Catecholamines = NE, E, D (NorEpinephrine, Epinephrine, dopamine)
  - "I'm SYMPATHETIC if you NEED to run away from a mountain CAT in the woods at night" can help you remember sympathetic actions (dilated pupils, ↑ HR, ↑ respirations, bronchodilations, etc.)
- Vagus nerve controls parasympathetic
- Postpartum hemorrhage want to ↑ uterine contraction = Pitocin (oxytocin)
- NTG is vasodilator
- SVT not responding to adenosine = Verapamil or Cardizem
- On-line physician = strongest medical control (over protocols)
- Personal MD must accompany patient to override ER MD on-line
- SQ does NOT work in shock
- IM best in deltoid—does NOT work in shock
- Prolonged CPR = metabolic acidosis
- BP = CO (SV × HR) × PVR
- 1 pint blood = 500 cc
- Chemical mediator of sympathetic = NE
- Convert lb to kg
- Traumatic asphyxia scenario
- Sucking chest wound scenario
- 12-lead shows AMI—who is NOT fibrinolytic candidate
- Lasix = 0.5–1 mg/kg, give slowly
- Common placement for needle decompression
- Hypokalemia = low T wave
- Extreme mood swings = manic disorder
- Breech delivery = transport (may need a/w for baby)
- Prolapsed cord can cut off blood supply to fetus
- Stable angina scenario (exercise)
- Cushing's Triad
- Occipital lobe = sight
- Do NOT stop orifice bleeding in ↑ ICP—releases pressure
- Flat jugular veins = hypovolemia
- ADA for AIDS patient
- Informed consent most common and best
- Best protection from lawsuit = proper training
- Pathophysiology of shock
- EKG strips = 3rd degree, VF, VT
- PEA treatment
- Define primigravida
- Peds weight 20 kg—joules to defibrillate? (first and second)
- First medic on scene MCI = triage
- First signs of respiratory distress in child
- Atropine side effects = dry mouth, blurred vision
- PVCs with bradycardia = Atropine
- Charcoal 1 g/kg or 50 g for poisoning (adult)
- Side effects of diuretic = hypotension, hypokalemia
- LUQ = spleen
- RUQ = cholecystitis
- Anaphylaxis scenario

©2006 Prentice-Hall Inc.

- GCS 3 scenario
- Burns anterior chest, abdomen, and upper arms = 27%
- Dilute Epi 1:1,000 to make Epi 1:10,000
- Lead II has no P waves = SA node NOT initial pacemaker
- 3rd degree heart block = syncope
- VF = defibrillate (don't wait—defibrillate)
- Unstable VT (decreased LOC) = synchronized cardiovert
- Antepartum = before delivery of fetus
- Transport female abdominal pain in left lateral recumbent
- EOA/EGTA used in unconscious adult
- Presence of ↑ CO_2 stimulates normal respiration
- Pulse pressure = difference in systolic and diastolic
- Narrowing pulse pressure in shock and tamponade
- Widening pulse pressure in head injury
- In CHF decrease preload and afterload
- Patient slurred speech, left side paralysis—do NOT run D_5W wide open
- If monitor fails and you didn't check it = negligence
- Four necessities for successful suit = duty, breach, harm caused, proximate cause
- Sizing of ET tube (little finger)
- Hallmark of decompensated shock = drop in BP
- Difference between decompensated and irreversible shock—unknown when enough damage done to be irreversible organ failure
- Best stage to catch and treat shock = compensated
- Cause of hypovolemia in burn patient
- When opposite side of brain is bruised = contracoup (deceleration injury)
- Kinetic energy = weight, mass, *velocity* (most important)
- What are you measuring in ET tube? internal diameter
- Metabolic acidosis—preexisting = bicarb
- Cyanotic flail chest = BVM
- Pulse oximetry measures trends in oxygen saturation
- Hypoxemia = decreased oxygen in blood
- Collapsed alveoli = atelectasis
- Good Samaritan laws implemented by state, NOT EMS
- Ominous sign of respiratory failure in 6 y.o. = altered mentation
- When can medic start IV = standing orders/protocols, on-line med direction
- + JVD, no breath sounds on left = pleural decompression, BVM, IV, transport
- Abused child—report
- MCI 20 y.o. cardiac arrest = leave
- 20 kg = 40 j defibrillate in pediatric
- Duplex radio system—two way
- Multiplex for telemetry
- Routes for Valium in peds = IV, IO, rectal (some services now use nasal)
- Ethics = rules, standards, morals
- OSHA mandates workplace safety
- QA programs ID problems to ↑ standard of care
- Medic works by delegation of authority/what can do depends on local protocols
- Good Samaritan = off duty, met standard of care, patient consent, no reimbursement
- Civil law = tort (most medics sued under)
- Psych patient most likely to claim injury
- Living will for MD only; paramedic needs valid DNRO
- Base station at highest point

- FCC governs communication
- KKK = ambulance rules
- FM = frequency modulation = most common EMS (and UHF)
- 10 medical communication channels range 463–468 MHz
- Modulator transforms electrical energy into sound waves
- Safety (you) first—most rescuer deaths in confined space
- Assessment (begins at dispatch), gain access, emergency care, disentanglement, removal, transport (in order)
- Extrication = removal of victim from area of danger
- Windshield laminated glass = use fire ax
- Air chisel cuts skin or sheet metal
- Car battery disconnect negative first
- Preplanning and communication most important aspects of MCI
- START triage (30—2—can do)
- Mitochondria energy source of cell
- Microorganisms cause infection = fungus, bacteria, virus
- Homeostasis = maintain internal balance, equilibrium
- Radial/80, femoral/70, carotid/60 (minimum systolic)
- Battle's sign, raccoon eyes = basilar skull (late)
- Hyperresonant = tension, pneumothorax, emphysema, asthma (trapped air)
- Dull = hemothorax, pneumonia, tumor
- Cullen's, Kehr's, and Grey-Turner's signs
- AAO × 3 = person, place, time
- Pulse/rate, quality, regularity; newborn 140–160
- Respiratory rate = 12–20, newborn 40–60
- Temp/oral 98.6°/rectal 99.6°/axillary 97.6°
- Below glottis is sterile
- Epiglottis and glottic opening at vocal cords
- Carina = split (vagal stimulation if hit)
- Vallecula = Macintosh
- Brain stem = respirations/1st medulla, 2nd pons
- TV (tidal volume) = 500 cc
- MV (minute volume) = TV × RR
- Dead space = 125–150 cc
- Hypercarbia = ↑ carbon dioxide in blood
- Every COPD patient is on hypoxic drive for boards
- NC = 20–40%, mask = 40–60%, NRBM = 90+%
- TBW = 60% (75% ICF, 25% ECF/20%interstitial and 5–7% intravascular)
- Sodium = most common ECF cation
- Potassium = most common ICF cation
- Chloride = most common ECF anion
- Hypernatremia = ↑ sodium
- Hyperkalemia = ↑ potassium
- Hypercalcemia = ↑ calcium
- Blood removes waste, delivers oxygen, hormones, and regulates temp
- Plasma transports electrolytes, glucose, hormones
- RBC = erythrocyte—carries oxygen on Hgb
- WBC = leukocyte, infection
- Platelets = thrombocytes—clotting
- Hemotoxin = substance that destroys RBC

©2006 Prentice-Hall Inc.

- Controlled Substance Act of 1970 = schedule of addictive drugs (may not sell or use heroin, LSD, schedule I no medical use)
- Harrison Narcotic Act 1914
- Inotrope = contraction; chronotrope = rate
- Dopamine = 1–4 dopaminergic, 5–10 beta, 11–20 alpha
- tsp = 5 cc, Tbs = 15 cc, ounce = 30 cc
- IVP = PINCH tubing
- Definitions: cough, sneeze, hiccough, sigh (opens lower A/W), dyspnea, hemoptysis, hypoxia, anoxia, orthopnea (CHF), tactile fremitus, eupnea
- S/sx respiratory difficulty = nasal flaring, accessory muscle use, tracheal tugging (direction toward affected side), intercostal retractions
- COPD/pink puffer = pursed lips, barrel chest, hyperresonance, expiration is active, polycythemia (too many RBC)
- COPD/blue bloater = chronic bronchitis, cough, ↑ mucus, overweight, cyanotic
- Status asthmaticus = no relief from Epi
- Asthma = expiratory wheezing first, (1) albuterol, (2) Epi SQ, (3) Solu-Medrol
- Pneumonia = SOB, fever, gradual onset, elderly and young, viral pulmonary infection (can be bacterial)
- P.E. (pulmonary embolus) = sudden onset sharp chest pain, shock, respiratory distress, female/birth control pills (BCP), postop, postpartum, DVT, bedridden treatment = ↑ oxygen—can hear normal breath sounds
- Pituitary = pea-shaped, in brain, oxytocin and ADH
- Vasopressin = ADH, 40 units one time only
- Adrenal Glands = superior to kidneys, Epi and NE
- Pancreas—part abdominal, part retroperitoneal
- Ulcer = black tarry stools (melena) or coffee ground emesis (hematemesis)— ↑ GI
- Lower GI = bright-red blood or wine-colored stool (hematochezia)
- Kidney stone = renal calculus, flank pain, hematuria, pain may be groin or lower abdomen
- Gallbladder stores bile; liver produces
- Cholecystitis—RUQ pain, right shoulder pain, 5 Fs (female, fertile [multipara], forty years old, after fatty meal, flatulent, and fair [makes 6])
- Hepatitis—RUQ tender, sick for several days, jaundice, N/V, coke urine, clay stools
- Renal failure—dialysis = fluid overload caution
- Predialysis = pulmonary edema, hyperkalemia (use calcium) acidosis (bicarb)
- Postdialysis—electrolyte imbalance and hypovolemia
- AVPU
- OPQRST
- SAMPLE
- GCS
- APGAR
- ABG norms: pH 7.35–7.45, CO_2 35–45, O_2 80–100, bicarb 22–26
- Amiodarone (Cordarone) first line, (1) nonperfusing patient—300 mg/30 cc/30 seconds, (2) perfusing patient—150 mg/100 cc/10 minutes bolus or drip
- Thiamine = B1 = 100 mg
- Glucagon = 1 mg
- Kehr's Sign = left shoulder pain; may indicate ruptured spleen
- Benadryl for Haldol, Compazine OD—Narcan works on Darvon
- Procardia not approved for use as antihypertensive
- Pitocin—10–20 units in IV of 500–1,000 cc

SECTION 10
Pathophysiologies

Pathophysiology Checklist
Glossary

PATHOPHYSIOLOGY CHECKLIST

ID#	Pathophysiology	Done ✓
1.01	Normal/Healthy and Detrimental Reactions to Stress and Causes of Stress in EMS	
1.02	Normal/Healthy and Detrimental Reactions of Anxiety	
1.03	Circumstances when relatives, bystanders, and others should be removed from the scene	
1.04	Hemorrhage (a. Capillary, b. Venous, c. Arterial)	
1.05	Hemorrhage Management of Open Wound (a. Direct Pressure, b. ↑ (elevation), c. Pressure Dressing, d. Pressure Point, e. Tourniquet)	
2.01	Cheyne-Stokes Respirations/Biot's Respiration	
2.02	Spontaneous Pneumothorax	
2.03	Epiglottitis/Croup	
2.04	Allergy/Anaphylaxis	
3.01	Hyperventilation Syndrome	
3.02	COPD/Emphysema	
3.03	Bronchitis/Bronchiolitis/Laryngitis	
3.04	Chronic Bronchitis	
3.05	Bronchial Asthma	
3.06	Pulmonary Thromboembolism	
3.07	Pneumonia	
3.08	ARDS	
3.09	Neoplasms of the Lung	
4.01	Hypotension/Hypoperfusion	
4.02	Cardiogenic Shock	
4.03	Types and Stages of Shock and Hemorrhage	
4.04	Spinal Shock/Spinal Neurogenic Shock	
4.05	Compensated, Decompensated, and Irreversible Stages of Shock	
5.01	External Hemorrhage Management/Internal Hemorrhage Management	
5.02	Dislocations, Tendon Injury, Sprain, and Strain	
5.03	Fractures: Open and Closed/Different Types	
5.04	Pelvic Fractures	
5.05	Rib Fractures, Sternal Fracture, and Flail Segment	
5.06	Ruptured Globe/Orbital Fracture	
5.07	LeFort Fractures	
5.08	Closed Soft Tissue Injuries (a. Contusion, b. Crush, c. Hematoma)	
5.09	Open Soft Tissue Injuries (a. Amputation, b. Incision, c. Crush, d. Penetrations/Punctures, e. Impaled Object)	
5.10	Open Soft Tissue Injuries (OSTI) (a. Abrasion, b. Avulsion, c. Laceration, d. Major Arterial Laceration)	
5.11	Pulmonary Contusion/Myocardial Contusion	
5.12	Barotrauma, Air Embolism, and Decompression Illness	
5.13	Coarctation of the Aorta/Transection of the Aorta	
5.14	Thoracic Vascular Trauma (a. Aorta, b. Vena Cava, c. Pulmonary Arteries/Veins)	
5.15	Myocardial Rupture/Pericardial Tamponade	
5.16	Hemothorax/Hemopneumothorax	
5.17	Pneumothorax (a. Simple, b. Open, c. Tension)	
5.18	Fractured Larynx	
5.19	Traumatic Asphyxia	
5.20	Cerebral Contusion	
5.21	Intracranial Hemorrhage (a. SAH, b. SDH, c. Epidural, d. Intracerebral)	
5.22	Incomplete Cord Injury (a. Central Cord Syndrome, b. Anterior Cord Syndrome, c. Brown-Sequard)	
5.23	Basal Skull Fracture	
5.24	Crush Injury (a. Crush Injury, b. Crush Syndrome, c. Compartment Syndrome)	
5.25	Cervical Spine Fracture	

(continued)

ID#	Pathophysiology	Done ✓
5.26	Transection of Spinal Cord with Quad- and Paraplegia	
5.27	Abdominal Trauma to Solid Organs	
5.28	Abdominal Trauma to Hollow Organs	
5.29	Ruptured Diaphragm	
5.30	Define Thermal, Inhalation, Chemical, Electrical, and Radiation Burns	
5.31	Radiation Exposure (including Types and Characteristics)	
5.32	Chemical (with example of eye)/Electrical Burn	
5.33	Thermal Burn/Inhalation Burn	
5.34	General Management of Burn (including Airway and Ventilation, Circulation, Pharmacological Management, Transport, Psychological, and Parkland Formula)	
5.35	Local and Systemic Complications of Burns	
5.36	Burns: Depth Classification/BSA estimates (a. "9s," b. "Palms," c. other)	
5.37	Blast Injury within an Enclosed Space	
5.38	Assessment, Management, Legal Aspects, and Documentation of Abuse and Assault	
5.39	Categories of Abuse (spouse, elder, child) with examples of each	
5.40	Profile characteristics of spouse abuser, elder abuser, child abuser, and sexual assailant	
5.41	Profile characteristics of "at-risk" spouse, elder, and child	
6.01	Define behavior and give examples distinguishing normal and abnormal behavior	
6.02	Verbal techniques useful in managing the emotionally disturbed patient	
6.03	Describe Medical-Legal considerations for management and safe restraint of emotionally disturbed	
6.04	Depression/Suicide with risk factors for suicide and "at-risk" suicide behaviors	
6.05	Bipolar Personality Disorder/Schizophrenia	
6.06	Psychogenic Reaction	
6.07	Techniques of gathering information and assessing patients with behavioral problems	
6.08	Focused Abdominal Pain History, Questioning Technique and Specific Questions, Describe Exam Technique	
6.09	Esophageal Varices/Peptic Ulcer Disease (PUD)	
6.10	Upper GI Bleeding	
6.11	Lower GI Bleeding/Hemorrhoids	
6.12	Acute Gastroenteritis, Gastritis, and Colitis	
6.13	Diverticulitis, Crohn's Disease, and Irritable Bowel Syndrome (IBS)	
6.14	Appendicitis/Bowel Obstruction	
6.15	Pancreatitis	
6.16	Peritoneal Inflammation	
6.17	Cholecystitis	
6.18	Acute Hepatitis/A/B/C/D/E	
6.19	Acute Renal Failure/Chronic Renal Failure	
6.20	Renal Dialysis and Complications	
6.21	Renal Calculi	
6.22	Urinary Tract Infection (UTI)/Pyelonephritis	
6.23	Torsion Testicle/Prostatitis	
6.24	Influenza	
6.25	Sepsis/MRSA	
6.26	Tuberculosis (TB)	
6.27	Meningitis/Encephalitis	
6.28	Hypoglycemia/IDDM/NIDDM (including body's compensatory mechanisms to promote homeostasis)	
6.29	Correlate abnormal findings in the assessment with their clinical significance in patients with hypoglycemia	
6.30	Hyperglycemia/Diabetic KetoAcidosis (DKA)	
6.31	Differentiate between pathophysiology of normal glucose metabolism, diabetic glucose metabolism, and ketone body formation	
6.32	Alzheimer's Disease/Parkinson's Disease	

©2006 Prentice-Hall Inc.

6.33	Dementia/Organic Brain Syndrome (OBS)	
6.34	Delirium	
6.35	Identify and Define Routes of Entry of toxic substances and factors affecting decision to induce vomiting with poison ingestion	
6.36	S/Sx and Management of common ingested caustics, hydrocarbons, household substances, and bleach	
6.37	S/Sx and Management of common inhaled toxic substances	
6.38	S/Sx and Management of common injected toxic substances (including bites and stings)	
6.39	S/Sx and Management of common surface absorption toxic substances	
6.40	Acute ETOH Poisoning	
6.41	Define *poison by OD*, list most common ODs with pathophysiology, S/Sx, and Management (cyanide, CO, metals, plants, and mushrooms)	
6.42	Most commonly abused drugs (both chemical and street names) with patho, S/Sx, and Management (cocaine, cannabis, amphetamines, barbiturates, sedatives, opiates, sexual purposes/gratification)	
6.43	Most commonly abused drugs with patho, S/Sx, and Management (MAOIs, over-the-counter [OTC] pain meds, NSAIDS, TCAs, salicylates, acetaminophen, Theophylline, Lithium, serotonin syndromes, cardiac and psych meds)	
6.44	Food Poisoning (including causative organisms)	
6.45	ETOH Abuse and Withdrawal	
6.46	Cushing's Syndrome/Adrenal Insufficiency	
6.47	Heat Stroke: Classical/Exertional	
6.48	Leukemia	
6.49	Seizures: Major types with assessment findings and management	
6.50	Fever: Definition, Pathophysiologic Mechanism, and Management	
7.01	Starling's Law and Cardiac Output	
7.02	Coronary Artery Disease (CAD)/Peripheral Vascular Disease (PVD)	
7.03	Transient Ischemic Attack (TIA)	
7.04	Strokes: Types, Assessment, and Management	
7.05	Hypertensive Emergency	
7.06	Intracranial Hemorrhage: Types, Assessment, and Management	
7.07	Fibrinolytic Eligibility	
7.08	Myocardial Infarction	
7.09	Stable Angina/Unstable Angina	
7.10	Prinzmetal's Angina	
7.11	Palpitations	
7.12	Stokes-Adams Syndrome	
7.13	Indications and Possible Complications of Temporary and Permanent Artificial Pacemakers	
7.14	Sudden Onset Atrial Fibrillation	
7.15	Rapid Ventricular Response/Rate (RVR) Dysrhythmias	
7.16	Vasovagal Syncope/Vertigo	
7.17	Ventricular Dysrhythmias	
7.18	WPW	
7.19	Pericarditis	
7.20	Endocarditis	
7.21	Carotid Sinus Sensitivity	
7.22	Subclavian Steal Syndrome	
7.23	Sick Sinus Syndrome	
7.24	GastroEsophageal Reflux Disease (GERD)/Esophagitis	
7.25	Thoracic Aneurysm/Dissecting Thoracic Aneurysm	
7.26	Hiatal Hernia	
7.27	Pleuritis/Pleurisy	
7.28	Costochondritis	
7.29	Mitral Valve Prolapse	
7.30	Abdominal Aortic Aneurysm (AAA)/Dissecting AAA	

(continued)

		Done ✓
7.31	Paroxysmal Nocturnal Dyspnea (PND)	
7.32	Preload, Afterload, and Left Ventricular End-Diastolic Pressure (LVEDP) as they relate to Heart Failure	
7.33	Cocaine Induced Chest Pain	
7.34	CHF (differentiate early and late Left Ventricular Failure [LVF] and Right Ventricular Failure [RVF])	
7.35	Pulmonary Edema and Its Relation to Left Ventricular Hypertrophy (LVH)	
7.36	Pulseless Electrical Activity (PEA)	
8.01	Mittelschmerz/Pelvic Inflammatory Disease (PID)	
8.02	Sexual Assault (with examples)	
8.03	Sexually Transmitted Diseases (STDs) (including HIV)	
8.04	Vaginal Discharge, Bleeding, and Hemorrhage	
8.05	Types of Abortion (with Definition, S/Sx, and Management)	
8.06	Premature Labor	
8.07	Multiple Gestation/Premature Infant	
8.08	Preeclampsia/Eclampsia	
8.09	Placenta Previa/Abruptio Placenta	
8.10	Abnormal Presentations (with Definition, S/Sx, and Management)	
8.11	Meconium Aspiration/Hyaline Membrane Disease	
8.12	Maternal Drug Abuse: Effects on mother and neonate	
8.13	Prolapsed Cord/Uterine Inversion	
8.14	Ruptured Uterus/Ectopic Pregnancy	
8.15	Postpartum Hemorrhage	
8.16	URI/RSV	
8.17	Kawasaki Disease	
8.18	Sickle Cell Anemia/Sickle Cell Crisis	
8.19	Guillain Barre' Syndrome/Multiple Sclerosis/Muscular Dystrophy	
8.20	Myasthenia Gravis/Cerebral Palsy/Cystic Fibrosis	

©2006 Prentice-Hall Inc.

Pathophysiology: _____

Patho # _____

On disease/condition pathophysiologies be sure to include:

☐ Definition   ☐ Cause/Etiology/Mechanism   ☐ S/Sx (assessment findings)   ☐ Management

_____
_____
_____
_____
_____
_____
_____
_____
_____
_____
_____
_____
_____
_____
_____
_____
_____
_____
_____
_____
_____
_____
_____
_____
_____
_____
_____
_____
_____
_____
_____
_____
_____
_____
_____
_____
_____
_____
_____
_____
_____

Source: _____   Pages/Web Site: _____

GLOSSARY

Load and go—A phrase used in trauma situations with a patient who needs immediate transport. Only immediate life threats are taken care of on scene; all other assessments and treatments are done en route.

Stay and play—The opposite of load and go. A phrase indicating a trauma patient who is stable and can have a complete assessment and initial treatment on scene.

1°—First degree.

2°—Second degree or secondary to. . . .

2°I—A type of heart block; means second degree type 1 (Wenckebach).

2°II—A type of heart block; means second degree type 2.

3°—A type of heart block; means third degree block (or complete); also third degree as in a burn.

6 Rs—Six rights of medication administration.

A/W—Airway.

AAOx—Awake, alert, and oriented times _____. AAO × 3 would mean awake, alert, and oriented to person, place, and time; AAO × 4 would be to person, place, time, and event.

ABC—Airway, breathing, circulation.

ABG—Arterial blood gas.

ACh—Acetylcholine.

ACLS—Advanced cardiac life support.

ACS—Acute coronary syndrome.

ADA—Americans with Disabilities Act.

AED—Automatic external defibrillator.

ALS—Advanced life support.

AMI—Acute myocardial infarction.

APGAR—Appearance, pulse, grimace, activity, respirations.

ASA—Acteylsalicylic acid or aspirin.

ATV—Automatic transport ventilator.

AV fistula—Arteriovenous connection; a surgically implanted tube to connect an artery and vein used for hemodialysis.

AVPU—Alert, verbal, pain, unresponsive.

BBS—Bilateral breath sounds.

BGL—Blood glucose level.

BiPAP—A continuous positive airway pressure in which both inspiratory and expiratory pressures are set above atmospheric pressure.

BLS—Basic life support.

Bolus—An amount of fluid (or food) given all in one dose.

BP—Blood pressure.

©2006 Prentice-Hall Inc.

BPM—Breaths per minute (some texts also use this abbreviation for beats per minute).

BRB—Bright-red blood (bleeding).

BSA—Body surface area.

BSI—Body substance isolation.

BVM—Bag-valve-mask.

BVT—Bag-valve-tube.

Caudally—A directional term meaning toward the tail (coccygeal region).

cc—Cubic centimeters (equal to ml—milliliter).

CHARTED—A mnemonic for the narrative portion of a patient care report. It stands for complaint, history, assessment, Rx (treatment plan), transport, evaluation (of treatment), disposition (hospital, report).

CHF—Congestive heart failure.

cm—Centimeter.

cmH$_2$O—Centimeters of water.

CN—Cranial nerve.

CNS—Central nervous system.

CO—Cardiac output or carbon monoxide, depending on context or reference.

Constricting band—An elastic type band placed on an extremity in a manner to restrict venous return, but allow arterial flow (lets veins fill up).

CO$_2$—Carbon dioxide.

COPD—Chronic obstructive pulmonary disease.

CP—Chest pain.

CPAP—Continuous positive airway pressure.

CPR—Cardiopulmonary resuscitation.

CSM—Carotid sinus massage.

CTM—Cricothyroid membrane.

CVA—Cerebral vascular accident (stroke).

CVC—Central venous catheter.

D/C—Discontinue.

DCAP-BLS-TIC—Deformities, contusions, abrasions, punctures/penetrations, burns, lacerations, swelling, tenderness, instability, crepitus.

DKA—Diabetic ketoacidosis.

DOB—Date of birth.

DOC—Drug of choice.

DOPE—A mnemonic for ET check (dislodged, obstructed, pneumothorax, equipment).

DSD—Dry sterile dressing.

DTs—Delerium tremens.

DVT—Deep vein thrombophlebitis.

EBL—Estimated blood loss.

ECF—Extracellular fluid.

ECG/EKG—Electrocardiogram.

EGTA—Esophageal gastric tube airway.

EJ—External jugular.

EMS—Emergency medical services.

EOA—Esophageal obturator airway.

Epiglottis—"Trap door" of cartilage that flops down to cover trachea and protect from aspiration.

EPS—Extrapyramidal syndrome.

ET—Endotracheal.

ETA—Estimated time of arrival.

EtCO$_2$—End tidal carbon dioxide.

ETOH—Ethanol.

ETT—Endotracheal tube.

FBAO—Foreign body airway obstruction.

FCC—Federal Communications Commission.

FDA—Food and Drug Administration.

Foley—A catheter to be placed in the urinary bladder.

Fr.—French (a measurement of tube diameter).

ga—Gauge (a measurement of needle diameter).

GCS—Glasgow Coma Score.

GI—Gastrointestinal.

GI/GU—GastroIntestinal/genitourinary.

GT—Gastric tube.

GYN—Gynecology, a branch of medicine specific to women, involving the reproductive organs and the breast.

H$_2$O$_2$—Hydrogen peroxide.

Haz-mat—Hazardous materials.

HHN—Handheld nebulizer.

HR—Heart rate.

HTN—Hypertension.

Hypoperfusion—Below normal perfusion . . . SHOCK.

ICF—Intracellular fluid.

ICP—Intracranial pressure.

ICS—Incident command system.

IM—Intramuscular.

IMS—Incident management system.

Inner canthus—Inner corner of the eye (tear duct side).

IO—Intraosseus.

IV—Intravenous.

IVP—Intravenous push (bolus).

IVPB—Intravenous piggyback.

JVD—Jugular venous distension.

KVO—Keep vein open.

LBB—Long backboard.

LOC—LEVEL of consciousness (not loss).

LPM—Liters per minute.

LVH—Left ventricular hypertrophy.

MCI—Mass/multiple casualty incident.

MDI—Metered dose inhaler.

©2006 Prentice-Hall Inc.

MI—Myocardial infarction.

ml—Milliliter (cc).

ml/kg—Milliliters per kilogram.

mmHg—Millimeters of mercury.

MOI—Mechanism of injury.

MRSA—Methcillan (or multiple antibiotic) resistant *staphylococcus aureus*.

MSDS—Materials safety data sheet.

MVA—Motor vehicle accident.

MVC—Motor vehicle collision.

NG—Nasogastric.

NGT—Nasogastric tube.

NI—Nasointestinal.

NPA—Nasopharyngeal airway.

NRBM—Nonrebreather mask.

NS—Normal saline.

NTG—Nitroglycerine.

NTI—Nasotracheal intubation.

OB—Obstetrics.

OGT—Orogastric tube.

OPA—Oropharyngeal airway.

OPQRST—A mnemonic for obtaining information about pain (onset, provoking factors, quality, region/radiation, severity, time).

OSHA—Occupational Safety and Health Administration.

-ostomy—Surgically formed opening connecting internal structure to outside of body.

-otomy—Incision into.

Oxygenate—Provision of oxygen.

P—Pulse.

Parkland Formula—Formula for calculating fluid resuscitation needed in burn victims.

PASG—Pneumatic anti-shock garment.

PCA (pump)—Patient controlled administration.

PCR—Patient care report (run sheets).

PEA—Pulseless electrical activity.

PERRL—Pupils equal round and react to light.

PID—Pelvic inflammatory disease.

PMS—Pulse, movement, sensation (CSM—circulation, sensation, movement, can be confused with carotid sinus massage).

PO—Per os, by mouth.

PPE—Personal protective equipment.

PPV—Positive pressure ventilation.

PRN—As needed.

PUD—Peptic ulcer disease.

QA—Quality assurance.

RN—Registered nurse.

RSI—Rapid sequence induction.

RSV—Respiratory synctial virus.

SAMPLE—A mnemonic for history (symptoms, allergies, medications, past/pertinent history, last oral intake, event(s) leading up to 9-1-1 call).

SDH—Subdural hematoma/hemorrhage.

Sellick's—A maneuver applying cricoid ring pressure to occlude esophagus.

Septum—Wall.

SHS—Supine hypotensive syndrome.

Signs—EMS provider can see, feel, smell, taste, etc.

SL—Sublingual.

SMR—Spinal motion restriction.

SOAPED—A mnemonic for charting narrative (symptoms, objective [signs], assessment, plan, evaluation, disposition).

SOB—Shortness of breath.

SQ—Subcutaneous.

SSN—Social security number.

SSS—Sick sinus syndrome.

START—Simple triage and rapid transport.

Stoma—Artificially created opening (opening into trachea, for example).

SubQ—Subcutaneous.

SV—Stroke volume.

Sx—Symptoms.

TBW—Total body water.

TCA—Tricyclic antidepressant.

TCP—Transcutaneous pacer.

TK—Tourniquet (obstructs venous AND arterial flow).

TKO—To keep open.

Trach—Tracheostomy/tracheotomy.

TV—Tidal volume (V_T).

URI—Upper respiratory infection.

UTI—Urinary tract infection.

UVC—Umbilical vein catheter/cannula.

VAD—Venous access device.

Ventilate—BREATHE—get air IN and OUT.

VF—Ventricular fibrillation.

VT—Ventricular tachycardia.

Whistle-tip—Suction catheter with small hole that applies suction when covered.

WO—Wide open.

©2006 Prentice-Hall Inc.